A Clinician's Handbook of Child and Adolescent Psychiatry

This authoritative clinical handbook provides a comprehensive overview of the main disorders encountered by child and adolescent psychiatrists in clinical practice, ranging from eating, sleep and affective disorders to substance abuse, gender identity disorder and sexual abuse. The approach is evidence based and emphasis is on good clinical practice and quality control of patient care. In contrast to other books in the field, the authors' intention is not to cover exhaustively all the relevant science, but rather to present in condensed form any research findings that are significant for clinical practice.

For coherence, each chapter is constructed in the same way: introduction, definition and classification, epidemiology, the clinical picture, aetiology, treatment and outcome. The disorders covered are based on the ICD-10 and DSM-IV classifications, and appendices include documents for assessment of intervention planning and evaluation.

Christopher Gillberg is Professor of Child and Adolescent Psychiatry at Göteborg University, Sweden.

Richard Harrington was Professor of Child and Adolescent Psychiatry at the University of Manchester.

Hans-Christoph Steinhausen is Professor of Child and Adolescent Psychiatry at the University of Zurich.

A Clinician's Handbook of Child and Adolescent Psychiatry

Edited by

Christopher Gillberg
University of Göteborg, Sweden

Richard Harrington
University of Manchester, UK

Hans-Christoph Steinhausen
University of Zurich, Switzerland

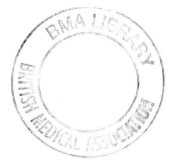

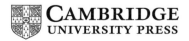

CAMBRIDGE
UNIVERSITY PRESS

CAMBRIDGE UNIVERSITY PRESS
Cambridge, New York, Melbourne, Madrid, Cape Town, Singapore, São Paulo

Cambridge University Press
The Edinburgh Building, Cambridge CB2 2RU, UK

Published in the United States of America by Cambridge University Press, New York

www.cambridge.org
Information on this title: www.cambridge.org/9780521819369

© Cambridge University Press 2006

First published 2006

Printed in the United Kingdom at the University Press, Cambridge

A catalogue record for this publication is available from the British Library

ISBN-13 978-0-521-819367 hardback
ISBN-10 0-521-81936-9 hardback

Cambridge University Press has no responsibility for the persistence or accuracy of URLs for external or third-party internet websites referred to in this publication, and does not guarantee that any content on such websites is, or will remain, accurate or appropriate.

Every effort has been made in preparing this publication to provide accurate and up-to-date information that is in accord with accepted standards and practice at the time of publication. Nevertheless, the authors, editors and publisher can make no warranties that the information contained herein is totally free from error, not least because clinical standards are constantly changing through research and regulation. The authors, editors and publisher therefore disclaim all liability for direct or consequential damages resulting from the use of material contained in this publication. Readers are strongly advised to pay careful attention to information provided by the manufacturer of any drugs or equipment that they plan to use.

Contents

Preface

Child and adolescent psychiatry is a rapidly expanding branch of medicine. Important research gains have been made in the past decades, and there is now a firm knowledge basis for many of the psychiatric disorders with child or adolescent onset. This knowledge has taken some time to filter through to clinical child and adolescent psychiatric services.

The aim of this book is to provide a comprehensive overview of the relevant objectives of child and adolescent psychiatry in clinical practice. The approach is decisively evidence based as far as this is possible with the current status in the field and thus avoids the consideration of various theoretical or even speculative approaches. Rather, the emphasis is on guidance for good clinical practice and help with the quality control of patient care. The various chapters have been written by experts in the respective fields. In contrast to other textbooks, the major objective is not to cover all relevant research findings exhaustively but rather to condense the scientific knowledge that is significant for clinical practice. Thus, the present deskbook deals with clinical disorders only.

The list and order of contents is guided by the ICD-10 and the various chapters also comment on the DSM-IV classification. A clear common structure for the chapters enforces the coherence of the monograph. After an introduction, definition and classification, epidemiology, the clinical picture, aetiology, treatment and outcome are specifically outlined for each disorder. Tables, figures and flowcharts, serve as additional sources of information and highlight special messages. Various appendices include important documents for assessment of intervention planning and evaluation.

The book is intended for child and adolescent psychiatrists, and for other specialists working in, or at the borders of, child mental health, including community and developmental pediatricians, school health doctors, child neurologists and adult and forensic psychiatrists. The language and writing style are such that it should also be a valuable source of clinical guidance for psychologists, social workers, nurses and other paramedical professionals working in the field.

The authorship is international with a strong European and North American orientation. The editors are grateful for the willingness and effectiveness of the authors to adopt the special structure and the intended message of this textbook and to bring in their expertise in order to provide an accurate and comprehensive account of the current state of knowledge of the various child and adolescent psychiatric disorders. Special thanks are also due to the publisher, most notably to Pauline Graham, Jo Bottrill and Mary Sanders for the assistance in producing this book.

Sadly, Richard Harrington died shortly before finalization of the manuscript of this book. His death is a great loss to his family, his colleagues and his friends. Besides his outstanding scientific contributions to child and adolescent psychiatry, he was a most skilful and experienced clinician and a genuine and warmhearted personality. This book will serve as a commemoration to Richard Harrington.

Contributors

Tobias Banaschewski
Universität Göttingen
Abt für Kinder-und Jugend-
psychiatrie der Universität
von-Siebold Str. 5
D-37075 Göttingen, Germany

Joseph H. Beitchman
Child and Family Studies Centre
Clarke Institute of Psychiatry
250 College Street
Toronto, Ontario
Canada M5G 1V7

Arnon Bentovim
The London Child and Family
Consultation Service
97 Harley Street
London W1G 6AG, UK

Oscar G. Bukstein
Western Psychiatric Institute and Clinic
Child and Adolescent
Psychiatry Division
3811 O'Hara Street
Pittsburgh, PA15213, USA

Marie Byatt
Child and Development Psychiatry
Royal Liverpool Children's Hospital
Alder Hey
Mulberry House
Eaton Road
Liverpool L12 2AP, UK

Andrew F. Clark
Prestwich Hospital
Adolescent Psychiatry
Service
Bury New Road
Prestwich
Manchester M25 3BL, UK

Peggy T. Cohen-Kettenis
Academisch Ziehenhuis
Utrecht Department of Child and
Adolescent Psychiatry
Po Box 85500
NL-3508, GA Utrecht
The Netherlands

Elena Garralda
Child and Adolescent
Psychiatry (Academic Unit)
Faculty of Medicine
Imperial College
St Mary's Campus
Norfolk Place
London W2 1PG, UK

Christopher Gillberg
Department of Child and
Adolescent Psychiatry
University of Göteborg
Kungsgatan 12
SE 411 19 Göteborg
Sweden

Richard Harrington (deceased)
Department of Child and Adolescent
Psychiatry
Royal Manchester
Children's Hospital
Hospital Road, Pendlebury
Manchester M27 4HA, UK

Jonathan Hill
Child Mental Health Unit
Royal Liverpool Children's Hospital
Alder Hey
Mulberry House, Eaton Road
Liverpool L12 2AP, UK

Peter Hill
Department of Psychological Medicine
Great Ormond Street
Hospital for Sick Children
London WC1N 3JH, UK

Patricia Hughes
Department of Psychiatry
Jenner Wing
St George's Hospital
Medical School
London SW17 ORE, UK

Carla J. Johnson
Dept of Speech and Language Pathology
University of Toronto
500 University Avenue
Toronto, Ontario
Canada M5G 1V7

Barbara Maughan
Institute of Psychiatry
De Crespigny Park
Denmark Hill
London SE5 8AF, UK

Martin Newman
William Harvey Clinic
313–315 Cortis Road
London SW116 6XG, UK

Thomas H. Ollendick
Virginia Polytechnic Institute and
State University
Child Study Center
Department of Psychology
Blacksburg, Virginia 24061-0355,
USA

Aribert Rothenberger
Universität Göttingen
Abt für Kinder-und Jugend-
psychiatrie der Universität
von-Siebold-Strasse 5
D-37075 Göttingen,
Germany

Stephen Scott
Department of Child and Adolescent
Psychiatry
Institute of Psychiatry
Denmark Hill
London SE5 8AF,
UK

Laura D. Seligman
Department of Psychology
University of Toledo
No 948
Toledo, OH 43606
USA

Margaret J. Snowling
Department of Psychology
University of York
York YO10 5DD, UK

Paul Stallard
Department of Child and
Family Psychiatry
Royal Hospital
Combe Park
Bath BA1 3NG, UK

Hans-Christoph Steinhausen
Department of Child and Adolescent
Psychiatry
University of Zurich
Neumünsterallee 9
Postfach CH 8032 Zurich
Switzerland

Gregory Stores
Department of Psychiatry
University of Oxford
Univ Section
Park Hospital, Old Road
Headington, Oxford OX3 7LQ, UK

Michaela Swales
Child and Development Psychiatry
Royal Liverpool Children's Hospital
Alder Hey
Mulberry House
Eaton Road
Liverpool L12 2A, UK

Eric Taylor
Department of Child and Adolescent
Psychiatry
Institute of Psychiatry
Denmark Hill
London SE5 8AF,
UK

Per Hove Thomsen
Department of Child and Adolescent
Psychiatry
University Hospital Aarhus
Harald Selmersvej 66
8240 Risskov
Denmark

Alexander von Gontard
Department of Child and Adolescent
Psychiatry
University of Homburg
D-66421 Homburg
Germany

Brain disorders

Hans-Christoph Steinhausen and Christopher Gillberg

University of Zurich, Switzerland University of Göteborg, Sweden

Introduction

All mental functioning, be it normal or abnormal, is mediated by the brain. Thus, no child and adolescent psychiatric disorder can be thought of as not being brain related. However, there is a separate category of disorders in which the structure of the brain itself is disordered or in which the basic neurological functions are altered so that normal mental functioning may not result. This is most obvious in those disorders that result from morphological alterations of the brain structure due to a noxious agent or event, or due to a neurobiological deficit that seriously affects the organization and development of the brain.

Classification of brain disorder in childhood and adolescence is not very satisfactory. The major classes of brain disorders as set out in the ICD-10 are derived mainly from manifestations of disorders in adulthood with insufficient consideration of developmental aspects in childhood and adolescence. Thus, in contrast to most of the remaining chapter in this volume both ICD-10 and DSM-IV are not considered as the relevant framework for classification of brain disorders in childhood and adolescence.

In this chapter the following major brain disorders with a basic neurological alteration of brain structures and functions will be described: injury, infectious disorder, cerebral palsy, epilepsy and brain tumours. In an additional section the concept of minor brain dysfunction syndromes will be discussed. This concept has been very influential in the past and has largely been ignored in the more recent academic debate in child and adolescent psychiatry. Given its remaining relevance in practical child and adolescent psychiatry, an attempt will be made to identify those elements in the concept that reflect the notion fruitfully and validly that there is a continuum of brain-related symptoms between neurologically

A Clinician's Handbook of Child and Adolescent Psychiatry, ed. Christopher Gillberg,
Richard Harrington and Hans-Christoph Steinhausen. Published by Cambridge University Press.
© Cambridge University Press 2005.

defined structural brain disorders, and the concept of minor brain dysfunction syndromes.

Given the similarities of psychopathological features and mechanisms in the various brain disorders, some repetition cannot be avoided in the present chapter. However, it was decided to have relatively complete descriptions of the various phenomena and issues of each brain disorder so that the busy clinician will get sufficient information from each section of this chapter.

Brain injury

Definition and classification

Traumatic head and brain injury results from an extended force that insults the brain and leads to a transient or persistent impairment of physical, cognitive, behavioural or emotional functions. It may be divided into open and closed head injuries. Open head injury is defined by penetration of the brain, e.g. a depressed skull fracture with underlying cerebral laceration. Usually localized brain damage is involved. Closed head injury is more common, secondary to traffic accidents or to a fall. The resulting damage may be marked by contusions, intracranical hematomes, intra-ventricular, subarachnoid, subdural and epidermal hemorrhages and contrecoup injuries opposite to the initial impact. Furthermore, diffuse damage of the brain may be a sequel.

A common classification of the severity in the acute stage distinguishes mild, moderate and severe brain injury. The differentiation usually is based on the extent or duration of coma and the posttraumatic amnestic period. Derived from adult traumatology, the Glasgow Coma Scale (GCS) has also been used most frequently in the population of children and adolescents. The GCS measures eye opening, verbal response and hand or leg movement by rating each response on a scale of 1 to 5 and aggregating all three items. Higher scores represent better responsiveness and prognosis.

According to the GCS mild brain injury is defined by a score of 13 or more, posttraumatic amnesia of less than 12 hours or a loss of consciousness for 5 minutes or less. Moderate brain injury is defined by a GCS score of 9 to 12, a post-traumatic amnestic period of 12 to 24 hours, or a loss of consciousness between 5 and 60 minutes (or even more in some studies). Finally, severe brain injury is associated with a GCS score of less than 9, or post-traumatic amnesia lasting more than 24 hours. However, the GCS has been criticized for being often too crude a measure for children. Comparisons of the research literature are hampered by different definitions of the depth and length of coma as a measure of severity. Several studies in children converge in using the above-mentioned GCS total scores as an indicator of the depth of coma and extending the length of post-traumatic amnesia to 7–14 days in order to define severe brain injury.

Epidemiology

Incidence and prevalence rates

Traumatic brain injury is a very frequent cause of morbidity and mortality in childhood and adolescence. Estimated incidence rates range from 185 per 100 000 children from infancy to age 14 per annum to 295 per 100 000 adolescents and young adults aged 15 to 24 per annum in the United States. With a rate of 550 per 100 000 and per annum, the risk is highest among the 15–19 year olds. Figures around 45 000 children under 16 years with the number of deaths per annum being around 300 have been established in the United Kingdom. British figures document that 10% of children admitted to accident and emergency departments will have a moderate brain injury, and 1 per cent will have a severe injury. As many as 2.5 per cent of children may have sustained a head injury leading to admittance to accident and emergency departments during childhood.

Sex ratios

In terms of prevalence of brain injury, boys outnumber girls 2:1 with a lower rate in young children up to 5 years of age. The gender discrepancy emerges in infancy and is most prominent during school age and adolescence.

Implications for clinical practice

Head and brain injury is a leading cause of mortality and disability in young people and one of the most common causes of chronic brain syndromes in children. In some cases the injury results in transient or even permanent physical and/or cognitive and/or behavioural and emotional deficits. Highly sophisticated professional skills, including expert knowledge in psychopathology, are needed in order to assist the children who are victims of head and brain injury.

Clinical picture

Main features and symptoms

The symptoms due to brain injury vary considerably depending on cause, severity and type of head injury (open vs. closed), additional pre-morbid functioning and age of the child, post-traumatic coping and quality of the psychosocial environment. The various symptoms may be grouped on three functional levels as shown in Table 1.1.

On the neuropsychiatric level the clinical picture differs according to the phase of the disorder.

Table 1.1. Functional sequelae in brain injury

A. Neuropsychiatric
- Acute symptoms
  - Loss of consciousness, agitation, loss of orientation, short attention span
- Transient symptoms
  - Amnesia, slowing of impulse, affective lability, irritability, hallucinations, thought disorder
- Chronic symptoms
  - Psychopathology: agnosia, apraxia, dementia, disinhibition, hyperactivity, attention deficits, personality changes
  - General psychopathology: emotional and conduct disorders, adjustment disorders

B. Neurologic
- Headaches
- Sleep disturbances
- Epilepsy
- Hydrocephalus
- Spasticity
- Movement disorders
- Apallic syndrome

C. Endocrine
- Hormonal disturbances due to
  - Posterior pituitary deficiencies
  - Anterior pituitary deficiencies
  - Hypothalamic pituitary axis dysfunctions

D. Neurocognitive
- Impaired intellectual functions
- Reduced speed of information processing
- Language and communication skills impairment
- Impaired learning and memory
- Attention deficits
- Perceptual deficits
- Executive functions deficits

E. Educational
- Impaired progress in school
- Failing a grade
- Special education provision
- Scholastic skills deficit

F. Psychosocial
- Dysfunctional individual adaptation
- Dysfunctional family adaptation
- Social disintegration

- In the acute phase varying degrees of depth of coma dependent on the severity of the trauma are noticeable with a loss of consciousness even missing in some children. Mild head injury typically is associated only with transient symptoms of dizziness, headaches, confusion and fatigue with no loss of consciousness or a loss of consciousness not exceeding 20 minutes. A diagnosis of delirium may be stated when agitation, loss of orientation and short attention span are evident.

- There may be a transient phase of relatively short-lived psychopathological features due to a post-traumatic impairment of mental functioning including memory, impulse, affects and thought. Minor transient psychopathological syndromes include slowing of impulse, loss of initiative, forgetfulness, emotional lability and irritability. Moderate to severe transient psychopathological syndromes may include prolonged amnesia and even psychotic symptoms, like formal thought disorder, hallucinations and paranoid symptoms.

- In the chronic phase various specific impairments may become evident. In some children localized deficits leading to the syndromes of agnosia, apraxia and aphasia may result from the injury. A persistent intellectual impairment may justify a diagnosis of childhood dementia and a persistent behavioural pattern resembling a frontal lobe syndrome in adults may be emerging. This syndrome of social disinhibition is marked by a lack of impulse control, hyperactivity and attention deficits and may be accompanied by forgetfulness, talkativeness and carelessness. Owing to the persistent change in the child's behavioural features, a post-traumatic personality change may become noticeable.

  Even more common in the chronic phase are symptoms of general psychopathology. With the well-established increased risk of any child psychiatric disorder in brain disorder, there may be an interaction between neurological and behavioural factors in addition to separate paths for the two factors contributing to specific psychopathologies. These interactions may result in oppositional defiant and conduct disorders, anxiety disorders or affective disorders or rather than creating symptoms *de novo* may amplify a pre-existing hyperkinetic disorder. Among the adjustment disorders the possibility of some symptoms or, less common, the full picture of post-traumatic stress disorder should be considered.
  In addition to the various neuropsychiatric features, there is a wide range of symptoms on the neurologic level.

- Various post-traumatic headaches resemble other chronic headaches like migraine and tension headaches, cluster, cervicogenic and myofacial pain headaches. In association with dizziness, nausea or vomiting, other problems of the trauma like hematomas, arterial dissection or aneurysm have to be ruled out.

- A sizeable proportion of patients with head injury experience sleep disturbances. The most frequent early symptom after head injury is hypersomnolence. It is assumed that hypersomnolence results from damage of the reticular formation or the posterior hypothalamus. Insomnia is less common after brain trauma.

- Post-traumatic seizures at the time of the impact do not increase the risk of epilepsy necessarily. However, this is the case for seizures occurring later in recovery. In contrast to adults, children are more prone to develop early seizures and status epilepticus.
- Another potential complication of head injury is hydrocephalus, especially when there is subarachnoial or intraventicular hemorrhage. Hydrocephalus occurs only rarely when there is massive hemorrhage. The typical manifestation is months later.
- Only in the most severe head trauma does spasticity occur. Resulting from an impairment of corticospinal pathways, fine and gross motor co-ordination and dexterity are affected. Spasticity is marked by an increased tone associated with hyperreflexia.
- Appearing only months to years following the injury movement disorders are a relatively rare complication. Most frequently, the symptoms are due to damage of the basal ganglia or the nigrostriatal pathways leading, for instance, to dystonia of a hemiplegic limb or choreoathetosis. Tremor may follow even mild traumatic brain injury.
- Severe brain trauma may result in rare cases in the apallic syndrome characterized by a functional disconnection of the cortex and the brainstem. The main symptom is the so-called coma vigile with the patient having a markedly reduced consciousness without content and activities while being awake and reduced to a few basal autonomous functions.

Also, the endocrine system may be affected by traumatic head injury in various ways.

- The involvement of the posterior pituitary may lead either to excessive retention of free water or to diabetes insipidus with inappropriate or insufficient secretion of antidiuretic hormones.
- Damage to the anterior pituitary may result in dysfunction of various target organs. Thus, short stature may result from deficiencies in growth hormone, hypothyroidism from a deficit of thyroid-stimulating hormone, hypogonadism from deficiencies in follicle-stimulating and luteinizing hormone, and hypoadrenalism from adrenocorticotropic hormone deficits.
- Excessive appetite and also anorexia may be the consequence of post-traumatic hypothalamic dysfunction, and precocious puberty may result from dysfunction of the hypothalamic–pituitary axis.

Further sequelae of head and brain injury are evident on the neurocognitive level.

- Depending on the severity of damage, there is a varying degree of impaired intellectual functions, with a decrement between performance and verbal scale scores in standardized tests. Non-verbal functioning is more closely correlated to severity of injury than are verbal scores. The former is more dependent on speech, dexterity and problem-solving skills whereas verbal skills rely on retrieval of information that may be overlearnt. The impairment of the general level of functioning may manifest as a loss of skills, a failure to make any progress or a slower rate of learning.

- Another very frequent neuro-cognitive sequel is reduced speed of information processing affecting various other neuro-cognitive functions, i.e. language, learning and memory, attention and perceptual and motor tasks. Functionally, the affected children may be slower in everyday life, including school and leisure time activities, where fast and complex information processing is needed.

- Problems of naming and with expressive and written language and a deficit in verbal fluency will point to language and communication skills impairment. Sometimes the impact of the trauma may also result in transient mutism. Depending on the age of the child, grammar and syntax may be affected in pre-schoolers whereas higher-level language skills may become deficient in older children and in adolescents. Persistent problems may include a lack of prosody, slowed rate of speech or articulation deficits.

- Further problems stem from impaired learning and memory leading to slowed down knowledge and skills acquisition processes, forgetfulness and absent-mindedness that can be seen both in the classroom and at home. Verbal memory deficits may result in failure to recall instructions, or failure to remember can lead to the necessity of repetitions.

- Frequently encountered problems include attention deficits and distractibility. Children with head injuries have problems with both sustained and focused attention and are easily distracted by extraneous events going on around them. Keeping them on task at school or engaging them in activities for a long time at home is not an easy task.

- Among perceptual deficits visual–perceptual motor skills may be affected soon after the injury and these deficits may persist over longer periods in severe injuries. These functional difficulties may be the result of partial loss of visual fields or double vision in a few children.

- Owing to the high vulnerability of the frontal lobes to traumatic brain injuries, executive functions frequently are disturbed. These functions comprise basic attention and orientation, working memory, meta-representation skills, semantic representation skills and a monitoring system. They involve the capacity for self-determination, self-direction, self-control and regulation. Deficits in these areas impair limitations on the child's capacity to adapt appropriately to changes in environmental demands.

The various neurocognitive deficits lead to various problems on the educational level.

- A large proportion of children with head injuries do not make normal progress in school, fail a grade or need special education provision due to less capable performance at school.
- Educational achievement in these children may be hampered by specific scholastic skills deficits in terms of reading backwardness or sometimes even dyslexia, problems with written language and/or deficits in arithmetic skills with dyscalculia in the most severe cases.

Finally, there are various important consequences on the psychosocial level.

- In each instance of brain injury the child and adolescent has to cope with the impairment resulting from the trauma. Thus, a process of individual adaptation has to start that is based on the individual resources and pre-morbid personality features. Depending on these qualities, there may be both risk and protective factors that either contribute to the heightened risk of general psychopathology in brain disordered patients or buffer against it.
- Family resources are of similar importance. A lack of support from the family may stem from dysfunctional adaptation. Usually families, and most specifically parents, undergo a process of adaptation that starts from an initial shock phase with limited understanding and potential for goal-directed actions. An intermittent phase is then marked by various feelings of anxiety, guilt, anger and blame and finally a relatively stable phase of adaptation is reached. Dysfunctional processes of adaptation may be marked by insufficient care of the patient and/or his siblings, increased family disagreements, partnership problems or even break-up of the family. These problems may be even more pronounced if there is grief and loss for another family member who has died in the accident, a parent or sibling suffering from post-traumatic stress disorder as a consequence of witnessing the injury or an injured parent or sibling.
- Beyond the family, the wider psychosocial environment with relatives, friends and peers reacts to the handicapping condition of the child and exerts an influence on the psychosocial adaptation of the affected child. The reactions may vary between isolation and rejection on the one hand and integration and support on the other. The individual child and his family may both be affected by those either negative or positive processes.

Differential diagnosis and comorbidity

The main question of differential diagnosis in brain injury is whether or not a given symptom or syndrome may be delineated directly or only indirectly from the brain disorder. There is little doubt that very early signs of delirium that can be observed, for instance, in the emergency department, i.e. loss of consciousness, agitation and loss of orientation are related directly to the impact on the brain. However, in the case of lacking information on history, it may not be clear whether there is a closed head injury or an infectious disorder or an intoxication or another noxious agent exerting an influence on the brain. These various causes will have to be ruled out by careful physical examination including laboratory assessments and neuroimaging.

Similarly, transient psychotic features may pose the question whether or not symptoms of schizophrenia may also explain the clinical picture. Owing to the similarity of the main features in the two conditions, differentiation may be difficult in the absence of clear anamnestic data. Most commonly, the transient psychotic features in brain disorders are marked by hallucinations that are closer to reality and less bizarre and strange and by more concrete and trivial paranoid symptoms.

In the absence of a clear history and/or the exclusion of other aetiologies the localized symptoms of agnosia, aphasia and apraxia also deserve careful examinations assisted by neuroimaging in order to rule out causes other than injury, i.e. brain tumours or anomalies of brain vessels.

With the dominant manifestations of general psychopathology, there is less of a question of differential diagnosis or co-morbidity than an attempt to differentiate the various factors that may have contributed both separately and in interaction with the brain injury to the clinical symptoms.

Various sequelae of the brain injury on the neurologic and endocrine level that may lead to the development of orthopaedic disorders (e.g. scoliosis, contractures, arthritis) may be viewed as co-morbid disorders.

Diagnostic instruments and assessment

The main source of diagnosis in brain injury is clinical examination by the use of history taking, observation and neurological assessment. Neuroimaging by the use of computed tomography (CT), magnetic resonance imaging (MRI) and electroencephalogram (EEG) is mandatory in order to get a full and comprehensive picture of the brain injury.

Neuropsychiatric examination of acute symptoms in brain injury will take place only in the emergency room and transient symptoms will also be noticeable most probably in intensive care units, where examination has to be performed in collaboration with neuropeadiatricians and neurosurgeons. Continuous and repeated observations within relatively short intervals of time are needed in order to examine the fluctuating course of symptoms.

The main domain of neuropsychiatric assessment are the chronic sequelae of brain injury that have to be followed over years in some cases with a very protracted course. The majority of symptoms are represented by neuropsychological deficits in the areas of intellectual functioning, speed of information processing, language and

Table 1.2. Areas of assessment, interview questions, and neuropsychological tests (adapted from Middleton 2001)

Area of assessment	Interview questions	Neuropsychological tests
1. Intellectual functioning	Loss of skills Failure to make any progress Slower rate of learning	Wechsler Intelligence Scale for Children (WISC-III) Wechsler Primary and Preschool Scales of Intelligence (WIPPS-R)
2. Speed of information processing Motor speed Thinking speed	Time to carry out everyday living tasks (e.g. getting dressed) Grasp what is going on around them (e.g. in general conversation) Process information in unpressed situations Gather and express thoughts Respond to questions or requests Carry out motor tasks	Peg boards, Coding and Symbols (WISC-III)
3. Language and communication skills Expressive language Receptive language Word finding Written language	Ability to initiate conversations Clarity of speech and intonation Word finding Grammatical structure of speech Ability to express ideas Ability and flexibility to follow general conversation Understanding of jokes, ambiguity, and abstract concepts Writing, reading and spelling	Standardized Speech and Language Tests Picture Vocabulary Tests Verbal Scale of WISC-III
4. Learning and memory Visual and verbal memory Immediate and delayed memory Recall and recognition	Forgetting simple instructions Losing belongings Forgetting homework Forgetting plans for the next day Forgetting what happened yesterday Forgetting where things have to be put down in the home Need for many repetitions	Children's Memory Scale Test of Memory and Learning Wide Range Assessment of Memory and Learning Rivermead Behavioural Memory Test

5. Attention	Attention span	Attentional task batteries
Vigilance and attention	Distractibility	Continuous performance test (CPT)
Sustained attention	Deficits in organization of tasks	
Divided and focused attention		
6. Visual-perceptual skills	Trips over or bumps into things	Rey–Osterieth Complex Figure
Spatial awareness	Ignores things on one side of the field of vision	Performance Scale WISC-III
Visuo-construction	Has difficulties with writing, drawing or copying	Tests of Visuo-Motor Integration
Visual organization	Has problems doing puzzles or playing with constructional toys	
Visuo-motor integration	Has poor aims in ball games, etc.	
7. Executive functions	Self-organize (for school, clothes, bedroom)	Wisconsin Card Sorting Task
Verbal fluency	Plan homework and other activities	Stroop Test
Working memory: planning and execution	Keep to plans and not to be distracted by peripheral information	Tower of London
Ability to shift set	Initiate activity	
Ability to inhibit responding to peripheral information	Evaluate own work objectively	
8. Educational achievement	Progress in school	Standardized Achievement Test
Reading	Failing a grade	Standardized Scholastic Skills Tests
Spelling	Special education	
Writing	Scholastic skills	
Arithmetic		

communication skills, learning and memory, attention, visual–perceptual skills and executive functions. As a consequence, educational achievement may be hampered considerably.

Assessment of these neuropsychological deficits needs both exploration and testing. Table 1.2 provides an overview of the area of assessment, probes of interview questions and recommendations for neuropsychological tests. For various functions, recommendations for specific tests have to remain rather general when national standardization is needed for individual assessment.

The process of assessing multiple areas of function over years of follow-up must be regarded in a developmental context. With changes of the child's functions in these areas, problems will not only disappear but also will take some time to emerge, e.g. only after months and years. Thus there may not be only remission of symptoms but also a process where the child partially grows into functional deficits.

Aetiology

The causes of brain injury vary with age. The majority of head injuries in infants are caused by falls or abuse. In older children and adolescents traffic accidents, sports and leisure-time activities account for the majority of injuries. Children and adolescents with pre-existing disorders, in particular hyperkinetic disorder and children from disadvantaged psychosocial environments are at increased risk of head injury.

The severity of damage in open head injury is related to the kinetic energy of the penetrating object. Thus, the shot of a gun or rifle results in more damage than a hit with an object. Open head injuries result in more localized damage than closed head injuries. The pathophysiology of closed head injuries and the severity of the damage are related to the translational and rotational forces involved. Contusions most commonly involve the inferior frontal and temporal lobe surfaces. Rotational forces most often affect the subcortical white matter, the upper brainstem, the superior cerebellar peduncle and the basal ganglia by axonal shearing, leading to diffuse damage in these areas. Shearing effects are also observed by the use of neuroimaging in the hippocampus, corpus callosum and at interfaces between the brain and the dura. Injury of the cell membrane and intracellular swelling leads to cerebral oedema.

The neuropsychiatric sequelae may be mediated via organic pathways or via psychosocial pathways. There is a direct link between brain injury and impaired neurocognitive processing. However, brain injury can also lead to various adverse psychosocial consequences. As stated above, it may be assumed that many common psychiatric disorders in brain-injured children result from an interaction of organic and psychosocial risk factors.

Treatment

Clinical management and treatment setting

Depending on the severity of brain injury, the affected children and adolescents require multidisciplinary intervention. Open head injuries will require neurosurgical interventions and pharmacological measures against the accompanying cerebral oedema. Whereas mild head injuries may not require more than psychiatric consultation, moderate to severe forms of head injuries deserve intensive and often long-standing rehabilitation. Starting with the consultation in the emergency room or intensive care unit, the child and adolescent psychiatrist will be part of an interdisciplinary team consisting of neuropaediatricians, neurosurgeons, orthopaedists, psychologists, physiotherapists, speech and language therapists, occupational therapists, nurses and teachers. Frequently, highly specialized rehabilitation units are required for long-term care of brain-injured children.

Within this interdisciplinary team, the child and adolescent psychiatrist are responsible mainly for the promotion of positive psychosocial adaptation of the patient and his family. The measures of intervention include psychotherapy, behaviour modification, family and team counselling and psychopharmacotherapy.

Psychological interventions

Both the patient and his or her family require professional assistance in their process of adaptation. Supportive psychotherapy may be used to help the child coping with the burden of the disorder. Behavioural interventions including contingency management or skills training may assist the process of redeveloping lost skills or provide intervention schedules for the rehabilitation team in specialized units in order to control for behavioural excesses or deficits. Furthermore, educational achievements have to be recalibrated according to the child's current potential. Accordingly, the school has to be informed and counselled in order to adapt the curriculum to the individual needs of the child.

Owing to the above-mentioned problems in adaptation, the family also will need specific professional attention. Family counselling, including clear and honest information about the patient's present status and the problems of clearly defining prognosis, is helpful and will be appreciated by the family. Usually, the family will find it stressful to live with uncertainty so that at least the discussion of fears and worries with the parents can be useful and supportive. Additional information on getting the necessary extra help in school or about local or national support groups in order to have contact with families in a similar life situation are needed and valued by the parents. Family counselling also will allow an additional focus on mental suffering of other family members, problems with the healthy siblings or within the parents' partnership so that psychotherapeutic and behavioural interventions directed at these problems may be installed.

Psychopharmacotherapy

Various target symptoms can be altered successfully with psychopharmacological interventions. Table 1.3 provides a list of medications, their possible clinical indications and common and less common side effects. With the exception of the stimulants and typical neuroleptics, the safety and efficacy of these medications have not been tested thoroughly for children. However, stimulants, lithium, anticonvulsants, anxiolytics, selective serotonin-reuptake inhibitors, neuroleptics, β-blockers and α-adrenergic agonists are frequently used in acute or chronic rehabilitation of children with traumatic brain injury.

The treating expert needs to be aware of the fact that children with traumatic brain injury may react differently to certain drugs when compared with children without evidence of brain injury. For instance, the responsiveness to stimulants is less favourable than in attention deficit hyperactivity disorder (ADHD) unrelated to trauma. Children with brain injury may also be more sensitive to untoward side effects so that drugs that usually cause drowsiness only may result in somnolence during the day, cognitive blunting and insomnia at night. Similarly, medication-induced anorexia may affect weight gain and growth negatively.

Monitoring and evaluation of treatment

Since the rehabilitation process in children suffering from moderate to severe brain injury may be long-lasting, constant monitoring of the child's development and progress is essential. Besides expert examination of neuropsychiatric symptoms also behavioural and emotional functioning may be assessed by use of standardized parental checklists like the Child Behaviour Checklist (CBCL) or its companion instrument, the Teacher Rating Form (TRF), or the Strengths and Difficulties Questionnaire (SDQ, see Appendix to the chapter on conduct disorders). With more severe manifestations of brain injury and the accompanying intellectual impairment, more specific checklists developed for handicapped and mentally retarded populations may be more appropriate (see chapter on mental retardation).

One of the cornerstones of evaluation of treatment is repeated neuropsychological testing of various domains that may be affected and have been described above. The areas of assessment and recommended tests have been collected in Table 1.2. Furthermore, drug treatment needs careful monitoring of effects and side effects, and behavioural interventions specifically are apt to evaluation given the fact that clearly defined behavioural symptoms and targets are addressed.

Table 1.3. Medication used to treat brain-injured patients (adapted from Guthrie *et al.*, 1999)

Medication	Possible clinical indication	Common side effects	Less common side effects
Stimulants			
Methylphenidate	Inattention	Anorexia	Tics
Dextroamphetamine	Impulsivity	Insomnia/Irritability	Weight loss
	Hyperactivity	Headache/Tachycardia	Depression
			Hypertension
	Aggression w/above	Tremor, weight gain	Nystagmus,
			Acne
Lithium	Mood lability	Polydipsia, polyuria	Hypothyroidism
Tricyclics			
Amitryptiline	Headache	Sleepiness	Cardiac effects
Anticonvulsants			
Valproic acid	Episodic dyscontrol	Drowsiness	Hepatotoxicity
Carbamazepine	Aggressive outbursts	Weight gain	Blood dyscrasias
Gabapentin	Mood lability		
Selective serotonin-reuptake inhibitors			
Fluoxetine	Depression	Insomnia	Akathisia
Sertraline	Obsessive–compulsive symptoms	Agitation	Disinhibition
Paroxetine	Self-mutilation	Anorexia	
Fluvoxamine	Pathologic laughter/crying	Drowsiness	
		Weight gain	
Anxiolytics			
Lorazepam	Agitation	Drowsiness	Tolerance
Clonazepam	Anxiety	Cognitive slowing	Dependence
		Disinhibition	
		Drowsiness	
		Gastrointestinal complaints	
Neuroleptics			
Chlorpromazine	Psychosis	Hyperprolactenemia	Tardive dyskinesia
Haloperidol	Violent outbursts	Extrapyramidal symptoms	Malignant hyperthermia
Risperidone		Anticholinergic symptoms	Agranulocytosis
Olanzapine		Photosensitivity	
β-Blockers			
Propranolol	Aggression w/sympathetic arousal	Bradycardia	Arrhythmias
		Hypotension	Agranulocytosis
		GI disturbances	Bronchospasm
		Depression	
α-Adrenergic agonists			
Clonidine	Hyperactivity	Sedation	Hypotension
Guafacine	Inattention	Nightmares	Anxiety
	Impulsivity	Restlessness	Hallucinations
		Depression	

Problematic issues

Strong ethical problems may arise in a few cases of prolonged apallic syndromes where continuation of intensive care may be put in question by the parents. These situations require counselling in a highly sensitive way by very skilful and reflective doctors and should be embedded in a setting of continuous and intensive psychological care of the entire family.

Outcome

The short- and long-term outcomes strongly depend on the severity of the head injury. A thorough review of studies in mild head injuries that had been published between 1970 and 1995 found no adverse effects on academic and psychosocial outcome nor on neuropsychological outcome at the more extreme tail of the mild injury distribution.

The outcome with moderate to severe brain injury is less favourable. Educational achievement was impaired with GCS scores <13 and duration of coma >20 min in some follow-up studies. Attention deficits may be observed even in children with better scores. Post-traumatic amnesia >1 week has been established as an important cut-off point for lasting memory problems. Impaired dexterity and visual–motor copying have been observed even $2\frac{1}{2}$ years after severe injuries. Severely injured children have also been found to be less socially integrated.

Despite the relatively unfavourable findings of follow-up studies, it should be noted that, even in the moderate to severe injury groups, there is sizeable individual variation and that outcome is also related to environmental and not only to organic factors so that a close-response relationship between severity of the trauma and long-term sequelae does not fully describe a varying picture embedded in a developmental process.

Infectious disorders

Definition and classification

Infectious disorders are important in child psychiatry because they can (a) directly cause and/or trigger psychiatric symptoms, (b) cause permanent brain lesions that may lead indirectly to such symptoms, and (c) change the symptoms of an already existing child psychiatric disorder. Clinically, the most relevant distinction is that between meningitis and encephalitis with additional subclassification according to the class of the infectious agent, i.e. bacterial or viral subtype. These subgroups may be broken down further by the specific infectious agent, e.g. herpes encephalitis, CMV (cytomegalovirus) encephalitis, or HIV encephalitis.

Epidemiology

Prevalence and incidence rates and sex ratio

Infectious disorders of the brain are quite common in childhood. No overall figures can be given. In accordance with their higher vulnerability boys are affected more frequently than girls. The rate at which infectious disorders of the brain lead to major psychiatric disorders in children and adolescents is unknown.

Clinical implications

The more common manifestations of meningitis and encephalitis can have important psychiatric sequelae and cause handicapping conditions. Furthermore, there are some specific, though rare, associations between certain types of infections and psychiatric disorders, e.g. between streptococcal infections and tic disorders or obsessive compulsive disorder (OCD) and between rubella or herpes with autism, autistic-like conditions or mental retardation.

Clinical picture

Main features and symptoms

The clinical presentation of an infectious brain disorder varies considerably interindividually and depending on agent and timing of infection. The pattern of clinical symptoms in brain infections is shown in Table 1.4 with a differentiation between symptoms in the acute state and chronic sequelae.

- In the acute state the presenting symptoms are caused by local central nervous system (CNS) manifestations. Nearly all patients suffering from either meningitis or encephalitis develop fever, nuchal rigidity and altered mental state. The latter is marked by various intensities of altered consciousness, symptoms of delirium, disorders of impulse and, in some instances, even psychotic features. A wide range of neurological features result from the infection. Generalized seizure activity occurring during the acute state of meningitis is not associated with subsequent development of epilepsy, whereas focal seizures tend to have a worse prognosis.

- The chronic sequelae may include various behavioural symptoms and it is not uncommon for the symptoms constellation to be one of fairly typical hyperkinetic disorder, autism or even depression and schizophreniform psychosis. Frequent sequelae include mental retardation and neurological complications. During the several weeks to months following the infection, physical impairments such as communicating hydrocephalus, gait disturbances, incontinence, deafness and blindness may develop. Even the endocrine and the autonomous systems may be affected. In contrast to bacterial meningitis, neurologic sequelae are rare in viral meningitis, whereas they are very common in viral encephalitis.

Table 1.4. Clinical symptoms of brain infections

Acute state

- Headache, nausea, vomiting, nuchal rigidity, fever
- Altered consciousness of varying intensity
- Delirium including disorientation, agitation, illusions
- Disordered impulse including lethargy and overactivity
- Psychotic symptoms including hallucinations and changes in affect
- Neurological symptoms including Brudzinski's or Kernig's sign, seizures, cranial nerve dysfunction, sensory impairment, paresis, ataxia
- Disturbance of sleep–wake cycles

Chronic sequelae

- Behavioural symptoms
  - Attention deficits
  - Disorders of impulse
  - Changes in affect and emotions
  - Problems in social relating
  - Aggression
- Cognitive impairment
- Epilepsy
- Neurological impairment including paresis, hypotonia, movement disorders, sensory impairments, speech and language disorder
- Physical symptoms including endocrine disorders (growth delay, precocious puberty), autonomous dysfunctions, disturbed sleep–wake cycles

Various types of infectious diseases may be associated with the development of distinct psychiatric disorders.

- Streptococcal infections can lead to, trigger, or exacerbate symptoms that are inseparable from those shown by individuals suffering from tic disorders including Tourette syndrome (see chapter) and obsessive compulsive disorders (see chapter).
- Congenital infections occasionally lead to brain lesions in areas which are believed to represent susceptibility regions for particular neuropsychiatric syndromes. Cytomegalovirus and rubella may be the underlying cause of, or a major risk factor in, certain cases of autistic disorder.
- Also herpes encephalitis has been shown convincingly to lead occasionally to full-blown autism in individuals who have not had any autistic symptoms prior to onset of the infectious disorder.
- Mycoplasma encephalitis has been reported to be associated with the onset of schizophreniform psychosis that, albeit of a transient nature, has persisted for a year or more after the first symptoms emerged.

- Acute infections, such as infectious mononucleosis, or a influenza-like syndrome with protracted course may lead to the chronic fatigue syndrome with severe and chronic fatigue, depression, inability to concentrate, decreased memory and multiple other complaints.
- The main behavioural and cognitive features of human immunodeficiency virus (HIV) infections in children include deterioration in academic progress, subtle neurocognitive deficits in the areas of attention, motor, memory and perception, social withdrawal and increased emotional lability in the early stages. Often, there is a paucity of facial movements, as is found in diseases of the basal ganglia. Other symptoms include those of ADHD and conduct disorders. In the advanced stages of CNS–HIV psychomotor slowing, apathy and neurologic seizure such ataxia and spasticity in the legs are indicative of encephalopathy.
- Owing to persistence in tissue for long periods, infections with *Borrelia burgdorferi* may lead to chronic Lyme disease. The illness is characterized by three stages. In the first stage, the characteristic erythema migrans (bullseye rash) is visible. In the second stage, 1 to 4 months after the tick exposure, aseptic meningitis is the most common manifestation with associated mild encephalitis and further neurological complications. The third stage, developing years to months after the tick, is marked by tertiary neuroborreliosis with severe neurological sequelae. The most common form of chronic Lyme disease is a subacute encephalopathy with focal CNS deficits, motor disorders, seizures, headaches and various neurocognitive deficits. Children tend to have minor complications of shorter duration.

Differential diagnosis and assessment

Careful history taking, neurological and laboratory assessment of the inflammatory and infectious process including blood and cerebrospinal fluid (CSF) tests and neuroimaging are essential in order to establish the correct diagnosis since mental state abnormalities show large variations and insufficient specificity for various disorders. The clue to the underlying cause is often the acute/subacute onset or some associated physical symptoms including eye, ear, spleen, liver and skin anomalies in congenital infections, and fever, headache and other neurological symptoms in postnatal syndromes.

Aetiology

The pathogenesis of acute bacterial meningitis results from a rapid accumulation of granuloctes in the CSF, which is associated with several inflammatory mediators. The enhanced brain–blood barrier (BBB) permeability leads to a number of pathophysiological sequelae including cerebral oedema, increased intracranical pressure and ventriculitis as potential complications. In later stages decreased blood flow and vascular impairment secondary to inflammation may lead to cerebral ischemia and infarction.

In viral meningitis the pathogenesis involves hematogenous spread to the CNS. Enteroviruses are the most significant causal agents of this, most commonly in the summer and fall months.

Among more than 100 infectious agents causing acute viral encephalitis herpes simplex type 1 is the most common. Other causally related viruses include enteroviruses, arboviruses, Epstein–Barr virus, CMV and rabies. The direct infection of neuronal cells, predominantly of the grey matter, is the most likely pathogenic mechanism with inflammatory reactions playing an additional role.

HIV produces CNS symptoms by migration of infected macrophages from outside the CNS through the BBB into the brain. In addition, microglia, multinucleated giant cells and various neurotoxic factors with a predominance in the basal ganglia are involved. Most of the children are infected intrauterinally, through the mother.

The underlying cause of the psychiatric disorder is either the infectious agent alone (such as is likely to be the case in autism following herpes encephalitis) or an interaction between the brain lesion caused by the agent and some genetic susceptibility (such as in the case of exacerbation of tics in Tourette syndrome). In the case of herpes encephalitis it appears that the frontal and temporal brain lesions caused by the virus are responsible for the neuropsychological deficits that lead on to the syndromal presentation of autism. In Tourette syndrome, the hypothesis is that antibodies against streptococcal agents cross-react with basal ganglia nerve cell tissue to exacerbate the symptoms of tics and obsessive–compulsive behaviours.

Long-term psychosocial adaptation is dependent on various factors. Besides direct effects resulting from the brain disorder, there are various indirect effects including developmental status, coping capacities and resources of the child, support from parents and siblings and assistance from relatives, peers and school. The process of interaction of these various factors may either be helpful in adjusting to the sequelae of the basic disorder or may even aggravate a burdensome illness.

Treatment

Clinical management and treatment setting

In the acute state most children suffering from infectious disorders of the brain will have to be admitted to a paediatric hospital. Close co-operation between a neuro-paediatrician and a liaison child psychiatrist may be helpful. More frequently, the child and adolescent psychiatrist will be responsible for the treatment of the chronic behavioural sequelae of the infection of the brain.

Psychological interventions

Chronic behavioural and cognitive sequelae due to the handicapping conditions and severity deserve intensive rehabilitation including measures of psychotherapy, behaviour modifications, speech and language therapy, physiotherapy and special education. A multidisciplinary team approach is mandatory and sometimes only highly specialized rehabilitation centres can meet the requirements. Both the needs of the patient and the family have to be considered if the mental and physical state of the child has changed dramatically from the premorbid development, and a process of major re-adjustment has to be assisted and guided.

Pharmacotherapy

Acute or subacute infections of the brain should be treated according to guidelines for such infections in collaboration with a doctor with expertise in this area. The definite treatment for bacterial meningitis is early administration of antibiotics. No specific antiviral therapy currently is available for treatment of enteroviruses, the most common causal agents of the small group of viral meningitis. The treatment of choice for viral encephalitis is acyclovir and AZT is indicated in HI infections due to its good CNS penetration.

Psychiatric symptoms may well respond to neuroleptics and stimulants according to the indications for these drugs. Interactions with antiepileptic drugs (AED) have to be considered if the patient is receiving AEDs. These interactions are shown in Table 1.9.

Monitoring and evaluation of treatment

Besides continuous physical assessment including neurological and laboratory assessment, behavioural and emotional changes have to be recorded. Psychopathological features should be described carefully. In addition, behavioural features may be evaluated by various informants including parents, therapists of different kind, and special education teachers. Standardized rating scales and questionnaires may be used (e.g. the Child Behaviour Checklist (CBCL) or the Strengths and Difficulties Questionnaire (SDQ)). Neuropsychological testing of various cognitive functions including general intelligence, speech and language, memory, learning, perception and attention is a major cornerstone of the evaluation of treatment. Specific recommendations for neuropsychological assessment are given in Table 1.2 in the section on brain injury.

Information of patients and parents

Psychoeducation and guidance of patients and parents is of high importance, given the fact that the chronic sequelae of infectious brain disorders may be extremely burdensome. Especially the high mortality rate of meningitis caused by arboviruses

and the increased rate of severe handicaps in the survivors makes intensive counselling and guidance of the parents mandatory. Close co-operation between the
child psychiatrist and the rehabilitation team is essential in order to provide accurate information and assistance to the patient and the parents. Reactions of grief
and depression should be identified and lead to the installation of appropriate
treatment.

Outcome

The outcome of infectious brain disorders varies a lot. Congenital infectious syndromes and herpes encephalitis appear to carry a gloomy prognosis unless treatment can be started early and brain tissue destruction be minimized. Mycoplasma
encephalitis may run a protracted course (over 6 to 18 months) but neuropsychiatric symptoms may eventually resolve. The outcome for most cases of viral
encephalitis is poor. Treatment of streptococcal disorders in connection with tics
eventually may prove to be a fruitful avenue for improving the outcome in some
cases of tic disorders, but the evidence to date is too limited to draw any definitive
conclusions. Patients with focal epilepsy as a result of bacterial meningitis tend to
have a worse prognosis.

Cerebral palsy

Definition and classification

Cerebral palsy is a heterogeneous group of non-progressive, but often changing,
motor impairment syndromes secondary to lesions or anomalies of the brain ori-
ginating in the early stages of its development. Often, the motor disabilities are
accompanied by other clinical manifestations of brain disorders, including epilepsy,
learning problems, sensory impairments, and not least, behavioural and emotional
problems.

The type and distribution of spasticity forms the basis of subclassification of
cerebral palsy. In spastic hemiplegia just one side of the body is affected whereas
in spastic diplegia both legs are affected to a severe extent and both arms to a
mild extent. Quadriplegia or tetraplegia denotes the severe spastic affection of all
four limbs. Less frequently, ataxia, or dyskinesia (athetosis) dominate the motor
problems of cerebral palsy.

Epidemiology

Prevalence rates

The prevalence rates for cerebral palsy reported in the world literature since 1990
are quite stable at approximately 0.2–0.25 per cent. The percentages of cerebral palsy

attributed to prenatal risk factor vary between 8 and 43%. This variation may be due to differences in defining exposure to risks. Prevalence rates of the subtypes of cerebral palsy also differ considerably. An English register study of more than 1000 children with cerebral palsy found 35 per cent to have quadriplegia, 31 per cent to have hemiplegia and 22 per cent to have diplegia. A further 5–10 per cent have ataxia (including atactic diplegia) and some variants are considered unclassifiable.

Implications for clinical practice

With 2 in 1000 children and adolescents, cerebral palsy is not a frequent though very handicapping condition and is the single largest course of severe physical disability in childhood.

Clinical picture

Main features and symptoms

Epidemiological and clinical studies of children with cerebral palsy have shown the following characteristics with regard to psychiatric disorders.

- The prevalence of psychiatric problems is higher than in normal children amounting to half and more of the population of children with cerebral palsy. It is increased significantly if two common accompanying factors of cerebral palsy are there, namely, mental retardation and specific reading retardation. This tends to be true also for accompanying seizures. All three factors indicate that there is a relation between organic severity and rate of psychiatric problems.
- In general, there is no distinctive association of cerebral palsy with any type of psychiatric disorder except hyperkinetic disorders. In hemiplegia, with its relatively mild physical disability and little or no intellectual impairment, around half of all affected children have at least one psychiatric disorder. Among these children conduct and emotional disorders each affect one-quarter, hyperkinetic disorders another 10 per cent, and autism around 3 per cent.
- The most common emotional disorders in children with hemiplegia are specific phobias, separation anxiety and generalized anxiety. Some patients also develop depressive disorders. Also, frequently these children show markedly defiant and negativistic behaviour also leading in some cases to marked aggression. A considerably larger number of children with hemiplegia than healthy children show some autistic features. Also in this subgroup IQ, which is associated with degree of neurological impairment, is the best predictor of psychiatric problems. The latter are again more common if specific learning difficulties are present.
- Children with hemiplegia encounter an increased risk of social isolation due to teasing, victimization, marginalization and lack of friendships. These problems

may be due in part to constitutional problems with social understanding and relatedness.

- Psychiatric and behavioural problems are often very persistent and may be seen for many years.

Aetiology

The causes of cerebral palsy are largely unknown. However, some associations are known, namely, between cerebrovascular accidents and hemiplegia, between a variety of generalized brain insults and quadriplegia, and between severe rhesus disease and athetosis. There is a hereditary component in ataxia and prematurity is an important risk factor for various forms of cerebral palsy, most notably for diplegia.

The determinants of psychiatric disorders are multifactorial. Certainly, the underlying brain disorder implies a heightened vulnerability with limited cognitive potential (in many cases) and a lack of personal and psychosocial resources adding to the risk of developing psychiatric problems. Among the latter, social rejection and isolation among peers and within the family are powerful sources of individual maladjustment. In hemiplegia, some degree of bilateral involvement, the presence of seizures and lower IQ have been shown to be associated with a higher rate of psychiatric disorder.

Treatment

The basic condition of cerebral palsy requires competent neurological and orthopaedic treatment with physiotherapy being the major cornerstone. Additional mental retardation and/or sensory impairment may imply that the child with cerebral palsy may not be educated in the mainstream schooling system but, rather, need special education.

With the high probability of developing additional psychiatric problems, there is not only the need for careful monitoring and assessment but also for early intervention or even for the development of preventive approaches. In principle, all sorts of psychological interventions including brief and supportive individual psychotherapy, behavioural interventions, counselling and psycho-education are applicable. Since the families are subjected to the burden of sometimes very distressing and enduring care, a family approach in counselling and guiding is indicated. All these efforts should be started early and be continued over years.

Some of the psychiatric problems such as the frequent hyperkinetic disorders may require standard psychopharmacological treatment. There is a lack of well-controlled studies on the efficacy and effectiveness of drug treatment in children with cerebral palsy. Thus, very careful titration processes and monitoring of effects and side effects are mandatory. If there is co-existent epilepsy, the application of psychotropic medication may lead to interactions with antiepileptic drugs. Potential interactions are outlined in Table 1.9. However, improved control of seizures also may in some instances improve behaviour and cognitive status. Similarly, stimulant medication can result in improved learning if there is a hyperkinetic disorder, and the application of SSRI can help with depression, obsession and compulsion.

Outcome

Cerebral palsy itself is a chronic condition, marked by persistent physical disability of interindividually varying degree. Concomitant mental retardation and sensory impairment may have an additional impact on the course of the disorder. However, it has to be emphasized that many affected individuals experience a satisfying and productive lifestyle with normal psychosocial adaptation.

There is a very limited body of empirical research on the longitudinal stability of psychiatric problems in children suffering from cerebral palsy. A recent British study of a representative sample of children with hemiplegia found a remarkable stability of psychiatric problems in these children. After a follow-up period of 4 years, 70 per cent of the former psychiatric cases were still fulfilling criteria of psychopathology. In the pre-school years, extending symptoms were predictive of later conduct and hyperactivity problems, and in the school years, hyperactivity was particularly predictive of continuing psychiatric problems. The continuity of psychiatric problems was mainly dependent on the severity and the type of the initial psychiatric problems, whereas neurological, cognitive, demographic and family factors did not contribute much to the persistence of the problems.

Despite the high rate of psychiatric disorders in childhood, hemiplegia does not seem to lead to a particularly raised frequency of adult psychiatric disorders. Some childhood problems may persist as maladaptive personality traits and rather restricted lifestyles with limited social activities and professional careers.

Epilepsy

Definition and classification

Epilepsy is a chronic condition of recurrent unprovoked seizures. The latter can be defined as sudden, involuntary, transient alterations in cerebral function due to abnormal discharge of neurones.

The sub-classification of the various types of epilepsy by the International League Against Epilepsy (ILAE) is based on three factors, namely: (a) clinical seizure mani-festations, which define the seizure, (b) electroencephalogram (EEG) ictal patterns, and (c) EEG interictal pattern. According to Table 1.5 either partial or generalized and, in addition, unclassified seizures are differentiated. A partial seizure begins in

Table 1.5. Classification of epilepsy according to the International League Against Epilepsy (ILAE)

I. Partial (focal, local) seizures
    Definition: The first clinical and/or EEG changes indicate initial involvement of part of one hemisphere.
    Partial seizures are classified on the basis of an impairment of consciousness
    A. Simple partial seizures (no impairment of consciousness)
    B. Complex partial seizures (with impairment of consciousness)
    C. Partial seizures with secondary generalization
II. Generalized seizures
    Definition: The first clinical and/or EEG changes indicate initial involvement of both hemispheres.
    Consciousness is impaired
    A. Absence/atypical absence
    B. Myoclonic
    C. Clonic
    D. Tonic
    E. Tonic–clonic
    F. Clonic–tonic–clonic
    G. Atonic

one area or has a focus, whereas a generalized seizure has an initial bihemispheric involvement both clinically and on EEG. Unclassified seizures include those with insufficient information available and neonatal seizures.

Epidemiology

Prevalence rates

Epilepsy in terms of recurrent seizures affects 0.5–1 per cent of the population and up to 10 per cent of individuals have at least one affable seizure at some time in their life. Three-quarters of all epilepsies originate before 20 years of age. By the same age, 5 per cent of all children and adolescents will have experienced a seizure but fewer than one in five of these will develop epilepsy. Within 5 years of seizure onset, 80 per cent of children will be expected to be seizure free. Approximately 2–5 per cent of children will have febrile seizures.

A recent nationwide British study found a prevalence rate for psychiatric disorders of 37 per cent, with a rate of a 56 per cent for complicated epilepsy and 26 per cent for uncomplicated epilepsy. Scandinavian studies suggest that, if epilepsy is combined with mental retardation, then the risk of psychiatric disorder is higher still.

Implications for clinical practice

Epilepsy is a very common disorder in children and adolescents. The rate of non-recurrent afebrile and febrile seizures without progression into epilepsy is much higher. The majority of children and adolescents with epilepsy will become seizure free. However, a sizeable proportion of patients remain with a severe and handicapping condition. The prevalence rate for accompanying psychiatric disorders is elevated significantly and asks for additional provision of mental health services.

Clinical picture

Main feature and symptoms

A full description of the clinical symptomology of the epilepsies is beyond the scope of this chapter. This section will concentrate on (a) epileptic syndromes with psychiatric manifestations and (b) a more general discussion of the association between epilepsy and mental functioning.

Epileptic syndromes with psychiatric manifestations

Certain epileptic syndromes have significant psychiatric or neurobehavioural problems. These include temporal lobe epilepsy (complex partial seizures), infantile spasms, the Lennox–Gastaut syndrome, the Landau–Kleffner syndrome (LKS), and the syndrome of continuous spike-waves during slow-wave sleep (CSWS) also known as Electric Status Epilepticus during Slow sleep (ESES).

- The large majority of patients with temporal lobe epilepsy marked by odd movements, postures, dreamy states, prolonged absences, automatisms and vocalizations show psychiatric disorders. There are specific associations with hyperkinetic disorders and excessive rage outbursts. The risk for a schizophrenia-like psychosis in later life is elevated. Complex partial seizures are one of the most common epileptic syndromes in autism.
- There is a strong association between infantile spasms characterized by brief jack-knife spasms and hypsarrhythmia on the EEG, on the one hand, and mental retardation on the other since many cases have their origin in tuberous sclerosis or a brain malformation. The most common psychiatric disorders are hyperkinetic disorders and autism.
- In the Lennox–Gastaut syndrome, which presents in young children with frequent myoclonic, tonic and atonic seizures (stare, jerk and fall seizures), the great majority of affected children has severe mental retardation. In prolonged episodes of minor states the child is socially unresponsive, aggressive, less articulate and may show minor twisting of hands and face.
- The Landau–Kleffner syndrome is a rare epileptic syndrome characterized by language regression (usually associated with verbal auditory agnosia, and sometimes

referred to as acquired aphasia) and an abnormal EEG/seizures. Hyperactivity is common as are autistic features. The classical LKS occurs in a previously normal child usually in the 3–7-year-old age range. LKS variants include children without clinical seizures but with abnormal EEGs, children with autism with language regression and abnormal EEGs, and children with congenital aphasias, also called developmental language disorders with epileptiform EEGs.

- The syndrome of CSWS is characterized by spike and wave activity that occurs during at least 85 per cent of slow-wave sleep and commonly is accompanied by infrequent seizures. The affected children had been normally developing prior to onset usually between 6 and 10 years and experience regression in mental, language, and behavioural functions. Main psychiatric manifestations include hyperkinetic features, aggressiveness, affective lability, transient psychosis and regressive behaviour features. LKS and CSWS sometimes are considered to exist on the same spectrum of epileptic behaviour syndromes.

The association between epilepsy and mental functioning

As outlined above in the section on epidemiology, there is a significantly heightened rate of general psychopathology in children suffering from epilepsy. Overall, the most frequently observed psychiatric disorders are hyperkinetic disorders, autism spectrum disorders and mental retardation. There is a clear association between complicated epilepsy, as indicated by additional neurological abnormalities, and further increase of psychiatric morbidity.

The traditional concept of an epileptic personality has been discredited and replaced by more detailed analyses of behaviour problems and personality features. The latter have found that dependency, suicidal behaviour, an external rather than an internal locus of control, lack of self-esteem and feelings of anxiety and fears are more common among children with epilepsy.

The term paradoxical or forced normalization, denotes a specific phenomenon of an abrupt worsening of behaviour in patients with epilepsy when seizures are controlled and the EEG improves. The behaviours do not only include symptoms of psychosis but also dyslexia and affective disorders, histrionic features and hypochondrial symptoms. Usually, paradoxical normalization occurs with a change in anticonvulsant drugs. It is more frequent in adults but may also be observed in children.

Whereas most children with uncomplicated epilepsy show cognitive functioning in the normal range of intelligence, the IQ is lowered in complicated epilepsy. A high proportion of children with epilepsy show mental retardation and, the greater the degree of pro-existing mental retardation, the higher the risk of developing epilepsy. Only in a small number of children intellectual functioning is deteriorating as a result of the disorder and/or deficits in appropriate care.

However, there are several ways in which epilepsy can create learning problems of various size. An extreme is prolonged, brain-damaging status epilepticus. Via state-dependent learning also a non-convulsive status epilepticus accompanied by generalized spike-wave discharges or frequent absence seizures may contribute to disability. Frequent epileptiform discharges without convulsions may also have an impact in terms of so-called transitory cognitive impairment, leading to frustrating experiences, which may affect learning. Similar effects may stem from frequent local or frequent hemispheric discharges, e.g. on the basis of congenital brain malformations.

In addition, there also may be underestimated post-ictal effects in terms of state-dependent learning disability if, in very frequent seizures, there is not sufficient time for the affected child to recover from one seizure before another. The same principle of post-ictal effects applies also to frequent nocturnal seizures or CSWS.

Finally, antiepileptic drug treatment also may contribute to impairment of cognitive functioning. Sedative effects of the wrong type of anticonvulsant may affect learning adversely. Drugs such as phenobarbital, the benzodiazepines and vigabatrin may show a paradoxical effect in children by mimicking the symptoms of hyperkinetic disorders. Children with autism and epilepsy often show particularly adverse behavioural toxicity during treatment with clonazepam and other benzodiazepines.

Unfortunately, research on the cognitive adverse effects of chronic antiepileptic drug treatment in general is plagued by a multitude of methodological shortcomings, so that currently no satisfactory statement can be given. The overall conclusion is that, in relation to cognition, some children benefit significantly, a middle group does not appear to be affected and a third group is made worse by the antiepileptic medication.

A more detailed analyses of the determinants of both cognitive impairment and behavioural problems will be provided in the section on aetiology below.

Differential diagnosis and co-morbidity

From a psychiatric point of view, there is a need to differentiate various disorders from epilepsy as shown in Table 1.6. These disorders are also called non-epileptic paroxysmal events or non-epileptic periodic events and need to be considered in patients with intractable epilepsy or persistently normal EEG. However, it should be kept in mind that many patients with epilepsy have a normal EEG and diagnosis of epilepsy does not require an abnormal EEG. Furthermore, the high rate of psychopathology in epilepsy does also allow the possibility that epilepsy and one of these disorders may coincide in terms of co-morbidity. Medical history and careful description of symptoms are more important than an EEG in diagnosis and differential diagnosis in epilepsy.

Table 1.6. Differential diagnosis of epilepsy

- Pseudoseizures
- Movement disorders
  - Tics and Tourette syndrome
- Sleep disorders
  - Night terrors
  - Somnambulism
  - Hypersomnia
  - Narcolepsy
- Panic attacks
- Rage attacks or episodic dyscontrol
- Migraine
- Munchhausen's syndrome (by proxy)

The following implications derived from differential diagnosis are outlined in Table 1.7.

- Pseudo-seizures may combine with true seizures. Indicators of pseudo-seizures include situations when the child is being observed rather than staying alone, a gradual rather than a sudden onset, uncontrolled flailing paroxysms rather than true clonus, theatrical movements accompanied by loud shouting or screaming, avoidance of painful stimuli and injury during an attack, sudden offset with an immediate return to an alert and responsive state and lack of paroxysmal discharges on the EEG during an episode.
- Tics and especially ocular tics, including Tourette syndrome, may sometimes evoke the question whether myoclonic jerk are present. Again, the lack of paroxysmal discharges in the EEG will allow differential diagnosis.
- Various sleep disorders including night terrors, somnambulism, hypersomnia and narcolepsy will have to be excluded not only by the different phenomenological features but also by the lack of specific epileptiform activity in the EEG.
- Panic attacks with their sudden onset of fear occur usually without alteration of awareness but can be confused with simple partial seizures because the latter can also be associated with a sensation of panic or fear.
- Rage attacks or episodic dyscontrol represent episodes of severe conduct or violent behaviour. Usually, they are associated with some provocation or a precipitating event, although some may develop spontaneously. Rage attacks may be more common in children and adolescents with epilepsy, hyperactivity or personality disorder. During an attack, the EEG does not show epileptiform activity. However, due to the underlying disorder, the inter-ictal EEG may be abnormal.

- Migraine, especially when accompanied by benign paroxysmal vertigo, visual hallucinations, olfactory auras, déjà vu, acute confusional states or transient global amnesia may be diagnosed erroneously as epilepsy. The lack of hypersynchronous epileptic discharges on the EEG, again, will allow distinction.
- Factitious creating or false reporting of symptoms as in Munchhausen's syndrome when the patient originates the symptoms or in Munchhausen's syndrome by proxy, with a parent creating the symptoms in the child, represent very rare instances of differential diagnosis of epilepsy.

Diagnostic instruments and assessment

The main source of diagnosis in epilepsy is careful history taking. Thus, the clinical interview is the main diagnostic instrument. Neuroimaging, especially MRI and EEG may assist the diagnostic process, but may be normal. However, neuroimaging may be very helpful for excluding underlying causes for the seizures, such as a tumour. Observation and description of the event determine classification of the seizure type.

An inter-ictal EEG may show signs of an underlying epileptic tendency, which is present in many patients with epilepsy. However, many patients with epilepsy also show a normal EEG, most particularly between seizures. Thus, a normal EEG does not exclude the diagnosis of epilepsy.

In addition to the basic neurologic examination, the neuropsychiatric assessment is based primarily on the clinical interview and requires expertise in general psychopathology in children and adolescents. Information by caretakers and other educators may be obtained either by interview or standardized checklists, allowing for the screening of a large variety of behavioural abnormalities. The latter include the Child Behaviour Checklist (CBCL) for parents, the Teacher Rating Form (TRF) or the Strengths and Difficulties Questionnaire (SDQ, see Appendix to chapter on conduct disorders). Various more specific checklists for the handicapped are available and may be helpful specifically in identifying problems due to the frequent accompanying mental retardation (see chapter on Mental Retardation).

Both the epilepsy itself and the evaluation of drug treatment in terms of effects and side effects require careful and continuous monitoring. Neuropsychological testing should be used in order to assist this process. Recommendations can be found in Table 1.2, indicating the areas of assessment, related clinical questions and selected neuropsychological tests.

Aetiology

The causes of the epilepsy itself will be discussed only briefly in this chapter. Clearly, hereditary and/or brain-related factors are involved. However, in children and adolescents, as in adults, the largest group of approximately two-thirds represent idiopathic or cryptogenic cause, 20 per cent have congenital causes, 5 per cent result from trauma, 4 per cent from infection, 2 per cent have neoplastic and 1 per cent show degenerative causes. Age at onset is important insofar as perinatal injury, metabolic disorder or congenital malformations are more common causes in the young age, whereas vascular diseases or tumours are more likely to have an impact in adults. Recently, a genetic source has been found for some types of epilepsy, e.g. an association of juvenile myoclonic epilepsy to chromosome 6 or autosomal dominant nocturnal frontal lobe epilepsy to chromosome 20.

The mechanisms involved in the psychopathology of epilepsy are complicated and need to consider at least three main categories of risk factors and their interaction: (a) brain-related factors – the epilepsy itself and further neurological factors, (b) non-brain-related factors – chronic illness, developmental and subject variables, and (c) treatment-related factors – antiepileptic treatment, surgery and quality of care.

Among the brain-related factors it is, first, the epilepsy itself that has a strong impact on psychopathology. The peri-ictal disturbances of prodome, aura and automatism each present with behavioural phenomena including disturbed mood, feelings of anxiety and symptoms of conduct disorder. In the immediate post-ictal phase confusion, tiredness, irritability, depression and even paranoid states may manifest themselves. Among the inter-ictal disturbances there is the above-mentioned reciprocal phenomenon of behavioural abnormalities and epilepsy that goes along with the paradoxical normalization in the EEG. Other previously mentioned epilepsy-related factors include focal temporal or frontal discharges, frequent absence seizures or non-convulsive status epilepticus that have a direct impact on behaviour by producing various symptoms such as socially withdrawn behaviour or attention deficit disorder.

Further epilepsy-related factors include age at onset and chronicity. The aetiological significance of early onset and long duration of epilepsy may be at least partly due to the third factor of mental retardation because infantile spasms and the Lennox–Gastaut syndrome account largely for this association. High seizure frequency and poor seizure control may be entangled similarly with other factors, such as brain damage, so that the effect on cognitive and behavioural functioning may not be direct. Also the relationship between seizure type and psychopathology and intelligence may be quite inconclusive due to the fact that most studies have concentrated on TLE or primary generalized epilepsies.

In addition to the epilepsy itself, other factors reflecting the associated brain damage or dysfunction play a major role. This may be independent of the epilepsy or be caused by the epilepsy. Injury of the frontal lobe can result in specific neurocognitive dysfunction, or damage to the dominant temporal lobe may result in speech and language disorder. Mediated effects from the brain damage may also become effective by rendering the child more liable to stresses and strains that may impair the development.

Various non-brain-related factors contribute to the heightened risk of developing psychiatric disorders in epilepsy. As in other chronic illnesses, epilepsy poses a major challenge to the resources of the individual and the family. Deficient coping, parental psychopathology, disturbed family relationships, problem with the healthy siblings or teasing and social isolation outside the family may each have an additional detrimental effect on psychosocial adaptation of the child with epilepsy. The interactive association between epilepsy and these factors is evident in as much as the latter can be both the cause and the consequence of the former.

Finally, treatment-related factors can have an impact on the development of behavioural and cognitive abnormalities. The need for continuous antiepileptic drug treatment renders the child with epilepsy particularly vulnerable to side effects. Among the older and well-established drugs, phenobarbital and benzodiazepines may cause sedation, irritability and disruptive behaviour disturbances mimicking hyperkinetic disorder. Gabapentin can exacerbate pre-existing hyperactivity and learning problems and topiramate has been associated with general slowing of cognition and behaviour. Cognitive and behavioural side effects of polytherapy, the often necessary combination of different drugs may be underestimated and brain surgery may occasionally result in worsening rather than improvement of the behaviour. Deficient quality of care and lack of compliance may also add to abnormal behavioural functioning in the child with epilepsy.

Treatment

Clinical management and treatment setting

The appropriate treatment of children and adolescents with epilepsy requires special expertise. A multidisciplinary team of neuropaediatricians, child and adolescent psychiatrists, and psychologists with specialization in child neuropsychology and behavioural interventions should join forces for the basic care of a patient with epilepsy. Depending on indication, this team should be supplemented by the neurosurgeon.

Support should also come from various experts dealing with varying degrees of disability, i.e. from physiotherapists, speech and language therapists, occupational therapists and special education teachers. Many patients with uncomplicated epilepsy can be treated in ordinary services or practices, whereas the more complicated cases need to be continuously cared for by specialized units in the tertiary sector of services.

Drug treatment plays a major role in the core of epilepsy. Due to the protracted and often chronic course, continuous counselling of the patient and the family and

Table 1.7. Efficacy of standard antiepileptic drugs, according to seizure type (Thiele *et al.*, 1999)

Drug	Seizure type					
	GTC	Absence	Focal/II general	Tonic	Atonic	Myoclonic*
Phenobarbital	+	–	+	+	+	+
Phenytoin	+	–	+	+	–	–
Carbamazepine	+	–	+	–	–	–
Valproic acid	+	+	+	+	+	+
Ethosuximide	–	+	–	–	–	–
Trimethadione	–	+	–	–	–	–
Primidone	+	–	+	+	+	+
Ethotoin	+	–	+	+	–	–
Methsuximide	+	+	+	+	+	–
Benzodiazepines, especially clonazepam	+	+	+	+	+	+
Felbamate	+	+	+	+	+	+
Gabapentin	–	–	+	–	–	–
Lamotrigene	+	+	+	+	+	+
Topiramate	+	+	+	+	+	+
Tiagabine	–	–	+	–	–	–

GTC = generalized tonic clonic seizures; + = efficacious; – = not efficacious.
*Infantile spasms are a certain type of myoclonic, tonic, or mixed type of seizure. Medications used for these include adrenocorticotropic hormone (ACTH), vigabatrin, valproate, benzodiazepines and perhaps topiramate or tiagabine.

various psychosocial interventions are warranted. The specific psychiatric problems of this clientele make both psychological and psychopharmacological treatment mandatory in a large proportion of affected patients A team approach in delivering the various interventions should be followed.

Psychological interventions

Besides prevention of seizures, the major aims of treatment include compliance with treatment strategies, prevention of additional disability due to behavioural problems, psychosocial adaptation to the disorder and social integration of the child. The major forms of intervention in order to meet these goals include individual and family counselling, behaviour modification with the child in his or her natural environments (i.e. home, school, outdoor activities), supportive psychotherapy for emotional and adaptive problems, individual or couple therapy for parents with emotional and/or relationship problems, and family therapy if indicated for the entire family. Besides the child and adolescent psychiatrist, various other therapists may share this complex task.

Table 1.8. Doses, pharmacokinetics and side effects of anticonvulsant drugs (Thiele *et al.*, 1999)

Anticonvulsant	Dose (mg/kg/day)	Therapeutic range		Half-life (hours)	Side effects
Phenobarbital	5	10–30;	15–40	40–75	Sedation, irritability, learning and sleep problems, hyperactivity, ataxia
Primidone	10–25	5–12		5–11	Sedation, nausea, vomiting, diplopia, dizziness, ataxia
Phenytoin	5	10–20		5–18	Gingival hyperplasia, hirsutism, cognitive dysfunction
Carbamazepine	20–30	4–12		8–25	Diplopia, blurred vision, ataxia
Valproate	30–40	50–100		12	Nausea, vomiting, anorexia, weight gain, hepatotoxicity, alopecia, pancreatopathy thrombocytopenia
Ethosuximide	25	50–100		24–36	Nausea, vomiting, anorexia, headaches
Felbamate	45–60	50–100		16–23	Anorexia, weight loss, insomnia, aplastic anaemia, liver failure
Gabapentin	45–60	2–10	(20)	6	Fatigue, weight gain, behavioural problems, disinhibition
Lamotrigene	5–10	2–10	(20)	12–25	Rashes, Stevens–Johnson syndrome, TEN
Topiramate	5–24	–		20	Lethargy, weight loss, anorexia, ataxia, mood disorders
Tiagabine	–	–		5–8	Dizziness, lethargy, anxiety, tumour, concentration problems

–, not established.

Pharmacotherapy

Antiepileptic drug treatment

Only recurring seizures according to the definition of epilepsy or the presence of multiple risk factors for the re-occurrence of seizures are clear indications for antiepileptic drug (AED) treatment. Seizure type, seizure activity and the efficacy and side-effect profile of a drug determine the choice of drug. The efficacy of the various AEDs is documented in Table 1.7.

First-line AEDs include carbamazepine, ethosuximide, phenobarbital, phenytoin, valproic acid and clonazepam. Non-responders to these drugs may be treated with second-line AEDs including chlorazepate, methuximide, acetazolamide and ethotoin. Recently newly developed AEDs include felbamate, gabapentin, lamotrigene, topiramate, tiagabine and vigabatrin. Doses for the most frequently used AEDs, together with pharmacokinetics and side effects are shown in Table 1.8.

Treatment should always be started with a single AED and be titrated slowly. If the single AED is not effective, a second is to be substituted with maintenance of the dosage of the first drug until seizures are controlled and slow discontinuation thereafter. If possible, polytherapy should be avoided due to the risk of drug interactions, more side effects, higher costs and lower compliance.

Alternative therapies include the ketogenic diet, which is composed of high-fat, low-carbohydrate and low-protein food. This intervention has been proved to lead to a significant reduction of seizure activity in children with difficult-to-control seizures. Side effects include weight loss, dehydration, acidosis, abdominal pain and lethargy. Surgical implantation of a vagel nerve stimulator may also be a very effective method of controlling seizures.

Psychopharmacotherapy for associated psychiatric disorders

The reluctance to use psychotropic medication in children with epilepsy is not in the best interests of these children. Indications can be divided broadly into (a) autism spectrum and developmental disorders, (b) disruptive disorders including hyperkinetic disorders and conduct disorders, (c) internalizing disorders including affective and anxiety disorders and (d) psychosis.

Psychotropic medication can have pharmacodynamic and pharmacokinetic interactions with AEDs that need special consideration. The most common pharmacodynamic effect is additive sedation. Pharmacokinetically increased or decreased plasma levels of both substances can result. The most common known and theoretic interactions between psychotropics and AEDs are shown in Table 1.9. Starting with low doses, adding slowly, and monitoring plasma levels and toxicity will contribute to safe use of psychotropics in children with epilepsy and control for lowering of the seizure threshold, which can result from psychotropics.

Treatment of the main psychiatric disorders in children with epilepsy, with an emphasis on psychotropic medication, will now be summarized.

- Autism spectrum disorders or severe developmental disorders predominantly require behavioural interventions and special education. However, in some instances (e.g. severe obsessionality interfering with functioning) neuroleptics or even serotonin re-uptake inhibitors (SRI) with cautious dose titration may be indicated.
- Hyperkinetic disorder (attention deficit hyperactivity disorders) can be treated effectively and safely with stimulants. The traditional concern that stimulants could result in more seizures is no longer valid. However, for children still having seizures while receiving AED, more caution is warranted. If stimulants fail, clonidine or guanfacine can be used cautiously. Tricyclic antidepressants have a pronounced effect on seizure threshold and should thus be avoided or

Table 1.9. Pharmacodynamic interactions of psychotropic medications with antiepileptic drugs (adapted from Thiele et al., 1999)

Psychotropic class	Specific compounds	Interactions
Stimulants	Methylphenidate, dextroamphetamine, adderall	Use cautiously with active seizure disorders; methylphenidate infrequently raises phenytoin, primidone and phenobarbitol levels
		Increased risk of hepatotoxicity when combined with hepatically metabolized AEDs
α-Adrenergic agonists	Clonidine, guanfacine	Variable effects on seizure threshold, usually benign
Antidepressants		
Selective serotonin re-uptake inhibitors	Fluoxetine	Increased carbamazepine, valproate, phenytoin, mephenytoin, ethosuximide, trimethadione, benzodiazepine and methsuximide levels; decreased fluoxetine levels with phenobarbitol, carbamazepine
	Paroxetine	No interactions found
	Fluvoxamine	Increased carbamazepine, phenytoin, mephenytoin, benzodiazepine, methsuximide levels
	Sertraline	Increased lamotrigine due to inhibition of glucoronidation; increased phenytoin and diazepam levels
	Citalopram	Decreased citalopram levels with carbamazepine, phenobarbitol, primidone
Unique compounds	Nefazadone	Increased carbamazepine, ethosuximide, trimethadione and benzodiazepine levels; decreased nefazadone levels with carbamazepine phenobarbitol, primidone
	Trazodone	Decreased trazodone levels with phenobarbitol, carbamazepine, primidone, case report of phenytoin toxicity with trazodone
	Mirtazepine, venlafaxine, bupropion, buspirone	Decreased levels with phenobarbitol, carbamazepine, primidone. Decreased buspirone plasma levels with phenytoin and carbamazepine
Tricyclics	Imipramine	Increase in carbamazepine levels; decreased imipramine levels with phenobarbitol, carbamazepine, primidone
	Nortriptyline	Decreased nortriptyline levels with phenobarbital; increased levels with valproate
	Desipramine	Decreased desipramine levels with phenobarbitol, carbamazepine
	Amitriptyline, clomipramine	Decreased tricyclic antidepressant levels with phenobarbitol, carbamazepine, primidone; increased tricyclic antidepressant levels with valproate
Mood stabilizers	Lithium	Case reports of neurotoxicity at therapeutic lithium levels with carbamazepine co-administration

(cont.)

Table 1.9. (cont.)

Psychotropic class	Specific compounds	Interactions
	Valproate	Increases levels of lamotrigine, phenobarbitol, diazepam, lorazepam, carbamazepine epoxide, primidone; displaces phenytoin and carbamazepine from protein binding sites; phenytoin decreases and felbamate increases valproate levels; uncommonly can produce absence seizures when combined with clonazepam
	Carbamazepine	Carbamazepine decreases levels of valproate, clonazepam, ethosuximide, lamotrigine, topiramate, tiagabine, primidone, antidepressants, neuroleptics; in combination with felbamate or lamotrigine increased carbamazepine epoxide and variable carbamazepine level effects; reports of ataxia and blurred vision when combined with lamotrigine; increased risk of neurotoxicity with lithium; decreased carbamazepine levels with phenobarbitol, phenytoin, primidone; variable effects on phenytoin levels with carbamazepine
Benzodiazepines	Clonazepam	Increased levels of primidone. Variable effects on phenytoin and carbamazepine levels; additive sedation with other sedating agents
	Alprazolam, lorazepam, zolpidem	Additive sedation with other sedating agents
	Chlorpromazine	Increased phenytoin and valproate levels, theoretical increase in lamotrigine levels
Atypical neuroleptics	Risperidone	Increase in extrapyramamidal symptoms with phenytoin
	Olanzepine	No interactions found
	Clozapine	Decrease in clozapine with carbamazepine, phenobarbitol; case reports of asterixis induced by clozapine with carbamazepine and lithium; case reports of delirium when benzodiazepines added
	Quetiapine	Potential changes in plasma level with phenytoin, carbamazepine, phenobarbitol, primidone due to CYP 3A4 interactions
Classic neuroleptics	Haloperidol	About 50% decreased haloperidol levels with carbamazepine, increased carbamazepine levels with haloperidol
	Loxapine	Increased carbamazepine epoxide levels with loxapine
	Thioridazine	Decreased levels with phenobarbitol; phenobarbitol levels variably affected; rare variable effect on phenytoin levels

reserved for patients for whom other treatments have failed. If frequent epileptiform discharges are responsible for poor attention or overactivity, the appropriate treatment should be effective antiepileptic medication.

- Intermittent explosive disorders or episodic dyscontrol syndromes can also be a direct manifestation of seizure discharge. Ictal violence is likely to be non-directed and stereotyped, whereas organized violent behaviour is directed at specific targets. A patient may also be violent during post-ictal confusion.

- Non-ictal violence is associated more frequently with mental retardation and psychosis. The use of atypical neuroleptics such as risperidone, olanzapine or quetiapine can be effective for intermittent explosive disorder. However, given the often long-standing administration of these drugs, there is a concern of side effects including tardive dyskinesia.

- Depression and anxiety disorders are common among children with epilepsy. If psychological interventions are not feasible or have failed, antidepressant medication may be initiated. In line with current approaches in the general population, the selective serotonin re-uptake inhibitor (SSRI) represent the drugs of first choice (see chapter on Affective Disorders). If the patient does not respond to the first SSRI, a second should be tried. Furthermore, augmentation by use of other drugs is possible. Buproprione is to be avoided in epileptic children because it increases the number of seizures. Possible interactions between SSRI and AED are listed in Table 1.9.

- Panic affects or other anxiety disorders can also be treated briefly with benzodiazepines. However, the development of tolerance and the risk of withdrawal symptoms, including increased seizures, limit the administration of benzodiazepines for the short term until SSRI take effect. Also, the behavioural toxicity of benzodiazepines in children with brain disorders needs to be kept in mind.

- Mood instability can be seen as a symptom of bipolar disorder, severe ADHD or intermittent explosive disorder. Mood stabilizers such as carbamazepine or valproic acid, or the recently developed AEDs, can have significant effects including better tolerance of stimulant treatment of ADHD. Among the mood stabilizers lithium is most proconvulsive, whereas the other mentioned drugs can have significant interactions with other AEDs (see Table 1.9).

- Psychotic symptoms and illogical thinking are more common in children than previously believed. First-line medication is represented by the atypical neuroleptics risperidone, olanzapine and quetiapine. Clozapine should be avoided because of its pronounced proconvulsive effects or be reserved for psychoses that have been refractory to other drugs.

Monitoring and evaluation of treatment

The essential role that AED treatment plays in symptom control, and the common indications for the administration of psychotropic drugs, makes continuous monitoring of effects and side effects mandatory. Laboratory checks need to control for plasma levels and toxicity. In addition, careful observation of symptoms, especially of seizures, is essential for the titration process of AED treatment.

Any intervention for psychiatric problems, be it psychological or pharmacological, needs to be evaluated for its outcome. Both the clinical interview, and the administration of standardized questionnaires and checklists, serve these purposes. Examples for checklists were given above in the section on diagnostic instrument and assessment.

Problematic issues

There is a sizeable proportion of medically refractory epilepsy, which has been recently estimated to include 10–20 per cent of new patients per year with seizures. These patients could be candidates for epilepsy surgery. Presurgical examination has to determine whether or not there is an epileptogenic zone in the brain that is apt for cortical resection. Invasive monitoring has to exclude, via critical stimulation, that no so-called eloquent cortex tissue is removed that would leave the patient with an unacceptable neurological handicap. Focal resection would only be appropriate if the epileptogenic zone is not in eloquent cortex.

In severe cases with a large epileptogenic zone, localization to one hemisphere, and a contralateral neurological deficit, hemispherectomy can be considered. If the epileptogenic zone cannot be identified and the patient suffers from multifocal seizures, especially with generalized seizures that lead to drop attacks, a corpus callosotomy, leading to a disconnection of the two hemispheres, can be performed. The corpus callosotomy is only a palliative procedure, whereas both focal cortical resection and hemispherectomy are curative.

Recent evaluations of surgical treatment of epilepsy in children, adolescents and adults have provided favourable results. Good outcome was particularly associated with the resection of tumours, temporal lobe surgery before the age of 15 years and less than 10 years' duration of epilepsy. Psychosis is no longer considered to be an absolute contraindication to neurosurgery. Some children, e.g. those suffering from the rare Landau–Kleffner syndrome improve dramatically in their learning ability after surgery. In temporal lobectomy the complete removal of abnormal tissue containing the epileptogenic zone should lead to better outcome. With early onset of seizures, there is a good chance that brain plasticity will have ensured that most useful cognitive functions reside in the normal tissue.

Outcome

The general outcome of epilepsy varies with the type of seizures. Infantile spasms mainly occur as a result of pre-existing brain damage and therefore carry a poor prognosis. The same also applies to the Lennox–Gastaut syndrome. In contrast, absence seizures respond well to adequate anticonvulsive treatment and do not lead to handicapping long-term developments.

Also temporary lobe epilepsy (TLE) has a better long-term prognosis than once considered. This statement applies particularly for the simple partial seizures rather than for the complex practical seizures in which the persistence into adulthood is associated with poor social outcome. Most children with TLE become adults without psychiatric disorder. Risk factors for an unfavourable outcome include low IQ, early onset of epilepsy, high frequency of seizures, a left-sided EEG focus, hyperkinetic disorders, rage attacks and a history of special education.

Prognosis for intellectual function is good in uncomplicated epilepsies where there is only one seizure type, which responds promptly to a simple anticonvulsant regimen. This applies especially for onset of epilepsy later in childhood or in adolescence.

Brain tumours

Definition and classification

The major brain tumours in childhood comprise medulloblastoma, astrocytoma, brainstem glioma and ependymoma. Other less frequent brain tumours in childhood include mesodermal tumours (e.g. meningioma) and tumours of the pituitary (e.g. craniopharyngioma). In children, over two-thirds of the primary brain tumours arise below the tentorium, whereas in adults tumours tend to arise above the tentorium. Less than 45 per cent of brain tumours are malignant with an exceptionally poor prognosis, such as high-grade glioma, ependymoma, high risk primitive neuroctodermal tumours (an inclusive term for medulloblastoma and other histologically similar CNS tumours) and brain tumours in infants.

Epidemiology

Incidence rates

Recent statistics from the United States have calculated an annual incidence rate of 22 cases per million. Similar rates have also been estimated in other countries. Astrocytoma make up 45 per cent of the relative incidence rate, followed by medulloblastoma with 20 per cent, and brainstem glioma and ependymoma each with 10 per cent.

Implications for clinical practice

Brain tumours in childhood are relatively rare. However, both the malignancy of certain types of tumours, and the high impact on quality of life of others in long-term survivors, imply high demands on care and expertise. Only in highly specialized teams of the tertiary services will child and adolescent psychiatrists see sufficient numbers of patients to build up special expertise. However, many surviving patients will return to the community and will require child psychiatric care and treatment there.

Clinical picture

Main features and symptoms

The determinants of clinical symptoms in brain tumours are age at onset, location of the tumour, rate of growth and the presence of metastatic disease. In school-age children clinical syndromes mainly depend on the neuroanatomic location (i.e. infratentorial vs. supratentorial) and whether or not they result in raised intracranial pressure.

- The posterior fossa or intratentorial compartment is the most common neuroanatomic location for brain tumours in children. Frequent expansion of growth results in a variety of neurological symptoms. A full description of these symptoms is beyond the scope of this chapter. Suffice it to say that the neurological sequelae of cerebellar astrocytomas, ependymomas or brainstem tumours include a variety of severely handicapping symptoms, such as hydrocephalus, hemiparesis, vomiting, headache, ataxia, diplopia, dysphagia and dysarthria to name just a few major symptoms.

- The supratentorial tumours originate either from the dicencephalon or from the cerebral hemispheres. Craniopharyngiomas or germ cell tumours may result in endocrine dysfunction with growth failure, precocious puberty, obesity, hypothermia and may cause hydrocephalus and raised intracranial pressure. Tumours arising in the cerebral hemispheres usually are associated with seizures of focal neurological deficits. Most of these tumours are astrocytomas and mixed glial tumours.

- Psychiatric symptoms sometimes may precede gross neurological abnormalities. A change in behaviour or personality and cognitive deficiencies may be the primary manifestation of a frontal lobe tumour. Difficulty in performing simple, repetitive procedures in terms of apraxia may be noticeable before major neurological symptoms are apparent. Cerebellar tumours may present with lethargy and irritability and tumours causing endocrine dysfunction such as craniopharyngioma may be accompanied by affective lability, depression, anorexia, disorders of impulse and sleep disturbances. Also in brainstem tumours such as diffuse pontine glioma behavioural symptoms including attention deficits, irritability and even personality changes may be present as very first indicators. Depending on the location, cerebral tumours may be associated by visual hallucinations if the occipital lobe is affected, and agnosia and apraxia if the locus is the parietal and temporal lobe. Due to the raised intracranial pressure, cerebral tumours frequently produce disordered consciousness.

- As a result both of the tumour itself and treatment intervention, various cognitive impairments may result. In medulloblastoma long-term effects of neurocognitive deficits in attention, memory, language comprehension and acquisition, and academic achievement depend on age of diagnosis, type and duration of symptoms, tumour extent, cranial radiotherapy (CRT) and duration of survival. CRT generally results in cognitive impairment, i.e. in deficits in fine motor, visuo-motor, visuo-spatial and memory functions and is associated with a drop in IQ and needs for special assistance in school.
- In addition to disease-related factors, psychosocial adaptation is challenged by a variety of further risk factors. Hospitalization, multiple painful and medical procedures, alteration of physical appearance, isolation from peers, and the wide range of possible deficits in senses, mobility, emotional and behavioural functioning may overstress the coping resources of the child. Also, the family may be overwhelmed by the multitude of psychological stresses as evidenced by the initial shock of the diagnosis, the uncertainty of prognosis, the stress of decision making, the disruption of family life and the disruption of normal social activities that almost inevitably result from the severe disorder of the child. Thus, social isolation, alienation and disruption may result both for the child and for the family and may coincide with, or lead to, various behavioural abnormalities.
- Finally, additional medical therapy involving anti-epileptic drugs (AED) and steroids can have an impact on both cognitive and behavioural functioning. AEDs can alter attention and may cause mood changes. Steroids with higher doses can result in irritability, excitation, insomnia and also psychosis, most particularly in the postoperative phase, but also later on.

Differential diagnosis and co-morbidity

With the rather unspecific first behavioural signs, many manifestations of brain tumours may be mistaken as abnormalities resulting from other than brain-related factors. Recurrent vomiting, anorexia or chronic weight loss may imply gastroenterologic dysfunction. Affective lability, frequent mood swings or depression might, at first sight, raise the question as to whether a primary affective disorder is present. Tumours of cerebral hemispheres with presenting hallucinations might also imply the differential diagnosis of schizophrenic psychosis. Various neurological syndromes (e.g. aphasia) and endocrine disorders should be considered as consequences of brain tumours rather than as co-morbidities. Differential diagnosis rests mainly on a complete neurological examination and neuroimaging of the brain, preferentially by MRI. For ordinary child and adolescent psychiatric practice, it is essential to exclude a primary brain tumour in various symptoms of psychopathology.

Diagnostic instruments and assessment

The psychiatric contribution to the interdisciplinary examination of brain tumours in children is primarily based on observation and exploration of the various symptoms of psychopathology across a long-term period. Symptoms will be varying not only as a function of tumour location and raised intracranical pressure but will also alter across time due to tumour development, intervention effects, developmental effects and environmental conditions.

In long-term survivors, and with the aim of evaluating medical interventions, neuropsychological testing is of great importance. The often progressive deficits over time in intellectual functioning and learning make cognitive assessment mandatory at regular intervals after therapy in order to institute appropriate interventions. Various functions in the area of intelligence, language, motor, attention, perception and executive functions need to be assessed. Some guidance with regard to clinically related questioning and recommendations for suitable tests is given in Table 1.2.

The question of behavioural and emotional functioning can also be assessed by standardized questionnaires and checklists like the Child Behaviour Checklist (CBCL) for parents, the Teacher Rating Form (TRF), or the Strengths and Difficulties Questionnaire (SDQ, see the Appendix to chapter on conduct disorders). Questionnaires for the assessment of quality of life may also provide valuable insights into the stresses and strains of the child and the family. These instruments assess domains such as activity and mobility, psychological well-being, social integration, comfort or pain, achievement and others.

Aetiology

The large majority of brain tumours in children arise without any obvious predisposing condition. However, there are a few hereditary syndromes that can lead to central or peripheral nervous tumours. They include neurofibromatosis-1, which is an autosomal dominant disorder with a mutation on the long arm on chromosome 17, neurofibromatosis-2, which is due to a mutation on the long arm of chromosome 22, and tuberous sclerosis, which is an autosomal dominant disorder.

As in other brain disorders, the aetiology of psychiatric symptoms in brain tumour is multidetermined. The various factors include tumour-related risks (e.g. tumour location, raise of intracranial pressure), treatment-related risks (e.g. CRT, AED, steroids), general disease-related risks (e.g. chronicity, progressive nature, hospitalization), individual risks (e.g. developmental factors, coping deficits) and environmental risks (e.g. lack of family support, social isolation). Deficits in psychosocial adaptation and psychiatric symptoms may vary inter-individually depending on the interaction of these risk factors.

Treatment

Clinical management and treatment setting

The principles of therapy of brain tumours include radical surgical resection wherever possible, assisted by cranial radiotherapy and chemotherapy when indicated. The broad spectrum of early and late effects, including various neurological deficits, hormonal deficiencies as well as cognitive and behavioural dysfunction, requires an extended and highly specialized clinical team. In particular, experts in neuro-surgery, anaesthesia, neuro-oncology, neuropsychology, psychiatry, rehabilitation and social work are needed to provide the necessary specialized care. Tertiary service centres are needed for the provision of these programmes.

Psychological interventions

The need for psychiatric assistance may be articulated repeatedly in the course of care for children with brain tumours. In the first 48 hours after operation, pain syndromes, mood disturbances, withdrawal and suicidal ideation require assessment and intervention. During hospitalization and after discharge, many of these problems may persist and may be supplemented by additional symptoms such as phobias, anxiety and anger.

During the various phases of clinical treatment, psychological preparation for various examinations and surgery is necessary. Expertise in behavioural techniques, imagery or hypnosis can be used in order to prepare the child for the management of pain, anxiety, needle phobias as well as nausea and vomiting associated with chemotherapy. The recovery process of the child will be assisted greatly by these interventions.

Any pre-morbidly existing or post-diagnosis developed co-morbid psychiatric problem can also be addressed by various interventions of the child and adolescent psychiatrist including brief and supportive psychotherapy, crisis intervention, behaviour modification or long-term care and counselling. The family should receive similar guidance and assistance during the various phases of adaptation with an initial shock phase and later on in developing stable adaptation processes.

Further goals include the professional reflection of feelings and reactions of the rehabilitation team. Members of the team that cares for children with malignant disorders may themselves develop feelings of depression, anxiety and burn-out so that team counselling is another important task of the experienced child and adolescent psychiatrist. Finally, he or she is also an important mediator and counsellor to the school system in establishing appropriate expectations for achievement and academic progress.

Psychopharmacotherapy

Indications for drug treatment include the use of SSRI and mood stabilizers with affective disorders and of atypical neuroleptics with psychotic symptoms and severe aggressive outbursts. Stimulants may not only be helpful for the treatment of ADHD symptoms but also in the so-called post-radiation syndrome, which can last for as long as 6 months after radiotherapy and is characterized by increased somnolence and fatigue and by marked attention deficits.

In general, medications with use in brain-injured patients can be administered similarly in children with brain tumours. An outline is given in Table 1.3. In the case of co-existing epilepsy and treatment with AEDs, the same caveat regarding interactions between AEDs and psychotropic medication applies that has been articulated in the section on the treatment of epilepsy and co-morbid psychiatric disorders (see Table 1.9).

Monitoring and evaluation of treatment

Careful observation of the patient for any change of the target symptom of intervention, and continuous monitoring of any side effect including toxicity are mandatory for any implementation of drug treatment. Neuropsychological testing may also be helpful in order to detect subtle changes in cognitive impairment. In some instances it may be difficult to differentiate between intervention effects by pharmacotherapy or CRT or direct effects of the tumour.

Psychological interventions may be evaluated by use of structured questionnaires for the assessment of personality features, behavioural and emotional abnormalities, quality of life and satisfaction of the client, be it the patient, the family or the rehabilitation team.

Problematic issues

Both the fatality of a brain tumour and treatment failure represent major problems in the care of children with brain tumours. Malignant tumours can only be insufficiently cured. Thus counselling the child and his family in the process of dying is one of the most difficult tasks in psychological care. It requires a most sensitive, reflective and honest guidance by the professional in order to assist the patient and his family in a process of mourning and grief that may start early in the disease process and continue after the death of the child.

Treatment failure can result from the inability to achieve local control either because of surgical inaccessibility or because of lack of therapeutic intent at the initial surgical resection. Often, radical surgical resection could be achieved only at the cost of neurological morbidity. Only new technologies that increase the ability to more safely resect brain or more effective medical therapies will solve this dilemma.

Outcome

Long-term survival after developing a brain tumour in childhood is different for the various types of tumours. The overall 5-year survival rate is 70 per cent in medulloblastoma of standard risk and 40% in high risk medulloblastoma. Low grade astrocytoma has the highest 5-year overall survival rate with 90% of the affected children, whereas it is only 30% in high grade astrocytoma. The figure is lowest for brainstem glioma (7%) and amounts to 50% for ependymoma. The rates for progression-free survival is lower than the reported overall figures.

As described above, long-term survivors show a high rate of cognitive impairments and limited educational experiences. Psychological maladjustment is prominent and has been shown empirically to depend on low socio-economic standards, young mothers and single-parent families, younger age of the patient, physical stigmatization, functional impairment and low IQ.

Syndromes attributed to minimal brain dysfunction

Definition and classification

The concept of minimal brain damage (MBD) emerged in the early twentieth century, years after George Still described a syndrome that he linked to 'moral dyscontrol' and that comprised attention deficits, impulsivity, motor restlessness, clumsiness and various types of learning problems. It became rooted firmly after an epidemic of encephalitis around 1920 had left many previously purportedly well-functioning children affected by similar symptoms. In the late 1940s and the 1950s it became one of the most common 'diagnoses' in child psychiatry. However, criticism against the concept mounted in the 1960s when it became clear that not all children with the problems referred to had 'minimal' brain damage, but widespread brain dysfunction, and that others had no documented brain damage at all. The meaning of MBD then changed to minimal brain dysfunction. In the early 1980s, two influential papers by Sir Michael Rutter – highlightling again the criticism from the 1960s and adding that children with various kinds of proven minimal brain damage did not show necessarily any of the symptoms believed to be diagnostic of MBD – seemed to put the concept to rest. It soon became superseded by other labels and combinations of labels such as attention deficit disorder, hyperkinetic disorder, deficits in attention, motor control and perception syndrome (DAMP), and specific developmental disorders (including developmental coordination disorder or DCD).

The research literature has had little to say about MBD in the past 20 years. However, in clinical practice, the term has remained in many centres, usually as an umbrella term for various combinations of problems in the areas of attention, activity control, impulsivity, motor control, perception and learning (including speech and language).

A survey of all the many synonyms, acronyms and partly overlapping concepts used in this field is beyond the scope of this chapter. However, a list of some of the most common diagnostic labels is appropriate (Table 1.10). The Table provides a brief introduction to the symptom profiles encountered in children who have been given the, sometimes incorrect, label of MBD over the past 50 years.

Epidemiology

Prevalence rates

The prevalence rates for 'MBD' have varied from a few per cent to as many as one in five children, even though most estimates have been below 10 per cent of all children at school age. The figure has varied most of all with the definition used. Unfortunately, many of the studies in the field have not used operationalized criteria at all. One of the very few studies actually to have used strict criteria found a minimum rate of 4 per cent in the 1970s in Sweden, with one in four of these being regarded as severe. That study referred to 7 year-old children with the combination of the problem now subsumed under the label of DAMP (meaning the combination of AD(H)D and DCD). Boys are about three times more often affected than girls.

Implications for clinical practice

The MBD label is still used sometimes in clinical practice to describe children who usually have ADD or ADHD in combination with various kinds of developmental and learning disorders. In Scandinavia, such combinations are diagnosed frequently under the descriptive label of DAMP. This 'condition' affects a few to several per cent of all school-age children.

Clinical picture

Main features and symptoms

Epidemiological and clinical studies of children with DAMP have shown the following characteristics with regard to psychiatric disorders.

- The prevalence of psychiatric problems is very much higher than in children without DAMP amounting to two-thirds of the population of children with the syndrome. It is increased significantly if DAMP is combined with psychosocial

Table 1.10. Syndromes attributed to minimal brain dysfunction

Diagnostic label	Comments
MBD	Once referred to minimal brain damage, since *c.* 1960 to minimal brain dysfunction. Almost universally used label in child psychiatry up until *c.* 1980. Still in clinical use in many countries. Usually refers to various combinations of attention and motor/learning problems. Inappropriate in that it implies brain dysfunction on phenotypical grounds and in its use of the word 'minimal'
ADD (Attention deficit disorder)	DSM-III-label (APA 1980). Still in use in the US, usually to refer to the inattentive subtype of AD/HD (see below). Semantically confusing (should be 'deficit' *or* 'disorder', not both). Diagnostic criteria in the DSM-III loose and subjective. Pervasiveness not required. With or without motor/learning problems
ADHD (Attention deficit hyperactivity disorder)	DSM-III-R-label (APA 1987). Does not account for cases without clear hyperactivity. Pervasiveness required for cases classified as 'severe'. With or without motor/learning problems
AD/HD (Attention-deficit/hyperactivity disorder, predominantly inattentive, predominantly hyperactive–impulsive, or combined subtypes)	DSM-IV-label (APA 1994). Accounts for cases without clear hyperactivity, but does not make it clear how the two predominant subtypes are inter-related (if at all). Requires a measure of pervasiveness. With or without motor/learning problems
DAMP (Deficits in attention, motor control and perception)	Accepted term in Nordic countries. Umbrella concept covering various combinations of attentional/activity problems in conjunction with motor control and perceptual problems. Recently harmonized with DSM-IV to mean AD/HD with DCD (see below). Probably the concept that resembles George Still's original descriptions most closely
Hyperkinetic disorder	ICD-10-label (WHO, 1993). Mostly used in the UK. Refers to a syndrome that must include all of inattention, impulsivity and hyperactivity. In the past, this diagnosis was often made only if there were no major oppositional or conduct problems. The syndrome was then considered very rare. As used currently it is believed to be not very rare, that oppositional and conduct problems are extremely common, and that motor/learning problems are the rule in severe cases
Clumsy child syndrome	UK concept. Highlights only one aspect of what is usually a multifaceted syndrome
MPD (Motor perception dysfunction)	Nordic concept. Attention problems, autistic features and other specific learning problems are common in this group
DCD (Developmental coordination disorder)	DSM-IV-label (APA 1994). Synonymous with Nordic concept of MPD
MND (Minor neurological dysfunction)	Sometimes used to describe summary score for minimal motor/neurological problems or 'soft neurological signs'
MCD (Minimal cerebral dysfunction)	Rarely used term. Usually refers to overriding concept of cerebral dysfunctions rather than to any specific clinical syndrome
Organic brain syndrome	Central European concept. Highlights certain behavioural features, but essentially similar to MBD-concept
OBD (Organic brain dysfunction)	Used particularly by European groups highlighting the importance of neonatal reflexes in the pathogenesis of attentional and motor/learning problems

adversity. However, the link with autism spectrum problems (see below) is associated with the severity of the symptoms of DAMP and not at all with psychosocial conditions.

- In general, there is no distinctive association of DAMP with any type of psychiatric disorder except for ADHD (which is usually included in the DAMP/MBD diagnosis *per se*), autism spectrum disorders, depression and conduct disorder. In DAMP, with its relatively mild physical disability and little or no intellectual impairment, around two-thirds of affected children have at least one psychiatric disorder. Autism spectrum disorders (including full-blown Asperger syndrome) occur in more than half of all those with severe DAMP (children with severe DAMP usually have all of the following: attention deficits/hyperactivity, fine motor problems, gross motor problems, perceptual dysfunction and speech and language deficits). It is not uncommon for a child to present with DAMP around the age of 3 or 4 years and then to be 're-diagnosed' some years later as having an autism spectrum disorder. Conversely, some children are suspected of suffering from an autism spectrum disorder at a very young age and then develop the typical symptoms of DAMP (attention deficits and motor clumsiness and an uneven pattern of abilities in the field of learning). Depression is present in about one-third of all children with DAMP, regardless of degree of severity. The highest rate appears to be around the age of 8–12 years, and may be associated in many cases with feelings of always being unsuccessful at school and in peer relationships. Oppositional defiant problems are present in about 35–40 per cent of all pre-school children with DAMP. When present, it is usually symptomatic from a very young age and does not develop later in childhood. Conduct disorder and later antisocial personality disorder develop in about half of these cases with severe oppositional and defiant behaviours.
- The most common emotional disorders in children with DAMP are specific phobias, separation anxiety and generalized anxiety. Some patients also develop depressive disorders (see above). Frequently, these children with DAMP and emotional disorders also show markedly defiant and negativistic behaviour, leading in some cases also to marked violent behaviours.
- Children with DAMP encounter an increased risk of social isolation due to teasing, victimization, marginalization and lack of friendships. These problems may, in part, be due to constitutional problems with social understanding and relatedness. In severe cases, autism spectrum disorders may be present (see above).
- Psychiatric and behavioural problems are often very persistent and may be seen for many years. Over the years, the additional ('co-morbid') psychiatric problems are often those that contribute to the very poor psychosocial outcome seen in so many cases with DAMP. As children with DAMP grow up, many will meet criteria for one or more of the so-called 'personality disorders'. However, it is unclear

whether it is helpful or not to make 'additional' diagnoses of these conditions in people with DAMP, given that they provide little in the way of explaining the underlying problems or in terms of suggesting avenues for appropriate interventions.

Aetiology

The causes of DAMP are not known in any detail, but familiality is extremely common and there is a high rate of associated pre- and perinatal problems. Most of the available indirect evidence (such as that from the study of attention deficits and hyperactivity, which are universal phenomena in DAMP) suggests that the familiality is due to genetic factors. The meaning of the high rate of pre- and perinatal problems is less clear. These problems could be a reflection of an underlying genetic abnormality in the child, an index of psychosocial adversity (which is also common in the DAMP syndrome) or a factor indicating a risk for structural brain damage. The few studies that have looked at these factors in any detail suggest that the DAMP syndrome is often caused by genetic factors, either alone or in combination with some degree of brain damage. Psychosocial factors themselves appear not to contribute to the presentation of the DAMP syndrome as such but may be strongly associated with co-morbid conditions such as oppositional defiant disorder and conduct problems.

Treatment

The basic condition of DAMP cannot be cured at the present time. Nevertheless, attention deficits and hyperactivity are amenable to the same kind of interventions that are helpful in treating ADHD (see chapter on hyperkinetic disorders). Many families of children with DAMP benefit greatly from having the diagnosis made and explained to them in some detail. The children will usually derive considerable benefit from having their teacher gaining a better understanding of the child's specific needs in terms of the educational setting. Training of working memory is probably important in many cases. A training programme for the motor deficits that are part and parcel of the DAMP syndrome is sometimes a key intervention that may have to be drawn up by a physiotherapist or by an occupational therapist. Physical education teachers usually have to be informed in detail about the child's motor control problems. Some children with DAMP need the additional input of speech–language therapists. Those who do not seem to develop in a hopeful manner in spite of these kinds of interventions may be candidates for treatment with a stimulant or another drug effective in the treatment of ADHD. Associated psychiatric problems usually need the same approach when it comes to interventions as is useful for children with the particular psychiatric problem without DAMP.

With the high probability of developing additional psychiatric problems, there is not only the need for careful monitoring and assessment but also for early intervention or even for the development of preventive approaches. In principle, all sorts of psychological interventions are applicable. A family approach in counselling and guidance is always indicated. All these efforts should be started early and often be continued over many years.

Outcome

DAMP/MBD itself is a chronic condition marked by persistent psychosocial disability of varying degree. Probably no more than one in three does well in terms of education, vocational skills, daily living skills, psychosocial interactions and independent living in their mid-twenties. A limited database suggests that diagnosis in childhood, and interventions as outlined in the foregoing (particularly psychoeducational approaches), may contribute significantly to a better outcome. Concomitant psychiatric disorders of various kinds – perhaps particularly autism spectrum disorders and conduct disorder – contribute to a worse outcome. Learning disability/mental retardation and severe executive function deficits may have an additional impact on the course of the disorder. However, it has to be emphasized that some affected individuals experience a satisfying and productive life with normal psychosocial adaptation.

There is a very limited body of empirical research on the longitudinal stability of psychiatric and academic problems in children suffering from DAMP. One longitudinal prospective study from Göteborg, Sweden, suggested that, if untreated, DAMP may be associated with a poor psychosocial outcome in more than 50 per cent of the cases. 'Poor outcome' in that study referred to the presence in early adult age of one or more (usually two or more) of the following: full-time sick pension, severe criminality, severe drug or alcohol abuse, persistent major psychiatric disorder (such as bipolar disorder and schizophrenia), or the persistence of a disabling autism spectrum disorder. No more than a few per cent of all cases had had a successful academic career.

SUGGESTED READING

F. M. C. Besag, Childhood epilepsy in relation to mental handicap and behavioural disorders. *Journal of Child Psychology and Psychiatry* **43** (2002), 103–31.

S. Davies, I. Heyman & R. Goodman, A population survey of mental health problems in children with epilepsy. *Developmental Medicine and Child Neurology* **45** (2003), 292–5.

C. Gillberg, *Clinical Child Neuropyschiatry* (Cambridge: Cambridge University Press, 1995).

R. Goodman, Brain disorder. In M. Rutter & E. Taylor, eds. *Child and Adolescent Psychiatry – Modern Approaches*. 4th edn. (Oxford: Blackwell 2002).

E. Guthrie, J. Mast, P. Richards, M. McQuaid & S. Pavlakis, Traumatic brain injury in children and adolescents. *Child and Adolescent Psychiatric Clinics of North America* **8** (1999), 807–26.

J. A. Middleton, Practitioner review: psychological sequelae of head injury in children and adolescents. *Journal of Child Psychology and Psychiatry* **42** (2001), 165–80.

P. Satz, K. Zaucha, C. McCleary, R. Light, R. Asarnow & D. Barker, Mild head injury in children and adolescents: a review of studies (1970–1995). *Psychological Bulletin* **122** (1997), 107–31.

J. Siffert, M. Greenleaf, R. Mannis & J. Allen, Paediatric brain tumours. *Child and Adolescent Psychiatric Clinics of North America* **8** (1999), 879–903.

H.-C. Steinhausen & C. Rauss-Mason, Epilepsy and anticonvulsive drugs. In M. Rutter & P. Casaer, eds.: *Biological Risk Factors for Psychosocial Disorders.* (Cambridge: Cambridge University Press 1991).

E. Thiele, J. Gonzales-Heydrick & J. J. Riviello, Epilepsy in children and adolescents. *Child and Adolescent Psychiatric Clinics of North America* **8** (1999), 671–94.

2

Substance use disorders

Oscar G. Bukstein

Western Psychiatric Institute and Clinic, Pittsburgh, PA, USA

Introduction

Substance use and abuse by children and adolescents remain critical problems for modern developed countries. Although tolerance and public policy for substance use vary among Western countries, the use of psychoactive substances and other harmful of abuse is common among adolescents. The use of such psychoactive agents can lead to a variety of negative consequences for youth. The risk for substance use and abuse, the acquisition of use behaviours, and development into substance use disorders and interventions for such problems should be considered in a comprehensive manner that considers neurobiology, development and the adolescent's environmental ecology.

This chapter presents essential background information for the clinician in order to understand the presentation, risk, prevention and treatment of adolescents with substance use problems. While written primarily from the perspective of clinical and research experience in the United States, the processes of addictive behaviours are similar for all adolescents. Modifications for assessment and treatment should be made for cultural and ethnic differences when relevant.

Definition and classification

According to the *International Classification of Disease*, 10th edition (ICD-10), the pathological use of substances is classified under the heading of 'Mental and behavioural disorders due to psychoactive substance use'. In addition to the clinical conditions of acute intoxication with or without various complications, withdrawal states, psychotic disorders and amnestic disorders; the primary diagnoses are 'harmful use' and 'dependence syndrome', which correspond closely to the *Diagnostic and Statistical Manual of Mental Disorders – IV*, 4th edition (DSM-IV) diagnoses of

A Clinician's Handbook of Child and Adolescent Psychiatry, ed. Christopher Gillberg,
Richard Harrington and Hans-Christoph Steinhausen. Published by Cambridge University Press.
© Cambridge University Press 2005.

'substance abuse' and 'substance dependence'. The term 'substance use disorders' encompasses both substance abuse and substance dependence, under the DSM-IV category of substance-related disorders. Substance use disorders are defined for alcohol, amphetamine or amphetamine-like, caffeine, cannabis, cocaine, hallucinogens, inhalants, nicotine, opioids, phencyclidine (or phencyclidine-like) and sedative-hypnotic- or anxiolytics. Although these parameters were written to apply to both children and adolescents, adolescents are referred to most frequently due to the less frequent occurrence of SUDs in prepubertal children.

In ICD-10, 'harmful use' is defined as a pattern of psychoactive substance use that is causing damage to health. The fact that use or a pattern of use is disapproved of by another person or by culture, or may have led to socially negative consequences such as arrest (e.g. for use or possession) or family arguments is not in itself evidence of harmful use. For the ICD-10 Dependence Syndrome, the central descriptive characteristic is the often strong desire to take psychoactive substances. The syndrome also may include a physiological withdrawal state, evidence of tolerance and persisting use despite overt negative consequences.

The diagnosis of DSM-IV 'substance abuse' requires evidence of a maladaptive pattern of substance use with clinically significant levels of impairment or distress. Substance abuse is characterized by a maladaptive pattern of substance use. Recurrent use in adolescents who abuse substances results in an inability to meet major role obligations, leading to impaired functioning in one or more major areas of their life, and an increase in the likelihood of legal problems due to possession, risk-taking behaviour and exposure to hazardous situations. Substance dependence requires a substantial degree of involvement with a substance as evidenced by the adolescent meeting at least three criteria, including such symptoms as withdrawal, tolerance and loss of control over use. Adolescents commonly exhibit tolerance (i.e. requiring increasing amounts of a substance to achieve the same effect), which is one criterion for dependence, but show withdrawal or other symptoms of physiological dependence much less frequently. Tolerance, in the case of adolescent alcohol use, appears to have a low specificity for a diagnosis of alcohol dependence among adolescents, while withdrawal symptoms and medical problems as a consequence of use are much less common than in adults. However, increasing research points to a high prevalence of withdrawal symptoms in adolescents with cannabis and opiate use disorders. Preoccupation with use is often demonstrated by giving up previously important activities, increasing the time spent in activities related to substance use, and using more frequently or for longer amounts of time than planned. The adolescent may use despite the continued existence or worsening of problems caused by substance use. For adolescents, it is important to include criteria such as alcohol-related blackouts, craving and impulsive sexual behaviour when determining if criteria are met. Polysubstance use by adolescents appears to be the rule rather than the exception; therefore, adolescents often present with multiple SUD diagnoses.

Although these diagnoses of substance abuse and substance dependence assist clinicians in identifying adolescents with pathological patterns of substance use, the ICD-10 and DSM-IV criteria, developed for adults, have not been established as applicable to adolescents. For adolescents these diagnoses probably define a heterogeneous population and communicate insufficient information in terms of natural history and treatment response. While ICD-10 and DSM-IV remain the guides for determining substance-use-related pathology in adolescents, it is important to recognize the frequent differences between the most common manifestations of the diagnoses of substance abuse and dependence in adolescents vs. adults. While substance use is a necessary prelude to abuse or dependence, and regular use further increases the risk for SUDs, substance use *per se* is not sufficient for a diagnosis of abuse or dependence. Through the remainder of this chapter, I will use the term substance use disorders (SUDs).

Epidemiology

Prevalence and incidence rates

In the United States, substances such as opiates, LSD, inhalants and steroids have shown periodic epidemics among youth in the past several decades. In 2000, nearly a quarter of eighth graders report having taken an alcoholic beverage in the past 30 days and half of twelfth graders report having done so. A third of twelfth graders report having been drunk in the past 30 days. Almost 12 per cent of eighth graders and almost a quarter of high school seniors report having used any illicit drug in the preceding 30 days. In community studies, lifetime diagnosis of DSM-IV alcohol abuse ranges from 0.4 per cent to 9.6 per cent. Lifetime diagnosis of alcohol dependence range from 0.6 per cent to 4.3 per cent in the Oregon Adolescent Depression Project. The lifetime prevalence of drug abuse or dependence has ranged from 3.3 per cent in 15-year olds to 9.8 per cent in 17 to 19-year olds. Other than alcohol, 54 per cent of 12 graders and almost 27 per cent (26.8%) of eighth graders report ever having used any illicit drug. Marijuana is the most widely used of the illicit drugs with about a third of high-school students indicating some use in the preceding 12-month period. Six per cent of high-school seniors report daily marijuana use.

Overall, school surveys show that the lifetime prevalence of illicit drug use is highest in the USA and Australia (>40%) and high in Canada (>35%), but less than 20–25 per cent in Europe. In the late 1990s, the lifetime prevalence of illicit drug use rose 40% in Europe, while an increase in the USA over the 1991–7 period was followed by a decrease during 1997–2001. The increase in Europe appears to be the result of a doubling of prevalence rates in Eastern Europe. There are important differences between European countries. For example, in 1999, the lifetime prevalence of all illicit drug use was 36 per cent and 12 per cent for use of drugs other than cannabis in the United Kingdom (UK). During the same period, in Scandinavian countries, the lifetime prevalence ranged from 9–13 per cent for all illicit drugs and 3–6 per cent for drugs other than cannabis. The vast majority of students in Europe have drunk alcohol at least once in their lives, ranging from 61 per cent in Turkey to 95 per cent in the Czech and Slovak Republics and Denmark. The proportion of students reporting having drunk alcohol more than 40 times include Denmark at 49 per cent and the UK at 42 per cent. Binge drinking within the past 30 days was reported by 58 per cent of students in Denmark, 51 per cent in Finland, 48 per cent in the UK and 46 per cent in Iceland. Generally, teenagers in a group of northern countries reported the highest rates of heavy drinking and intoxication (drunkenness). Teenagers in southern Europe reported much lower levels of such behaviours and experiences.

As of 2000, cigarette smoking among adolescents in the USA has continued a decline from a peak in the mid-1990s. An almost 50 per cent increase in the rate of smoking among younger adolescents (eighth and tenth graders) in the early 1990s. In 2000, 14.6 per cent of eighth graders reported current smoking (defined as smoking at least once in the preceding 30 days) while 23.9 per cent of tenth graders and 31.4 per cent of twelfth graders reported current cigarette use. Approximately a quarter (24.7 per cent) of students nationwide reported having smoked a cigarette before the age of 13 years.

Sex ratios and ethnicity

For all substances, males use more than females, although the gap appears to be closing during the past two decades. Similarly, the gap is closing between lower levels of substance use in rural areas and higher levels in urban areas. This smaller gap may be due to increasing accessibility to all youth whether or not they live in urban or rural areas.

In the USA, white and Hispanic students report a lifetime prevalence of about 82 per cent for alcohol use as compared with 74 per cent for African-American youth. Heavy episodic use prevalence rates are 35, 37.7 and 18.8 per cent for white, Hispanic and African American students, respectively.

African-American students are more likely to report both lifetime and current use of marijuana than white students. In other countries similar ethnic differences in the rates of substance use and problems associated with use may be present.

Implications for clinical practice

Substance use by adolescents is not distributed randomly among adolescents of different genders, ethnicity or other demographic characteristics. Clinicians need to be aware of both demographic and other high-risk characteristics in order to target the most vulnerable populations of adolescents for prevention and treatment interventions. The specific characteristics of an adolescent may also shape the types of interventions or emphasis within an intervention that are used. For example, urban or female adolescents may have special needs distinctive from the intervention needs of rural or male adolescents.

Clinical picture

Main features and symptoms

Patients who present with substance use, and frequently with resulting intoxication, often manifest significant levels of acute change in mood, cognition and behaviour. The manifestations of substance use and intoxication vary with the type of substance(s) used, the amount used during a given time period, the setting and context of use and a host of characteristics of the individual such as experience with the substance, expectations, and the presence or absence of other psychopathology.

- Behavioural changes may include disinhibition, lethargy, hyperactivity or agitation, somnolence and hypervigilance.
- Changes in cognition may include impaired concentration, changes in attention span, and perceptual and overt disturbances in thinking, such as delusion.
- Mood changes can range from depression to euphoria.
- A hallmark of SUDs in adolescents is impairment in psychosocial and academic functioning. Impairment can include family conflict or dysfunction, interpersonal conflict and academic failure.
- Associated characteristics include deviant and risk-taking behaviour, and co-morbid psychiatric disorders such as conduct, attention-deficit/hyperactivity, mood and anxiety disorders.

Almost all psychoactive substances, including those available to adults such as alcohol and nicotine, are illegal for adolescents to obtain, possess and use although the legal age for use varies among developed countries. Certain of the negative consequences of substance use for adolescents follow from the illegal nature of, rather than from the actual, use.

Medical consequences

- Accidents such as motor vehicle accidents and trauma in adolescents commonly occur under the influence of substances. This includes driving motor vehicles and even bicycles and skateboards while intoxicated. Alcohol is estimated to be involved in as many as 40 per cent of adolescent drownings. Adolescents who use and abuse substances are more likely to participate in other risk-taking behaviours such as driving a motor vehicle while under the influence. Adolescent victims and perpetrators of violence, both with and without weapons, are commonly under the influence or have histories of SUDs.

Substance use is often associated with other high-risk behaviours. Early and promiscuous sexual behaviour is common among adolescents with the early onset of substance use and abuse. Among currently sexually active students nationwide, about a quarter had used alcohol or drugs at last sexual intercourse. Overall, male students were significantly more likely than female students to have used alcohol or drugs at last sexual intercourse. The impairment in judgement, and the increase in impulsivity, often produced by an intoxicated state, may result in unprotected and/or unsafe sexual activity and subsequent pregnancy and/or sexual transmitted diseases. Unsafe sexual practices are also common among these populations of adolescents.

- While not all adolescents who use or even abuse substances are considered to be at high-risk status for Human Immunodeficiency Virus (HIV) infection, substance use by an adolescent should prompt a thorough inquiry into specific HIV risk factors and consideration of appropriate testing. Although adolescents constitute a small percentage of the total number of individuals with HIV disease, the often long latency between HIV infection and the onset of symptoms mean that many acquire HIV as adolescents. Intravenous (IV) drug and crack cocaine abusers are among the subgroups of adolescents with the highest risk for HIV.
- Medical complications of substance use are uncommon among adolescents. Long-term sequelae such as liver disease and memory problems from chronic substance use may not become apparent until well into adulthood. Those adolescents who frequently use very high quantities of substance use or who are using acutely toxic substances may be an exception. For example, inhalants such as aromatic or halogenated hydrocarbons or other organic solvents may produce varying levels of neurotoxicity (including acute and chronic encephalopathy) and, on occasion, cardiac arrest secondary to arrhythmia even during the initial episodes of use.

Differential diagnosis and co-morbidity

Given the varying tolerance of various countries and cultures, it is not surprising that the mere use of substances by adolescents might be seen as abnormal or pathological or normative by others. Clinicians need to consider the effect of substance use on the adolescent and his or her family before giving a diagnosis.

Many adolescents with SUDs also have co-existing psychiatric conditions that cannot be described adequately within a single DSM-IV diagnostic category. Some

Table 2.1. Differential diagnoses and co-morbid disorders

Disruptive behaviour disorders
- Conduct disorder
- Oppositional defiant disorder
- Attention-deficit hyperactivity disorder

Mood disorders
- Major depressive disorder: single episode vs. recurrent
- Bipolar disorder
- Dysrthymic disorder
- Cyclothymia

Anxiety disorders
- Social phobia
- Post-traumatic stress disorder
- Generalized anxiety disorder
- Panic disorder

Other disorders
- Schizophrenia
- Bulimia nervosa

Personality disorders

---

conditions, such as disruptive behaviour disorders (e.g. oppositional defiant disorder, conduct disorder and attention-deficit/hyperactivity disorder, ADHD) and mood disorders (e.g. major depressive disorder and bipolar disorder), co-exist with adolescent SUDs more often than not (see Table 2.1). Knowledge of the assessment and treatment of these disorders is essential for the adequate management of SUDs. In view of the frequency of co-morbidity in adolescents, the clinician should consider, but not be limited by, the practice parameters applicable to both the substance use and the co-morbid psychiatric disorder. However, the optimal treatment of adolescents with SUD and psychiatric co-morbidity involves an integration of treatment modalities rather than merely concurrent or consecutive treatment with specific modalities for either SUD or psychiatric disorder(s).

Significant rates of adolescents with co-existing SUD and psychiatric disorders (disruptive behaviour disorders, mood disorders and anxiety disorders) are reported in both clinical and general populations. Furthermore, the co-morbidity of psychiatric disorders, particularly conduct disorder and, to a lesser extent, major depressive disorder, may have an effect on the alcohol and substance use and related problems both at baseline and at follow-up and impair an adolescent's ability to engage effectively in treatment. Evidence suggests that depression increases the rate and rapidity of relapse.

Disruptive behaviour disorders are the most common psychiatric disorders diagnosed in adolescents with SUDs. Conduct disorder, including the component of aggression, usually precedes and accompanies adolescent SUDs. Clinical populations of adolescents with SUDs manifest rates of conduct disorder ranging from 50 to almost 80 per cent. Although attention deficit hyperactivity disorder (ADHD) is often present in substance using and abusing youth, the observed association may be due to the high level of co-morbidity between conduct disorder and ADHD. The early onset of conduct disorder, aggressive behaviour, in the presence of attention deficit hyperactivity disorder, may increase the risk for later substance abuse still further. Aggressive behaviours are present in many adolescents who have substance use disorders. The direct pharmacological effects resulting in aggression may be exacerbated further by the presence of pre-existing psychopathology (e.g. ADHD, mood disorders), the use of multiple agents simultaneously and the frequent, relative inexperience of the adolescent substance user. For example, a novice user may be more likely than an experienced user to react to specific psychoactive effects with anxiety. An inexperienced drinker may drink too rapidly, thus causing a rapid rise in blood alcohol level and thus further impairment in judgement and behavioural controls.

Mood disorders, particularly depression, frequently have onsets both preceding and consequent to the onset of substance use and SUDs in adolescents. The prevalence of depressive disorders in these studies of clinical populations ranged from 24 to more than 50 per cent. Substance use disorders among adolescents are also a risk factor for suicidal behaviours, including ideation, attempts and completed suicide. Possible mechanisms for these relationships include acute and chronic effects of psychoactive substances. Adolescents who commit suicide frequently have used alcohol or other substances at the time of suicide. The acute substance use episode may produce transient but intense dysphoric states, disinhibition, impaired judgement and increased level of impulsivity or may exacerbate pre-existing psychopathology, including depression or anxiety disorders. A number of studies of clinical populations show high rates of anxiety disorders among youth with SUDs. In clinical populations of adolescents with SUDs, the prevalence of anxiety disorder ranged from 7 per cent to over 40 per cent. The chronology of the onset of comorbid anxiety and SUDs is variable, depending on the specific anxiety disorder. Social phobia usually precedes abuse while panic and generalized anxiety disorder may more often follow the onset of abuse. Adolescents with SUDs often have a past history or current manifestation of post-traumatic stress disorder (PTSD). Bulimia nervosa is also associated frequently with adolescents having substance use disorders. SUDs are very common among individuals, especially young and chronically impaired, who are diagnosed with schizophrenia.

Diagnostic instruments

Clinicians often use a variety of rating scales or standardized interviews to assess SUDs and associated problems (see Appendix 2.1). Screening instruments include The Drug Use Screening Inventory – Adolescents (DUSI-A) and the Problem Oriented Screening Instrument for Teenagers (POSIT), which self-administered instruments that tap relevant functional domains of substance use, psychiatric symptoms, school and vocational functioning, family functioning, social competency and peer relations, leisure and recreation, medical problems. More detailed interview instruments tapping the same domains include Adolescent Drug Abuse Diagnosis (ADAD), the Adolescent Problem Severity Index (APSI), the Severity Index (T-ASI), and the Comprehensive Adolescent Severity Inventory for Adolescents (CASI-A). Several brief self-report instruments provide measures of alcohol and substance use severity and consequences in addition to quantity and frequency of use. The Alcohol Dependence Scale (ADS) is a self-report measure of severity of alcohol dependence over the past year. The Rutgers Alcohol Problems Inventory (RAPI) consists of 23 items that assess negative consequences due to alcohol use typically experienced by adolescents. Other comprehensive instruments that measure substance use problem severity as well as a range of psychosocial constructs include the Global Appraisal of Individual Needs (GAIN). The Minnesota Chemical Dependency Adolescent Assessment Package (MCDAAP) includes a structured diagnostic interview, the Adolescent Diagnostic Interview (ADI), a brief screening tool, the Personal Experience Screening Questionnaire and Personal Experience Inventory (PEI), a comprehensive assessment instrument that covers all substances and related problems. It provides a list of critical items that suggests areas in need of immediate attention by the treatment provider and summarizes problems relevant for planning the level of treatment intervention.

Assessment

In evaluating the child or adolescent, the first goal is to determine if a problem in using one or more psychoactive substances exists, what effects substance use has on various domains of the adolescent's psychosocial functioning, and whether such a problem fits diagnostic criteria for substance abuse or dependence. To be considered a problem, substance use must produce some level of dysfunction in one or more domains of the adolescent's life. These domains include substance use and associated problems, psychiatric/behavioural, family, school/vocational, recreational/leisure and medical.

Because of the covert nature of substance use, optimal assessment often requires information from a variety of sources including the adolescent, parents (or other caregivers), other family members, school, any involved social agencies and previous treatment records. Elements of the parent/caregiver interview include the reasons for referral, parental concerns, and details, when known, about the presenting problems (onset, duration, consequences and impairment/dysfunction). Parents may have limited knowledge of their child's substance use patterns, although whenever possible collateral informants are desired. The interview should enquire about the extent of the parent's knowledge of their child's use patterns and negative consequences. Aggressive and suicidal behaviour are common among adolescents with substance use disorders. A treatment history should consist of enquiry into past mental health and SUD interventions, including response to treatment and attitudes about past interventions.

- A comprehensive developmental, social and medical history is a part of any complete assessment involving adolescents. Particularly important is a review of HIV risk factors, including sexual and other high-risk behaviours. Inquiry into these variables can often provide important information into pre-morbid functioning and risk factors for the development of SUDs. The parent/guardian should be able to provide information about a family history of SUDs, family functioning, stressors and supports as well as community resources and risks. Because family involvement forms the cornerstone of many empirically proven treatments, optimal family assessment includes observing how family members, including siblings, interact with one another.

- The interview of the adolescent is much more problematic due to the common desire of the adolescent to deny or minimize problems with substance use and related behaviours as well as the consequences of the substance use. The attitude of the clinician should be non-judgemental and flexible in the order of the interview elements. The clinician may wish to start with less potential anxiety-provoking elements such as enquiry into school, peers and family and delay questions about substance use and other deviant behaviours until later in the interview. The clinician may attempt to 'normalize' use in an attempt to get an accurate report. While using words and concepts appropriate to the adolescent's cognitive, linguistic and emotional development, the clinician should avoid jargon and attempts to appear more like a peer than adult. In clarifying the purpose of the interview/assessment, the clinician should ask about the adolescent's perception of the reason for referral and attitude about the assessment.

- Detailed assessment of the adolescent's substance use behaviour is an essential element of the interview. Enquiry into patterns of use includes information about the age of onset and progression of use for specific substances, quality, frequency and variability of use and the types of agents used. The clinician should ask about both direct and indirect consequences of use in the domains of family, school/or vocational, social and psychological functioning and medical problems. The interview should also include enquiry about the context of use, which concerns information about the adolescent's view of substance use, expectancies of use, the usual time and places of substance use, peer attitudes and use patterns, common behavioural and or emotional antecedents and consequences of use and the adolescent's overall social milieu. Finally, the clinician should ask about the adolescent's view of the substance use as a potential problem, past or current attempts to control or stop substance use and a review of the criteria for substance abuse and dependence (substance specific).

- The differential diagnosis of adolescent SUDs requires consideration that the reported domains of dysfunction attributed to substance use may be actually due to premorbid or concurrent problems such as disruptive behaviour disorders or social/environmental factors such as family or academic problems. The frequent co-morbidity of SUDs and other psychiatric disorders necessitates a comprehensive review of past and present psychopathology, including a psychiatric review of symptoms and treatment history. A timeline approach is suggested in attempting to sort out the relationship between co-morbid psychopathology, substance use, and developmental events and to assist in formulating a differential diagnosis and comprehensive treatment plan.

Several standardized assessment instruments can assist the clinician in the screening and comprehensive assessment of the adolescent with SUDs (see Appendix 2.1). The alcohol use disorder identification test (AUDIT) and the CRAFFT, two screening instruments for adolescents' alcohol and substance use disorders are in Appendix 2.2 and 2.3, respectively.

Motivational interviewing or enhancement (MI/ME) techniques are increasingly used during the assessment and on into treatment. This non-judgemental, non-directive strategy is designed to move the adolescent to a 'stage of change' more receptive to treatment or to behaviour change. The interview with the adolescent also includes elements common to all assessments of emotional and behavioural problems of adolescents.

Aetiology

Development and maintenance of the disorders

A number of characteristics of the adolescents, their families and their environments are associated with increased rates of substance use and SUDs. These are risk factors for SUDs (see Table 2.2) and are subsumed under four broad areas of risk factors: individual, peer, family and sociocultural. No one set of risk

Table 2.2. Risk factors for the development of substance use disorders
in adolescents

Individual factors
  Early disruptive behaviour disorder, e.g. ADHD
  Early aggressive behaviour, e.g. conduct disorder
  Poor academic performance, school failure
  Positive beliefs, attitudes about substance use

Biological factors
  Neuropsychiatric markers (e.g. static ataxia, latency of brain-evoked potentials)
  Neurogenetic traits (e.g. impulsivity, mood dysregulation)
  Differential levels of reinforcement from specific substances

Peer-related factors
  Peer substance use
  Peer beliefs, attitudes about substance use
  Earlier involvement with peers and away from family

Familial factors
  Parental substance use
  Parental beliefs, attitudes about substance use
  Parent tolerance of substance use
  Lack of closeness, attachment between parent and child
  Poor parental supervision and monitoring of child/adolescent

Sociocultural factors
  Community or neighbourhood characteristics
    Low socio-economic status
    High population density
    Physical deterioration
    High crime
  Media messages about substance use

factors necessarily is predictive of a SUD outcome, rather the number of risk factors appears to be the best predictor. Understanding the types of risk factors present in an individual allows one to target prevention and treatment efforts to factors important in the development and maintenance of SUDs. Despite similarities to adults in physical size and abilities, most adolescents have not obtained mature levels of cognitive, emotional, social or physical growth. They are challenged by the developmental tasks of forming a separate identity, preparing for appropriate societal and individual relationships including job, marriage and family. Within this context, adolescents experiment with a wide range of attitudes and behaviours.

Among these experimental behaviours is the use of psychoactive substances. There appears to be a fairly predictable progression of stages of adolescent substance use. Almost all adolescents experiment with 'gateway drugs' such as alcohol and cigarettes, with progressively fewer adolescents advancing to later and more serious levels of substance use, including the use of marijuana and other illicit drugs. First experiences with substance use most often take place in a social context with the use of 'gateway' substances, which are legal for adults and readily available to minors. For some groups, African-Americans in the USA, for example, marijuana may serve as a gateway drug. Initial use may occur because of ordinary adolescent curiosity or the availability of a substance. The early onset of substance use and a more rapid progression through the stages of substance use are among the risk factors for the development of SUDs. Thus, experimenters who are more likely to progress to SUDs are youth with multiple risk factors. The literature on the development of substance use and SUDs in adolescents has identified an assortment of individual, peer, family and community risk factors. Put in a developmental context, genetic predispositions to affective, cognitive and behavioural dysregulation are exacerbated by family and peer factors and the developmental issues of puberty leading to substance use and pathological use. Both temperament and social interactions (i.e. family, peer relations) have a critical role in adolescent SUD outcomes.

Developmental factors that contribute to early use or to continuing use include common adolescent feelings of omnipotence, issues of autonomy, peer influences or 'peer pressure'. Children and pre-adolescents are particularly susceptible to cultural factors such as media promotion of substance use, which may influence the initial use of such gateway substances as tobacco. The risk for SUDs in adolescents and the development of these disorders are similar to many other problems that are noted in youth. Each child may inherit certain genetic traits that are influenced by their environment, most notably their families and later, toward adolescence, by their peers. Different types of risk factors may be more significant for adolescents at specific stages of substance use. For example, peer and family factors are more critical at earlier stages of use, while individual risk factors, such as deviant behaviours and psychopathology, are likely to exert more influence at later stages of substance use. While no particular risk factor or set of risk factors completely predicts substance use, or the development of use disorders in adolescents, the number of risk factors may be the best guide to prediction.

Substance use can disrupt the ability of adolescents seriously to handle adequately other developmental tasks. Generally, the quantity and frequency of substance use peak in late adolescence or early adulthood, thus suggesting a maturational process. Most adolescents or young adults find that they cannot negotiate the demands and roles of adulthood while continuing a sustained pattern of substance use. Life events such as marriage, parenthood and moving away from the adolescent subculture increase the likelihood of decreasing or discontinuation of substance use. However, because some adolescents who abuse substances enter into adult roles (e.g. marriage, child-bearing) earlier than their non-substance-abusing peers, they may experience more difficulty in successfully carrying out these adult roles or tasks.

Treatment

Clinical management and treatment setting

- The primary goal for the treatment of adolescents with SUDs is achieving and maintaining abstinence from substance use. While abstinence should remain the explicit, long-term goal for treatment, a realistic view recognizes both the chronicity of SUDs in some populations of adolescents and the self-limited nature of substance use and substance use-related problems in other adolescent populations.

- Given these considerations, harm reduction, that is, reduction in the use and adverse effects/consequences of substances, a reduction in the severity and frequency of relapses, and improvement in one or more domains of an adolescent's functioning may be an acceptable interim, implicit goal for treatment. Included in the concept of harm reduction is a reduction in the use and adverse effects of substances, a reduction in the severity and frequency of relapses and improvement in one or more domains of the adolescent's functioning (e.g. academic performance or family functioning).

- Despite an acceptance of harm reduction as an interim goal for treatment, clinicians should discourage 'controlled use' of any non-prescribed substance of abuse as an explicit goal in the treatment of adolescents.

- Abstinence or decreased substance use should not be the only goal of treatment. The broad concept of rehabilitation involves targeting associated problems and domains of functioning for treatment. Integrated interventions that deal concurrently with co-existing psychiatric and behavioural problems, family functioning, peer and interpersonal relationships and academic/vocational functioning will produce not only general improvements in psychosocial functioning, but most likely will also yield improved outcomes in the primary treatment goal of achieving and maintaining abstinence.

- Among the important characteristics of successful treatment are sufficient duration, intensiveness and comprehensiveness, the presence of after-care or follow up treatment(s), sensitivity to cultural, racial and socio-economic realities of adolescents and their families, family involvement, collaboration with social services agencies, promotion of pro-social activities and a drug-free lifestyle and consideration of involvement in peer-based self-support groups such as Alcoholics Anonymous (AA) or Narcotics Anonymous (NA).

- A controversial element of traditional treatment programmes is the widespread use of group treatment. There is substantial evidence that group treatment can have significant negative effects on outcomes. Further emerging data suggests this iatrogenic effect may be limited to more deviant, conduct-disordered youths who nevertheless make up a substantial portion of the adolescent SUD treatment population. Clinicians should take caution when formulating groups for treatment and should consider alternative family-based or other modalities for more deviant youths.

- Treatment of adolescents with SUDs can take place at one of several levels of care, reflecting intensity of treatment and restriction of movement. Factors affecting the choice of treatment setting include:
  (a) motivation and willingness of the adolescent and family to co-operate with treatment
  (b) the adolescent's need for structure and/or limit setting that cannot be provided in a less restrictive environment
  (c) the need to provide a safe environment and the ability of the adolescent to care for him/herself
  (d) the existence of additional medical and/or psychiatric conditions
  (e) the availability of specific types of treatment settings for adolescents
  (f) the adolescent's and family's preferences for a particular setting
  (g) treatment failure in a less restrictive setting or level of care.
  Although residential programmes, including therapeutic communities, have a place in the range of setting options, community intervention settings, if feasible, may offer optimal generalization of treatment gains.

- Attendance in aftercare treatment or self-support groups (e.g. AA or NA) is related to positive outcomes in several studies of adolescent SUD treatment. Adolescents attending more intensive aftercare programmes involving case management and community reinforcement were more likely than those who did not receive these services to be abstinent from marijuana and have reduced their alcohol use at 3 months post-discharge. Following the acute treatment for substance use, on-going attention should be paid to co-morbid psychopathology and other comprehensive needs of the adolescent and family.

- Programmes with more comprehensive services such as vocational counselling, recreational activities and medical services (including birth control) had better outcomes. As with the success of multi-Systemic therapy (MST), programmes that deal with the social ecology or total life circumstances of the adolescent are likely to produce more lasting benefits.

Having a supportive environment (parents and peers), especially parents and peers who do not use substances, is important for optimal outcomes. Among this support can be self-support groups. Twelve-step approaches, using Alcoholics Anonymous

(AA) and Narcotics Anonymous (AN) as a basis for treatment, are perhaps the most common approaches for treatment and treatment programmes in the USA. Adolescents attending AA/NA meetings were more likely to abstain. Although 12-step programmes appear to be effective, they do not show an inherent advantage over other treatments nor have they been subject to controlled clinical trials. They are used best as adjuncts to other modalities. Several other studies have found that attendance at self-help or aftercare groups is associated with higher rates of abstinence and other measures of improved outcome when compared with those not participating in such groups following treatment.

Psychological interventions

Family interventions are critical to the success of any treatment approach with adolescents with SUDs, since a number of family-related factors, such as parental substance use or abuse, poor parent–child relationships, low perceived parental support, low emotional bonding, and poor parent supervision and management of the adolescent's behaviour, have been identified as risk factors for the development of substance abuse among adolescents.

Three domains of predictors that have figured prominently in longitudinal studies of the aetiology of adolescent substance use and SUDs are particularly relevant:
(a) characteristics of the parent–child relationship
(b) parental effectiveness
(c) parental SUDs.
Conflict between parents and adolescents, insufficient parental monitoring, inconsistent or otherwise ineffective discipline and parental alcoholism or other substance abuse have all been found to be robust correlates and predictors of adolescent substance use and SUDs. Although there are many approaches to family intervention, for substance abuse treatment, they have common goals:
• providing psychoeducation about SUDs, which decreases familial denial and resistance to treatment
• assisting parents and family to initiate and maintain efforts to get the adolescent into appropriate treatment and to achieve abstinence
• assisting the parents and family in establishing or re-establishing structure with consistent limit setting and careful monitoring of the adolescent's activities and behaviour
• improving communication among family members.
Family therapy is the modality most studied in the treatment of adolescents with SUDs. Based on the limited number of comparative studies, outpatient family therapy appears to be superior to other forms of outpatient treatment. Among the forms of family therapy having support based on controlled studies are functional family therapy, brief strategic family therapy, multi-systemic therapy (MST), family

systems therapy, and multidimensional family therapy. Integrative behavioural and a family therapy (IBFT) model combining a family systems model and cognitive–behavioural therapy have shown efficacy in controlled clinical trials.

Engaging youth and their families in treatment is often critical to the success of treatment. Specific engagement procedures have been incorporated, as part of many family-based interventions offer empirical support for efforts to conduct specialized engagement interventions that work directly with the parent, as one way of engaging the teenager in treatment. Adolescent perceptions can also contribute to whether the youth will be engaged in treatment and therefore suggest that specialized, adolescent-focused engagement interventions are necessary.

Treatment completion is the treatment variable related most consistently to positive outcome. Related variables are motivation and compliance, which are also related to better outcomes. Treatment and treatment programmes should strive to improve motivation, engagement and compliance with treatment. Modifications of motivational interviewing (MI) or enhancement techniques for adolescents have shown preliminary promise. MI and other brief interventions may serve to heighten motivation, increase self-efficacy, and provide personalized feedback and education tailored to specific substances and co-morbid problems such as psychiatric disorders. Several forms of family therapy have developed and tested an engagement intervention based on the assumption that the same maladaptive family interactional patterns that are linked to the adolescent's drug-using behaviours are likely to keep families from engagement in treatment. Based on brief strategic family therapy principles, therapists use family therapy manoeuvres to overcome temporarily the adolescent/family resistance. This approach has also demonstrated considerable improvements in improved treatment retention. Other family-based treatments such as MDFT and MST also have strong engagement goals and components. Contingency management procedures, which involve the use of alternative (to drug and alcohol) reinforcers in the environment, and are established as effective in adults, are being piloted in adolescent populations.

Researchers and clinicians are adapting interventions for specific psychiatric disorders for adolescents with SUD and psychiatric co-morbidity. For example, a number of cognitive–behavioural treatments (CBT), including many previously used with adults (e.g. relapse prevention), have been adapted as treatment modalities for adolescents with substance use disorders. Many cognitive–behavioural modalities, such as parent training, social skills, anger control and problem-solving training, developed for, and effective with, adolescents with conduct disorder also are relevant for youths with co-existing SUDs. CBT has also shown efficacy when combined with family, group and other modalities.

Psychoeducational measures

While information about the nature of SUDs, the effects and consequences of substances of abuse form an important component of SUD treatment and prevention, psychoeducation alone should never be the sole intervention modality. Trials of psychoeducation vs. more extensive intervention have shown that psychoeducation is not an adequate single intervention.

Psychopharmacology

The presence of significant psychiatric co-morbidity in adolescent substance abusers suggests that psychotropic medications may be used in this population. Only recently has there been research evaluating the efficacy and safety of any psychotropic medication in the treatment of adolescents with SUDs. Open trials with pemoline and bupropion for ADHD and fluoxetine for depression have been conducted in a population of drug-dependent delinquents. More recently, a placebo-controlled trial of pemoline reported the efficacy of pemoline in improving ADHD symptoms in adolescents with co-morbid ADHD and SUD. This study also demonstrated that medication treatment of ADHD alone, without specific SUD or other psychosocial treatment, did not decrease substance use.

Potential targets for pharmacological treatment include depression and other mood problems, ADHD, severe levels of aggressive behaviour and anxiety disorders. There are studies in the literature demonstrating the efficacy of pharmacological agents prescribed for adolescents with SUDs and co-morbid psychiatric disorders. Some limitations do exist in the use of psychotropic medications for adolescents with co-morbid SUDs and psychiatric disorders. General considerations, while described in general here, are discussed in more detail in other reviews. Pharmacological approaches such as lithium and serotonergic re-uptake inhibitors have produced significant improvements in adolescents with SUDs and co-morbid mood disorders.

Medications used to target craving (e.g. naltrexone, bupronorphine, acamprosate and ondansitron) that are increasingly used among adults have been used in case reports in adolescents. Their value in adolescents has yet to be tested in controlled trials. These, and aversive agents such as disulfiram, could be considered for use in more severely affected or treatment-resistant adolescents.

Clinicians should use the same caution in considering pharmacological treatment for adolescents with co-morbid SUDs and psychiatric disorders as they do with youth with psychiatric symptoms alone. The presence of SUDs or substance use may increase the potential for intentional or unintentional overdose with certain psychotropic medications, especially in combination with some substances of abuse. Some commonly used pharmacological agents, such as psychostimulants and benzodiazepines, may have inherent abuse potential.

Assessing the risk of concurrent use of various substance(s) of abuse and the pharmacotherapeutic agent is critical before prescribing any medication for an adolescent with a SUD. Informed consent should include a description of possible dangers of concurrent use of agents. The risk of abuse of a therapeutic agent either by the adolescent, his peer group or family members should prompt a thorough assessment of the risk of this outcome (e.g. past history of abuse of the agent, family/parental history of substance abuse and/or antisocial behaviour). Often, parental or adult supervision of medication administration can alleviate concerns about potential abuse.

The clinician should also consider alternative agents with a lower potential for abuse. The newer long-acting stimulant preparations may offer less potential for abuse or diversion due to their form of administration and the ability to monitor more easily and supervise once a day dosing. However, their abuse potential has yet to be ascertained fully. Alternatives to psychostimulants (dextroamphetamine, methylphenidate; mixed amphetamine salts) for the treatment of attention-deficit hyperactivity disorder include pemoline, clonidine, tricyclic antidepressants, atomoxitine, venlafaxine and bupropion. Although many anxiety symptoms or disorders in adolescents can be treated successfully with psychosocial methods such as behaviour therapy, the use of tricyclic antidepressants, buspirone or selective serotonin re-uptake inhibitors are preferred over benzodiazepines.

Nevertheless, as the clinician should not dismiss the use of pharmacotherapeutic agents in the treatment of adolescents with SUDs, the use of any specific agent should not be discounted until a thorough consideration of the potential benefits vs. likely and possible risks is made. The clinician should monitor carefully the presence of adverse effects of pharmacotherapy and the potential relationship of these effects to on-going substance use.

Outcome

Although there are over 1000 studies on drug and alcohol treatment in adults, there are a relatively small number of adolescent treatment outcome studies. A decade-old review of adolescent treatment outcome in 16 studies concluded that treatment is better than no treatment.

- Pre-treatment factors associated with outcome were race, seriousness of substance use, criminality and educational status.
- The in-treatment factors predictive of outcome were time in residential treatment, involvement of family, use of practical problem-solving and provision of comprehensive services such as housing, academic assistance and recreation.

- Post-treatment variables, which were thought to be the most important determinants of outcome, included association with non-using peers, involvement in leisure time activities, work and school.

In more recent reviews of the literature, similar variables were reported to be related most consistently to successful outcome: treatment completion, low pre-treatment use, peer and parent social support and non-use of substances. These more recent reviews also found evidence that treatment was superior to no treatment. Although insufficient evidence was found to compare the effectiveness of treatment modalities, outpatient family therapy appeared to be superior to other forms of outpatient treatment.

The recent Drug Abuse Treatment Study for Adolescents (DATOS-A) in the USA is a multisite prospective treatment outcome study of 1732 adolescent admissions to 23 programmes in four US cities. In the year following treatment, patients reported decreased heavy drinking, marijuana and other illicit drug use and criminal involvement as well as improved psychological adjustment and school performance. Although the length of time in treatment was generally short, longer treatment stays were associated with several favourable outcomes. Nearly two-thirds (63%) of the sample reported at least one co-morbid DSM-IV disorder. At baseline when compared with non-co-morbid youths with SUDs, these youths with co-morbid disorders were more likely to be alcohol or other drug dependent and have more problems with family, school and criminal involvement. Although co-morbid youths reduced their drug use and problem behaviours after treatment, they were more likely to use marijuana and hallucinogens and engage in delinquent in the 12 months after treatment when compared with non-co-morbid adolescents.

In terms of controlled clinical trials, most studies have used various forms of family therapy. Initially, studies of family therapy involved comparisons of specific forms of family therapy with other intervention modalities based on less well-defined models than the family-based treatments. Since the mid-1990s, family therapy treatment studies of SUD adolescents have compared specific family therapies with manualized, specific treatments. Additional intervention trials have utilized cognitive–behavioural therapy (CBT), motivational enhancement (ME), and combinations of these with family therapies. Finally, pharmacotherapuetic research for adolescents with alcohol and other substance use disorders is still in its infancy.

In summary, there is evidence that treatment is better than no treatment and that, at least for adolescents, family-based treatments appear to have the best evidence to support their efficacy. However, we still have a poor sense of what types of therapies or modalities work better for specific populations of adolescents, such as those with specific psychiatric co-morbidities or racial/ethnic status, and we know little about the role of treatment intensity on outcome.

SUGGESTED READING

S. A. Brown, E. J. D'Amico, D. M. McCarthy & S. F. Tapert, Four-year outcomes from adolescent alcohol and drug treatment. *Journal of Studies on Alcohol* **62** (2001), 381–8.

O. G. Bukstein & R. E. Tarter, Substance use disorders in children and adolescents. In E. Coffey, ed., *Textbook of Pediatric Neuropsychiatry* (New York: American Psychiatric Press, 1998).

O. G. Bukstein & J. Kithas, Adolescent substance use disorders. In Rosenberg, D., Davanzo, P. A. & Gershon, S., eds. *Child and Adolescent Psychopharmacology* (Marcel-Dekker, 2002).

Y. Hser, C. E. Grella, R. L. Hubbard *et al.*, An evaluation of drug treatments for adolescents in 4 US cities. *Archives of General Psychiatry* **58** (2001), 689–95.

C. S. Martin & K. C. Winters, Diagnosis and assessment of alcohol use disorders among adolescents. *Alcohol Health and Research World* **22** (1998), 95–105.

P. M. Monti, S. M. Colby & T. A. O'Leary, *Adolescents, Alcohol, and Substance Abuse: Reaching Teens through Brief Interventions* (New York, NY, US: The Guilford Press, 2001).

R. E. Tarter, Evaluation and treatment of adolescent substance abuse: a decision tree method. *American Journal of Drug and Alcohol Abuse* **6** (1990), 1–46.

E. F. Wagner & H. B. Waldron, *Innovations in adolescent substance abuse interventions* (Amsterdam, Netherlands: Pergamon/Elsevier Science Inc., 2001).

H. B. Waldron, Adolescent substance abuse and family therapy outcome: a review of randomized trials. In T. H. Ollendick & R. J. Prinz, *Advances in Clinical Child Psychology* (New York: Plenum, 1997) vol. 19, pp. 199–234.

R. J. Williams & S. Y. Chang, A comprehensive and comparative review of adolescent substance abuse treatment outcome. *Clinical Psychology: Science and Practice* **7** (2000), 38–166.

Appendix 2.1. Selected instruments for screening and assessment of substance use problems in adolescents

Instrument	Reference	Type of instrument	Comments
Adolescent Drug Abuse Diagnosis (ADAD)	Friedman, A. S. & Utada, A. (1989). A method for diagnosing and planning the treatment of adolescent drug abusers (The Adolescent Drug Abuse Diagnosis, ADAD). *Journal of Drug Education* **19**: 285–312.	Assessment; interview	Provides severity ratings on multiple domains of functioning (substance use, family, psychiatric/behavioural, medical, school/ vocational, leisure time, peer relations)
Adolescent Problem Severity Index (APSI)	Metzger, A., Kushner, H. & McLellan, A. T. (1991). *Adolescent Problem Severity Index.* Philadelphia, University of Pennsylvania.	Assessment; interview	Provides severity ratings on multiple domains of functioning (substance use, family, psychiatric/behavioural, medical, school/ vocational, leisure time, peer relations)
CRAFFT	Knight, J. R., Sherritt, L., Shrier, L. A., Harris, S. K. & Change, G. (2002). Validity of the CRAFFT substance abuse screening test among adolescent clinic patients. *Archives of Pediatrics and Adolescent Medicine* **156**: 607–14.	Screening; brief interview	Six-item brief screen for primary care professionals
Comprehensive Adolescent Severity Inventory for Adolescents (CASI-A)	Meyers, M. Meyers, K., McLellan, A. T., Jaeger, J. L. & Pettinati, A. (1995). The development of the Comprehensive Addiction Severity Index for Adolescents (CASI-A): an interview for assessing multiple problems of adolescents. *Journal of Substance Abuse Treatment* **12**: 181–93.	Assessment: interview	Provides severity ratings on multiple domains of functioning (substance use, family, psychiatric/ behavioural, medical, school/vocational, leisure time, peer relations)

(cont.)

Appendix 2.1. (cont.)

Instrument	Reference	Type of instrument	Comments
The Drug Use Screening Inventory-Adolescents (DUSI-A)	Tarter, R. E., Mezzich, A. C., Kirisci, L. & Kaczynksi, N. (1994). Reliability of the Drug Use Screening Inventory among adolescent alcoholics. *Journal of Child Adolescent Substance Abuse* **3**:25–36.	Screening; self-administered	159-item: documents the level of involvement with a variety of drugs and quantifies severity of consequences associated with drug use
Global Appraisal of Individual Needs (GAIN)	Dennis, M. L. (1998). *Global Appraisal of Individual Needs (GAIN) manual: Administration, Scoring and Interpretation* (Prepared with funds from CSAT TI 11320). Bloomington, IL: Lighthouse Publications.	Interview	Documents SUD and other psychiatric diagnoses; placement criteria; health, mental distress and environment; and service utilization outcomes
Personal Experience Screening Questionnaire (PESQ)	Winters, K. (1992). Development of an adolescent substance abuse screening questionnaire. *Addictive Behaviors* **17**:479–90.	Screening; self-administered	40-items; screens for the need for further assessment of drug use disorders
Problem Oriented Screening Instrument for Teenagers (POSIT)	Rahdert, R. & Radhert, E. (1991). *The Adolescent Assessment and Referral System Manucl.* DHHS Publication No. (ADM) 91–1735 Rockville, MD: National Institute on Drug Abuse.	Screening; self-administered	139 items; designed to identify problems and potential treatment or service needs in 10 areas, including substance abuse, mental and physical health, and social relations.
Teen Addiction Severity Index (T-ASI)	Kaminer, Y., Bukstein, O. G. & Tarter, R. E. (1991). The Teen Addiction Severity Index (T-ASI): rationale and reliability. *International Journal of Addictions* **26**:219–26.	Assessment; interview	Provides severity ratings on multiple domains of functioning, including substance abuse, mental and physical health, and social relations.

Appendix 2.2. Alcohol use disorder identification test (AUDIT)

1. How often do you have a drink containing alcohol?

0	1	2	3	4
Never	Monthly or less	2–4 times a month	2–3 times a week	4 or more times a week

2. How many drinks containing alcohol do you have on a typical day when you are drinking?

0	1	2	3	4
1 or 2	3 or 4	5–6	7–9	10 or more

3. How often do you have 6 or more drinks on one occasion?

0	1	2	3	4
Never	Less than monthly	Monthly	Weekly	Daily or almost daily

4. How often during the last year have you found that you were not able to stop drinking once you had started?

0	1	2	3	4
Never	Less than monthly	Monthly	Weekly	Daily or almost daily

5. How often during the last year have you failed to do what was normally expected from you because of drinking?

0	1	2	3	4
Never	Less than monthly	Monthly	Weekly	Daily or almost daily

6. How often during the last year have you needed a first drink in the morning to get yourself going after a heavy drinking session?

0	1	2	3	4
Never	Less than monthly	Monthly	Weekly	Daily or almost daily

7. How often during the last year have you had a feeling of guilt or remorse after drinking?

0	1	2	3	4
Never	Less than monthly	Monthly	Weekly	Daily or almost daily

8. How often during the last year have you been unable to remember what happened the night before because you had been drinking?

0	1	2	3	4
Never	Less than monthly	Monthly	Weekly	Daily or almost daily

9. Have you or has someone else been injured as a result of your drinking?

0	1	2
No	Yes, but not in the last year	Yes, during the last year

10. Has a relative or friend, or doctor or other health worker been concerned about your drinking or suggested you cut down?

0	1	2
No	Yes, but not in the last year	Yes, during the last year

Score of 8 or more indicates possible problem drinking; further assessment is recommended.

Appendix 2.3.

The CRAFFT[*]

    C: Have you ever ridden in a *car* driven by someone (including yourself) who was 'high' or had been using alcohol or drugs?

    R: Do you ever use alcohol or drugs to *relax*, feel better about yourself, or fit in?

    A: Do you ever use alcohol or drugs while you are by yourself, *alone*?

    F: Do you ever *forget* things you did while using alcohol or drugs?

    F: Do your *family or friends* ever tell you that you should cut down on your drinking or drug use?

    T: Have you ever gotten into *trouble* while you were using alcohol or drugs?

Those who have scores of 2 or higher are recommended for further assessment

[*] Knight, J. R., Sherritt, L., Shrier, L. A., Harris, S. K. & Change, G. (2002). Validity of the CRAFFT substance abuse screening test among adolescent clinic patients. *Archives of Pediatrics and Adolescent Medicine* **156**, 607–14.

3

Schizophrenia and schizophrenia-like disorders

Andrew F. Clark

Prestwich Hospital, Manchester, UK

Introduction

Approximately 20 per cent of people with a lifetime diagnosis of schizophrenia date the first onset of their psychotic symptoms to before the age of 20 years. One of the key tasks therefore, of the child and adolescent psychiatrist is early recognition and treatment of the disorder notwithstanding its rarity in their overall practice. A much larger number of young people, however, are referred to child and adolescent mental health services with the key question 'might this young person be developing or suffering from the early stages of schizophrenia or some other psychotic disorder?'. The clinician must also therefore, possess expert knowledge of both its typical and atypical presentations and its differential diagnoses.

Other psychotic disorders presenting during adolescence (and more rarely during childhood) are those of acute or transient psychotic disorders not lasting long enough for a diagnosis of schizophrenia, schizoaffective disorders, delusional disorders, psychotic episodes occurring as part of an underlying affective disorder and psychotic disorders secondary to substance misuse or to general medical conditions.

In many instances the clinician will be able to arrive at a clear formulation and diagnostic understanding and to develop a specific treatment plan. In others, however, diagnostic uncertainty will remain despite a full and careful assessment, even one lasting over a period of weeks. In these cases it is important that the clinician is able to tolerate this uncertainty whilst continuing to take a problem-focused approach to the young person's difficulties. Similarly, for some individuals their psychotic episode will resolve relatively rapidly with no residual symptoms or impairments and therefore no need for on-going contact with mental health services, whilst for others it will continue a chronic or relapsing and remitting course necessitating a lifetime of psychiatric care. This chapter aims to give the

A Clinician's Handbook of Child and Adolescent Psychiatry, ed. Christopher Gillberg,
Richard Harrington and Hans-Christoph Steinhausen. Published by Cambridge University Press.
© Cambridge University Press 2005.

Table 3.1. Comparison of ICD-10 and DSM-IV classifications of schizophrenia and related disorders

ICD-10		DSM-IV	
Code	Diagnosis	Code	Diagnosis
F20	Schizophrenia sub-types	–	Schizophrenia sub-types
	Sub-types		Sub-types
F20.0	Paranoid	295.3	Paranoid
F20.1	Hebephrenic	295.1	Disorganized
F20.2	Catatonic	295.2	Catatonic
F20.3	Undifferentiated	295.9	Undifferentiated
F20.4	Post-schizophrenic depression	295.6	Residual
F20.5	Residual	295.4	Schizophreniform disorder
F20.6	Simple	298.8	Brief psychotic disorder
F20.8	Other	297.3	Shared psychotic disorder
F20.9	Unspecified	295.7	Schizoaffective disorder
F23	Acute and transient psychotic disorders	298.9	Psychotic disorder not otherwise specified
F24	Induced delusional disorder		
F25	Schizoaffective disorder		
F29	Unspecified non-organic psychosis		

clinician a framework for assessment and management that can be applied across all these complex clinical dilemmas.

Definition and classification

The basis for the classification of psychotic disorders rests primarily upon the recognition of constellations of symptoms rather than on any full understanding of the underlying pathologies. Both ICD-10 and DSM-IV take broadly similar approaches (Table 3.1) but with some significant differences both in the terminologies used and in the symptom constellations required for specific diagnoses.

Schizophrenia and schizophreniform disorder

The key features of schizophrenia are those of marked perceptual disturbances often accompanied by social and personal impairments but usually occurring in clear consciousness and without sustained accompanying depressive or elated mood disturbance. These symptoms are reflected in both the ICD-10 and the DSM-IV diagnostic criteria for schizophrenia (see Tables 3.2 and 3.3) albeit with slightly different emphases. DSM-IV, however, helpfully also makes explicit that, in children and adolescents, a failure of the individual to make expected interpersonal, academic or occupational progress during a period of illness represents for them a deterioration in functioning.

Table 3.2. Clinical diagnostic criteria for schizophrenia (F20) according to ICD-10

One of the symptoms (a)–(d) for at least 1 month:

(a) thought echo, insertion or withdrawal and thought broadcasting;

(b) delusions of control, influence or passivity, clearly referred to body or limb movements or specific thoughts, actions or sensations; delusional perception;

(c) hallucinatory voices giving a running commentary on the patient's behaviour, or discussing the patient among themselves or other types of hallucinatory voices coming from some part of the body;

(d) persistent delusions of other kinds that are culturally inappropriate and completely impossible, such as religious or political identity, or superhuman powers and abilities (e.g. being able to control the weather, or being in communication with aliens from another world);

or at least two of the symptoms e–h for at least 1 month:

(e) persistent hallucinations in any modality, when accompanied either by fleeting or half-formed delusions without clear affective content, or by persistent overvalued ideas, or when occurring every day for weeks or months on end;

(f) breaks or interpolations in the train of thought, resulting in incoherence or irrelevant speech or neologisms;

(g) catatonic behaviour, such as excitement, posturing, or waxy flexibility, negativism, mutism and stupor;

(h) 'negative' symptoms such as marked apathy, paucity of speech, and blunting or incongruity of emotional responses, usually resulting in social withdrawal and lowering of social performance; it must be clear that these are not due to depression or to neuroleptic medication;

or over a duration of at least 1 year

(i) a significant and consistent change in the overall quality of some aspects of personal behaviour, manifest as loss of interest, aimlessness, idleness, a self-absorbed attitude, and social withdrawal. (applies to simple schizophrenia only (F20.6))

all in the absence of major affective symptoms, overt brain disease or current state of drug intoxication or withdrawal.

Perhaps the most striking difference on first reading is that ICD-10 appears only to require an illness period of 1 month whereas DSM-IV requires an illness period of 6 months. However, the 6-month period referred to in DSM-IV (Criterion C) can include a prodromal period in which the only evidence of illness is alteration in social and personal functioning and increasingly odd or overvalued ideas or experiences before the onset of frank psychotic (Criterion A) symptoms. In contrast, the 1-month period required by ICD-10 can start only with the development of specific psychotic symptoms, and any prodromal phase is specifically excluded. In

Table 3.3. Diagnostic criteria for schizophrenia according to DSM-IV

A. *Characteristic symptoms:* Two (or more) of the following, each present for a significant portion of time during a 1-month period (or less if successfully treated):

  (1) delusions

  (2) hallucinations

  (3) disorganized speech (e.g. frequent derailment or incoherence)

  (4) grossly disorganized or catatonic behaviour

  (5) negative symptoms, i.e. affective flattening, alogia, or avolition

Note: Only one Criterion A symptom is required if delusions are bizarre or hallucinations consist of a voice keeping up a running commentary on the person's behaviour or thoughts, or two or more voices conversing with each other.

B. *Social/occupational dysfunction:* For a significant portion of time since the onset of the disturbance, one or more major areas of functioning such as work, interpersonal relations, or self-care are markedly below the level achieved prior to the onset (or when the onset is in childhood or adolescence, failure to achieve expected level of interpersonal, academic, or occupational achievement).

C. *Duration:* Continuous signs of the disturbance persist for at least 6 months. This 6-month period must include at least 1 month of symptoms (or less if successfully treated) that meet Criterion A (i.e. active phase symptoms) and may include periods of prodromal or residual symptoms. During these prodromal or residual periods, the signs of the disturbance may be manifested by only negative symptoms or two or more symptoms listed in Criterion A present in an attenuated form (e.g. odd beliefs, unusual perceptual experiences).

D. *Schizoaffective and mood disorder exclusion:* Schizoaffective and mood disorder with psychotic features have been ruled out because either (1) no major depressive, manic, or mixed episodes have occurred concurrently with the active-phase symptoms; or (2) if mood episodes have occurred during active-phase symptoms, their total duration has been brief relative to the duration of the active and residual periods.

E. *Substance/general medical condition exclusion:* The disturbance is not due to the direct physiological effects of a substance (e.g. a drug of abuse, a medication) or a general medical condition.

F. *Relationship to a pervasive developmental disorder:* If there is a history of autistic disorder or another pervasive developmental disorder, the additional diagnosis of schizophrenia is only made if prominent delusions or hallucinations are also present for at least a month (or less if successfully treated).

practice therefore, many young people even with relatively acute onset none the less fulfil criteria for schizophrenia within both systems. Those young people with a total illness duration of less than 6 months but otherwise fulfilling DSM-IV criteria (including active psychotic symptoms for a minimum duration of 1 month) receive a diagnosis of schizophreniform disorder. (Confusingly this term is used differently in ICD-10; see below under briefer psychotic episodes.)

Both ICD-10 and DSM-IV do describe a variety of sub-types of schizophrenia (paranoid, hebephrenic/disorganized, catatonic, undifferentiated, residual). Often, however, a young person's symptoms within a single episode will be drawn from two or more of these sub-types. Neither is there any convincing evidence that any sub-type is predictive of treatment response or prognosis. The clinical usefulness of these subtypes is therefore debatable. DSM-IV does also offer an alternative dimensional approach to sub-typing, rating severity of psychotic, disorganized and negative symptoms, which may be useful in some instances.

ICD-10 offers two additional sub-types, post-schizophrenic depression and simple schizophrenia. 'Post-schizophrenic depression' refers to a depressive episode arising in the aftermath of a schizophrenic illness but when acute symptoms of the initial illness are much reduced. The term 'simple schizophrenia' is used to describe a sustained global deterioration in personal functioning (lasting at least 1 year) but without ever the development of delusional beliefs, hallucinatory experiences, thought disorganization or catatonic features. It is a rarely made diagnosis within ICD-10 and one that is difficult to make with certainty, given the non-specific nature of the symptoms. Neither diagnosis is contained in the main body of DSM-IV, although research criteria for both are given in its Appendix.

Briefer psychotic disorders

The terms Acute and Transient Psychotic Disorders (ICD-10) and Brief Psychotic Disorder (DSM-IV) are used to describe psychotic episodes of sudden onset and no demonstrable organic aetiology that have relatively rapid resolution with full return to pre-morbid functioning. In DSM-IV the total duration from initial onset to full recovery with no residual impairments can be no more than 1 month, otherwise an alternative diagnosis becomes appropriate (e.g. schizophreniform disorder, psychosis NOS). In ICD-10, however, whilst brief schizophrenia-like episodes should be reclassified as schizophrenia if enduring beyond 1 month, other atypical acute onset psychoses are allowed to persist for up to 3 months. To add further confusion, in its description of the syndrome, ICD-10 refers to brief schizophreniform disorders as coming under this rubric.

Induced delusional or shared psychotic disorders

Very rarely, a situation develops wherein two individuals living in close emotional proximity share psychotic-like experiences and beliefs, although only one of them truly suffers from a genuine psychotic disorder (the folie à deux syndrome). This can occur in children living with either a psychotic parent or even, and much more rarely, a psychotic sibling. ICD-10 uses the term Induced Delusional Disorder to describe this, whilst DSM-IV prefers Shared Psychotic Disorder. Diagnostic criteria for the disorders are, however, identical.

Schizoaffective disorders

Both ICD-10 and DSM-IV classify schizoaffective disorders as a separate diagnostic group but the diagnostic criteria for the disorder differ significantly between the two systems. DSM-IV requires that the individual should meet the diagnostic criteria simultaneously for both schizophrenia and for a major depressive, manic or mixed episode (see Chapter 4 for diagnostic criteria for affective disorders). ICD-10, however, requires only that symptoms of both schizophrenia and an affective disorder be present concurrently but not necessarily that the individual should meet full diagnostic criteria for both disorders.

Mood disorders with psychotic features

Manic, depressive and mixed states can all have associated delusional beliefs and hallucinatory experiences as a part of their phenomenology. These are classified within the mood disorders but with a specific sub-category for the presence of psychotic features. (See Chapter 4 for greater discussion regarding the classification of mood disorders.)

Psychotic disorders induced by substance use or due to general medical conditions

In both ICD-10 and DSM-IV psychotic presentations secondary to physical disorder or to substance misuse are classified separately and according to the underlying organic aetiology. In the case of co-morbid substance misuse that is not considered to have an aetiological role in the psychotic episode, the two disorders should be coded separately. In practice, this distinction is not always easy to make (see Chapters 1 and 2 for a more detailed discussion of classificatory issues).

Epidemiology

Prevalence and incidence rates

Retrospective studies of adult sufferers of schizophrenia suggest that 20 per cent date the first onset of their overt psychotic symptoms to before the age of 20 years and 5 per cent to before the age of 15 years. Precise prevalence and incidence rates during childhood and adolescence for either schizophrenia or for psychotic disorders as a whole are not available, however. This is due to a combination of lack of truly population-based studies, inconsistency in diagnostic practices and instability of individual's symptom presentation and diagnosis over time. There is general agreement that the disorders are rare (prevalence ~0.2% of 13–19-year olds) and that their incidence and prevalence rates increase markedly over the teenage years.

Schizophrenia in childhood (onset before the age of 12 years) is exceptionally rare and the overwhelming majority of clinicians will not encounter any cases during their professional lifetime. From age 13 to 19 the disorder becomes progressively more common with estimates of a 50-fold difference in prevalence between those aged under 15 years and those above this age. In one study of all psychotic disorders (schizophrenia, schizophreniform disorder, atypical psychosis, affective psychosis and substance-induced psychosis; 41% schizophrenia) the prevalence rate of any psychotic disorder rose steadily from 0.9/10 000 at age 13 to 17.6/10 000 at age 19.

Sex ratios and ethnicity

Schizophrenia with adolescent onset appears to be more common in males than in females in most studies by a ratio of up to 2:1. However, this is not a finding consistent with a number of studies reporting a lower preponderance of males and some approaching equality between the sexes. These differences may reflect referral biases and again highlight the lack of robust epidemiological studies. There has been very little study of any variability in rates or presentations between adolescent sufferers from different ethnic and cultural groups, although consistent variations related to interactions between ethnic and cultural or societal factors have been shown in studies amongst adult sufferers.

Implications for clinical practice

Despite their rarity, clinicians do need to maintain an awareness and vigilance that schizophrenia and other psychotic disorders can present for the first time during the teenage years. Epidemiological variables are, however, of little use in guiding the clinician towards those young people most at risk of developing the disorders.

Clinical picture

Main features and symptoms

The core features of schizophrenia are those of distorted beliefs and perceptions ('positive symptoms'), of disorganization of thoughts and affect ('disorganized symptoms'), and of loss of drive, volition and emotional response ('negative symptoms'). These may manifest acutely or may develop insidiously with progressive greater abnormality of experience, thought and behaviour gradually becoming apparent. In a number of cases there is a prolonged period of increasing non specific behavioural abnormality and social and educational/vocational deterioration (the so-called 'prodromal period') which precedes evidence of more frank disturbance.

- Delusions and hallucinations may be characteristic in form (delusions – bodily, bizarre or impossible; auditory hallucinations – Schneiderian in nature (third person, running commentary, thought echo), although this is not always the case in adolescent onset cases. However, whilst the essential nature of phenomenology of schizophrenia is independent of the sufferer's age, the content of the abnormal beliefs and perceptions is not. Themes consonant with the development stage of adolescence are common, e.g. delusions and overvalued ideas regarding bodily appearance or disfigurement; delusions of great sporting or musical prowess or sexual desirability; hallucinatory experiences of abuse regarding personal, racial, gender or sexual identity. In younger adolescents, particularly those with borderline or mild learning difficulties, content may even relate more to childhood preoccupations of ghosts, monsters, animals and cartoon characters. The child's intellectual level and developmental stage will also influence the description of these experiences and it may, at times, be difficult to distinguish delusions from normal childhood fantasy or hallucinations from vivid imagery.

- Disorganization of thought processes may cause a marked inability to achieve educationally with a dramatic fall-off in performance. This may be associated with increased irritability as the young person struggles to mask or deny deficits. There may also be incongruity of emotional response with a young person displaying laughter or amusement inappropriately or, conversely, tears and sadness when pleasure would seem more suited. In some young people these may be the prime symptoms and it may be that referral to a psychiatrist is prompted by school concerns rather than by parents. This hebephrenic or disorganized sub-type tends to be a more common presentation in adolescence than in adulthood.

- 'Negative symptoms' also seem to appear more commonly and at an earlier stage in adolescent-onset cases than in adulthood. These may cause functional impairments in the young person's life such as social withdrawal, reduction in interests and declining school performance. They will be described frequently by parents or teachers as the young person having become 'lazy' or 'unmotivated' rather than being recognized as symptoms of an illness.

- A wide range of non-specific symptoms more associated with other disorders also may occur within a schizophrenic illness. Obsessive thinking and behaviours are common, anxious, elevated or low mood may occur (although should not predominate), and episodes of depersonalization and derealization are not uncommon.

Differential diagnosis and co-morbidity

The differential diagnosis for a first episode of schizophrenia is wide ranging and covers both psychiatric and physical disorders (see Table 3.4). Historically, the term 'childhood schizophrenia' was also used to describe infantile autism, although this has now long been abandoned. Young people with a pervasive developmental disorder (including Asperger's syndrome) should be diagnosed only as also suffering from schizophrenia when they are experiencing unequivocal delusions or hallucinations. This can cause some diagnostic difficulty in non-verbal children where

Table 3.4. Differential diagnosis for a first episode of schizophrenia

- Pervasive developmental disorders (including Asperger's syndrome)
- Affective disorders
- Schizoaffective disorders
- Substance-induced psychotic disorders (especially amphetamines, cocaine and ecstacy-like substances)
- Brief psychotic episodes
- General medical conditions (especially frontal and temporal lobe epilepsies, neurodegenerative disorders (e.g. Wilson's disease), metachromatic leukodystrophy and cerebral tumours)
- Non-psychotic conditions (conduct and emotional disorders, dissociative disorders, personality disorders (especially borderline personality disorder) and disturbances following sexual or physical abuse)
- Induced delusional disorder

one has to rely on externally observable behavioural changes suggestive of these. See Chapter 13 for a fuller discussion of pervasive developmental disorders.

Episodes of an affective disorder, irrespective of whether depressive, manic or mixed in state, can be confused with schizophrenia. Hallucinations, delusional beliefs and thought disorganization can all occur in a mood disorder associated with psychotic features. These are usually mood congruent and not associated with the presence of negative symptoms. Previous non-psychotic affective episodes can be helpful diagnostic pointers as can a positive family history for bipolar disorder. None the less the distinction can be hard to make in practice and the true nature of the disorder may only become evident over time. (For further discussion of affective disorders see Chapter 4.)

There continues to be considerable debate about the true nature of schizoaffective disorder (not least in the very different diagnostic criteria and thresholds set by ICD-10 and DSM-IV) but clinically it remains as a useful diagnostic entity. The concurrent co-existence in some individuals of classically schizophrenic symptoms with classically affective symptoms clinically is indisputable. There is also some prognostic utility in the diagnosis, as schizoaffective episodes appear to have a clinical course and outcome intermediate between those of schizophrenia and those of an affective disorder. There is some suggestion that episodes of schizodepression are perhaps more similar to schizophrenia in course and those of schizomania more similar to affective disorder, although evidence for this is not strong.

A substance-induced psychotic disorder must always be considered in the differential diagnosis, even where there is no overt history of substance use initially given.

Typically, these have an acute onset and relatively rapid resolution. The range of substances implicated in producing a psychotic episode is wide – amphetamines, cocaine, and ecstacy-like substances being perhaps the most commonly cited. However, increasing rates of poly-substance use and the development of ever newer 'designer' drugs can make identifying the putative causative agent impossible. Urine or hair analysis for illicit substances should be routine but this can merely demonstrate recent substance usage and not its relationship to the disorder, which could be causative, coincident, precipitating or self-medicating. (For further discussion of substance use disorders see Chapter 2.)

Brief psychotic episodes not fulfilling the symptomatic or duration criteria for a diagnosis of schizophrenia or affective disorder with psychotic features also occur relatively commonly amongst psychotic presentations. These are of an unknown nature with some individuals going on to have later episodes of more typical schizophrenia or affective disorder whilst others remain well with no further episodes of illness. When clear or unusual stressors are present, the clinician may be tempted to regard the psychotic episode as reactive to these (so-called 'brief reactive psychosis'), although this can by no means be presumed to be the case.

A wide range of general medical conditions can cause brain dysfunction leading to psychotic symptoms. These include frontal and temporal lobe epilepsies, neurodegenerative disorders (e.g. Wilson's disease), metachromatic leukodystrophy and cerebral tumours or other space-occupying lesions. Such presentations are rare but important to consider and exclude. (See Chapter 1 for a fuller consideration of brain disorders and their consequences.)

Hallucinations can also occur in a number of non-psychotic conditions in children and adolescents. These include conduct and emotional disorders, dissociative disorders, personality disorders (especially borderline personality disorder) and disturbances following sexual or physical abuse. In most instances, however, there will not be other core symptomatology suggestive of schizophrenia and the hallucinations will be non-Schneiderian in nature and the distinction will therefore be relatively easy to make. More difficult to distinguish but included in this group are also those young people with an induced delusional disorder consequent upon living in close emotional proximity to a truly psychotic individual.

Probably the most difficult diagnostic distinction to make is around those young people who show a non-specific change in functioning, coupled with development of increasing non-delusional odd ideas and magical thinking. It is clear that a proportion of these will go on to develop a frank psychotic episode within a relatively short period and will then be viewed retrospectively as having been suffering from 'prodromal schizophrenia'. However, even within groups of such individuals defined for maximal risk of developing schizophrenia (positive family history, marked change in functioning, quasi-psychotic symptoms) the 1-year conversion rate to frank schizophrenia is only 20–40 per cent with no clear discriminating or predictive factors. Whilst there are on-going studies of both pharmacological and psychological interventions in these groups these currently remain within the research domain. At present therefore, best clinical management probably is restricted to addressing any specific problems identified and to continued close monitoring so that, if a psychotic episode does develop, antipsychotic treatment can be started early.

Diagnostic instruments

The mainstay of diagnosis is a comprehensive clinical interview based upon multiple informants (young person, parents/carers, school), coupled with an appropriate physical assessment including examination and investigations. There are, however, some structured interview tools that can be helpful in clarifying the precise nature of psychotic symptoms. The Kiddie-SADS is an age-specific semi-structured diagnostic interview tool that maps directly onto DSM-IV diagnoses and consists of an initial screening interview followed by five diagnostic supplements, one of which (Supplement 2) is specific to psychotic disorders. This supplement (given at Appendix 3.1) probes in detail for evidence of delusional beliefs, hallucinatory experiences and evidence of motor, mood or thought abnormality. It therefore can provide a useful *aide memoire* for the clinician who encounters young people suspected of suffering from schizophrenia or other psychotic conditions only rarely.

Assessment

The initial stage of assessment of a young person with possible schizophrenia is a careful and detailed history obtained together and separately from both the young person and his parents and/or carers. Unless the family is strongly opposed to it, this should also be supplemented by information from school or college, particularly about cognitive and social functioning. The history should focus both upon current mental state and recent behavioural changes and upon obtaining a clear account of the young person's pre-morbid functioning and personality traits. At all times, the clinician should be focusing the assessment towards the two key questions 'what disorder(s), if any, is this young person suffering from?' and 'what treatment interventions, including psychological, social and educational, are likely to be indicated?'.

A comprehensive physical assessment, including a full neurological examination, is essential. Table 3.5 gives lists of those physical investigations which should be carried out in all suspected cases and those which should only be undertaken where there are specific abnormalities or indications found within the history or examination. In practice, the 'strike rate' for detection of significant abnormal investigation results is low (with the exception of urine toxicology, which

Table 3.5. Physical investigations in child or adolescent onset schizophrenia

First line (routine)	Physical examination including full neurological examination
	Full blood count
	Urea & Electrolytes
	Thyroid function
	Liver function
	Electroencephalogram
	Computed tomography (CT) or Magnetic resonance imaging (MRI) scan
	Drug screen (urine or hair analysis)
Second line (as indicated)	Autoantibody screen
	Serum calcium
	Chromosome studies
	Serum copper
	Arylsulphatase-A
	Cerebrospinal fluid examination

frequently reflects co-morbidity rather than causation). None the less a normal CT or MRI scan may reassure parents that all physical factors have been considered and thereby enable the progress of psycho-educational therapeutic interventions.

In addition to the mandatory psychiatric and physical assessment, formal psychometric assessment may also be helpful, although this will probably need to be deferred until the young person is less unwell and better able to collaborate in testing. This may reveal hitherto unrecognized general or specific learning difficulties and thereby inform future educational planning.

Family assessment is important with a dual emphasis upon both social care need and upon family relationships and levels of expressed emotion (EE). It is now well established that higher levels of expressed emotion (hostility, criticism, emotional overinvolvement and warmth) are associated with greater relapse rates and should be a target of therapy in their own right (see below under psychological treatments).

The goal of the assessment phase should be that, by its completion, the clinician has an understanding of the young person's presentation that encompasses the following:

(a) a full multiaxial diagnostic framework (I: Comorbid-disorders; II: Personality and developmental disorders; III: Intellectual abilities; IV: Physical disorders; V: Psychosocial circumstances; VI: Global functioning);

(b) a sense of the predisposing, precipitating and perpetuating factors operating around the young person's disorder and of the protective factors that may be harnessed in its treatment;

(c) an initial management plan, which includes consideration of the most appropriate setting for treatment and which is multimodal in nature.

Aetiology

The aetiology of schizophrenia is multifactorial and not precisely known.

• There is a substantial genetic component, most probably relating to the interactions of several different genes. First-degree relatives of someone suffering from schizophrenia have about a 15 per cent risk of developing the disorder themselves.

• Post-mortem studies and neuroimaging studies show increased rates of structural and functional brain abnormalities, particularly in cerebral volume and ventricular sizes, suggesting that at least some cases have a neurodevelopmental or neurodegenerative cause. There is some evidence that both these mechanisms may operate more strongly in early onset cases.

• Birth seasonality suggests that, in some cases, post-viral influences may be implicated but no single pathogen has been identified.

• Sufferers from schizophrenia appear to have experienced an excess of abnormal pre-natal and peri-natal events or complications but these could be secondary to pre-existing fetal neurodevelopmental abnormalities associated with the subsequent schizophrenia rather than causative of them.

• Substance misuse may act as a provoking or precipitating factor to an acute episode in an already predisposed individual but there is only limited evidence of its having a primary causative role. There is similarly no evidence that family environmental factors are causative, although they can play a significant part in the subsequent course of the disorder (see further below).

From a clinical perspective, these uncertainties combine to mean that the clinician is generally unable to answer satisfactorily the often-asked question 'why has my child developed this illness . . .?'. It is, however, important that, at an early stage, they do address in the negative the often unasked question '. . . and am I to blame for it?'. The greatly increased rates in first-degree relatives of sufferers does have implications for siblings, in particular, as parents, if not already affected, are likely to have passed the age of peak risk for developing a disorder.

Treatment

Clinical management

Following on from the comprehensive assessment process described above, the clinician's next task is to devise a treatment plan taking full account of the various predisposing, precipitating and perpetuating factors operating around the young person's disorder and of the protective factors that may be harnessed in its treatment. This should be multimodal, encompassing pharmacological, individual and family

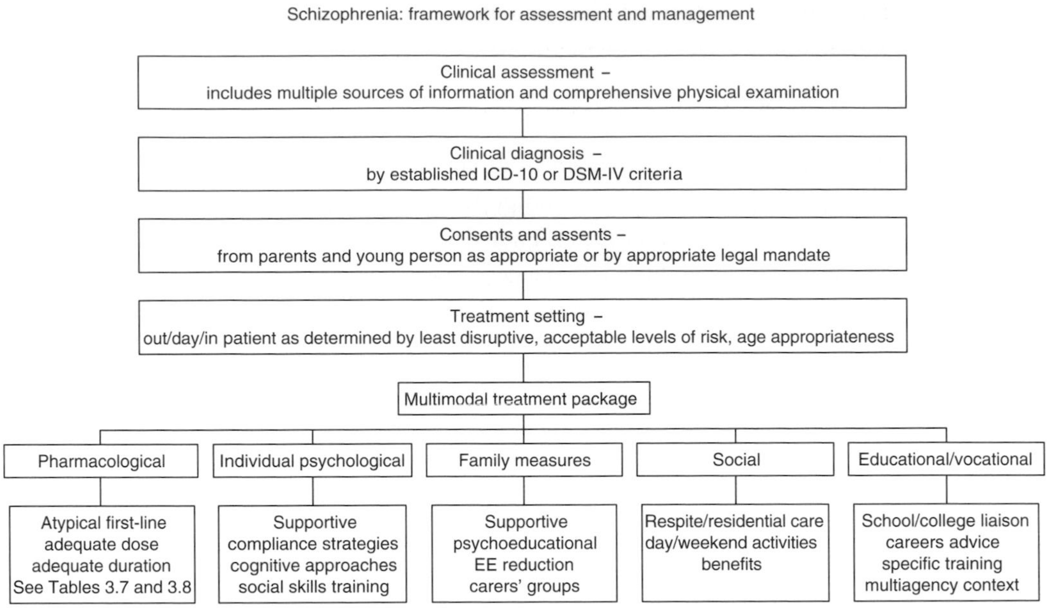

Schizophrenia: framework for assessment and management

Fig. 3.1.   Framework for management.

psychological, social and educational or vocational components (see Fig. 3.1 for an outline of this).

Consents and assents

So far as possible, the clinicians will seek the agreement and co-operation of both the young person and their parents/carers in any treatment plan. In some instances, however, either the parent or the child or both will not be in agreement. In these cases the first stage is careful explanation of the rationale behind the clinician's treatment plan and exploration of the reasons for the disagreement. This may lead to an agreed adoption of the initial plan, to an agreed adoption of an alternative treatment plan which although not the clinician's first choice is still within acceptable medical practice, or continued disagreement. In these last instances it may be necessary to consider whether a legal mandate to provide treatment is indicated, despite this being against the wishes of young person and parent or carer. The legal framework for this and for assessing the capacity or competence of the young person to give consent *vis-à-vis* reliance upon the consent of the parent will vary according to jurisdiction and practitioners are referred to their own legal advisors.

Treatment setting

The first question the clinician needs to consider is that of where the patient's care can be managed most appropriately. In general, the presumption in treatment of any

Table 3.6. Factors affecting treatment setting

Factors in favour of out-patient treatment
- Young person still maintaining family, school and social relationships
- Little/no evidence of risk to self
- Little/no evidence of risk to others
- Co-operative with assessment, investigations and treatments
- Supportive and well functioning family relationships
- Absence of other major home based psychosocial stresses
- Lack of age-appropriate in- or day-patient facilities

Factors in favour of day- or in-patient treatment
- Young person already withdrawn from social and school environments
- Significant evidence of risk to self (suicidality, unpredictability, self-neglect)
- Significant evidence of risk to others (violent or unpredictable behaviour or threat)
- Persecutory belief about current carers
- Unco-operative with assessment, investigations or treatments
- Problematic family relationships or high expressed emotion environment
- Psychosocial complexities
- Availability of age-appropriate setting

child psychiatric disorder should be of out-patient treatment as this maintains the young person in the usual family, social and educational environments. However, this may not be possible and in these cases it will be necessary to consider day- or in-patient treatment. Risk to self or others, likely co-operation in assessment or treatment and levels of family distress and supports are important considerations here (see Table 3.6). Admission to a child or adolescent in- or day-patient setting may also allow greater intensity and range of treatments – for example, reintegration into a peer group for a child who has withdrawn from most, or all, social contract. Ease of access and availability of admission to an age-appropriate in-patient setting may also play a part in decision making of both the clinician and the family, as in some instances the only in-patient option available may be the highly undesirable environment of an acute adult psychiatric admission ward. At times, however, this may be the only option in order to ensure the safety of the young person whilst a more appropriate setting is sought.

Pharmacotherapy (including drugs and dosages)

In contrast to most other psychiatric disorders occurring in children and adolescents, pharmacotherapy plays an essential part in the management of schizophrenia. There have been significant advances in recent years with the development of the newer 'atypical' antipsychotic drugs (amisulpiride, olanzapine, quetiapine, risperidone and zotepine), which have different side effect profiles to the older neuroleptic

Table 3.7. Incidence and severity of side effects of antipsychotic drugs

	Sedation	Acute extra-pyramidal	Dyskinesia	Weight gain	Hyper-prolactinaemia	Seizures
Haloperidol	**	****	****	*	****	**
Chlorpromazine	****	***	***	*	****	****
Amisulpiride	*	**			****	
Olanazapine	***	*	*	**	**	*
Quetiapine	***	*	*	**	*	*
Risperidone	**	**	**	**	****	*
Zotepine	****	***	*	****	***	****
Clozapine	****	*	*	****	*	****

*very low, **low, ***moderate, ****high.

medications that were previously the drugs of choice (see Table 3.7). These appear to be better tolerated and therefore are more likely to promote treatment concordance and better treatment outcomes, albeit that the scientific evidence bases for these are limited. This should mean that atypical antipsychotic drugs have now become the first-line drug of choice in all new-onset cases of schizophrenia.

There is no evidence of any difference in efficacy between the various atypical antipsychotic drugs (with the exception of clozapine in otherwise treatment-resistant cases – see below) and therefore clinician and patient preferences usually determine which is prescribed. This is usually by discussion of side effect profile and, if the patient were unfortunate enough to experience some of these, which would be least distressing to them. In most cases the clinical research underpinning the use of these drugs has been undertaken exclusively in adults and age-specific safety and efficacy data are not available. The clinician should discuss this 'off-label' usage with the sufferer and their family but should also place this in the context that this applies also to approximately 50 per cent of prescribing of medications to children for any indication.

Figure 3.2 outlines a framework for prescription of antipsychotic medication.

- In starting antipsychotic treatment the principle should always be to start with a low dose and gradually build up to a therapeutic level. Typical starting and maintenance dosages are shown in Table 3.8. Antipsychotic drugs usually do not exert a specific effect upon positive psychotic symptoms in less than 3–4 weeks, although many of them do show an anxiolytic or sedative effect much earlier. It is important to give any antipsychotic drug at a therapeutic dose for an adequate length of time (i.e. 6–8 weeks) before concluding it is ineffective.

Table 3.8. Recommended dosages of antipsychotic drugs

Drug	Starting dose	Usual therapeutic range	Maximal dose
Amisulpiride	100 mg twice daily	400–800 mg daily*	1200 mg daily*
Olanzapine	2.5–5 mg daily	10–15 mg daily	20 mg daily
Quetiapine	25 mg twice daily	300–450 mg daily*	750 mg daily*
Risperidone	0.5 mg twice daily	4–6 mg daily	10 mg daily*
Zotepine	25 mg thrice daily	75–300 mg daily*	300 mg daily*
†Clozapine	12.5 mg daily	300–450 mg daily*	900 mg daily*
††(*Haloperidol*	*1.5 mg twice daily*	*6 mg daily**	*10 mg daily**)
††(*Chlorpromazine*	*25 mg thrice daily*	*150 mg daily**	*300 mg daily**)

*given in divided dosages.

**manufacturer suggests as high as 16 mg permissible in some cases.

†treatment resistant cases only.

††*no longer recommended as first-line treatment.*

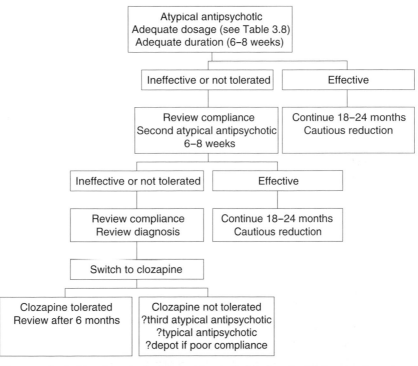

Drug treatment of adolescent onset schizophrenia

Fig. 3.2.   Pharmacological treatment of adolescent onset schizphrenia. All drug treatments only given in context of multimodal treatment package (see Fig. 3.1).

- If little or no effect is seen at therapeutic dosages at 4 weeks, then it is reasonable to increase the dosages, whilst of course remaining within recommended maximal levels. If little or no response is seen after 8 weeks of treatment with an adequate dosage, then the clinician should switch to a different drug. However, once two different antipsychotic drugs, given in adequate dosage and for adequate duration have proved ineffective, then the next step should be prescription of clozapine (see below under treatment resistant schizophrenia).

- Whilst the goal of drug treatment should always be monotherapy, in the acute stages it may be necessary to supplement the antipsychotic medication with adjunctive prescription of a benzodiazepine (e.g. lorazepam 1–2 mg or diazepam 5 mg repeated 6-hourly if necessary) for relief of acute distress and/or severely disturbed behaviour. It is important that this is reduced and stopped as the patient's psychosis improves so as to minimize dependency problems.

- Antipsychotic drug treatment should, however, be continued for a period of at least 18–24 months post-recovery and then only withdrawn gradually under close psychiatric oversight. The timing of this reduction should avoid concurrence with stressful life events and be determined in careful negotiation with the young person and their carers as it does carry an increased risk of relapse in the months immediately following cessation.

Psychological interventions

There is a range of psychological interventions relevant to the treatment of schizophrenia. In its acute phases the main focus is upon providing support and information both to the young person and to the family. The illness is a puzzling and often frightening one to the sufferer and the carers and it is important to allow both asking of questions and ventilating of anxieties. The timescale of action of antipsychotic drugs is slow and it is important that the family and young person are aware of this and feel held during this phase.

As the illness enters its recovery phase, more specific and targeted interventions become possible. Continued information giving to carers can move seamlessly into a more structured psychoeducational approach with an emphasis upon reducing any high levels of expressed emotion (excessive hostility, criticism or overinvolvement) that may be present. As the young person improves, it may be possible to involve them in this process through more formal family meetings. Such interventions with adult sufferers are now shown to have powerful and lasting effects in prevention of relapse and, although formal studies are lacking in childhood and adolescence, they should be regarded as an essential component of treatment. Individually focused psychological interventions at this stage include cognitive behavioural strategies aimed at challenging residual abnormal beliefs and perceptual experiences, problem-solving strategies aimed at developing better coping skills, and social skills training focusing upon both pre-morbid and illness-related social difficulties. Although not shown to prevent relapse, such cognitive behavioural approaches have, in adults, been shown to reduce symptoms and to improve general functioning.

Some individuals do make a full recovery from their psychotic episode but many others are left with some level of residual symptoms and deficits, failing to return to their previous level of personal or social functioning. This can leave a profound sense of loss both for the individual and for their family as hopes and aspirations for the future may have to be modified or abandoned. This sense of loss may usefully be addressed by bereavement counselling-style approaches with both the sufferer and their carers.

Compliance therapy and concordance enhancing strategies are useful through all stages of treatment, although do require the active collaboration of the individual. They consist of exploration of the gains and losses of treatment and through motivational techniques attempt to focus upon the positive benefits for the individual. Possible strategies to aid compliance include supervision of medication, dosing aids, single daily dosing where possible, and enlisting others in supporting medication compliance (e.g. at school or college).

Other interventions

The treatment of the young person's illness does not take place in a vacuum but rather in the context of their social and educational world.

- There should be an early assessment of the social care needs of the young person and the carers. This may highlight eligibility for additional benefits, a need for extra social or child care supports, a need for respite or holiday care, housing need or many other possibilities.
- There should also be active liaison with the young person's school, college or place of employment. Re-integration back into school will need to be managed carefully and it may be that a change or provision of additional supports is necessary.
- Finally, the potential role of the voluntary sector should not be overlooked. Many young people and their parents can draw significant help and support from attendance at support and self-help groups and the clinician should keep a reference file of local contacts for these, which can be given to sufferers and their families.

Monitoring and evaluation of treatment

Both schizophrenia and the drugs used to treat it can be life threatening and therefore close monitoring of the young person's mental and physical state during treatment is essential. This is easier if the patient is already in an in-patient or day-patient setting albeit at the cost of considerable personal and family disruption. If an out-patient,

Table 3.9. Internet sources of information for patients, parents and siblings

---

American Academy for Child and Adolescent Psychiatry: http://www.aacap.org
http://www.aacap.org/publications/factsfam/schizo.htm
One of a series of very useful fact sheets about mental health problems in childhood and adolescence

Royal College of Psychiatrists: http://www.rcpsych.ac.uk
http://www.rcpsych.ac.uk/info/mhgu/newmhgu23.htm
http://www.rcpsych.ac.uk/info/help/schiz/index.htm
http://www.rcpsych.ac.uk/campaigns/cminds/leaflets/sch/sch.htm
General and age-specific fact sheets about schizophrenia

@Ease (National Schizophrenia Fellowship): http://rethink.org
http://www.rethink.org/at-ease/siteindex.htm
A mental health information site designed for use by young people with specific information about schizophrenia

http://www.emental-health.com/schizophrenia.asp
Site with a wide range of information about schizophrenia although not specific to children and adolescents

---

contact should be frequent (at least weekly in the acute phases) with additionally a ready access to the treating psychiatrist for the family should the young person's mental or physical state deteriorate.

Regular evaluation and re evaluation of risk to both self and others should form a formal part of follow-up and it should be carefully recorded in the notes. As the acute phase resolves and the patient enters the recovery and rehabilitatory stages of the illness, the pace of change becomes slower and appointments may be less frequent. Serial assessments of overall functioning, at perhaps monthly or 3-monthly intervals, may be helpful in identifying areas of progress and change, possibly through use of easily rated instruments such as the CGAS or HoNOSCA scales (Appendices 3.2 and 3.3).

Information for patients and parents

It should already be clear that one essential in treatment is the provision of accessible accurate information that parents and young people can absorb and re-absorb at their own pace. There is a range of information sheets available to parents and young people prepared variously by professionals and by voluntary and self-help organizations. Many of these can be accessed via the Internet and it is useful for the professionals to maintain their own list of reliable (and less reliable) sites (see Table 3.9). The needs of siblings should not be overlooked, as they are likely to have many anxieties and questions, not merely about their brother's or sister's illness but also about its implications for their own future mental health.

Problematic issues

Co-morbid substance misuse

Many adolescents use alcohol, cannabis or other substances recreationally. The co-existence therefore of substance misuse and a psychotic illness presenting in a teenager is common. It does, however, pose particular diagnostic and treatment dilemmas. Not only can it be difficult to distinguish episodes of illness from those secondary to substance misuse but also it appears to carry a poorer prognosis in its own right. It is important therefore to address those factors promoting misuse from an early stage of treatment.

This is particularly so when it appears that a young person may be using cannabis in a misguided attempt at self-medication to relieve feelings of emptiness or boredom which, in reality, may reflect negative symptoms of the schizophrenic illness. Motivational interviewing techniques which focus upon the gains for a young person in staying well have been shown to be effective when used in treatment of adults with a dual diagnosis of a psychotic disorder and a substance misuse disorder. The specific management of the young person with substance misuse disorders is considered in detail in Chapter 2 (Bukstein).

Schizoaffective disorders

The concurrence of affective symptoms within an episode of schizophrenia is common. Symptoms of depression or low mood may derive from the young person's awareness of their illness, as a side effect of antipsychotic medication, or as an integral part of the schizophrenia. They need careful evaluation and monitoring as they may be associated with increased suicidal risk, particularly in those with a relatively severe form of the disorder but with preserved insight.

There is little evidence that adjunctive prescription of antidepressants is helpful, certainly in the acute stages, and psychological and environmental measures are more usually prescribed. Mood elevation, overactivity and other symptoms suggestive of a manic or schizomanic presentation again usually are treated with antipsychotic medication in the first instance. However, if they persist despite this, then adjunctive prescription of a mood stabilizer (e.g. sodium valproate, lithium, carbamazepine) may be of benefit. (See Chapter 4, Harrington, for fuller discussion of pharmacological treatments of affective disorders.)

Treatment resistance

The definition of treatment-resistant schizophrenia is a lack of satisfactory clinical improvement despite the sequential use of the recommended doses for 6 to 8 weeks of at least two antipsychotics, at least one of which should be atypical.

- In cases of apparent treatment resistance the clinician should first review the young person's history, current physical and mental state, any investigations undertaken and the treatment history to date in order to ensure that the diagnosis is correct and that appropriate treatment indeed has been prescribed.

• Secondly, they should be mindful of either lack of treatment concordance or of continuing co-morbid substance misuse as possible perpetuating factors of the illness. Other potential exacerbating factors such as regular prolonged contact with a setting of high expressed emotion should also be considered.

Poor treatment concordance should be addressed directly as soon as it is suspected. The reasons for it should be explored carefully with the patient (e.g. fear of, or actual, side effects, abnormal beliefs about the treatments themselves, an attachment to the illness itself, e.g. not wishing to lose special powers or attributes, non-acceptance of illness) and concordance-enhancing strategies discussed and attempted.

If these prove unsuccessful, then it may be necessary to give the medication as a long-acting 'depot' preparation – an oil-based injection given every 2 to 3 weeks. Currently, only risperidone of the atypical antipsychotics is available in such a preparation and it may therefore be necessary to give one of the older neuroleptic drugs with all their attendant short- and long-term side effect risks.

Presuming the diagnosis of treatment-resistant schizophrenia is sustained, then the next logical drug of choice is clozapine. This is the only antipsychotic drug shown to be effective in trials of treatment-resistant schizophrenia in both children and adults producing marked improvements in about two-thirds of sufferers but does have significant side effects. About 1 per cent of patients develop an agranulocytosis whilst on clozapine and therefore it should only be prescribed in the context of close hematological monitoring (in some countries, e.g. UK, this is a condition of its product licence). This should take place weekly for the initial 4 months, fortnightly for the remainder of the first year and monthly thereafter. Any falls in the white cell count should be followed carefully with increased frequency of monitoring and, if severe or persistent, it may be necessary to stop the drug. The agranulocytosis is usually reversible and the white cell count returns to normal within a short period. Once a patient has developed clozapine agranulocytosis, the drug should not be represcribed but rather they should be recommenced on whichever previous antipsychotic appeared to offer greatest benefit.

Other problematic side effects associated with clozapine are those of sedation (particularly on starting or increasing the drug), hypotension, excessive salivation and convulsive seizures in approximately 3 per cent of patients. The therapeutic dosage is usually in the range of 300–450 mg daily in divided doses. However, to avoid severe hypotension, the starting dose is more usually 12.5 mg daily with a gradual increase of 25–50 mg daily over the next 2–3 weeks until a therapeutic dose is reached. This should usually take place as an in-patient. In the event of a patient missing more than 48 hours of clozapine treatment for any reason, then a gradual restart is again necessary.

In some cases higher doses are necessary, the maximal dose being 900 mg daily. At doses above 600 mg daily, the risk of drug-induced seizures increases markedly and other side effects are also more common. In contrast to the other antipsychotic drugs, the action of clozapine can take some months to become apparent and, once started, it should not be stopped on grounds of lack of efficacy in less than 6 months.

Any consideration of prescription of clozapine needs careful explanation and discussion with the patient and their family. They need to be aware not only of the risks and benefits that it can bring but also of the need for treatment concordance and close and careful monitoring. They should be advised particularly to report any suspected infection or raised temperature as this may be the first sign of a developing agranulocytosis.

Psychological treatments should continue to be given alongside clozapine. There is some evidence amongst adult sufferers for the efficacy of cognitive approaches, particularly in enhancing coping strategies of those suffering from chronic or resistant illnesses.

Transition to adult services

Whilst some young people will have a single episode of illness from which they make a complete recovery, the majority will need ongoing psychiatric care and oversight beyond their teenage years. Their transition from child and adolescent mental health services into adult mental health services needs careful planning and management. Frequently, a young person's care plan will involve professionals from health, education, careers, social services and it is important that changes in personnel or agencies do not cause breakdown or failure in communication or planning. It is also undesirable that all professionals should change simultaneously (e.g. at an arbitrary age-related threshold), thereby leaving a young person and family bereft of any familiar professional figure and sense of continuity and consistency of approach. Rather a staged series of transitions should be aimed for, with a clear understanding shared amongst family and professional alike as to who is responsible for delivery and coordination of care at all times.

Outcome

Short and long term

It is important from the outset to be open and honest with young people and their families about the possible outcomes of their disorder. In the early stages of the illness, this means neither raising unrealistically high hopes of a total recovery nor giving too gloomy an outlook. Research studies provide outcomes for cohorts of individuals; young people and their families are interested solely in their own specific outcome – it is of little consolation to know that 80 per cent of individuals achieve some initial response to antipsychotic treatments if you or your son or daughter happens to be one of the 20 per cent who remain severely and unremitting ill.

In the short term many young people do show some response to antipsychotic treatment and make complete or partial recovery from their initial acute episode. However, the long term outlook is considerably poorer with outcome studies suggesting that most sufferers of early onset schizophrenia fare badly with over 50 per cent severely impaired and about 10% dying from suicide or other illness-related disorders (self-neglect, accident, drug-related complication from prescribed or non-prescribed medication).

Prognostic factors

The main predictors of outcome appear to be those of poor pre-morbid functioning and early development of negative symptoms, both of which predict a poorer prognosis. A prolonged duration of untreated psychosis also appears to be associated with a poorer outcome, although whether this is an independent effect or is related to pre-existing poor pre-morbid functioning is disputed. Co-morbid substance misuse, particularly if severe, is associated with higher rates of relapse and of a poorer outcome. Prominent affective symptoms, particularly if sufficient to fulfil a diagnosis of schizoaffective disorder, offer a relatively better prognosis than where there is no affective component.

SUGGESTED READING

American Academy of Child and Adolescent Psychiatry, Practice parameter for the assessment and treatment of children and adolescents with schizophrenia. *Journal of the American Academy of Child and Adolescent Psychiatry*, **40**(7) (2001), Suppl. 4S–23S. Standards and evidence base for current good practice in the assessment and treatment of children and adolescents with schizophrenia.

C. Barrowclough & N. Tarrier, Families of schizophrenic patients: cognitive behavioural intervention. In A practical guide to family intervention strategies. Cheltenham: Stanley Thornes, 1997).

A. F. Clark & S. W. Lewis, Practitioner review: treatment of schizophrenia in childhood and adolescence. *Journal of Child Psychology and Psychiatry*, **39** (1998), 1071–81. Practical overview of current treatment issues for young people with schizophrenia, albeit becoming dated in respect of advice regarding use of atypical antipsychotics.

J. Geddes, N. Freemantle, P. Harrison & P. Bebbington, Atypical antipsychotics in the treatment of schizophrenia: systematic overview and meta-regression analysis. *British Medical Journal*, **321** (2000), 1371–6. Systematic review casting doubts upon the evidence base for use of atypical antipsychotics as first-line drugs – the paper generated much subsequent correspondence expressing views for and against their use.

C. Hollis, Adolescent schizophrenia. *Advances in Psychiatric Treatment*, **6** (2000), 83–92. Contains outcome data on follow-up study of adolescents with schizophrenia admitted to Maudsley Hospital.

P. D. McGorry & H. J. Jackson, *The Recognition and Management of Early Psychosis: A Preventive Approach* (Cambridge: Cambridge University Press, 1999). Comprehensive discussion of issues and practice in first onset psychosis and early intervention services.

National Institute for Clinical Excellence, *Technology Appraisal No. 43: Guidance on the use of newer (atypical) antipsychotic drugs for the treatment of schizophrenia* (London: NICE, 2002). UK-based guidance derived from a systematic review of clinical and cost effectiveness of antipsychotic drugs in treatment of schizophrenia.

S. Pilling, P. Bebbington, E. Kuipers *et al.*, Psychological treatments in schizophrenia: 1. Meta-analysis of family intervention and cognitive behaviour therapy. *Psychological Medicine*, **32** (2002), 763–82. Concludes that both family interventions and CBT have proven efficacy and should be routinely offered as part of treatment programme.

S. Pilling, P. Bebbington, E. Kuipers *et al.*, Psychological treatments in schizophrenia: 2. Meta-analyses of randomized controlled trials of social skills training and cognitive remediation. *Psychological Medicine*, **32** (2002), 783–91. Concludes that neither social skills training nor cognitive remediation have yet been shown as effective for routine clinical practice.

H. Remschmidt, *Schizophrenia in Children and Adolescents* (Cambridge: Cambridge University Press, 2001). Comprehensive overview of all aspects of schizophrenia in children and adolescents.

D. Taylor, H. McConnell, D. McConnell & R. Kerwin, *The Maudsley 2001 Prescribing Guidelines* (London: Martin Dunitz, 2001). Regularly updated guidelines with useful algorithms. Specific section on psychosis but not to treatment of children and adolescents.

T. Wykes, N. Tarrier & S. Lewis, *Outcomes and Innovation in the Psychological Treatment of Schizophrenia* (Chichester: Wiley, 1998). Overview of range of psychological interventions appropriate to treatment of schizophrenia in adults.

Appendix 3.1. Key probe questions from K-SADS-PL Version 1.0: 10/01/96 # 2 Psychosis supplement

I. Hallucinations

Probes: In addition to the probes provided below for assessing the specific categories of hallucinations, use some of the following probes to further evaluate the validity of the reported hallucinations. *These voices you hear (or other hallucinations), do they occur when you are awake or asleep? Could it be a dream? Do they happen when you are falling asleep? Waking up? Only when it is dark? Do they happen at any other time also? Were you sick with fever when they occurred? Had you been drinking beer, wine, liquor? Or taking any drugs when it happened? Was it like a thought or more like a voice (noise) or a vision? Was it like you were imagining things? Did you have any control over it? Could you stop it if you wanted to? Were you having a seizure?*

1. Auditory hallucinations
   (a) Non-verbal sounds (e.g. music) *Do you hear music or other noises that other people cannot hear?*
   (b) Command hallucinations *Do the voices tell you to do anything? (What?) (Good or bad?) Have they ever told you to hurt or kill yourself? How? Have they ever told you to hurt or kill someone else? Who? How?*
   (c) Running commentary (commenting voice) *Do you hear voices that talk about what you're doing? Or feeling? Or thinking?*
   (d) Conversing voice *How many voices do you hear? What do they say? Do they talk with each other?*
   (e) Thoughts aloud *Do you ever hear your thoughts spoken aloud? If somebody stood next to you, could they hear your thinking? Is it a real voice outside your head?*
   (f) Other verbal hallucinations *Have there been other noises or voices you have heard that you have not told me about? Do the voices ever criticize you? Make fun of you? Say they are going to do bad things to you? Has God (Jesus), angels, demons, Virgin Mary, or saints ever talked to you? Are there any other people you know who had () talk to them?*
2. Location of voices/noises
   (a) Inside head only *Where did the voices come from? From inside your head? Was it your thoughts you heard? Could other people hear the voices?*
   (b) Outside head only *From outside your head, through your ears? Did it sound as clear as my voice does talking to you right now?*
   (c) Combination *Have the voices sometimes seemed to be inside your head, and other times outside your head? Sometimes like thoughts and other times like my voice now?*
3. Visual hallucinations
   Do you see things other children don't? What do you see? Did you see something real, or was it just like a shadow moving? How clear was it? Did you see it several times for several days in a row?
4. Tactile hallucinations
   Do you ever feel like someone or something is touching you, but when you look there is nothing there? Tell me about it?
5. Olfactory hallucinations
   Do you ever smell things other people don't smell? What is it?
6. Illusions
   False perceptions stimulated by a real perception which is momentarily transformed. They occur frequently due to poor perceptual resolution (darkness, noisy locale) or inattention and they are immediately corrected when attention is focused on the external sensory stimulus or perceptual resolution improves.

Have you ever seen things around your room at night that you thought were some-thing else? Like did you ever look at one of your stuffed animals or a shirt and think it was something that could get you? Have you ever looked at a rope and thought it was a snake? Other things?

7. Cultural acceptance of hallucinations

Does anyone else in your family or any members of your church experience the same (specify hallucination)?

II. Delusions

Probes: In addition to the probes provided below for assessing the specific types of delusions, use some of the following probes to further evaluate the validity of the reported delusions. *Are you sure that this (. . . ?) is this way? Could there be any other reason for it? How do you know that it happens as you say? Any other possible explanation? Is what you told me make believe or real?* **(You might suggest other possible explanations and see how the subject reacts to them).**

1. Grandiosity

Do you feel that you are a very important person or that you have special powers or abilities? What are they? Are you related to important people, like kings or the president or a sports figure? Do you have special powers like reading people's minds? Tell me more about it? Has God chosen you to perform any special tasks for him?

2. Guilt/sin

Do you ever feel like you did something terrible? What is the worst thing that you ever did? Do you deserve punishment?

3. Delusions of control

Do you have the feeling that you are being controlled by some force of power outside yourself? Whose power? Do you feel sometimes that you are a puppet or a robot and can't control what you do? Or that you are forced to move or say things that you don't want to?

4. Somatic delusions

Do you think you have any serious diseases? How do you know? Are you sure? Has something happened to your body or insides? Tell me about it. Maybe you just feel these things but nothing is wrong with you. Could that be?

5. Nihilism

Do you feel that something terrible will happen or has happened? What will happen? Have you felt that the world is coming to an end? When?

6. Thought broadcasting

Do you ever feel that your thoughts are broadcast out loud so that other people know what you are thinking? Like on a radio, so that anyone listening could hear them? Have you actually heard your thoughts spoken out loud? Have others heard them?

7. Thought insertion

Do you feel that thoughts are put into your mind that are not your own? Who put them there? How? Why?

8. Thought withdrawal
   Have you had thoughts taken out of your mind by someone or some special force? Tell me what happened.
9. Message from TV/radio
   Does the TV or radio ever talk about you or send you messages? What about songs?
10. Delusions of persecution
    Has anyone been making things hard, or purposely causing you trouble, or trying to hurt you, or plotting against you? How come?
11. Delusions that others can read his/her mind
    Can people know what you are thinking in some strange way? Is that because the way you look or is it just because they know what you are thinking because they can read your mind?
12. Delusions of reference
    Do people seem to drop hints about you? Do people say things with a double meaning? Do they do things in a special way to tell you something? Have things seemed especially arranged so only you understand the meaning?
13. Other bizarre delusions
    Any other special thoughts that you want to tell me about?
14. Subcultural or family delusions
    Do other people in your family also believe in what you say (ask the mother and if necessary other members of the family)? Do other members of your religion believe in that too? Do other children like your friends believe in what you believe?

III. Other psychotic symptoms
Rate based on observation during interview.

1. Affect
   (a) Flat affect
       Deficit in emotional contact not explainable by severe mood disturbance or preoccupation, i.e. even with adequate efforts on the part of the interviewer to establish appropriate emotional contact, the subject does not give back signs of emotional response such as occasional smiling, tearfulness, laughing, or looking directly at the interviewer. At the 'moderate' level or above, there is flatness of affect as indicated by monotonous voice, and facial expression lacking signs of emotion.
   (b) Inappropriate affect
       Affect is incongruous with content of speech, for example, giggles while discussing reason for hospitalization. Do not include mere embarrassment or excessively strong affect, as when subject cries when discussing a minor

disappointment. Incongruity does not mean excessive intensity but qualitative inconsistency with thought content and/or environmental circumstances.

2. Thoughts
   (a) Incoherence
      Speech that is generally not understandable, running together of thoughts or words with no logical or grammatical connection, resulting in disorganization.
   (b) Loosening of Associations
      Flow of thought in which ideas shift from one subject to another in a completely unrelated way.
3. Catatonic Behaviour
   Motor anomalies including immobility, stupor, rigidity, bizarre posturing, waxy flexibility and excited movements (purposeless and stereotyped excited motor activity not influenced by external stimuli).

IV. Impaired functioning during active illness
   1. Impaired school performance
   2. Impaired peer relations
   3. Impaired family relations
   4. Impaired self care

Appendix 3.2. Children's global assessment scale (CGAS)

Use intermediary levels (eg. 35, 58, 62). Rate actual functioning regardless of treatment or prognosis. The examples of behaviour provided are only illustrative and are not required for a particular rating.

100–91 Superior functioning in all areas (at home, at school, and with peers); involved in a wide range of activities and has many interests (e.g. hobbies or participates in extracurricular activities or belongs to an organized group such as Scouts, etc.); likeable, confident; 'everyday' worries never get out of hand; doing well in school; no symptoms.

90–81 Good functioning in all areas; secure in family, school, and with peers; there may be transient difficulties and 'everyday' worries that occasionally get out of hand (e.g. mild anxiety associated with an important exam, occasional 'blowups' with siblings, parents, or peers).

80–71 No more than slight impairment in functioning at home, at school, or with peers; some disturbance of behaviour or emotional distress may be present in response to life stresses (e.g. parental separations, deaths, birth of a sib), but these are brief and interference with functioning is transient; such children are only minimally disturbing to others and are not considered deviant by those who know them.

70–61 Some difficulty in a single area, but generally functioning pretty well (e.g. sporadic or isolated antisocial acts, such as occasionally playing hooky or petty theft; consistent minor difficulties with school work; mood changes of brief duration; fears and anxieties which do not lead to gross avoidance behaviour; self-doubts); has some meaningful interpersonal relationships; most people who do not know the child well would not consider him/her deviant but those who do know him/her well might express concern.

60–51 Variable functioning with sporadic difficulties or symptoms in several but not all social areas; disturbance would be apparent to those who encounter the child in a dysfunctional setting or time but not to those who see the child in other settings.

50–41 Moderate degree of interference in functioning in most social areas or severe impairment or functioning in one area, such as might result from, for example, suicidal preoccupations and ruminations, school refusal and other forms of anxiety, obsessive rituals, major conversion symptoms, frequent anxiety attacks, poor or inappropriate social skills, frequent episodes of aggressive or other antisocial behaviour with some preservation of meaningful social relations.

40–31 Major impairment in functioning in several areas and unable to function in one of these areas, is disturbed at home, at school, with peers, or in society at large, e.g. persistent aggression without clear instigation; markedly withdrawn and isolated behaviour due to either mood or thought disturbance, suicidal attempts with clear lethal intent; such children are likely to require special schooling and/or hospitalization or withdrawal from school (but this is not a sufficient criterion for inclusion in this category).

30–21 Unable to function in almost all areas, e.g. stays at home, in ward, or in bed all day without taking part in social activities or severe impairment in reality testing or serious impairment in communication (e.g. sometimes incoherent or inappropriate).

20–11 Needs considerable supervision to prevent hurting others and self (e.g. frequently violent, repeated suicide attempts) or to maintain personal hygiene or gross impairment in all forms of communication, e.g. severe abnormalities in verbal and gestural communication, marked social aloofness, stupor, etc.

10–1 Needs constant supervision (24-h care) due to severely aggressive or self-destructive behaviour or gross impairment in reality testing, communication, cognition, affect or personal hygiene.

The Children's Global Assessment Scale was adapted from the Global Assessment Scale for Adults (Shaffer, D., Gould, M., Brasic, J. *et al.*, Children's Global Assessment Scale (CGAS). *Arch. Gen. Psychiatry*, **40** (1983), 1228–31.)

Appendix 3.3. British Health of the Nation Outcome Scale for Children and Adolescents (HoNOSCA) Self-rated version of the British Health of the Nation Outcome Scales for Children and Adolescents

The patient is asked to assess the following items, selecting answers from the categories 'not at all', 'insignificantly', 'mild but definitely', 'moderately' or 'severely' (scored 0 (not at all) – 4 (severely)).

In the last 2 weeks

1. Have you been troubled by your disruptive behaviour, physical or verbal aggression?
2. Have you suffered from lack of concentration or restlessness?
3. Have you done anything to injure or harm yourself on purpose?
4. Have you had problems as a result of your use of alcohol, drugs or solvents?
5. Have you experienced difficulties keeping up with your usual educational attainments and abilities?
6. Has any physical illness or disability restricted your activities?
7. Have you been troubled by hearing voices, seeing things, suspicious or abnormal thoughts?
8. Have you suffered from self-induced vomiting, head/stomachaches/bedwetting or soiling, or other symptoms with no physical cause?
9. Have you been feeling in a low or anxious mood, or troubled by fears, obsessions or rituals?
10. Have you been troubled by a lack of satisfactory friendships or bullying?
11. Have you found it difficult to look after yourself or take responsibility for your independence?
12. Have you been troubled by relationships in your family or substitute home?
13. Have you stopped attending school/college/education sessions?

Gowers, S., Levine, W., Bailey-Rogers, S., Shore, A. Burhouse, E. Use of a routine, self-report outcome measure (HoNOSCA – SR) in two adolescent mental health services. *Br. J. Psychiatry* **180** (2002), 266–9.

4

Affective disorders

Richard Harrington

Royal Manchester Children's Hospital, UK

The defining characteristic of affective disorders is a change in affect or mood. In both the Tenth Revision of the International Classification of Diseases (ICD-10) and in the Fourth Edition of the *Diagnostic and Statistical Manual* (DSM-IV) there are many different categories of affective disorder. For example, as Table 4.1 shows, ICD-10 contains seven main categories of mood disorder, each with several sub-categories. Depressive conditions can also be classified in other parts of ICD-10, particularly under adjustment disorders, which include Brief Depressive Reactions (F43.20), Prolonged Depressive Reactions (F43.21) and Mixed Anxiety and Depressive Reactions (F43.22).

In clinical practice the most useful distinction is between disorders characterized by depression of mood (e.g. depressive episode, recurrent depressive disorder) and disorders in which there is a distinct period of elevated mood (e.g. manic episode, bipolar disorder). The present chapter is therefore divided into two sections, the first concerned with depressive disorders and the second with bipolar disorders (by convention, all patients with mania are classified in the bipolar group, whether or not they have had depression) (see Fig. 4.1).

Depressive disorder

Introduction

Until recently it was widely believed that depressive disorders were rare in young people. Young children were thought to be incapable of experiencing many of the phenomena that are characteristic of depressive disorders in adults. Affective disturbance in adolescents was often dismissed as adolescent 'turmoil'. Over the past 20 years, however, there has been a substantial change in the ways in which mood

A Clinician's Handbook of Child and Adolescent Psychiatry, ed. Christopher Gillberg, Richard Harrington and Hans-Christoph Steinhausen. Published by Cambridge University Press. © Cambridge University Press 2005.

Table 4.1. Mood (affective) disorders in ICD-10

F30	Manic episode
F31	Bipolar affective disorder
F32	Depressive episode
F33	Recurrent depressive disorder
F34	Persistent affective disorder
F38	Other mood (affective) disorder
F39	Affective disorder, unspecified

disturbance among the young has been conceptualized. The use of structured personal interviews has shown that depressive syndromes resembling adult depressive disorders can, and do, occur among both pre-pubertal children and adolescents. Indeed, clinical research in the UK has suggested that as many as one in ten referrals to child psychiatrists suffer from a depressive disorder. Depression may be becoming more prevalent among young people.

Definition and classification

ICD-10 and DSM-IV criteria

Most clinicians nowadays use one of the major adult schemes for diagnosing depressive disorder in both children and adolescents, DSM-IV or ICD-10. The schemes differ in many small ways, but at the core of both is the concept of an episodic disorder of varying degrees of severity that is characterized by depressed mood or loss of enjoyment that persists for several weeks and that is associated with certain other symptoms. Table 4.2 shows the DSM-IV criteria for Major Depressive Disorder and Table 4.3 the ICD-10 diagnostic research criteria for a Moderate Depressive Episode. In this chapter the DSM criteria will be used throughout because most treatment research has used DSM criteria.

Both DSM-IV and ICD-10 distinguish between mild, moderate and severe episodes of depression. The schemes take different approaches, however, in their definitions of severity. In ICD-10 severity is defined by symptoms, whereas in DSM-IV severity is defined in terms of symptoms and functional impairment. Classifying depression by severity is useful as severity is the single best predictor of response to treatment. As a general rule, a depressive episode that leads to complete cessation of functioning in any one domain (e.g. not going to school, complete social withdrawal) can be regarded as severe.

Both diagnostic schemes also distinguish between psychotic and non-psychotic episodes of depression. Psychotic depression, which is characterized by mood congruent delusions and hallucinations, is very uncommon before mid-adolescence.

Table 4.2. Criteria for major depressive episode in DSM-IV

A. Five (or more) of the following symptoms have been present during the same 2-week period and represent a change from previous functioning; at least one of the symptoms is either (1) depressed mood or (2) loss of interest or pleasure.
  (1) depressed mood most of the day, nearly every day, as indicated by either subjective report or observation made by others. Note: in children and adolescents can be irritable mood.
  (2) markedly diminished interest or pleasure in all, or almost all, activities most of the day, nearly every day
  (3) significant weight loss when not dieting or weight gain (e.g. a change of more than 5% body weight in a month), or decrease or increase in appetite nearly every day. Note: in children consider failure to make expected weight gains.
  (4) insomnia or hypersomnia nearly every day
  (5) psychomotor agitation or retardation nearly every day (observable by others, not merely subjective feelings of restlessness or being slowed down)
  (6) fatigue or loss of energy nearly every day
  (7) feelings of worthlessness or excessive or inappropriate guilt (which may be delusional) nearly every day
  (8) diminished ability to think or concentrate, or indecisiveness, nearly every day
  (9) recurrent thoughts of death (not just fear of dying), recurrent suicidal ideation without a specific plan, or a suicide attempt or a specific plan for committing suicide
B. The symptoms do not meet criteria for a mixed episode.
C. The symptoms cause clinically significant distress or impairment in social, occupational, or other important areas of functioning.
D. The symptoms are not due to the direct physiological effects of a substance (e.g. a drug of abuse, a medication) or a general medical condition.
E. The symptoms are not better accounted for by bereavement, i.e. after the loss of a loved one, the symptoms persist for longer than 2 months or are characterized by marked functional impairment, morbid preoccupation with worthlessness, suicidal ideation, psychotic symptoms, or symptoms of psychomotor retardation.

Nevertheless the concept is helpful because psychotic symptoms presage a worse adult prognosis and a greatly increased risk of conversion to bipolar disorder.

Other subtypes are less well established. DSM-IV and ICD-10 have a category for chronic mild depression lasting one or more years – dysthymia. However, longitudinal studies have shown that, in young people, there is much overlap of major depression and dysthymia and it is likely therefore that they are part of the same problem.

Co-morbidity between depression and other child psychiatric disorders is very common (see below) and DSM-IV and ICD-10 take different approaches to it. In ICD-10 it is assumed that a mixed clinical picture is more likely to be the result of a single disorder with different manifestations than of two or more disorders that happen to occur in the same individual at the same time. ICD-10 therefore has a

Table 4.3. Criteria for a moderate depressive episode in ICD-10

A. The general criteria for depressive episode must be met:
  G1. The depressive episode should last for at least 2 weeks.
  G2. There have been no hypomanic or manic symptoms sufficient to meet the criteria for hypomanic episode (F30-) at any time in the individual's life.
  G3. *Most commonly used exclusion clause.* The episode is not attributable to psychoactive substance use (F10-F19) or to any organic mental disorder (in the sense of F00-F09).

B. At least two of the following three symptoms (listed for F32.0, criterion B), must be present:
  (1) depressed mood to a degree that is definitely abnormal for the individual, present for most of the day and almost every day, largely uninfluenced by circumstances, and sustained for at least 2 weeks;
  (2) loss of interest or pleasure in activities that are normally pleasurable;
  (3) decreased energy or increased fatiguability.

C. Additional symptoms (from F32.0, criterion C), must be present to give a total of at least *six*:
  (1) Loss of confidence or self-esteem;
  (2) Unreasonable feelings of self-reproach or excessive and inappropriate guilt;
  (3) Recurrent thoughts of death or suicide, or any suicidal behaviour;
  (4) Complaints or evidence of diminished ability to think or concentrate, such as indecisiveness or vacillation;
  (5) Change in psychomotor activity, with agitation or retardation (either subjective or objective);
  (6) Sleep disturbance of any type;
  (7) Change in appetite (decrease or increase) with corresponding weight change.

category for mixed disorders, Mixed Disorders of Conduct and Emotions (F92), which includes the subcategory Depressive Conduct Disorder (F92.0). DSM-IV, by contrast, usually allows the investigator to diagnose several supposedly separate disorders, with the result that in surveys based on DSM it is quite common to find individuals with three or more diagnoses.

Clinical applicability

The application of adult diagnostic criteria to children and adolescents has been useful, but there are some limitations. First, adult criteria work less well in younger age groups, where it is often necessary to make assumptions about the meaning of some symptoms (for example, that a child who is negative and difficult to please has depressed mood). Secondly, current diagnostic systems have not really solved the problem of co-morbidity. Many children and adolescents with depressive disorder have other psychiatric problems, and it is often unclear in clinical practice which problem is primary (see below).

Epidemiology

Prevalence and incidence rates

Recent studies have estimated that the 1-year (or less) prevalence of major depressive disorder in adolescence is between 1 and 2 per cent. The prevalence is much lower in pre-adolescents, at around 1 per thousand. This increase in the incidence of depressive disorder occurs during early adolescence.

Sex ratios

Age trends in the incidence of depression are stronger in girls than in boys. Most studies have found that, in prepubertal children, there is either no gender difference in the prevalence of depression or there is a small male preponderance. In contrast, by late adolescence the female preponderance found in adult depression is well established.

Implications for clinical practice

The finding that young people can, and do, develop depressive disorders has had important implications for clinical practice. It has meant that clinicians are nowadays much more likely to recognize and treat depressive disorders among the young.

Clinical picture

Main features and symptoms

The main features of depressive disorder in young people are emotional changes, cognitive changes, motivational changes and neurovegetative symptoms.

Emotional symptoms

The main emotional symptom is depressed mood. Mood may be described as sad, blue or down. The child may cry more than usual but in some cases patients report that, although they feel like crying, they are unable to do so. Some children will deny feeling sad but will admit to feeling 'bad'. DSM-IV states that, in children, irritable mood may substitute for depressed mood. The young person no longer derives as much pleasure from life: this anhedonia may sometimes precede depression of mood.

Cognitive changes

These include feelings of low-self esteem with an exaggerated assessment of current life difficulties. Typically, depressed children or adolescents will have nothing to say when asked about their good points. There may be difficulties making decisions, either because of lack of confidence or because of subjective difficulty with thinking. When depression is severe the patient may feel that they are wicked or feel guilty for minor past misdemeanours, such as stealing. It should be noted, however, that it is normal for older children and adolescents to feel guilty about parental separation.

Hopelessness and helplessness may also be prominent. Suicidal ideas are particularly serious in the presence of such symptoms.

Motivational changes

Low energy, apathy, tiredness and poor concentration are all common in depressive disorder. Failure to complete tasks may make feelings of guilt and lack of confidence worse. School information may be crucial for a proper assessment of poor concentration.

Neurovegetative symptoms

These include changes in appetite, weight, sleep rhythm, libido, energy level and activity. In deciding whether these changes are abnormal, the clinician must take into account the young person's developmental stage (see Appendix 4.1). For example, 9-year olds on average sleep 1 hour more than 14-year olds. Somatic symptoms are particularly common in adolescents, who may present to the doctor with headache, abdominal pain or other regional pain. The clinician can be so distracted by these symptoms that the depressive syndrome, of which they are a part, goes unrecognized.

Differential diagnosis and co-morbidity (Fig. 4.1)

The first diagnostic issue is the differentiation between 'normal' mood and depressive disorder. Defining the boundaries between extremes of normal behaviour and psychopathology is a dilemma that pervades much of child psychiatry. It is especially problematic to establish the limits of depressive disorder in young people because of the cognitive and physical changes that take place during this time. Adolescents tend to feel things particularly deeply and marked mood swings are common during the teens. It can be difficult to distinguish these intense emotional reactions from depressive disorders. By contrast, young children do not find it easy to describe how they are feeling and often confuse emotions such as anger and sadness. They have particular difficulty describing the key cognitive symptoms of depression, such as hopelessness and self-denigration. Depressive disorder should therefore only be diagnosed when there is impairment of social role functioning, when symptoms of unequivocal psychopathological significance are present (such as severe suicidality), or when symptoms lead to significant suffering.

The next diagnostic issue concerns the distinction from other psychiatric disorders. Depression in this age group is associated with almost all the other child psychiatric disorders, including conduct disorder, anxiety states, learning problems, hyperactivity, anorexia nervosa and school refusal. In clinical samples co-morbidity with one or more of these disorders usually exceeds 75 per cent. Moreover, some of the symptoms that are part of the depressive constellation may arise as a symptom of other disorders. Thus, restlessness is seen in agitated depression, hypomania,

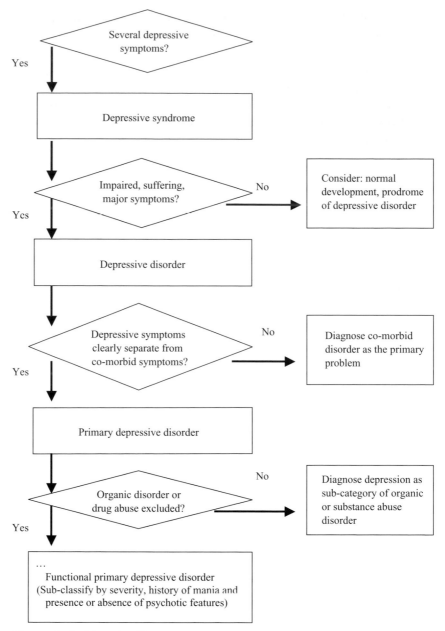

Fig. 4.1.   Diagnostic decision algorithm.

and hyperkinetic disorder. As a general rule, the double diagnosis should be made only when symptoms that are not simply part of another disorder clearly indicate the separate presence of a depressive disorder.

Although depression can occur in conjunction with any psychiatric problems, it is particularly common in the following:

- school refusal in adolescent girls;
- in adolescents with conduct disorder after a disciplinary crisis;
- in children or adolescents who have been abused or have experienced a very traumatic event;
- in children or adolescents who repeatedly harm themselves.

The final issue is whether the depressive disorder is part of an organic illness or substance abuse. Although it is very uncommon for organic illness to present with depression alone, any physical illness will increase the risk of depressive disorder, especially those that directly affect the brain (e.g. organic brain syndromes, endocrine disorders). Associations have been described with endocrine disorders and organic brain syndromes. There is growing evidence of an association between adolescent depression and substance abuse.

Measurement of depression

Table 4.4 shows the features of selected instruments that can be used to assess depression in young people. To choose between them the clinician must answer several key questions.

- *Question 1: what exactly do I want the measure for?* The most important issue is to define precisely what the measure needs to do. Pencil and paper measures are not good at making diagnoses as their diagnostic accuracy, compared with a gold standard structured interview, seldom exceeds 80 per cent. This means that, if the rate of disorder is 10 per cent or less, most cases with a 'high' score won't have depressive disorder. Their main uses are to screen for depression and as a quick way of obtaining data from multiple sources (e.g. parent and school). They may also be used to measure change, though scores on self-report depression questionnaires can fluctuate greatly from day to day. When choosing an interview, the main issue is whether to use a highly structured respondent interview (in which the structure resides in the question) and an investigator-based interview (in which the structure resides in the way the investigator has defined the phenomenon for study). The most widely used clinical interview for diagnosis and measuring change is the Kiddie Schedule for Affective Disorders and Schizophrenia (K-SADS). Appendix 4.1 shows an abbreviated version of the depression items. Diagnostic interviews and general questionnaires such as the CBCL can also assess co-morbidity, which is often an important issue with depressed youngsters.
- *Question 2: which personnel are available?* Experienced clinicians are not, in general, enthusiastic about using respondent-based interviews such as the Diagnostic Interview Schedule for Children (DISC). The DISC may, however, be very useful as a diagnostic aid for professionals without much clinical experience and its rigid script lends itself well to computerization.

Table 4.4. Selected measures of depression in young people

Measure	Type	Uses	Training (experience needed)	Completion time	Age range
Kiddie Schedule for Affective Disorders and Schizophrenia (K-SADS)	Investigator-based interview	Diagnosis (+++) Measure change (+++) Screening (−) Measure co-morbidity (+++)	Several weeks training (clinical experience helps)	1.5 to 2 hrs	9–18
Diagnostic Interview Schedule for Children (DISC)	Respondent-based interview	Diagnosis (++) Measure change (++) Screening (+) Measure comorbidity (+++)	Training in a few days (no clinical experience needed)	1.5 to 2 hrs	9–17
Children's Depression Rating Scale-Revised (CDRS-R)	Investigator-based interview	Diagnosis (++) Measure change (+++) Screening (+) Measure co-morbidity (−)	A day of training (clinical experience helps)	15 mins	10–18
Children's Depression Inventory (CDI)	Depression questionnaire	Diagnosis (−) Measure change (+) Screening (+++) Measure co-morbidity (−)	No training	10 mins	10–18
Mood and Feelings Questionnaire (MFQ)	Depression questionnaire	Diagnosis (−) Measure change (++) Screening (+++) Measure comorbidity (−)	No training	10 mins	10–18
Child Behaviour Checklist (CBCL)	General questionnaire	Diagnosis (+) Measure change (+) Screening (++) Measure comorbidity (++)	No training	20 mins	11–18
Berkley Puppet Interview (BPI)	Puppet interview	Diagnosis (++) Measure change (+) Screening (−) Measure comorbidity (++)	Several weeks training	1 hr	4–7

Use codes: (−) = Not useful; (+) = quite useful; (++) = definitely useful; (+++) = very useful.

- *Question 3: How much time is available?* Diagnostic interviews can take two or more hours in young people with significant psychiatric problems. Most questionnaires and interview-based measures of change take less than 20 minutes.
- *Question 4: What are the ages and developmental levels of my patients?* Assessment of depression usually requires that information is obtained directly from the young person. Although interviews such as the K-SADS are said to be used down to the age of 6 years, it is doubtful that full diagnostic interviews are suitable for face-to-face interviews until the child is aged 9 or 10 years. Similarly it is not until the age of 11 years and older that most children really can understand depression questionnaires. There are research techniques available for assessing depression in children as young as 4 years, using puppets or cartoons. However, at present these tools are not widely used in routine clinical work.
- *Question 5. Which source of information?* Most of the instruments shown in Table 4.4 also have parallel versions for parents. Information from parents is an essential part of any clinical assessment, but is particularly valuable in two clinical situations: first, in the assessment of depression in preadolescent children, who are often unable to give a clear account of some depressive symptoms; secondly, in assessing depression in young people with severe or psychotic depression, because such patients may downplay their symptoms.

Assessment

Although the accurate diagnosis of depressive disorder is an important part of clinical management, assessment only starts with the diagnosis; it does not stop with it. Depressed young people usually have multiple problems, such as educational failure, impaired psychosocial functioning, suicidal behaviour and co-morbid learning disorders. Moreover, they tend to come from families with high rates of psychopathology and may have experienced adverse life events. All these problems need to be identified and the causes of each assessed. Depression is a strong risk factor for both attempted and completed suicide, and in high risk cases the assessment should also indicate the degree of risk that patient poses to himself.

All patients with depression who are going to have antidepressants should have a medical history and examination. It is not usually necessary to conduct a physical examination in depressed adolescents, though one should be conducted if the history suggests a physical disorder could account for the depression. Relevant laboratory tests include hematology, biochemistry, urinary drugs screen and thyroid function tests.

The final part of the assessment involves the evaluation of the young person's personal and social resources. There is evidence that being successful at school or in other areas of life can protect young people from the effects of adverse life experiences. The best guide to the child's ability to solve future problems is his or her record in dealing with difficulties in the past. The ability of the family to support the patient should also be evaluated.

Aetiology

Depressive disorder is sometimes a reaction to a single severe stressor. Current aetiological theories suggest, however, that depression in young people more often arises from the accumulation and interaction over years of biological, psychological and social factors. These factors comprise the combination of (a) genetic influences, (b) the effects of chronic adversity, and (c) precipitating stressful events. They act through psychological and biochemical processes to produce the depressive syndrome. Once established, the syndrome is often prolonged by maintaining factors.

Genetic factors are probably less important in unipolar depressive conditions than in bipolar disorders, accounting for perhaps 50 per cent of the variation in depressive symptomatology in adolescents. Recent studies suggest that genetic effects are often indirect, acting through temperamental traits that increase vulnerability to stress. They may also act by increasing the risk of psychiatric disorders, such as anxiety and conduct disorders, which are themselves strong risk factors for depression.

Chronic adversities include both intrafamilial and extrafamilial factors. The most important familial factors are parental depression and other psychiatric disorders, family discord and parenting problems, including abuse. The most important extrafamilial factors are peer relationship problems (including bullying) and substance abuse.

Precipitating stressful events arise most commonly from the chronic stressors described in the previous paragraph, and include acute family problems (e.g. parental separation), a breakdown of a relationship with a peer and parental mental illness. The effects of acute stressful events depend to an important extent on their context and on the degree of threat that they pose to the child. For example, the death of a grandparent has much more impact on a child if the grandparent was the primary caretaker or an important source of support for that child.

Psychological processes are thought to play an important part in mediating the link between adversity and the development of depression. For example, in cognitive theory it is suggested that depressed people develop a distorted view of the world (such as the expectation that things will always go wrong), which is caused by earlier adversity. When the child experiences current adversity, these negative cognitions become manifest as automatic negative thoughts (e.g. the thought that 'it is hopeless, I knew I was no good at that') and this then leads to depression.

Biological theories have consisted, for the most part, of downward extensions of models first developed with adults. The best-known theory is the amine hypothesis, which proposes that depression is caused by underactivity in cerebral amine systems. Depression in young people may also be related to high levels of cortisol.

Maintaining factors can include (a) any of the above risk factors, (b) psychological or biological 'scarring' arising from the first depressive episode, or (c) the symptoms of depression itself (e.g. sleep disturbance leads to poor concentration, which in turn worsens negative thinking).

Treatment

Clinical management and treatment setting

The general principles of treatment follow from the description of the depressed young person's difficulties outlined above. Co-morbidity is frequent and there are many complications such as suicidal behaviour. Other types of adversity are part of the cause and may need intervention in their own right. Therefore, attention must be paid to biological, familial, educational and peer contributions. As with other child psychiatric disorders, it is important not only to treat the presenting problems but also to foster normal development. A treatment programme therefore has multiple aims: to reduce depression, to treat co-morbid disorders, to promote social and emotional adjustment, to improve self-esteem, to relieve family distress and prevent relapse.

The initial clinical management of depressed young people depends greatly on the nature of the problems identified during the assessment procedure. The assessment may indicate that the reaction of the child is appropriate for the situation in which he or she finds him- or herself. In such a case, and if the depression is mild, a sensible early approach can consist of the interventions outlined in Table 4.5. These include regular meetings, sympathetic discussions with the child and the parents and encouraging support. These simple interventions, especially if they are combined with measures to alleviate stress, are often followed by an improvement in mood. In other cases, particularly those with severe depression or suicidal thinking, a more focused form of treatment is indicated.

It is important that the clinician considers a number of key questions early on in the management of depressed young people. The first is whether the depression is severe enough to warrant admission to hospital. Indications for admission of depressed children are similar to those applicable to their adult counterparts and include severe suicidality, psychotic symptoms or refusal to eat or drink. A related question is whether the child should remain at school. When the disorder is mild, school can be a valuable distraction from depressive thinking. When the disorder is more severe, symptoms such as poor concentration and motor retardation may add to feelings of hopelessness. It is quite common in such cases to find that ensuring that the child obtains tuition in the home, or perhaps in a sheltered school, improves mood considerably.

Table 4.5. Components of early clinical management

Eliciting symptoms	Careful enquiry about the symptoms of depression
Explaining the diagnosis	Developmentally appropriate explanation of the diagnosis of depressive disorder and its symptoms, e.g. How irritability with the parent might not reflect the relationship but is a symptom of depression.
Explaining the causes	Developmentally appropriate explanation of the likely causes of the child's depressive disorder.
Establishing the focus of treatment	The process of translating the patient or parent's major complaints into solvable focused target problems. Choose symptoms that are important to the patient *and* are most likely to improve quickly (e.g. sleep problems rather than low self-esteem).
Optimistic reassurance	Whilst not being over-optimistic, the clinician must from an early stage get the idea over that depression in young people commonly remits and that coming for therapy (of whatever kind) will lead to positive changes. Also, that if one treatment does not work then another will follow.
Conveying expertise	Clinicians can convey expertise either directly or indirectly. An example of direct competence would be '*I am very familiar with the symptoms you are describing as I have worked quite a bit with young people who are depressed. I am sure that I can help you through some of these things*'.
Managing context	It may be possible to identify an important stressor/s that is likely to be relevant to the depression and which can be modified by a simple intervention

The second question is whether the depression is complicated by other disorders such as behavioural problems. If it is, then as a general rule it is best to sort out these complications before embarking on treatment for the depression.

The third question concerns the management of the stresses that are found in many cases of major depression. It is sometimes possible to alleviate some of these stresses, as shown in Table 4.6. However, in the majority of cases, acute stressors are just one of a number of causes of the depression. Moreover, such stressors arise commonly out of chronic difficulties such as family discord, and may therefore be very hard to remedy. Symptomatic treatments for depression can therefore be helpful even when it is obvious that the depressive symptoms occur in the context of chronic family or social adversity that one can do little to change.

Table 4.6. Managing the context of juvenile depression

Context	Management
Bullying at school	Encourage parent/s to discuss with the school, or phone school
Parental depression	Identify and treat, or actively encourage parent to seek treatment
Parental discord or divorce	Refer to local counselling service; information leaflet
Substance abuse	Refer to local drugs service
Academic problems	Discuss with parent/s and adolescent

Treatment algorithm

Figure 4.2 shows an algorithm for the treatment of moderately severe depression (depressive disorder that has not led to complete cessation of functioning in at least one domain). Findings from the control arms of pharmacological and psychological treatment trials suggest that around one-third of adolescents with major depression will remit given the basic clinical management outlined in the previous section, which should therefore be the first approach in most cases.

The best first-line treatment for moderately severe depressive disorder that persists despite initial clinical management has not yet been firmly established in comparative randomized trials. Many authorities suggest however that action-orientated psychological treatments, such as cognitive-behaviour therapy or interpersonal psychotherapy, are usually the interventions of first choice. If these fail, or are not available, then a trial of antidepressant medication should be considered (see below).

Severe major depression, in which there is complete inability to function in at least one major social domain (e.g. not going to school or not seeing friends

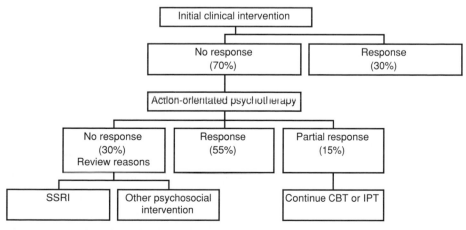

Fig. 4.2.   Management of moderately severe depression.

because of depression) is much less likely to respond to psychological treatment than mild or moderate depression. The first choice intervention is therefore likely to include antidepressant medication. Severely depressed youngsters often need intensive support, such as through a day unit or assertive outreach programme.

Psychological interventions

The most widely used psychological interventions with depressed young people are action-orientated here-and-now individual psychological treatments, particularly cognitive-behaviour therapy and interpersonal psychotherapy.

Many slightly different cognitive–behavioural approaches have been developed for depressed children and adolescents. Most programmes have the following features. First, the therapy often begins with a session or sessions on emotional recognition and self-monitoring. The aim is to help the young person to distinguish between different emotional states (e.g. sadness and anger) and to start linking external events, thoughts and feelings. Secondly, behavioural tasks may be used to reinforce desired behaviours and thence to help the young person to gain control over symptoms. Self-reinforcement is often combined with activity scheduling, in which the young person is encouraged to engage in a programme of constructive or pleasant activities. Patients are taught to set realistic goals, with small steps towards achieving them, and to reward themselves at each successful step on the way. At this stage, it is quite common to introduce other behavioural techniques to deal with some of the behavioural or vegetative symptoms of depression. For example, many depressed youngsters sleep poorly and will often be helped by simple sleep hygiene measures. Thirdly, various cognitive techniques are used to reduce depressive cognitions. For example, adolescents may be helped to identify cognitive distortions and to challenge them using techniques such as pro-con evaluation. Techniques to reduce negative automatic thoughts, such as 'focus on object', are also employed.

CBT has been used in both school and clinical settings. There have been at least six randomized controlled studies of CBT in samples of children with depressive symptoms recruited through schools and, in three of them, CBT was significantly superior to no treatment. A meta-analysis of randomized trials with clinically diagnosed cases of depressive disorder found that CBT was significantly superior to comparison conditions such as remaining on a waiting list or having relaxation training (pooled odds ratio of 2.2).

Interpersonal psychotherapy (IPT) is based on the premise that depression occurs in the context of interpersonal relationships. Like CBT, IPT is a brief time-limited therapy. The two main goals are to identify and treat, first, depressive symptoms and, secondly, the problems associated with the onset of depression. Two randomized trials have shown significant benefits from IPT in depressed adolescents.

There have been at least four randomized controlled trials of family therapy in adolescent depressive disorder. Two involved a family intervention only and two examined the value of parental sessions given in parallel with individual CBT. None has found a significant benefit of the family treatment. It would be premature though to conclude that family interventions have no place in managing juvenile depression. The association between juvenile depression and family dysfunction is so strong that family interventions should be considered sometimes. However, they should not, in general, be first-line treatments.

Other interventions

Depressed patients often have many different kinds of problems and therefore a clinician treating a depressed young person will need access to the full range of child mental health services, including social work and special educational provision.

Pharmacotherapy

The first-line pharmacological treatments are the serotonin-specific re-uptake inhibitors (SSRIs) such as fluoxetine and paroxetine. Three recently published randomized trials have produced positive results, with response rates of between 50 and 70 per cent. It should be noted, however, that placebo response rates in these studies have usually exceeded a third, which means that four or five patients must be treated with an SSRI to obtain one who has actually benefited from the SSRI. Once again, this underlines the importance of offering non-specific treatments before medication in most cases.

Once the decision is taken to prescribe medication, it is very important that an adequate course is given. This means ensuring not only that the correct dose is prescribed but also that every effort is taken to ensure compliance. Figure 4.3 shows an 'adequate course' of an SSRI.

As Table 4.7 shows, there are many different types of antidepressant. There is little evidence that any one drug is better than another. The main differences between them are their half-lives, their ability to inhibit the cytochrome P_{450} (CYP450) system in the liver, and their active metabolites. These differences sometimes can be important clinically. For example, the long half-life of fluoxetine means that there may have to be a delay of several weeks before an antidepressant that can interact with it (e.g. a monoamine oxidase inhibitor) can be given. On the other hand, the shorter half-life of paroxetine may account for its greater association with discontinuation reactions than some other antidepressants. The P_{450} cytochrome is important because many of the SSRIs are inhibitors of one of the enzymes that metabolizes tricyclics and other psychotropic drugs, CYP2D6. This means that potentially toxic levels can occur if the tricyclics and SSRIs are given together.

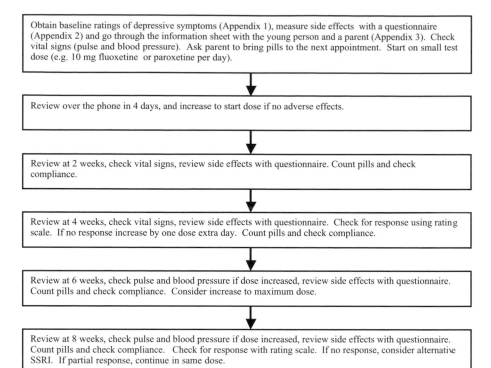

Obtain baseline ratings of depressive symptoms (Appendix 1), measure side effects with a questionnaire (Appendix 2) and go through the information sheet with the young person and a parent (Appendix 3). Check vital signs (pulse and blood pressure). Ask parent to bring pills to the next appointment. Start on small test dose (e.g. 10 mg fluoxetine or paroxetine per day).

Review over the phone in 4 days, and increase to start dose if no adverse effects.

Review at 2 weeks, check vital signs, review side effects with questionnaire. Count pills and check compliance.

Review at 4 weeks, check vital signs, review side effects with questionnaire. Check for response using rating scale. If no response increase by one dose extra day. Count pills and check compliance.

Review at 6 weeks, check pulse and blood pressure if dose increased, review side effects with questionnaire. Count pills and check compliance. Consider increase to maximum dose.

Review at 8 weeks, check pulse and blood pressure if dose increased, review side effects with questionnaire. Count pills and check compliance. Check for response with rating scale. If no response, consider alternative SSRI. If partial response, continue in same dose.

Fig. 4.3.   An 'adequate course' of an SSRI for adolescents with major depression.

Table 4.7. Anti-depressants

Name	Dose mg/day	Half-life	Form	Inhibits P_{450} system
Citalopram	20–60	36 h	Tablet or liquid	2D6 – some
Fluoxetine	20–60	9 days[a]	Tablet or liquid	2D6 – yes
Paroxetine	20–50	24 h	Tablet or liquid	2D6 – much
Sertraline	50–150	26 h	Tablet	2D6 – yes
Venlafaxine	75–375	11 h (slow release)	Tablet	2D6 – weak

[a] active metabolite has a very long half-life.

SSRIs seem to have fewer side effects than tricyclics and do not usually require specific cardiovascular monitoring. However, symptoms such as dry mouth and gastrointestinal upset can be a problem and there has been concern about the so-called 'serotonin syndrome'. This 'syndrome', which is probably better regarded as the extreme end of the continuum of toxicity, is characterized by alterations in cognition, behaviour, autonomic and central nervous system function as a result of increased postsynaptic serotonin receptor agonism. Abrupt discontinuation of SSRIs can lead to symptoms such as dizziness, nausea and lethargy, which may raise parental concerns about addiction. SSRIs should generally be tapered slowly over 4 weeks. If the patient still has difficulties coming off SSRIs with a shorter half-life (e.g. paroxetine), then a switch to a longer-acting SSRI (e.g. fluoxetine) may be helpful.

Monitoring and evaluation of treatment

The first step is to measure depressive symptoms carefully, using a diagnostic interview such as the depression section of the K-SADS (see Appendix 4.1). If a drug is to be prescribed, it is useful to measure 'side effects' before treatment starts, as parents and patients may confuse anxiety or depressive symptoms with side effects. Appendix 4.2 gives an example of a side effects questionnaire for SSRIs. Response to treatment should be reviewed approximately 8 weeks after it has started. If there has been no response at this point, then it is unlikely that the initial treatment (either psychological or pharmacological) will work and another line of treatment should be pursued.

There are many published studies on the rate of response of depressed young people to both psychological and pharmacological treatments, so it is now possible to compare the performance of a service with external standards. For example, for moderately severe major depression, one would normally expect a response rate at 8–10 weeks ('response' being defined as no longer meeting DSM criteria for major depression – see Table 4.2 and Appendix 4.1) to either CBT or an SSRI of between 55 and 65 per cent. Failure to achieve a response rate of more than 50 per cent should trigger a review of referral pathways, treatment protocols and staff training.

Problematic issues

The most important clinical problem is failure to respond to the initial treatment. As a general rule, failure to respond to psychological treatment is an indication for starting an SSRI. In patients who fail to respond to an adequate course of SSRI, there should be a review of the possible reasons. Non-compliance can be a major issue in this age group, and blood levels (if available) may help to identify this problem. There should also be a review of the diagnosis, and of any possible co-morbid problems such as abuse, family discord, bipolar disorder, drug dependence or physical illness.

As Fig. 4.4 shows, in patients who fail to respond to one SSRI the Texas Consensus Conference recommended a trial of another (e.g. paroxetine, increasing by 10 mg increments to 50 mg daily), on the grounds that some of the SSRIs are distinct chemically. If the young person fails to respond to a second SSRI, then monotherapy with another antidepressant should be considered, such as venlafaxine (modified release, up to 225 mg daily). Failure to respond to a third antidepressant should trigger a review of the clinical state. In many services it would be at this point that

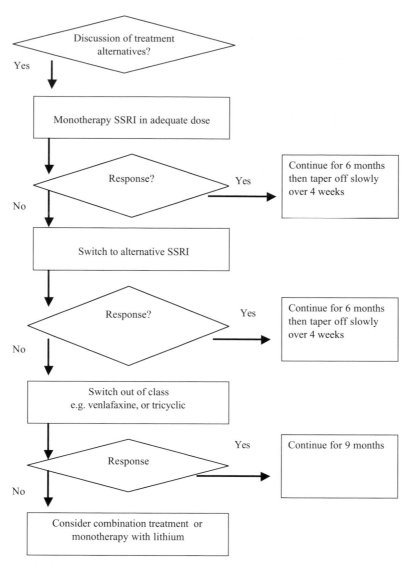

Fig. 4.4.   Medication algorithm.

other forms of therapy might be considered, such as admission to an inpatient unit. Augmentation with another agent might also be an option, but only if the patient has derived at least some benefit from the first treatment. Combination treatments can however be associated with toxicity. For example, SSRIs such as fluoxetine can increase blood levels of other psychotropics such as risperidone. The clinician should always remember that not every problem has a medical solution.

From time to time the clinician will encounter major depressive conditions in preadolescent children. These conditions tend to show more co-morbidity with other psychiatric disorders than adolescent depressive disorders and a stronger association with adversity, particularly family problems. The first-line treatments therefore are usually directed at these problems. If these treatments fail, then one or more of the treatments outlined above might be considered.

Information for patients and parents

Patients and parents often request information about depressive disorder and its treatment, especially if medication is to be prescribed. Appendix 4.3 shows an example of an information sheet about fluoxetine.

Outcome

Short- and long-term outcome

- In the short term, major depressive disorder in adolescents has a good prognosis, with about an 80 per cent chance of remission within a year.
- However, among those who recover, there is an increased risk of another episode, of around 40 per cent.
- This increased risk of further depression extends into adult life.
- A high proportion of depressed cases show other psychiatric disorders later in life, including anxiety disorder, conduct disorder and personality disorder.
- In comparison with non-depressed young people, there is a greatly increased risk of suicide, approximately 4 per cent over the following 15 years.

Prognostic factors

A worse outcome is associated with increased severity of depression, greater impairment at the time of the index episode, family discord, a family history of depression and co-morbidity with conduct disorder. The prognosis of conduct problems is no different in the presence of depression, so young people with depressive conduct disorder are at risk of all the adverse outcomes of conduct disorder, including criminality and antisocial personality disorder.

Bipolar disorders

Introduction

The concept of mania in pre-adolescent children has followed a similar course to that of depression. For many years it was believed that pre-adolescents did not develop adult-like manic states. Then about 15 years ago, several investigators reported substantial numbers of preadolescents who seemed to meet full adult criteria for mania. There is no doubt that these children have severe psychiatric problems,

Table 4.8. Criteria for a manic episode **in DSM-IV**

A. A distinct period of abnormally and persistently elevated, expansive, or irritable mood, lasting at least one week (or any duration if hospitalization is necessary).

B. During the period of mood disturbance, three (or more) of the following symptoms have persisted (four if the mood is only irritable) and have been present to a significant degree:
   1) inflated self-esteem or grandiosity
   2) decreased need for sleep (e.g. feels rested after only three hours of sleep)
   3) more talkative than usual or pressure to keep talking
   4) flight of ideas or subjective experience that thoughts are racing
   5) distractibility (i.e. attention too easily drawn to unimportant or irrelevant external stimuli)
   6) increase in goal-directed activity (either socially, at work or school, or sexually) or psychomotor agitation
   7) excessive involvement in pleasurable activities that have a high potential for painful consequences (e.g. engaging in unrestrained buying sprees, sexual indiscretions, or foolish business investments)

C. The symptoms do not meet criteria for a mixed episode.

D. The mood disturbance is sufficiently severe to cause marked impairment in occupational functioning, or in usual social activities or relationships with others, or to necessitate hospitalization to prevent harm to self or others, or there are psychotic features.

E. The symptoms are not due to the direct physiological effects of a substance (e.g. a drug of abuse, a medication, or other treatment) or a general medical condition (e.g. hyperthyroidism).

Note: Manic-like episodes that are clearly caused by somatic anti-depressant treatment (e.g. medication, electroconvulsive therapy, light therapy) should not count toward a diagnosis of Bipolar I Disorder.

---

but many uncertainties remain about the validity of the concept of pre-adolescent mania and about its links with 'classical' bipolar disorder in adults. This section will therefore focus on typical bipolar conditions in adolescents.

Definition and classification

ICD-10 and DSM-IV criteria

In both ICD-10 and DSM-IV bipolar affective disorder is characterized by repeated episodes in which mood and activity levels are disturbed. On some occasions there is elevation of mood and activity (mania or hypomania) and on other occasions lowering of mood and activity (depression). By convention, all patients with mania are classified in the bipolar group, whether or not they have had depression. Table 4.8 shows the diagnostic criteria for a manic episode in DSM-IV.

Both diagnostic systems emphasize that there should be clear shifts between these phases and that periods of elevated or depressed mood should be distinct. However, the concept of bipolar disorder has expanded from one in which there are major pathological variations in mood of an extreme form to one in which there may be relatively subtle variations in mood that merge imperceptibly with normal mood variation. These so-called sub-syndromal bipolar disorders include hyperthymia, dysthymia and cyclothymia. Moreover, phenomenological studies suggest that there is a great deal of overlap between depression and mania and that mixed states are relatively common. DSM-IV therefore has a category for mixed states.

Clinical applicability

These adult criteria for mania seem to work reasonably well in adolescents. As noted above, the use of adult diagnostic criteria for mania among preadolescents is still at an early stage. The criteria have often been modified, for example by dropping the requirement that there should be discrete episodes.

Epidemiology

Prevalence and incidence rates and sex ratios

Severe 'typical' bipolar disorder appears to be uncommon in adolescence. For example, in a large North American study only two of the 1500 adolescents who were evaluated met full diagnostic criteria for bipolar disorder. None of the published epidemiological studies has found any cases of bipolar disorder in preadolescents. Bipolar disorder shows an equal sex ratio in adolescents.

Clinical picture

Main features and symptoms

The main features of mania in young people are elevation of mood, increased activity and grandiose ideas.

Elevation of mood

This may range from mild euphoria to elation, and in some cases there may be infectious gaiety. In some cases mood may be irritable rather than euphoric, but the clinician should bear in mind that irritability is a very common symptom in young people.

Increased activity

This may involve motor behaviour, speech, or appetite, with sleep being reduced correspondingly. At first, the adolescent may actually get more done but as mania worsens the patients moves restlessly from one activity to another. Speech is rapid and thoughts speed up. Eventually ideas become loosely connected with punning and jumping from one topic to another using rhythms – clang associations. Appetite may be increased at first, but eventually declines.

Grandiose ideas

In the early stages of mania the adolescent may make tactless remarks in social situations, make inappropriate sexual advances or go on spending sprees. As mania worsens, they may embark on hare-brained schemes and become grandiose. They may believe they are on a special mission and develop delusion-like ideas. First-rank symptoms of schizophrenia can occur, including passivity experiences. Hallucinations may also occur, but are usually mood congruent.

Differential diagnosis

Mild forms of mania are confused easily with problems such as conduct disorder and attention deficit disorder. However behavioural disorders tend to be persistent, without the relapsing and remitting course of bipolar disorder. Severe, psychotic manic states can be difficult to distinguish from schizophrenia. Bipolar disorder tends to have a more sudden onset than schizophrenia and is less often associated with pre-morbid social dysfunction. Manic symptoms can occur when susceptible subjects have been prescribed antidepressants and there is also an association with substance abuse. Rarely, manic conditions may be seen with neurological disorders such as brain tumours.

Diagnostic instruments

Mania cannot be diagnosed by questionnaire and the diagnosis must therefore be made by an interview combined with direct observations of the young person's behaviour and by a careful history from the parent/s. Almost all of the major diagnostic interviews contain questions on manic symptoms. However, there is evidence that lay interviewers using highly structured respondent-based interviews tend to overdiagnose psychosis in young people. The best way of diagnosing mania is with a semi-structured diagnostic interview such as the K-SADS or the Child and Adolescent Psychiatric Assessment (CAPA), administered by a clinician or by an interviewer who has had specific training in the assessment of psychotic patients.

Assessment

As with any psychiatric disorder, bipolar disorder requires a thorough psychiatric assessment including the history of the presenting problem, impairment, developmental history and family functioning including a family history of bipolar disorder.

- The history of depressive and manic symptoms requires careful assessment in order to establish the diagnosis of bipolar disorder. Careful enquiry should be made into the degree of recovery between episodes as this is important in the differential diagnosis. Although chronic mania can occasionally occur in adolescents, failure to recover should alert the clinician to alternative diagnoses.
- The events surrounding the episodes should be documented carefully.
- It is also important to assess co-morbid problems, especially behavioural problems and substance abuse.
- Patients with mania require a medical history and physical examination.
- Blood should be taken for routine biochemistry and haematology, and for thyroid function tests. A urinary drug screen should also be conducted. Since mania-like states can occur with a variety of organic brain disorders, an electroencephalogram or magnetic resonance imaging scan may be indicated.
- Pre-morbid temperamental features include emotionality and poor attention.
- Family risk factors include major affective disorder and substance abuse.

Aetiology

About 60 per cent of the liability to bipolar disorder in adults is genetic, which means that, although there is a strong genetic component, other factors are also important. The mode of inheritance is unclear but it is likely that the majority of bipolar disorder involves complex genetic mechanisms interacting with environmental factors. Linkage findings have been difficult to replicate but recent reviews have implicated regions on several chromosomes, notably 18q, 21q, 4p and Xq.

Little is known about the aetiology of juvenile bipolar disorder. There have, for instance, been no large genetically informative studies of bipolar disorders in young people. However, there is no reason for thinking that juvenile bipolar disorder is any less genetic than it seems to be in adults. Adolescent bipolar disorder is familial and shows a distribution of affective illness in relatives that is compatible with genetic factors.

Treatment

Clinical management and treatment setting

The grandiose ideas and lack of judgement of adolescents with mania can get them quickly into serious trouble and therefore, in most cases, they will require admission to hospital. If the parents are in agreement, this can usually be achieved voluntarily, but in some instances compulsory detention under the law may be required. Other indications for admission include treatment resistance, lack of insight and acute danger to self or others. It is much better that admission is to a specialized adolescent service, as the aim is not only to contain behaviour but also to begin a long-term therapeutic process and to foster normal development.

In most cases, treatment is multimodal and involves pharmacotherapy, psychological treatment, family work and education.

Psychological treatment

Individual supportive work may help the patient to explore the implications of the diagnosis and to regularize lifestyle and sleeping patterns. Family work may also be helpful, as bipolar disorder often has a major impact on family life. It is often helpful to educate both the adolescent and the family about the early signs of relapse.

Pharmacotherapy

Pharmacological treatment of bipolar disorder can be divided into two phases: acute treatment of mania or depression and prophylaxis.

In the acute phase of mania, treatment usually comprises the combination of low potency neuroleptics such as chlorpromazine (200 to 400 mg per day in adolescents in four daily doses) and a mood stabilizer. The neuroleptic helps to maintain behavioural control and allows time for the mood stabilizer to work. In classic euphoric mania, the first-line mood stabilizer is lithium (0.8 to 1.2 mmol/l). Rapid cycling mania may be treated with carbamazepine (7–10 µg/ml). Severe manic excitement may also require the addition of a benzodiazepine, such as lorazepam.

The first-line treatment for depression in bipolar disorder is a thymoleptic such as lithium. Subsequently, SSRIs are recommended as they are less likely to cause manic switching than the tricyclics.

In adults, lithium has been shown to be effective for the prevention of manic and depressive episodes. Much less is known about its use in children or adolescents but there is some evidence that it is effective. As in adults, the blood lithium range for prophylaxis should be lower than for the acute phase, in the range from 0.6 to 1.0 mmol/l. Lithium is not metabolized, it is excreted by the kidneys. Young people have a faster elimination rate than adults, which results in the achievement of a steady state sooner. The easiest way to achieve this is to give a test dose of lithium 300 mg, then a daily dose of about 900 mg with adjustments following periodic blood tests every 5 days or so.

Problematic issues

The main problems are side effects, poor compliance and failure to respond, which are often interconnected.

Common side effects of lithium are nausea, headaches and tremor. Weight gain and acne are common in adolescents. Signs of lithium toxicity include confusion, drowsiness, slurred speech and muscle twitching. They can occur with normal serum levels and should lead to lithium being stopped immediately. Lithium is associated with thyroid problems and renal abnormalities, so creatinine and thyroxine should be measured every 6 months. Side effects of carbamazepine include rashes, ataxia and gastrointestinal disturbance. Blood dyscrasias are rare but require that a full blood count is done before treatment and every 6 months thereafter.

Poor compliance is very common, occurring in up to one-third of cases. It can be reduced by psychoeducation and by keeping side effects to a minimum.

Failure to respond to treatment for the acute phase of mania should trigger a review of compliance, blood levels, use of substances or alcohol, diagnosis and concurrent stress or physical illness. If there has been no response after 6 weeks, the most commonly used strategies are either to switch to another thymoleptic (e.g. from lithium to carbamazepine) or to combine thymoleptics (e.g. lithium plus carbamazepine).

Outcome

Relatively little is known about the outcomes of adolescent bipolar disorders, but the available data suggest that:
- bipolar disorders that occur in adolescence tend to follow the remitting and relapsing course of adult cases;
- there is a 50 per cent risk of relapse within 5 years even with treatment and there is a markedly increased risk of suicide and serious suicidal attempts;
- however, the adult prognosis is much better than with schizophrenia;
- in community samples only 1 per cent of adolescents with major depression go on to bipolar disorder, but in clinical samples the risk of switching is about 5 per cent;
- the best predictors of switching from depression to mania are psychotic features during the index depressive episode, a family history of bipolar disorder and premorbid cyclothymia.

Acknowledgements

Thanks to Joan Kaufman for permission to reproduce parts of the Kiddie-Sads-Present and Lifetime Version.

SUGGESTED READING

American Academy of Child and Adolescent Psychiatry. Practice parameters for the assessment and treatment of children and adolescents with bipolar disorder. *Journal of the American Academy of Child and Adolescent Psychiatry*, **36** (1997), 138–57.

American Academy of Child and Adolescent Psychiatry. Practice parameters for the assessment and treatment of children and adolescents with depressive disorders. *Journal of the American Academy of Child and Adolescent Psychiatry*, **37**(10 Suppl.) (1998), 63S–83S.

G. Clarke, P. Lewinsohn & H. Hops, *Leaders Manual for Adolescent Groups. Adolescent Coping with Depression Course.* (Eugene, OR: Castalia Publishing Company, 1990) (see also: www.kpchr.org/acwd/).

R. C. Harrington, J. Whittaker & P. Shoebridge, Psychological treatment of depression in children and adolescents: a review of treatment research. *British Journal of Psychiatry*, **173** (1998), 291–8.

R. Harrington, Affective disorders. In *Child and Adolescent Psychiatry: Modern Approaches. Fourth Edition*, ed. M. Rutter & E. Taylor. (Oxford: Blackwell Scientific, 2002), pp. 463–85.

C. W. Hughes, G. J. Emslie, M. L. Crimson *et al.* & The Texas Consensus Conference Panel on Medication Treatment of Childhood Major Depressive Disorder. The Texas Children's Medication Algorithm Project: report of the Texas Consensus Conference Panel on Medication Treatment of Childhood Major Depressive Disorder. *Journal of the American Academy of Child and Adolescent Psychiatry*, **38** (1999), 1442–54.

A. James & Javaloyes, Practitioner review: the treatment of bipolar disorder in children and adolescents. *Journal of Child Psychology and Psychiatry*, **42** (2001), 439–49.

N. D. Ryan, V. S. Bhatara & J. M. Perel, Mood stabilizers in children and adolescents. *Journal of the American Academy of Child and Adolescent Psychiatry*, **38** (1999), 529–36.

Assessment measures

J. C. Ablow, J. R. Measelle, H. C. Kraemer *et al.*, The MacArthur three city outcome study: evaluating multi-informant measures of young children's symptomatology, *Journal of the American Academy of Child and Adolescent Psychiatry*, **38** (1999), 1580–90.

A. Angold, M. Prendergast, A. Cox, M. Rutter & R. Harrington, The Child and Adolescent Psychiatric Assessment (CAPA). *Psychological Medicine*, **25** (1995), 739–53 (website: devepi.mc.duke.edu/).

A. Angold, E. J. Costello, S. C. Messer, A. Pickles, F. Winder & D. Silver, The development of a short questionnaire for use in epidemiological studies of depression in children and adolescents. *International Journal of Methods in Psychiatric Research*, **5** (1995), 237–49. (Mood and Feelings Questionnaire: available from J. Duncan, Duke University Medical Center, Box 3454, Durham, North Carolina 27710 (website: devepi.mc.duke.edu/).

M. Kovacs, Rating scales to assess depression in school aged children. *Acta Paedopsychiatrica*, **46** (1981), 305–15. (Children's Depression Inventory: available from A. D. D. WareHouse, Email sales@addwarehouse.com).

E. O. Poznanski, L. N. Freman & H. B. Mokros, Children's depression rating scale-revised. *Psychopharmacology Bulletin*, **21** (1985), 979–89 (website: www.psychtest.com).

J. Puig-Antich & W. Chambers, *The Schedule for Affective Disorders and Schizophrenia for school-aged children.* (New York State Psychiatric Institute, 1978), unpublished interview schedule (1996 version available from the Department of Psychiatry, University of Pittsburgh website: www.wpic.pitt.edu/ksads).

D. Shaffer, P. Fisher, C. Lucas, M. Dulcan & M. Schwab-Stone, NIMH Diagnostic Interview Schedule for Children version IV (NIMH DISC-IV): description, differences from previous versions, and reliability of some common diagnoses. *Journal of the American Academy of Child and Adolescent Psychiatry*, **39** (2000), 28–38 (website: www.c-disc.com/).

Appendix 4.1. Abbreviated version of the depression items from the Kiddie–Sads–Present and Lifetime Version (K-SADS-PL) (Kaufman et al., 1996).

Depressed Mood

Refers to subjective feelings of depression based on verbal complaints of feeling depressed, sad, blue, gloomy, very unhappy, down, empty, bad feelings, feels like crying. Excludes suicidal thinking, ideational items (e.g. hopelessness) and irritability. NOTE: an initial negative answer by the child may be changed if the child seems sad and the parent confirms depression.

Do you feel sad, blue, down or empty? Do you feel like crying? Over the past week, how often have you felt like that? How long does it last? When did these feelings start?

	P C BE	
	0 0 0	No information
	1 1 1	Not at all or less than once a week
	2 2 2	Subthreshold: often experiences dysphoric mood at least three times a week for more than 3 hours each time
	3 3 3	Threshold. Feels 'depressed' most of the day more days than not.

Duration: ———— Weeks

Irritability and anger

Subjective feelings of irritability, anger, crankiness, bad temper, short tempered, resentment or annoyance, whether expressed overtly or not. Rate the intensity and duration of such feelings.

Do you get annoyed, irritated or cranky at little things? Do you lose your temper too easily? Over the past week, how often have you felt like that? How long does it last? When did these feelings start?

	P C BE	
	0 0 0	No information
	1 1 1	Not at all or less than once a week
	2 2 2	Subthreshold: Feels definitely more angry or irritable than called for by the situation, at least three times a week for more than 3 hours each time
	3 3 3	Threshold. Feels irritable/angry daily, or almost daily, at least 50% of the time. Or often shouts, loses temper.

Duration: ———— Weeks

Anhedonia, lack of interest, or apathy, or boredom

Anhedonia refers to loss of ability to get pleasure, enjoy, or have fun by participating in activities with other children. **Boredom** is a term frequently used by children to refer to loss of enjoyment or loss of interest.

	P C BE	
	0 0 0	No information
	1 1 1	Not at all.
	2 2 2	Subthreshold: Several activities less pleasurable or interesting. Or bored at least 3 times a week.

(cont.)

Appendix 4.1. (cont.)

	P C BE	
What sorts of things do you do out of school? (get examples, computer games, sports, friends, etc). Do you look forward to doing these things? Do you still enjoy them? Do they interest you? (if stopped) When did you stop doing X? Why? Do you get bored? How often? When? When did these feelings start?	3 3 3	Threshold. Most activities much less pleasurable or interesting. Or bored daily.

Duration: _____ Weeks

Suicidal thinking or morbid thoughts or suicidal behaviour

	P C BE	
Suicidal thinking or morbid thoughts: this includes preoccupation with thoughts of death or suicide and plans to commit suicide. Also includes auditory hallucinations of a voice telling the child to kill himself. Do not include fear of dying.	0 0 0	No information.
	1 1 1	Not at all.
Suicidal behaviour: includes deliberate overdose of drugs, frequent or serious cutting, hanging and so on.	2 2 2	Subthreshold: transient thoughts of death or suicide, but not thought of a method. One or two trivial cuts.
Have you thought you might be better of dead? Have you thought about killing yourself? How would you do it? Have you actually tried to kill or hurt yourself? How?	3 3 3	Threshold. Often thinks of death or suicide, or has thought of a specific method, or has engaged in suicidal behaviour since the onset of depression.

Sleep disturbance

	P C BE	
Sleep disorder, including initial, middle, or terminal difficulty in getting to sleep or staying asleep. Also hypersomnia. Do not rate if the child feels no need for sleep. Take into account developmental variations in sleep: a 6–8 year-old sleeps about 10 hours, a 9–12 year-old about 9 hours, and a 12–16 year-old about 8 hours (all +/− an hour).	0 0 0	No information
	1 1 1	Not present
	2 2 2	Subthreshold: any sleep difficulties not reaching threshold
How has your sleep been? How long does it take you to get to sleep? Do you wake in the night? What time do you wake up? Or, have you been sleeping longer than usual?	3 3 3	Threshold. Two hours or more of initial insomnia or more than 30 minutes of middle or terminal insomnia most nights. Hypersomnia 2 hours more than usual, most days.

Concentration, inattention, or slowed thinking

Complaints (or evidence from teacher) of diminished ability to think or concentrate, which was not present to the same degree before the episode.

Do you know what it means to concentrate? (if no, it means like not being able to keep your mind on things) Have you had that kind of trouble? Is your thinking slowed down? Does it take you longer to do your school work, or other activities?

	P	C	BE	
	0	0	0	No information
	1	1	1	Not present
	2	2	2	Subthreshold: definitely aware of limited attention span but causes no major difficulties.
	3	3	3	Threshold: interferes with school work or other activities.

Change in appetite or weight

Appetite decreased or increased compared to usual or to peers if episode is long.

Total weight loss or weight gain from usual weight. Failure to gain 1.5 kgs over a 6-month period counts as weight loss in children aged 5–11 years.

How has your appetite been? Has it decreased, or increased? Do you eat snacks? How often? And your weight? Has that increased, or decreased? When were you last weighed? How much did you weigh?

	P	C	BE	
	0	0	0	No information
	1	1	1	Not present
	2	2	2	Subthreshold: Decrease or increase in appetite most days (e.g. misses snacks or has extra snacks). Weight loss or weight gain of 3–4%.
	3	3	3	Threshold: Moderate decrease or increase in appetite (e.g. misses meals or has extra meals). Weight loss or gain of 5% or more.

Psychomotor disturbances

Agitation: includes inability to sit still, pacing, wringing of hands, or non-stop talking. Do not include if it occurs during manic syndrome. The rating can include observations made by the interviewer or parents.

Retardation: visible, generalized slowing down of physical movements, reactions and speech. The rating can include observations made by the interviewer or parents.

	P	C	BE	
	0	0	0	No information
	1	1	1	Not present
	2	2	2	Subthreshold: Occasionally unable to sit quietly. Or conversation is noticeably slowed or there is slowed body movement.

(cont.)

Appendix 4.1. *(cont.)*

	P	C	BE	
Have you found it difficult to sit still or you have to keep moving? Do you walk up and down? Or wring your hands (demonstrate). *Or have you found that you cannot move as fast as before? Or found it hard to start talking? Or has your speech been slowed down?*			3 3 3	Threshold: Often unable to sit still, much fidgeting. Or, conversation is somewhat difficult to maintain, or moves very slowly.
Worthlessness or guilt				
Worthlessness includes feelings of inadequacy, inferiority, failure and self deprecation.	0	0	0	No information
Guilt is self-reproach for things done or not done, including delusions.	1	1	1	Not present
	2	2	2	Subthreshold: occasionally feels inadequate, or guilty about past actions.
How do you feel about yourself? Do you like yourself? What are your good points?How often do you feel like this? Do you feel bad about anything you have done? What about? How often do you feel like this?			3 3 3	Threshold: Often feels like a failure, or often feels guilt which he cannot explain.

Notes: Like any clinical interview the depression section should start with an unstructured introductory interview. The interview is conducted with the child (**C**), parent (**P**) and then combined into a best estimate (**BE**) which includes all sources of information (including case records, school and so on). The interviewer is not obliged to recite the probes verbatim. Rather, the objective is to establish whether the criteria set out in the definitions have been met.

All ratings apply to the past month. A 'definite' DSM episode requires five 'threshold' symptoms, one of which must be depressed mood, anhedonia or irritability. 'Probable' major depression can be diagnosed with four threshold symptoms and one subthreshold.

In most clinical trials the average score (total score divided by the number of scales completed is usually about 2.8 at the time of the first assessment, dropping to an average of about 1.5 to 1.8 after 12 weeks of treatment.

The full version of the K-SADS is available from the Department of Psychiatry, University of Pittsburgh.

Appendix 4.2. Health questionnaire – child

Your name . . . .   Date . . . . ./. . . . ./. . . . .
Over the past week, have you had any of the following symptoms?

		Put a ring round the answer	
Drowsiness or feeling tired	No	A little	A lot
Blurred vision	No	A little	A lot
Dry mouth	No	A little	A lot
Headaches	No	A little	A lot
Feeling restless	No	A little	A lot
Muscle twitching (tics)	No	A little	A lot
Pain in the arms or legs	No	A little	A lot
Loss of appetite	No	A little	A lot
Feeling sick	No	A little	A lot
Poor sleep	No	A little	A lot
Loose stools (diarrhoea)	No	A little	A lot
Feeling faint or fainting	No	A little	A lot
Rashes	No	A little	A lot
Creeping feeling on the skin	No	A little	A lot
Feeling easily upset	No	A little	A lot

Appendix 4.3. Fluoxetine and depressive disorder: commonly asked questions

What is depressive disorder?

Depressive disorder is a condition in which the patient suffers from feelings of depression and other symptoms such as poor sleep, lack of energy, loss of appetite and loss of concentration. Depressed young people often feel bad about themselves and hopeless about the future.

Many young people who suffer from depression will get better without medical treatment. However, in some instances, medication is required to reduce the depression.

What is fluoxetine?

Fluoxetine has been used to treat a variety of mental health problems in both adults and adolescents. You will be taking it to treat your depression. It is also known as Prozac.

How does fluoxetine work?

Young people usually get depressed for several reasons. These include bad experiences, such as bullying or problems at home, the hormonal changes of adolescence and genetic factors. It is believed that these factors can all alter the balance of chemicals in the brain and that this then leads to feelings of depression. It is thought that fluoxetine helps to increase the levels of some of these chemicals and this in turn reduces depression.

What do I have to do?

You will need to take fluoxetine once a day, usually in the mornings. We will start you on a low dose, sometimes as a syrup, and increase it slowly. You do not have to have blood tests, but these may very occasionally be necessary if you suffered from any serious illnesses in the past.

How long will I need to take it?

You should discuss this with your doctor. At first you will be given fluoxetine for about 2 months, so that we can find out if it helps you. If fluoxetine is helpful, the patient should continue taking it for at least 6 months. This is necessary because research studies suggest that patients who stop treatment sooner run the risk of becoming depressed again. Do not stop taking fluoxetine suddenly, talk to your doctor first.

What are the side effects?

Fluoxetine is one of the newer anti-depressants and has fewer side effects than the older anti-depressants. However, some side effects may occur. More common side effects include feelings of nausea, mild stomach pains, and sometimes diarrhoea or loss of appetite. These symptoms are usually relieved effectively by reduction in dosage. Some young people experience drowsiness, dry mouth and headache. If you have any concerns about possible side effects, please contact your doctor immediately. You should not take them if you are pregnant or you are thinking of becoming pregnant. Girls who could become pregnant must use an effective contraceptive whilst they are taking fluoxetine. You should avoid drinking too much alcohol, or taking other drugs whilst on fluoxetine.

Some people may develop symptoms such as dizziness, nausea, lethargy, headache, anxiety and poor sleep if they stop taking fluoxetine too quickly. Your doctor will explain to you how to avoid these symptoms.

Like many other drugs, in some countries fluoxetine is not licensed for use with children and the information leaflet sheet that comes with the medication may state that it is not recommended for use with children. However, fluoxetine has been tested in several clinical trials with children and these have shown that it is both effective and safe.

Are there any long-term side effects of taking fluoxetine?

Very little is known about the long-term effects of taking fluoxetine in adolescence. We do know, however, that depression can sometimes cause long-term problems and this is one of the reasons it must be treated promptly.

Who can take fluoxetine?

Anyone who is physically fit can take fluoxetine. However, you should not take the tablets if you have ever developed a rash or possible allergy to fluoxetine, if you have a serious medical condition, or if you suffer from any serious liver or kidney complaint.

When will I start to feel better and what are the chances of it working?

Research studies have shown that depressed adolescents who take fluoxetine or similar drugs are more likely to improve than depressed adolescents who are not given fluoxetine. This improvement does not usually start until between 2 and 4 weeks after the medication has started.

No treatment will work in every case, and around one-third of depressed adolescents given fluoxetine will still have difficulties after their course of treatment. It is important that fluoxetine is given a proper chance to work, so in our clinic it is given at full dosage for at least 8 weeks. If it has not worked after that, then other kinds of treatments will be given. There is a very good chance that you will be feeling better within 6 months.

What other treatments are available for depression in adolescents?

Your doctor will talk with you about this. In our clinic, fluoxetine and other medications will not normally be given unless non-medical treatments have been tried. Thus, in all instances, we will try to work with the adolescent and their family, to resolve the problems that are often associated with depression in this age group, such as family difficulties, bullying, etc. In some cases you will be offered a form of counselling.

What if I have any more questions?

If you have any further questions, in the first instance, please discuss them with the doctor who has prescribed fluoxetine for you. If you would like to speak to the consultant, then you should contact Dr XXX, Tel. YYY.

5

Anxiety disorders

Thomas H. Ollendick[1] and Laura D. Seligman[2]

[1] Department of Psychology, Virginia Polytechnic Institute and State University, USA
[2] Department of Psychology, University of Toledo, OH, USA

Introduction

The anxiety disorders constitute a broad spectrum of syndromes ranging from very circumscribed anxiety to pervasive, sometimes 'free-floating' anxiety or worry. As such, they are the most common group of psychiatric illnesses in children and adolescents (as well as adults). With the most recent editions of the *Diagnostic and Statistical Manual of Mental Disorders* (DSM-IV; APA, 1994) and, similarly, the *International Statistical Classification of Diseases and Related Health Problems* (ICD-10; WHO, 1992), the symptoms of children, adolescents and adults can be categorized by eight major but separate diagnostic syndromes associated with anxiety: panic disorder with agoraphobia, panic disorder without agoraphobia, agoraphobia without history of panic, specific phobia, social phobia, obsessive-compulsive disorder, post-traumatic stress disorder and generalized anxiety disorder.

Additionally, the DSM-IV and ICD-10 specify one anxiety disorder specific only to childhood: separation anxiety disorder. Earlier versions of the DSM included two additional anxiety diagnoses specific to childhood, namely avoidant disorder and overanxious disorder. In the most recent revision, however, avoidant disorder and overanxious disorder have been subsumed under the categories of social phobia and generalized anxiety disorder, respectively. Considerable evidence suggests that avoidant disorder and overanxious disorder are not distinct syndromes nor sufficiently different from their adult counterparts to merit separate diagnostic categories. For example, it has been shown that children and adolescents with avoidant disorder are no different from those with social phobia on a variety of sociodemographic variables including race, socioeconomic status or age at intake. Furthermore, neither rates of co-morbidity with affective disorders and

A Clinician's Handbook of Child and Adolescent Psychiatry, ed. Christopher Gillberg,
Richard Harrington and Hans-Christoph Steinhausen. Published by Cambridge University Press.
© Cambridge University Press 2005.

other anxiety disorders nor self-reported depression or fears were different for the two groups of children and adolescents. Similarly, no appreciable differences have been found between overanxious disorder and generalized anxiety disorder.

Although diagnostic systems such as the DSM and ICD describe anxiety as falling into several distinct syndromes or categories, there is also a rich body of literature examining anxiety at the symptom level. Rather than defining categorical distinctions, this view embraces a dimensional approach, examining the number of anxiety symptoms experienced by children and adolescents and the frequency or severity of such symptoms. This tradition is best illustrated in the work of Achenbach and his colleagues who have developed standardized measures such as the Child Behaviour Checklist, Teacher Report Form and Youth Self-Report. A broad index of anxiety is obtained from these measures.

As is evident, a wide range of topics is subsumed under the heading of anxiety disorders in childhood. This chapter will be limited to that perspective which examines anxiety as syndromes or disorders and, more specifically, to the examination of separation anxiety disorder, generalized anxiety/overanxious disorder, panic disorder, social phobia and specific (isolated) phobias. Obsessive-compulsive disorders and post-traumatic stress disorders are considered separately in Chapters 6 and 8 of this volume.

Separation anxiety disorder (SAD)

Definition and classification

The main feature of SAD is an excessive and unrealistic fear of separation from a major attachment figure that is unusual for the individual's developmental level. The DSM-IV and ICD-10 include a similar list of eight specific indicators of SAD (see Table 5.1).

In general, both classification systems include symptoms related to:

- recurrent distress upon or in anticipation of separation
- worries about harm to the attachment figure or the child him or herself that would result in separation
- difficulties in attending school or being alone or without the attachment figure in other settings, problems sleeping alone
- nightmares about separation and
- physical symptoms either upon or in anticipation of separation.

Both require that the symptoms result in some degree of impairment; ICD-10 specifies that impairment is in the social domain whereas DSM-IV indicates that symptoms may result in impairment not only in social domains but also in academic, family and other domains. DSM-IV and ICD-10 differ in terms of requirements for

Table 5.1. Diagnostic criteria for separation anxiety disorder

DSM-IV	ICD-10
A. Developmentally inappropriate and excessive anxiety concerning separation from home or from those to whom the individual is attached, as evidenced by three (or more) of the following: 1. recurrent excessive distress when separation from home or major attachment figures occurs or is anticipated 2. persistent and excessive worry about losing, or about possible harm befalling, major attachment figures 3. persistent and excessive worry that an untoward event will lead to separation from a major attachment figure (e.g. getting lost or being kidnapped) 4. persistent reluctance or refusal to go to school or elsewhere because of fear of separation 5. persistently and excessively fearful or reluctant to be alone or without major attachment figures at home or without significant adults in other settings 6. persistent reluctance or refusal to go to sleep without being near a major attachment figure or to sleep away from home 7. repeated nightmares involving the theme of separation 8. repeated complaints of physical symptoms (such as headaches, stomachaches, nausea, or vomiting) when separation from major attachment figures occurs or is anticipated	The key diagnostic feature is a focused excessive anxiety concerning separation from those individuals to whom the child is attached (usually parents or other family members) that is not merely part of a generalized anxiety about multiple situations. The anxiety may take the form of: (a) an unrealistic, preoccupying worry about possible harm befalling major attachment figures or a fear that they will leave and not return; (b) an unrealistic, preoccupying worry that some untoward event, such as the child being lost, kidnapped, admitted to hospital, or killed, will separate him or her from a major attachment figure; (c) persistent reluctance or refusal to go to school because of fear about separation (rather than for other reasons such as fear about events at school); (d) persistent reluctance or refusal to go to sleep without being near or next to a major attachment figure; (e) persistent inappropriate fear of being alone, or otherwise without the major attachment figure, at home during the day; (f) repeated nightmares about separation; (g) repeated occurrence of physical symptoms (nausea, stomach ache, headache, vomiting, etc.) on occasions that involve separation from a major attachment figure, such as leaving home to go to school; (h) excessive, recurrent distress (as shown by anxiety, crying, tantrums, misery, apathy, or social withdrawal) in anticipation of, during, or immediately following separation from a major attachment figure.

Table 5.1. (*cont.*)

DSM-IV	ICD-10
B. The duration of the disturbance is at least 4 weeks. C. The onset is before age 18 years. D. The disturbance causes clinically significant distress or impairment in social, academic (occupational), or other important areas of functioning. E. The disturbance does not occur exclusively during the course of a Pervasive Developmental Disorder, Schizophrenia, or other Psychotic Disorder and, in adolescents and adults, is not better accounted for by Panic Disorder With Agoraphobia. **(a) Specify if:** (a) Early Onset: if onset occurs before age 6 years	Many situations that involve separation also involve other potential stressors or sources of anxiety. The diagnosis rests on the demonstration that the common element giving rise to anxiety in the various situations is the circumstance of separation from a major attachment figure. This arises most commonly, perhaps, in relation to school refusal (or 'phobia'). Often, this does represent separation anxiety but sometimes (especially in adolescence) it does not. School refusal arising for the first time in adolescence should not be coded here unless it is primarily a function of separation anxiety and that anxiety was first evident to an abnormal degree during the preschool years. Unless those criteria are met, the syndrome should be coded in one of the other categories in F93 or under F40–F48. Excludes: * mood [affective] disorders (F30–F39) * neurotic disorders (F40–F48) * phobic anxiety disorder of childhood (F93.1) * social anxiety disorder of childhood (F93.2)

age of onset. While DSM-IV specifies an age of onset anytime prior to 18 years, the ICD-10 indicates that separation concerns must be present during the preschool years and SAD is only diagnosed during late childhood and adolescence when symptoms are a continuation of concerns first manifested during early childhood. DSM-IV is also more specific in that it requires symptoms to occur for a minimum of 4 weeks; ICD-10 includes no specific criterion for minimum duration.

Finally, DSM-IV includes an early onset specifier. This applies in cases in which symptom onset occurs prior to age six; this is not relevant for the ICD-10 diagnosis since onset must be early. Little is known about the clinical implications of early onset or whether youth with an early onset represent a distinct group.

Epidemiology

Prevalence and incidence rates

Most community surveys estimate the prevalence rate of SAD to be around 3.5–5 per cent. Young children mostly account for these cases as the rate in adolescence decreases to less than 1 per cent. However, in prepubertal children SAD tends to be the most commonly reported anxiety disorder in epidemiological as well as referred clinical samples.

Sex ratios and ethnicity

SAD tends to be somewhat more common in girls than boys though in young children the difference tends to be quite small and with older children and adolescents discrepancies may be partially accounted for by the hesitancy of boys to report separation fears.

The degree to which separation from attachment figures early in life is valued or expected varies to a great degree across cultures. This may affect both the degree to which separation concerns are interpreted as symptomatic and the amount of distress and impairment engendered by the symptoms. Additionally, youth from various ethnic backgrounds may present with somewhat different clinical pictures. For example, some evidence suggests European-American youth are more likely to present with school refusal as part of SAD while African-American youth may more typically present with specific fears.

Implications for clinical practice

Prior to adolescence SAD is one of the most common anxiety disorders seen in clinical practice, with roughly equal numbers of boys and girls seeking treatment. Although the disorder may persist into adolescence and even adulthood, it is relatively rare in post-pubertal children.

Clinical picture

Main features and symptoms

The main feature of SAD is excessive distress either before or during separation from an attachment figure, usually the mother. Often this is manifested in tantrums when separation is attempted. Somatic complaints in order to prevent separation or in response to separation are also common.

School refusal is a particularly debilitating symptom and one that often serves as the impetus for families to seek treatment. However, SAD is not the sole cause of school refusal or school phobia and other causes such as social phobia and oppositional behaviour must be considered.

Children with SAD may complain of sleep difficulties either because they are unable to sleep alone or because they experience nightmares when they sleep. Perceptual distortions, especially at night or surrounding bedtime may also be reported. For example, these children may interpret noises or shadows as burglars. In addition, the refusal to separate may interfere with academic performance and some children with SAD may have missed significant amounts of schooling before coming for treatment. Similarly, because of the reluctance to engage in social activities that result in separation, especially overnight activities, youth with SAD may have significantly limited opportunities for socialization and many report at least some degree of social problems.

The added parenting responsibilities that often come along with having a child with SAD may cause conflict and distress among family members and in some cases the parent (or other attachment figure) may also report anxiety around separating from the child.

Differential diagnosis and co-morbidity

SAD is often co-morbid with other anxiety disorders and depression. Although it is thought that SAD may develop into panic disorder (PD) later in life, concurrent comorbidity is rare in that SAD is evident mostly in young children and panic disorder rarely manifests itself until adolescence. Children with SAD may, however, experience panic attacks upon, or in anticipation of, separation. This condition can be distinguished from PD in that the child is fearful of separation or an event, such as kidnapping, that would result in separation and not the panic attack itself.

SAD may also be confused with generalized anxiety disorder (GAD), given that children may express numerous fears; however, in SAD the fears revolve around the theme of separation or a threat that would result in separation whereas in GAD there may be no unifying theme or numerous, broad or overarching themes. Children with GAD may also dwell on worries about past events while this would be less typical of children with SAD.

When school refusal is a primary symptom, SAD must be differentiated from social phobia, oppositional defiant disorder, or even a specific phobia.

- It must be determined whether the child is motivated to avoid characteristics of the school environment itself, in which case a diagnosis of social or specific phobia may be more appropriate.
- If the child refuses to go to school because this enables him or her to engage in activities that are more reinforcing than schoolwork or if the refusal is used as a form of retaliation, a diagnosis of Oppositional Defiant Disorder (ODD) should be considered. It may be helpful to keep in mind that SAD may be seen more often in younger children while more serious manifestations of ODD are more likely in older children.
- If the child would experience little or no discomfort at school if the primary attachment figure was there or when the child's concerns centre around harm befalling the attachment figure or the child him or herself a diagnosis of SAD is most likely.

Assessment

Most diagnostic interviews designed for use with young children contain sections for the assessment of SAD and can be used in conjunction with a clinical interview. The Anxiety Disorders Interview Schedule for Children (ADIS-IV/C+P) was designed specifically to assess for anxiety disorders and, as such, it may be the most appropriate when anxiety is the primary concern. Other useful diagnostic interviews include the NIMH Diagnostic Interview Schedule for Children (DISC) and the Diagnostic Interview for Children and Adolescents–Revised (DICA-R).

Many questionnaires exist to assess anxiety in youth and some of the more recent ones have items that map directly onto the SAD diagnostic criteria. Recommended self-report instruments include the Multidimensional Anxiety Scale for Children (MASC), the Screen for Child Anxiety Related Emotional Disorders (SCARED), the Spence Children's Anxiety Scale (SCAS) and the Fear Survey Schedule for Children – Revised (FSSC-R, see Appendix 5.1). A list of recommended interviews and questionnaires can be found in Table 5.2. Although these instruments are not specific to SAD in that they assess for other anxiety disorders or the physiological, cognitive and subjective components of anxiety in general, they can be helpful in obtaining information about SAD and differentiating it from related disorders.

In order to assess for co-morbidity and to assist in differential diagnosis, a thorough assessment for depression should be conducted. The Children's Depression Inventory (CDI) might be considered under such circumstances. When school refusal is present, the School Refusal Assessment Scale (SRAS) can be a useful aid for differential diagnosis.

Generalized anxiety disorder

Definition and classification

Both the DSM-IV and the ICD-10 identify the main features of GAD as:
- excessive free-floating worry
- somatic symptoms associated with the worry or as a result of the worry (e.g. tension headaches).

The complete diagnostic criteria for GAD according to both classification systems are presented in Table 5.3. All of the symptoms of GAD specified in ICD-10 are included in the DSM-IV diagnostic criteria, although they are separated and the conceptual organization is somewhat different. In addition, DSM-IV goes further in that it specifies that the worry must be difficult to control. The DSM-IV is also more specific in terms of the duration of symptoms required (i.e. 6 months) and the number of somatic symptoms that must be present (i.e. three for adults and

Table 5.2. Representative assessment options: description and psychometric properties

Instrument	Description	Subscales/procedural comments	Psychometric properties
Anxiety Disorders Interview Schedule – Child / Parent (ADIS-C/P). *Source:* Silverman, W. K. & Albano, A. M. (1996). *Anxiety Disorders Interview Schedule for DSM-IV, Child and Parent Versions.* San Antonio, TX: Psychological Corporation.	Structured diagnostic clinical interview, child and parent versions.	Screens for all childhood internalizing and externalizing disorders of DSM-IV but especially useful for the anxiety and phobic disorders.	– Inter-rater reliability 0.98 ADIS-C, 0.93 ADIS-P; – Retest reliability 0.76 ADIS-C, 0.67 ADIS-P; – Sensitivity to treatment effects for childhood anxiety and phobias.
Behavioural avoidance tests (BAT; in vivo, exposure-based assessment of approach/avoidance of a phobic stimulus) *Source:* Ollendick, T. H. & Cerny, J. A. (1981). *Clinical Behavior Therapy with Children.* New York: Plenum Press.	Although heterogeneity for BAT procedures exists in the literature, typically a child is asked to enter a room containing the relevant phobic stimulus. The child's approach toward the stimulus is recorded and a percentage of steps or stages completed out of the total number of steps is calculated.	Differing opinions regarding the number of steps, as well as differing steps for different stimuli. For example, our phobia project currently uses 10 steps for dog phobia and 13 steps for snake phobia.	– BAT performance seems to be reliable for any one type of BAT for any one given child; – However, the heterogeneity of procedures makes large comparisons difficult across studies; – Issues of test-retest reliability and standardization of procedures are currently being addressed by our phobia project.
Child Anxiety Sensitivity Index (CASI). *Source:* Silverman, W. K., Fleisig, W., Rabian, B. & Peterson, R. (1991). Childhood Anxiety Sensitivity Index (CASI). *Journal of Clinical Child Psychology,* **20,** 162–8. App. B	Self-report measure consisting of 18 items, Likert scale (3-point: none, some a lot). Assesses fear of anxiety symptoms or 'fear of fear.' Useful for ages 7–16.	Consists of a total score and three subscale scores: physical concerns, mental incapacitation concerns and social concerns.	– Excellent to satisfactory retest reliability (0.76 for clinical sample and 0.79 for non-clinical sample at 2-week interval); – Internal consistency 0.87; – Anxious children have significantly higher total and subscale scores than non-clinical matched controls.

(cont.)

Table 5.2. (cont.)

Instrument	Description	Subscales/procedural comments	Psychometric properties
Child Behaviour Checklist (CBCL); *Source:* Achenbach, T. M. (1991). *Integrative guide for the 1991 CBCL/4–18, YSR, and TRF profiles.* Burlington: University of Vermont.	Measure typically filled out by a child's parent or caretaker. Inquires generically into a child's skills, behaviours, interactions, and hobbies. Age range 4 to 18 years.	Separates internalizing and externalizing difficulties into various problem scales which can be useful: withdrawn, somatic complaints, anxious/depressed, social problems, thought problems, attention problems, delinquent behaviour and aggression	– Satisfactory to excellent retest reliability (approx 0.89 at 1 week, 0.75 at 1 year, 0.71 at 2 years; – Inter-rater agreement approx 0.65 to 0.75 for parents; – Scaled scores can be interpreted such that there is an 89.1% correct classification rate.
Direct Observation of Anxiety (DOA). *Source:* Ollendick, T. H. & Cerny, J. A. (1981). *Clinical Behavior Therapy with Children.* New York: Plenum Press.	A child's anxious behaviours (e.g. shaking, sweating, clinging, trembling, crying) are typically coded by an observer based upon a predetermined observation system.	Various protocols exist for the observation of many different types of anxiety. These differing methodologies also incorporate differing numbers of behaviours to be recorded.	– Diverse methodologies and coding systems exist. – Reliabilities are reported to range from low to very high depending on the coding protocol.
Fear Survey Schedule for Children–Revised (FSSC-R). *Source:* Ollendick, T. H. (1983). Reliability and validity of the Revised Fear Survey Schedule for Children (FSSC-R). *Behaviour Research and Therapy,* **21** 685–92. App. A.	Self-report, measure consisting of 80 specific phobia items, Likert scale (3-point: none, some, a lot). Useful for ages 7–16.	Consists of a total score and five subscales: fear of failure, fear of the unknown, fear of injury and small animals, fear of danger and death, and medical fears.	– Excellent to satisfactory retest reliability (approx. 0.82 at 1 week and 0.55 at 3 months), Alpha = 0.95; – School phobic children have significantly higher total scores than matched controls, as do children with specific phobias; – Discriminates significantly between different types of specific phobia when completed by parent or child.

Measure and source	Description	Reliability and validity
Multidimensional Anxiety Scale for Children (MASC). *Source:* March, J., Parker, J., Sullivan, K., Stallings, P. & Conners, C. K. (1997). The MASC: Factor structure, reliability, and validity. *Journal of the American Academy of Child and Adolescent Psychiatry,* **36**, 554–65.	Measures wide range of anxiety symptoms, Likert scale (4-point) self-report, 39-items, age range 8 to 18 years. Four factors with subfactors including – physical symptoms (tense/somatic), harm avoidance (anxious coping/perfectionism), social anxiety (humiliation/performance) and separation anxiety.	– Internal reliability of total score is 0.90; – Satisfactory to excellent retest reliability (0.79 at 3 weeks, 0.93 at 3 months); – Good convergent validity with RCMAS (0.63); – Excellent discriminative validity between anxious and normal controls with 87% correct classification.
Revised Children's Manifest Anxiety Scale (RCMAS). *Source:* Reynolds, C. R. & Richmond, B. O. (1985). *Revised Children's Manifest Anxiety Scale manual.* Los Angeles: Western Psychological Services.	Self-report, measure consisting of 37 items related to anxiety; age range 6 to 19 years, response is 'yes' or 'no'. Consists of a total anxiety score and four subscale scores: physiological anxiety, worry/oversensitivity, concerns/concentration, social and lie/social desirability.	– Satisfactory retest reliability (approx. 0.68 at 9 months); – Discriminates significantly between state and trait anxiety when compared to the STAIC (RCMAS scores associated with 'chronic manifest or generalized anxiety'.
Screen for Child Anxiety Related Emotional Disorders – Revised (SCARED-R). *Source:* Muris, P., Merckelbach, H., Schmidt, H. & Mayer, B. (1999). The revised version of the SCARED-R: Factor structure in normal children. *Personality and Individual Differences,* **26**, 99–112.	Self-report measure consisting of 66 items related to DSM-IV anxiety disorders, age range 8 to 18 years, response is on a 3-point Likert scale. Consists of a total scale score and seven subscale scores: separation anxiety disorder, generalized anxiety disorder, panic disorder, social phobia, obsessive-compulsive disorder, traumatic stress disorder and specific phobias.	– Internal reliability of total score is 0.94; – Internal reliability of specific phobia scale is 0.58– 0.71; – Good convergent validity with FSSC-R (total Scale correlates 0.64; – Discriminates significantly between anxious and disruptive disorders.
Spence Child Anxiety Scale (SCAS). *Source:* Spence, S. H. (1997). Structure of anxiety symptoms among children: a confirmatory factor-analytic study. *Journal of Abnormal Psychology,* **106**, 280–97.	Self-report measure consisting of 38 items related to DSM-IV anxiety disorders, age range 8 to 16 years, response is on a 4-point Likert scale ranging from never to always. Consists of a total scale score and six subscale scores: separation anxiety, generalized anxiety, panic, social phobia, obsessive-compulsive and fears/phobias.	– Internal reliability of total score of 0.93; – Internal reliability of subscales all above 0.80; – Good convergent validity with RCMAS and internalizing score of CBCL but not Externalizing Score; – Discriminates significantly between anxious and disruptive behaviour disorders.

(*cont.*)

Table 5.2. (cont.)

Instrument	Description	Subscales/procedural comments	Psychometric properties
Spider Phobia Questionnaire Source: Kindt, M., Brosschot, J. F. & Muris. P. (1996). Spider phobia questionnaire for children (SPQ-C): a psychometric study and normative data. *Behaviour Research and Therapy*, **34**, 277–82.	Self-report measure consisting of 29 spider phobia related items, response is 'true' or 'not true'.	Scores on all items are summed to create a total score that suggests the degree of spider fear.	– Satisfactory test – retest reliability (approx 0.61 at 6–7 weeks); – Discriminates significantly between spider phobic and non-phobic girls.
Teacher Report Form (TRF). *Source:* Achenbach, T. M. (1991). *Integrative Guide for the 1991 CBCL/4–18, YSR, and TRF Profiles.* Burlington: University of Vermont.	Measure typically filled out by a child's teacher. Inquires generically into a child's skills, interactions, and hobbies, as well as maladaptive behaviours.	Separates internalizing and externalizing difficulties into various problem scales which can be useful: withdrawn, somatic complaints, anxious/depressed, social problems, thought problems, attention problems, delinquent behaviour and aggressive behaviour.	– Satisfactory to excellent retest reliability (approx. 0.9 at 2 weeks, 0.75 at 2 months, 0.66 at 4 months); – Inter-rater agreement approx 0.54 for teachers seeing students in different settings; – Scaled scores can be interpreted such that there is a 79.3% correct classification rate.
Youth Self-Report (YSR). *Source:* Achenbach, T. M. (1991). *Integrative Guide for the 1991 CBCL/4–18, YSR, and TRF Profiles.* Burlington: University of Vermont.	Measure typically filled out by the child. Inquires generically into a child's skills, interactions, and hobbies, as well as problematic behaviours.	Separates internalizing and externalizing difficulties into various problem scales which can be useful: withdrawn, somatic complaints, anxious/depressed, social problems, thought problems, attention problems, delinquent behaviour and aggressive behaviour.	– Satisfactory retest reliability (approx. 0.72 at 1 week, 0.49 at 7 months); – Scaled scores can be interpreted such that there is a 71.9% correct classification rate.

Table 5.3. Diagnostic criteria for generalized anxiety disorder

DSM-IV	ICD-10
A. Excessive anxiety and worry (apprehensive expectation), occurring more days than not for at least 6 months, about a number of events or activities (such as work or school performance).	The sufferer must have primary symptoms of anxiety most days for at least several weeks at a time, and usually for several months. These symptoms should usually involve elements of:
B. The person finds it difficult to control the worry.	(a) apprehension (worries about future misfortunes, feeling 'on edge', difficulty in concentrating, etc.);
C. The anxiety and worry are associated with three (or more) of the following six symptoms (with at least some symptoms present for more days than not for the past 6 months). *Note:* Only one item is required in children.	(b) motor tension (restless fidgeting, tension headaches, trembling, inability to relax); and (c) autonomic overactivity (lightheadedness, sweating, tachycardia or tachypnoea, epigastric discomfort, dizziness, dry mouth, etc.).
1. restlessness or feeling keyed up or on edge	In children, frequent need for reassurance and recurrent somatic complaints may be prominent.
2. being easily fatigued	The transient appearance (for a few days at a time) of other symptoms, particularly depression, does not rule out generalized anxiety disorder as a main diagnosis, but the sufferer must not meet the full criteria for depressive episode, phobic anxiety disorder, panic disorder, or obsessive-compulsive disorder.
3. difficulty concentrating or mind going blank	
4. irritability	
5. muscle tension	
6. sleep disturbance (difficulty falling or staying asleep, or restless unsatisfying sleep)	
D. The focus of the anxiety and worry is not confined to features of an Axis I disorder, e.g. the anxiety or worry is not about having a panic attack (as in panic disorder), being embarrassed in public (as in social phobia), being contaminated (as in obsessive-compulsive disorder), being away from home or close relatives (as in separation anxiety disorder), gaining weight (as in anorexia nervosa), having multiple physical complaints (as in somatization disorder), or having a serious illness (as in hypochondriasis), and the anxiety and worry do not occur exclusively during post-traumatic stress disorder.	Includes: *anxiety neurosis *anxiety reaction *anxiety state
E. The anxiety, worry, or physical symptoms cause clinically significant distress or impairment in social, occupational, or other important areas of functioning.	Excludes: *neurasthenia
F. The disturbance is not due to the direct physiological effects of a substance (e.g. a drug of abuse, a medication) or a general medical condition (e.g. hyperthyroidism) and does not occur exclusively during a mood disorder, a psychotic disorder, or a pervasive developmental disorder.	

adolescents, 1 for children). DSM-IV also requires clinically significant impairment as a result of the symptoms.

A significant difference between the two classification systems is that the ICD-10 does not allow for the dual diagnosis of GAD with Depression, Panic Disorder, Obsessive-Compulsive disorder, or a phobic disorder. DSM-IV, on the other hand, specifies that the worry must not be limited to a theme that would be better accounted for by another disorder; however, if this criterion is met, it does allow for comorbid diagnoses.

GAD now subsumes the diagnosis of Overanxious Disorder of childhood, present in DSM-III-R and ICD-9. The primary difference between GAD and Overanxious Disorder is in the greater emphasis on somatic symptoms in the GAD diagnosis. However, DSM-IV does specify modifications to the number of somatic symptoms that must be present in children. In addition, the worry described by GAD is a future focused worry or anxious apprehension whereas the criteria for Overanxious Disorder indicated that children may worry about their performance and behaviour during past events as well.

Epidemiology

Prevalence and incidence rates

If it is assumed that children who had previously met diagnosis for Overanxious Disorder would meet the current GAD diagnostic criteria, prevalence rates for GAD in community samples is around 6 per cent. Some studies, however, suggest a much lower rate, even below 1 per cent.

Sex ratios and ethnicity

The disorder appears to be somewhat more common in girls than boys and more frequently affects older children and adolescents.

Although some form of GAD seems to be present across many cultures, the ways in which anxiety and apprehension are expressed may vary. For example, although some children may openly express and verbalize anxious concerns, for others this may be manifested as perfectionism or numerous somatic complaints.

Implications for clinical practice

GAD is not uncommon in help-seeking samples but may masquerade as a physical complaint for some time before the emotional component of the disorder is recognized. Frequently, GAD co-occurs with both SAD and the depressive disorders. As a result, differential diagnosis is critical.

Clinical picture

Main features and symptoms

Youth presenting with GAD may first come in with physical complaints and may have sought medical treatment numerous times before being recognized. These children may be perfectionist and, although some children and adolescents with GAD express age-consistent worries such as concerns about school and athletic performance, others will express concerns that appear to be beyond their years, such as the state of world affairs and the possibility of war or concerns about family economics or parental job security. Often concerns focus on health issues both for the child and other family members. Children may seek excessive reassurance or comfort from family members, or in some cases, the child, may have limited activities in order to avoid information that has the potential to lead to additional worries. For example, some parents of GAD children will not allow the child to watch television in order to avoid any news stories that could cause or exacerbate the child's concerns.

Anxiety disorders and depression are not unusual in family members of children with GAD so the clinical picture may be complicated by impairment or limited functioning in the child's care providers.

Differential diagnosis and co-morbidity

Differential diagnosis and co-morbidity will vary with the diagnostic system used. Without restrictions, GAD is often co-morbid with depression and other anxiety disorders, particularly SAD.

Because of the somatic complaints present in GAD and the physical disorders that may cause tension or mimic anxiety, it is important that a thorough physical examination is conducted to differentiate GAD from physical disorders such as hyperthyroidism. Moreover, if somatic complaints coupled with worries about health and disease limited to the child him or herself are the only concern, a somatoform disorder should be considered.

Additionally, if numerous worries are present but revolve around a unified theme such as social embarrassment or separation, the more specific anxiety disorder diagnosis is appropriate. GAD must also be distinguished from eating disorders (see Chapter 10) if the worries are solely related to weight or appearance; concerns about appearance are often present in youth with GAD but are part of a larger picture of more diffuse worries. In addition, given the nature of obsessional worry in GAD it can be difficult to distinguish from OCD. In GAD the worry tends to be around realistic or everyday concerns although the degree of worry is excessive; in OCD, the worry tends to be of a less realistic nature and is typically ego-dystonic.

For young children the latter distinction, however, may either not be true or can be difficult to assess.

Assessment

Although no specific instruments to assess GAD in youth are in widespread use, the diagnostic interviews and questionnaires listed in Table 5.2 provide information for the diagnosis of GAD and associated symptomatology. In addition, the Revised Children's Manifest Anxiety Scale (RCMAS) is frequently used to measure generalized or 'manifest' anxiety, even though it is becoming somewhat outdated at this time.

Panic disorder

Definition and classification

The primary diagnostic features of PD according to both the DSM-IV and the ICD-10 are:
- recurrent, intense but time-limited periods of fear
- the attacks must be unexpected or at least initially not associated with a specific situation
- the attacks involve autonomic and/or cognitive symptoms such as fears that one will go crazy or die.

The DSM-IV and ICD-10 criteria for PD are listed in Table 5.4. In addition, the DSM-IV criteria for a panic attack and for agoraphobia are listed in Tables 5.5 and 5.6, respectively. Both the DSM-IV and the ICD-10 require that multiple panic attacks occur within a period of 1 month to meet criteria for PD. In general, as with the other anxiety disorders, the diagnostic criteria included in DSM-IV are somewhat more specific. For instance, DSM-IV requires a minimum of four attacks within a 1-month period and a minimum of 4 of 13 specified autonomic or cognitive symptoms to constitute a full-blown panic attack. DSM-IV also recognizes that the attacks, although initially unpredictable, may become associated with certain situations or cues over time.

Despite the similarities in the two classification systems, two important conceptual differences exist. First, the DSM-IV requires at least a 1-month period in which there is a change in behaviour pursuant to the attacks or that the individual develops a fear of additional attacks or their implications. Thus, in the DSM system, the core of the disorder is what is commonly termed 'the fear of fear', whereas in the ICD system the presence of panic attacks – not the fear of fear – constitutes the disorder. This is an important distinction in that panic attacks can and do occur with other disorders and, while many individuals experience panic attacks, those who

Table 5.4. Diagnostic criteria for panic disorder

DSM-IV	ICD-10

Panic Disorder With Agoraphobia
A. Both (1) and (2)
  (1) recurrent unexpected panic attacks
  (2) at least one of the attacks has been followed by 1 month (or more) of one (or more) of the following:
    (a) persistent concern about having additional attacks
    (b) worry about the implicaton of the attack or its consequences (e.g. losing control, having a heart attack, 'going crazy')
    (c) a significant change in behaviour related to the attacks
B. The presence of agoraphobia
C. The panic attacks are not due to the direct physiological effects of a substance (e.g. a drug of abuse, a medication) or a general medical condition (e.g. hyperthyroidism).
D. The panic attacks are not better accounted for by another mental disorder, such as social phobia (e.g. occurring on exposure to feared social situations), specific phobia (e.g. on exposure to a specific phobic situation), obsessive-compulsive disorder (e.g. on exposure to dirt in someone with an obsession about contamination), post-traumatic stress disorder (e.g. in response to stimuli associated with a severe stressor), or separation anxiety disorder (e.g. in response to being away from home or close relatives).
	In this classification, a panic attack that occurs in an established phobic situation is regarded as an expression of the severity of the phobia, which should be given diagnostic precedence. Panic disorder should be the main diagnosis only in the absence of any of the phobias in F40.
	
	For a definite diagnosis, several severe attacks of autonomic anxiety should have occurred within a period of about 1 month:
	  (a) in circumstances where there is no objective danger;
	  (b) without being confined to known or predictable situations; and
	  (c) with comparative freedom from anxiety symptoms between attacks (although anticipatory anxiety is common).
	
	Includes:
	*panic attack
	*panic state

Note: The criteria for panic disorder without agoraphobia are identical with the exception of criteria B which states 'The Absence of Agoraphobia'.

interpret them as dangerous or become preoccupied with a possible reoccurrence appear to constitute the PD group that experiences considerably more associated impairment.

The second difference is that in the DSM-IV agoraphobia is always considered in the diagnosis of PD. Three possible diagnoses are available, PD without Agoraphobia, PD with agoraphobia, and agoraphobia without history of panic,

Table 5.5. DSM-IV definition of a panic attack

A discrete period of intense fear or discomfort, in which four (or more) of the following symptoms developed abruptly and reached a peak within 10 minutes:

1. palpitations, pounding heart, or accelerated heart rate
2. sweating
3. trembling or shaking
4. sensations of shortness of breath or smothering
5. feeling of choking
6. chest pain or discomfort
7. nausea or abdominal distress
8. feeling dizzy, unsteady, lightheaded, or faint
9. derealization (feelings of unreality) or depersonalization (being detached from oneself)
10. fear of losing control or going crazy
11. fear of dying
12. paresthesias (numbness or tingling sensations)
13. chills or hot flushes

Table 5.6. DSM-IV definition of agoraphobia

A. Anxiety about being in places or situations from which escape might be difficult (or embarrassing) or in which help may not be available in the event of having an unexpected or situationally predisposed panic attack or panic-like symptoms. Agoraphobic fears typically involve characteristic clusters of situations that include being outside the home alone; being in a crowd or standing in a line; being on a bridge; and traveling in a bus, train, or automobile.

   Note: Consider the diagnosis of specific phobia if the avoidance is limited to one or only a few specific situations, or social phobia if the avoidance is limited to social situations.

B. The situations are avoided (e.g. travel is restricted) or else are endured with marked distress or with anxiety about having a panic attack or panic-like symptoms, or require the presence of a companion.

C. The anxiety or phobic avoidance is not better accounted for by another mental disorder, such as social phobia (e.g. avoidance limited to social situations because of fear of embarrassment), specific phobia (e.g. avoidance limited to a single situation like elevators), obsessive-compulsive disorder (e.g. avoidance of dirt in someone with an obsession about contamination), post-traumatic stress disorder (e.g. avoidance of stimuli associated with a severe stressor), or separation anxiety disorder (e.g. avoidance of leaving home or relatives).

although this latter diagnosis is less commonly applied, especially in children. No such link is made in the ICD-10. This is because the DSM-IV considers agoraphobia to be avoidance of situations or excessive anxiety about being in situations in which a panic attack might take place or in which it would be difficult to escape should an attack occur. In contrast, ICD-10 considers agoraphobia to be the fear of open or crowded places or a fear of situations in which escape might be difficult. Although ICD-10 provides diagnostic codes to indicate the presence or absence of PD when agoraphobia is the main diagnosis, no explicit conceptual link is made.

Epidemiology

Prevalence and incidence rates

PD is rare in prepubertal children and some believe that the condition does not exist prior to puberty. Others, however, have shown that panic attacks certainly occur prior to pubescence, and that PD itself can and does occur (although infrequently). Typical onset is either in adolescence or young adulthood. In adolescence, PD is less common than many of the other anxiety disorders, occurring in about 1 per cent of youth.

Sex ratios and ethnicity

PD is seen more commonly in girls than boys, as is the associated agoraphobic avoidance. Currently, no data are available about ethnic or cultural differences.

Implications for clinical practice

Although PD is not seen commonly in paediatric community samples, the degree of impairment engendered by the disorder, especially when it is accompanied by agoraphobic avoidance, can often cause those who are affected to seek treatment. It is critical that it be differentiated from medical conditions such as hyperventilation syndrome and asthma in such instances.

Clinical picture

Main features and symptoms

Youth seeking treatment may present because of intense fear about the meaning of the attacks or because of the interference in functioning engendered by the agoraphobic avoidance. Many times, families will have sought medical treatment or may believe that the attacks have a serious underlying physiological cause that has not been discovered.

By the time treatment is sought, the child may have missed significant amounts of school as a result of the panic attacks. Agoraphobic avoidance of places such as shopping malls, sporting events, and theatres and restaurants may result in severely restricted social opportunities and development.

Often separation concerns may accompany the PD or may have preceded it. Significant anxiety between attacks is not unusual and depressive symptoms and hopelessness may accompany the panic attacks particularly if the family has been unsuccessful in obtaining adequate treatment, resulting in a prolonged period of symptoms.

Differential diagnosis and co-morbidity

PD is often accompanied by other anxiety disorders or symptoms, especially early onset SAD. However, it should be noted that some studies have found a high rate of co-morbid separation anxiety in youth with PD whereas others have not. Affective disturbances are common.

Panic attacks may occur in the context of other anxiety disorders such as social or specific phobias. In this case the attacks are situationally cued from the onset and the diagnosis of PD would not be appropriate. Additionally, PD can be differentiated from other anxiety disorders, such as GAD, in that those with PD experience discrete periods of intense anxiety. That is, while there is some debate on this issue, panic attacks are thought to last for a period of minutes, not days or hours. Worry about the reoccurrence of the attacks, on the other hand, continues long after the attack has subsided. In disorders such as GAD, the patient typically reports no discrete periods of worry but rather constant worry perhaps with periods of varying intensity.

Given the nature of the physical symptoms of panic attacks, PD must be differentiated from potentially serious medical conditions such as asthma, hyperventilation disorder, irregular heart rhythms, mild myocardial infarctions and thyroid dysfunction. PD can, however, accompany or be exacerbated by a medical condition.

Assessment

In addition to the general measures listed in Table 5.2 (e.g. MASC, SCARED, SCAS, FSSC-R), the Children's Anxiety Sensitivity Index (CASI, see Appendix 5.2) has been found to be useful. This instrument measures sensitivity to the actual cues of anxiety (i.e. the 'fear of fear'). In addition, individually tailored self-monitoring forms can be useful in diagnosis and treatment planning as well as monitoring treatment progress. Ideally, the panic attack symptoms, as well as the situations in which they occur and their severity, should be noted. Frequency of attacks as well as frequency of agoraphobic avoidance (or approach towards previously avoided situations) should also be recorded.

Due to the physical nature of the complaints involved in PD, it is important that a thorough physical examination with accompanying laboratory tests be conducted in order to rule out a medical condition that could account for the symptoms (e.g. hyperventilation disorder, asthma).

Social phobia (social anxiety disorder)

Definition and classification

The main diagnostic feature of social phobia, also referred to as social anxiety disorder by some, is the fear of social situations in which there exits the potential or perceived potential for negative evaluation by others. As a result, the situations are either avoided or endured with great distress (ICD-10 requires that avoidance predominate). Behavioural expressions of the distress can include panic attacks, more limited autonomic symptoms, or children may exhibit tantrums.

The ICD-10 includes two diagnostic categories for social phobia, one specific to childhood, with an onset before age 6 (See Tables 5.7 and 5.8). The DSM no longer has a child specific equivalent of Social Phobia; instead the diagnostic criteria include qualifying notes for the application of the diagnosis to children (see Table 5.7). The DSM-IV also notes that, with the exception of children, the patient must be able to recognize that their fear is excessive. DSM-IV criteria require that social anxiety in children is not limited to situations involving adults. No such limitation exists in the ICD-10 criteria. In fact, in the diagnosis specific to childhood, ICD-10 notes that the symptoms may be limited to situations involving only adults, other children, or both.

DSM-IV includes a specifier to indicate situations in which the disorder is generalized. This applies in cases in which the individual is fearful of most social situations. DSM-IV is also more specific in that it requires symptoms continue for a minimum of 6 months before a diagnosis of social phobia is considered.

Another distinction between the DSM-IV and ICD-10 concerns the scope of the social phobia diagnosis. DSM-IV recognizes that, in contrast to situations in which the generalized specifier applies, socially phobic individuals may become fearful of very specific situations. If the focus of the fear is the potential for negative evaluation by others, the social phobia diagnosis applies in the DSM system. Common examples include public speaking fears and test/examination anxiety. According to the ICD-10 the latter is considered a specific and not a social phobia (see Specific Phobias).

Epidemiology

Prevalence and incidence rates

Epidemiological studies suggest that the prevalence rate for Social Phobia is approximately 1 per cent. Estimates vary widely, however, and it may be that these figures are underestimates given that many socially phobic youth become embarrassed if someone discovers their anxiety and therefore may be reluctant to report symptoms.

Sex ratios and ethnicity

Studies with adults suggest that social phobia is slightly more prevalent in women than in men; little data are available for children and adolescents, however.

The degree to which social extraversion is valued varies from culture to culture and therefore the impairment associated with social anxiety could also be expected

Table 5.7. Diagnostic criteria for social phobia

DSM-IV	ICD-10
A. A marked and persistent fear of one or more social or performance situations in which the person is exposed to unfamiliar people or to possible scrutiny by others. The individual fears that he or she will act in a way (or show anxiety symptoms) that will be humiliating or embarrassing. *Note:* In children, there must be evidence of the capacity for age-appropriate social relationships with familiar people and the anxiety must occur in peer settings, not just in interactions with adults.	All of the following criteria should be fulfilled for a definite diagnosis:
	(a) the psychological, behavioural, or autonomic symptoms must be primarily manifestations of anxiety and not secondary to other symptoms such as delusions or obsessional thoughts;
	(b) the anxiety must be restricted to or predominate in particular social situations; and
	(c) avoidance of the phobic situations must be a prominent feature.
B. Exposure to the feared social situation almost invariably provokes anxiety, which may take the form of a situationally bound or situationally predisposed panic attack. *Note:* In children, the anxiety may be expressed by crying, tantrums, freezing, or shrinking from social situations with unfamiliar people.	Includes:
	*anthropophobia
	*social neurosis
C. The person recognizes that the fear is excessive or unreasonable. *Note:* In children, this feature may be absent.	
D. The feared social or performance situations are avoided or else are endured with intense anxiety or distress.	
E. The avoidance, anxious anticipation, or distress in the feared social or performance situation(s) interferes significantly with the person's normal routine, occupational (academic) functioning, or social activities or relationships, or there is marked distress about having the phobia.	
F. In individuals under age 18 years, the duration is at least 6 months.	
G. The fear or avoidance is not due to the direct physiological effects of a substance (e.g. a drug of abuse, a medication) or a general medical condition and is not better accounted for by another mental disorder (e.g. panic disorder with or without agoraphobia, separation anxiety disorder, body dysmorphic disorder, a pervasive developmental disorder, or schizoid personality disorder).	
H. H. If a general medical condition or another mental disorder is present, the fear in Criterion A is unrelated to it, e.g. the fear is not of Stuttering, trembling in Parkinson's disease, or exhibiting abnormal eating behaviour in anorexia nervosa or bulimia nervosa.	
Specify if: Generalized: if the fears include most social situations (also consider the additional diagnosis of avoidant personality disorder)	

Table 5.8. ICD-10 criteria for social anxiety disorder of childhood

Note: This diagnostic category is used only for disorders that arise before the age of 6 years, that are both unusual in degree and accompanied by problems in social functioning, and that are not part of some more generalized emotional disturbance.

Children with this disorder show a persistent or recurrent fear and/or avoidance of strangers; such fear may occur mainly with adults, mainly with peers, or with both. The fear is associated with a normal degree of selective attachment to parents or to other familiar persons. The avoidance or fear of social encounters is of a degree that is outside the normal limits for the child's age and is associated with clinically significant problems in social functioning.

Includes: Avoidant disorder of childhood or adolescence

to vary. Children's social roles also vary across cultures to a large extent, and this may be particularly true when it comes to the ways in which children are expected to interact with adults as well as the rigidity of social norms and the importance placed on proper compliance. Therefore, in some cultures children may be expected to behave in ways that may at first appear to be consistent with a diagnosis of social phobia and the degree of distress experienced by the child as well as the deviation from cultural norms needs to be carefully assessed. In some cultures children with social phobias may be fearful of offending others, particularly adults, or may fear that they will bring dishonour or embarrassment to their family as a result of inappropriate behaviour in public.

Implications for clinical practice

Some degree of social anxiety in youth is not unusual particularly during adolescence; however, social phobia can lead to significant impairment across most areas of child's life and may impact the family. Social phobia may also be seen with GAD and depression.

Clinical picture

Main features and symptoms

Children with social phobia may be reluctant to report their symptoms and much information may have to be gathered through parent and teacher reports. School-age children with social phobia may be most anxious in performance situations such as giving speeches or having to perform in an athletic event or musical recital; however, these events may be relatively rare and, as such, may not engender the same degree of impairment as the informal social interactions that children encounter everyday.

Some children with social phobia may have accompanying social skills deficits that need to be addressed. Others possess age-appropriate social skills but their anxiety interferes with the ability to demonstrate these skills and some socially anxious children will demonstrate good social skills but will either perceive that they are not performing properly when in social situations or they may fear that, although they do not have a history of social skills problems, they may be unable to behave appropriately in any future social situation.

Differential diagnosis and co-morbidity

Social phobia may also be seen with co-morbid depression and GAD and it is not unusual for these conditions to be present in family members.

Socially phobic individuals may experience panic attacks or symptoms of panic attacks when in social situations; however, if the panic attacks are limited to situations in which there is the perceived possibility of negative evaluation and this is the focus of the anxiety, social phobia is a more appropriate diagnosis than PD. Similar considerations must be taken in differentiating social phobia from a specific phobia.

The avoidance of social situations seen in social phobia may also be confused with the apathy experienced by depressed youth. When avoidance of social situations co-occurs with hopelessness and apathy rather than anxious apprehension, the diagnosis of depression should be considered.

Assessment

In addition to the general measures listed in Table 5.2, the Social Phobia Anxiety Inventory for Children and the Social Anxiety Scales for Children and Adolescents have been developed specifically to assess for social anxiety. Behavioural avoidance/approach tests, described under specific phobias, can also be useful in the assessment of social phobia.

Specific (isolated) phobias

Definition and classification

The primary feature of specific phobias is the intense and unrealistic fear of specific objects or situations. Both ICD-10 and DSM-IV specify that the feared object is avoided whenever possible, or the DSM-IV also suggests that intense distress when contact with the phobic stimulus occurs is diagnostically equivalent (see Table 5.9 for diagnostic criteria). The ICD-10 also includes a diagnostic category specific to childhood (see Table 5.10).

Table 5.9. Diagnostic criteria for specific phobia

DSM-IV	ICD-10
A. Marked and persistent fear that is excessive or unreasonable, cued by the presence or anticipation of a specific object or situation (e.g. flying, heights, animals, receiving an injection, seeing blood).	All of the following should be fulfilled for a definite diagnosis:
B. Exposure to the phobic stimulus almost invariably provokes an immediate anxiety response, which may take the form of a situationally bound or situationally predisposed panic attack. *Note:* In children, the anxiety may be expressed by crying, tantrums, freezing, or clinging.	(a) the psychological or autonomic symptoms must be primary manifestations of anxiety, and not secondary to other symptoms such as delusion or obsessional thought;
C. The person recognizes that the fear is excessive or unreasonable. *Note:* In children, this feature may be absent.	(b) the anxiety must be restricted to the presence of the particular phobic object or situation; and
D. The phobic situation(s) is avoided or else is endured with intense anxiety or distress.	(c) the phobic situation is avoided whenever possible.
E. The avoidance, anxious anticipation, or distress in the feared situation(s) interferes significantly with the person's normal routine, occupational (or academic) functioning, or social activities or relationships, or there is marked distress about having the phobia.	Includes: *acrophobia *animal phobias *claustrophobia *examination phobia *simple phobia
F. In individuals under age 18 years, the duration is at least 6 months.	
G. The anxiety, panic attacks, or phobic avoidance associated with the specific object or situation are not better accounted for by another mental disorder, such as obsessive-compulsive disorder (e.g. fear of dirt in someone with an obsession about contamination), post-traumatic stress disorder (e.g. avoidance of stimuli associated with a severe stressor), separation anxiety disorder (e.g. avoidance of school), social phobia (e.g., avoidance of social situations because of fear of embarrassment), panic disorder with agoraphobia, or agoraphobia without history of panic disorder.	

Specify type:
• **Animal type**
• **Natural Environment type** (e.g., heights, storms, water)
• **Blood-injection-injury type**
• **Situational type** (e.g. airplanes, elevators, enclosed places)
• **Other type** (e.g. phobic avoidance of situations that may lead to choking, vomiting, or contracting an illness; in children, avoidance of loud sounds or costumed characters)

Table 5.10. ICD-10 criteria for phobic anxiety disorder of childhood

This category should be used only for developmental phase-specific fears when they meet the additional criteria that apply to all disorders in F93 [emotional disorders with onset specific to childhood], namely that:

(a) the onset is during the developmentally appropriate age period;

(b) the degree of anxiety is clinically abnormal; and

(c) the anxiety does not form part of a more generalized disorder.

Excludes: Generalized anxiety disorder

Aside from the more specific criteria included in DSM-IV and the requirement that the symptoms cause significant impairment in functioning; the two systems also differ in that DSM-IV specifies five specific types of specific phobias: animal type (e.g. fear of dogs, snakes, spiders), natural environment type (e.g. fear of thunderstorms, heights, fires), situational type (e.g. fear of flying, fear of elevators), blood-injection-injury type (e.g. fear of seeing blood, receiving an injection) and other type (e.g. fear of choking) whereas ICD does not. ICD-10 also specifies that the criteria for GAD cannot be met to receive the specific phobia diagnosis whereas DSM-IV does not make this stipulation; moreover, ICD fails to specify a duration criterion whereas DSM-IV indicates duration of at least 6 months. The implications of these diagnostic differences for prevalence and incidence as well as assessment and treatment currently are not known.

Epidemiology

Prevalence and incidence rates

Community surveys suggest that approximately 2.5 per cent of children and adolescents have specific phobias that engender significant impairment (using DSM criteria). Rates across studies vary, however, and seem to be somewhat higher when children provide information than when parent report is used as the basis for diagnosis.

Sex ratios and ethnicity

Little epidemiological data exist comparing the rate of specific phobias in boys and girls; however, it appears that girls are slightly more likely to develop a specific phobia than boys. However, the degree to which this is accurate varies widely across the different types of phobias, with BII occurring more frequently in boys than girls. Also self-reported fears tend to occur equally frequently in some cultures (e.g. Africa) but more frequently in girls than boys in others (e.g. USA, United Kingdom, Australia and China). Reasons for these differences are thought to be determined culturally but the exact mechanisms are understood poorly at this time.

Implications for clinical practice

Although specific fears are common throughout childhood and adolescence, it is less common for these to reach the intensity and to cause the level of impairment at which families seek treatment. However, treatment may be sought when the child is unable to take part in a specific event or if the phobia interferes with social activities. Often, specific phobias seen in clinical practice may be accompanied by other anxiety problems.

Clinical picture

Main features and symptoms

Youth presenting with Specific Phobias may be embarrassed about their fears but may seek treatment when an upcoming event increases motivation for treatment. Alternatively children with specific phobias may be seen when there are multiple fears or phobias that together are causing considerable limitations. This may also be the case when specific phobias are seen as part of a larger clinical picture that may include other anxiety disorders or depression.

Differential diagnosis and co-morbidity

Panic attacks may occur as part of the symptom picture in a specific phobia; however, with a phobia the panic attacks are situationally bound and fear remains focused on the phobic stimulus and not the panic attacks. Specific phobias also need to be differentiated from social phobia. If an object or event is feared because of the possibility that it may be associated with public embarrassment or the negative evaluation by others rather than the properties of the object or event itself, the diagnosis of social phobia is more appropriate.

In some cases specific phobias can be confused with OCD. A phobic individual will attempt to avoid the feared stimulus or become distressed upon contact but will not usually engage in compulsions that are not realistically connected to avoiding harm from the feared stimulus. In addition, unless the phobic individual is anticipating having to come into contact with the feared object there is not the intrusive obsessive quality to the fear as seen in OCD.

As noted previously, specific phobias may be seen with other anxiety disorders.

Assessment

In addition to the interviews and questionnaires listed in Table 5.2, especially the FSSC-R, behavioural avoidance/approach tests (BATs) can be useful in evaluating specific phobias and in monitoring treatment response. In a BAT the phobic individual is confronted with the feared object and asked to approach as close as he or she is able. In this way the individual's comfort in approaching the feared stimulus can be monitored easily by measuring the distance between the individual and the object at the conclusion of each trial.

Self-monitoring can also be helpful in assessing the degree of interference caused by avoidance of the feared object. Data collected can be simply frequency counts of the number of times the feared stimulus is approached or avoided.

Aetiology

There is a growing body of evidence that suggests that the development and maintenance of the anxiety disorders in children occur as a function of synergistic processes involving genetic, biological, familial, learning, and environmental forces. Data supporting this position come from multiple sources including familial concordance studies, twin studies, longitudinal studies of anxiety and temperament, and experimental laboratory and behavioural studies. A number of familial studies, for example, clearly reveal high concordance rates of anxiety among first-degree relatives of anxiety-disordered patients. In addition, children of anxiety-disordered parents and parents of anxiety-disordered children have been found to have far higher rates of anxiety disorders than controls. Finally, the concordance rates of anxiety symptoms and disorders have been shown to be higher in MZ than DZ twins. Although these studies support a familial transmission of anxiety, the differences in concordance rates between MZ twins relative to DZ twins are relatively low compared to other disorders, suggesting the importance of shared genetic and environmental factors. Thus, the genetic predisposition to the development of an anxiety disorder can be said to be only a general one.

The exact nature of this genetic predisposition is not understood fully. However, some data suggest that behavioural inhibition to the unfamiliar – a characteristic of temperament – may be genetically based and may serve as a risk factor for the development of an anxiety disorder. Behavioural inhibition is characterized by the tendency to respond to novel situations with hesitancy, fear, reticence, and restraint. Generally, children who are inhibited behaviourally are shy and fearful as toddlers, quiet and withdrawn in unfamiliar situations in childhood, and introverted and anxious as teenagers. Behavioural inhibition has been shown to be a relatively stable characteristic that is associated with signs of sympathetic arousal (including elevated heart rates and higher norepinephrine values), even in very young children. In one study, children (2 to 7 years of age) of parents with PD were found to be more likely to demonstrate this characteristic than children of parents with MDD or other psychiatric disorders. In another study, children identified as behaviourally inhibited were found to have higher rates of anxiety disorders than uninhibited children. It is thus possible that this temperamental characteristic is a marker for a predisposition that is genetically based and that serves to increase the vulnerability for an anxiety disorder.

Although it is clear that anxiety disorders are familial, and it is possible that a general predisposition for anxiety (rather than say a predisposition for a specific anxiety disorder) is based genetically, the expression of any one anxiety disorder is undoubtedly related to a transaction between life circumstances and developmental processes that occur throughout development and across the lifespan. Children universally experience transient fears and anxieties over the course of development that both are normal and evolutionarily adaptive. However, as this normal developmental process unfolds, certain perturbations occur and pathological fears and anxieties may emerge. Developmental periods of increased vulnerability (e.g. separation from parents, entry into school, onset of puberty), in concert with certain life events, may lead to the expression of any one specific anxiety disorder (say SAD vs. PD versus GAD).

These life events and experiences affect, and undoubtedly are affected by, learning experiences that shape particular anxiety responses and the subsequent development of specific disorders. Through the processes of classical, operant and vicarious conditioning, children learn that certain stimuli are associated with aversive consequences, and that fearful and avoidant behaviours result in certain consequences that may, at times, be reinforcing. Children of anxious parents may also be more likely to observe overly anxious behaviour in their parents, and be more likely to have fearful behaviour reinforced (inadvertently perhaps) by their parents (who themselves may be averse to unpleasant and embarrassing situations than less anxious parents). Just as the child's anxious behaviours are shaped inadvertently by their parents, the parents' behaviour may be reinforced negatively by their anxious child becoming less upset and calm under such circumstances.

Thus, in brief, the aetiology of anxiety disorders in childhood is likely to be a function of genetic, biological, familial, learning and environmental processes. Life circumstances and events, in combination with the individual's genetic and biological predisposition and developmental transitions, may then determine the development, expression, and form of any one anxiety disorder.

Treatment

Psychosocial interventions

The status of evidence-based practice for anxious and phobic children supports primarily the use of cognitive–behaviour therapy (CBT) interventions. Several major factors distinguish CBT for children from other psychosocial interventions for youth:

- The focus of treatment is on maladaptive learning histories and erroneous or overly rigid thought patterns.

- Treatment is focused on the here and now rather than orientated toward uncovering historical antecedents of maladaptive behaviour or thought patterns.
- Treatment goals are clearly determined and parents and youth seeking treatment are asked to delineate the types of changes they wish to see as a result of treatment.
- Progress is monitored throughout treatment using objective indicators of change, such as monitoring forms and the rating devices such as those discussed above and described in Table 5.2.
- CBT is a skills-building approach.
- Because the goal of treatment is to develop skills that can be used outside of treatment sessions and eventually independent of the therapist, CBT is often action-orientated, directive, and educational in nature. Also for this reason, CBT typically includes a homework component in which the skills learned in treatment are practised outside the therapy room.
- CBTs for children often incorporate skills components for parents, teachers, and sometimes even siblings or peers. For example, parents might be trained in how to reward courageous behaviour and how to ignore (i.e. extinguish) excessive reports of anxiety in their children.
- CBT is designed to be relatively short term, rarely extending beyond 6 months of active treatment.
- In addition to the active treatment phase, CBT for anxious children may incorporate spaced-out 'booster sessions' that extend over a longer period of time (i.e. another 4 to 6 months) to ensure maintenance and durability of change.

Table 5.11 lists some of the most common CBT treatment strategies for anxiety disorders in youth. (In addition, a relaxation script for use with children is included in Appendix 5.3.) These strategies are often used first in sessions and then practised in related homework assignments outside of session by both the child and his or her parents. A workbook is often provided to assist with these homework assignments. Additionally, weekly monitoring of gains is pursued.

In summary, CBT interventions have been shown to be highly effective with anxiety disorders in children. It should be noted that these treatments have been used primarily with anxious children between 7 and 14 years of age and, as with other problem areas and disorders, additional research is required to determine whether these treatments will be effective with adolescents and younger children. Still, it is obvious that they show considerable promise and recent work with PD adolescents and preschool youngsters with SAD suggests their utility. Given their proven effectiveness, they constitute the first line of treatment for anxious children.

Table 5.11. Components of CBT treatments for anxiety disordered children and adolescents

Child components		Parent components	
Behavioural	Cognitive	Behavioural	Cognitive
• Exposure to anxiety producing stimuli	• Cognitive restructuring in anxiety provoking situations	• Reinforcement of child's non-anxious behaviour	• Problem solving
• Self-reinforcement for non-anxious behaviour	• Coping self-talk	• Planned ignoring for anxious behaviour	• Cognitive restructuring around own anxiety related to child's fears
• Relaxation training	• Recognizing and reinterpreting somatic sensations	• Model problem solving non-anxious behaviour for child	
• Role plays to practise skills in anxiety provoking situations	• Cognitive restructuring of self-evaluations		

Pharmacological interventions

There are few adequately designed studies available that establish the safety and efficacy of any class of medication for the childhood anxiety disorders, with the exception of OCD. Still, medication treatments have been used frequently and the major options include the benzodiazepines, the tricyclic antidepressants (TCAs), and serotonin re-uptake inhibitors (SSRIs). All have demonstrated efficacy in adult anxiety disorders such as PD, GAD, and social phobia, although their efficacy with children has not been well established. Moreover, these agents are not as typically effective as CBT and appear to have reduced long-term favourable outcomes.

As recommended by many clinicians and researchers, a detailed medical and family history should be obtained, as well as laboratory measures, before beginning any pharmacological regimen. For example, if a patient complains of feeling heat intolerance with warm, moist skin, weight loss, and rapid heart rate, it would be desirable to complete baseline thyroid studies. The prescribing clinician, with the consent of parent and child, should consult with the child's primary care physician to be aware of any additional medical issues, and to determine if the child has had a recent physical examination. Both the parent and child need to be informed about the risks and benefits of medication treatment. It is also important to be clear with the child and parent what target symptoms will be monitored to determine effectiveness of the medication.

Benzodiazepines

The benzodiazepines bind to the γ-aminobutyric acid receptor (GABA) membrane chloride channel complexes, which lead to enhanced CNS inhibition through the neurotransmitter GABA. Besides the anxiolytic effect, benzodiazepines are also used for their anticonvulsant, hypnotic and muscle relaxant properties. Although an extensive literature exists regarding the effectiveness of benzodiazepines in adult anxiety disorders, there have been only a few studies, with small sample sizes, that have examined them in the childhood anxiety disorders. Most of the studies involve children and adolescents who are co-morbid with other disorders such as major depression and school refusal. The results of these studies, though limited, suggest:

- Benzodiazepines can be effective.
- However, it is unclear whether the benefits from the benzodiazepines can be fully accounted for by placebo effects.
- Moreover, the side effects can be significant and considerable.

The most common side effects from benzodiazepines include:

- drowsiness
- headache
- nausea
- fatigue.

The side effects are dose related and can lead to tremor, slurred speech and ataxia. There have also been reports of 'paradoxical reactions' where the child experiences overexcitement, irritability and perceptual disorganization. Another concern is the potential risk of dependence and withdrawal associated with the benzodiazepines – such concerns rule them out as a front-line treatment for the anxiety disorders.

If children and adolescents are treated with benzodiazepines, it is recommended that it be for a limited amount of time and at the lowest possible dose. As clinically indicated, the dose should be increased every three to four days. Once treatment is complete, the benzodiazepine should be tapered gradually to avoid any risk of withdrawal symptoms, including insomnia, gastrointestinal complaints, rebound anxiety and concentration difficulties.

Tricyclic antidepressants

Dysregulation of both the noradrenergic and serotonin system of the central nervous system is thought to be related to the development of anxiety disorders. In general, the effectiveness of the tricyclic antidepressants appears to be through the metabolism and/or the re-uptake of the monoamine neurotransmitters. The significant and often hard to tolerate side effects are due to the TCAs blockade at the muscarinic/cholinergic, histamine (H1) and α-adrenergic receptors. The most common side effects are constipation, nausea, orthostatic hypotension, sedation and weight gain. The majority of clinical trials performed using TCAs did not have children and adolescents with anxiety disorders alone, but rather the much more complicated co-morbid group of 'school refusing' children. The placebo-controlled studies of tricyclic antidepressants for anxiety-based school refusal children have provided conflicting results.

An issue of grave concern with tricyclic antidepressant use in children is associated with a growing recognition of cardiac risk. There have been reports of children who died suddenly while being treated with appropriate dosages of desipramine. Given the uncertain clinical efficacy of TCAs for anxiety-disordered children plus the significant side effects, particularly the cardiac risk, this class of medication is also not the first choice of action.

However, if these medications are used, the treating clinician should obtain baseline vital signs including sitting and standing blood pressure with pulse, as well as a baseline EKG. Once the therapeutic dose is reached, the EKG should be repeated and serum levels should be checked. This should be repeated with each significant dose adjustment.

Serotonin re-uptake inhibitors

The current state of the data regarding psychopharmacology leaves the SSRI antidepressants as the leading pharmacological candidate for the treatment of childhood anxiety disorders. The safety of the SSRIs recommends them as a choice, as does their effectiveness in treating depression, which is frequently co-morbid with childhood anxiety disorders. Moreover, the SSRIs have shown preliminary efficacy in the treatment of adult anxiety disorders including GAD, PD and social phobia.

There is limited but good evidence available for the use of SSRIs to treat childhood anxiety disorders. Again, the majority of the studies include a mix of patients with GAD, SAD, social phobia, PD, selective mutism and anxiety disorder not otherwise specified.

- Open trials and one randomized trial suggest that fluoxetine has preliminary benefit in the treatment of youth with OAD/GAD, SAD and social phobia.
- Sertraline has been shown to more effective in treating GAD in youth than a placebo.
- The main side effects found with sertraline treatment were dry mouth, drowsiness, leg spasms and restlessness. All of these side effects were more likely in children treated with sertraline than with a drug placebo.
- Fluvoxamine has also been shown to be more effective than a placebo in treating GAD, SAD and social phobia with or without co-morbid externalizing disorders.
- The main side effects found with fluvoxamine were increased motor activity or agitation, which appears to be dose related, and abdominal discomfort.

In prescribing SSRIs, it is recommended that the medication be initiated at a low dose, for example, with sertraline, 25 mg for the first 7 days, and then increased to 50 mg, increasing slowly as clinical response dictates. Once a therapeutic dose is reached, this dose should be maintained for 6–8 weeks to determine its efficacy.

Withdrawal symptoms have been reported with the discontinuation of SSRIs, including nausea, headache, dizziness and agitation. Therefore, these medications should not be abruptly discontinued. From the available evidence on the effects of medications, it appears that the SSRIs are a first-line psychopharmacological treatment for childhood anxiety disorders.

Combining treatments in a multidisciplinary framework

Disease management model

It was clear by the late 1970s that a disease management model based on a psychosocial approach was as powerful a change strategy in psychiatry as it was in other areas of medicine. Consistent with this approach, combined treatment is the rule rather than the exception across most of medicine, cf. the treatment of hypertension with antihypertensives and weight reduction or the treatment of juvenile rheumatoid arthritis with ibuprofen and physical therapy. In this regard, the treatment of the anxious child can be thought of as partially analogous to the treatment of juvenile-onset diabetes, with the caveat that the target organ, the brain in the case of the anxiety disorders, requires psychosocial interventions of much greater complexity. The treatment of diabetes and anxiety disorder both involve medications, insulin in diabetes and in anxiety, typically, a serotonin re-uptake inhibitor. Each also involves an evidence-based psychosocial intervention that works in part by biasing the somatic substrate of the disorder toward more normal functioning. In diabetes, the psychosocial treatment of choice is diet and exercise, and in anxiety, cognitive change and exposure-based CBT. However, not everybody recovers completely even with the best of available treatments, so some interventions need to target coping with residual symptoms, such as diabetic foot care in diabetes and helping patients and their families cope skilfully with residual symptoms in the anxiety disorders.

Combined psychosocial and pharmacological treatments

Psychosocial treatments usually are combined with medication for one of three reasons.

- In the initial treatment of the child – especially the severely ill child – two treatments may provide a greater 'dose' and thus may promise a better and perhaps speedier outcome. For this reason, many patients with SAD, GAD, or PD opt for combined treatment even though CBT alone may offer equal benefit.

- Co-morbidity frequently but not always requires two treatments, since different targets may require different treatments. For example, treating an 8-year old who has ADHD and SAD with a psychostimulant and CBT is a reasonable treatment strategy. Even within a single anxiety disorder, important functional outcomes may vary in response to treatment. For example, acute anticipatory anxiety in the SAD child may be especially responsive to a benzodiazepine and reintroduction to school with graduated exposure.
- In the face of partial response, an augmenting treatment can be added to the initial treatment to improve outcome. For example, CBT can be added to an SSRI for PD to improve PD-specific outcomes. In an adjunctive treatment strategy, a second treatment can be added to a first one in order to impact one or more additional outcome domains positively. For example, an SSRI can be added to CBT for GAD to handle co-morbid depression or panic disorder.

A stages-of-treatment model

As a general rule, it is best to use the simplest, least risky and most cost-effective treatment intervention available and to do so within a stages-of-treatment model in order to identify key decision points in the everyday treatment of patients with anxiety disorders. In particular, to be useful to clinicians, a treatment review should address the following.

Selection of initial treatment

Given evidence-based psychotherapy and pharmacotherapy, and very few studies of combined vs. unimodal treatment, the clinician must make a judgement about the relative benefits and risks of single vs. combined treatment over the short and long term. Besides relative effectiveness, the feasibility, acceptability and tolerability of the treatment must also be considered. With these caveats in mind, some rough guidelines for treatment selection are suggested in Fig. 5.1. In addition, to those conditions depicted in Fig. 5.1, which suggest CBT as a first line of treatment, clinicians may also want to turn to medication treatment if a sufficient trial of CBT has not been successful. However, given that most readily available psychotherapies do not typically use CBT procedures (particularly exposure), it would need to be determined whether an adequate trial had taken place. Additionally, clinicians may want to try medication as a first line treatment when developmental disorders or cognitive limitations on the part of the child suggest that he or she may not be able to fully engage in CBT treatment.

The management of partial response

Most patients improve substantially with current unimodal treatments. However, it is likely that most will not normalize, especially when functional outcomes rather

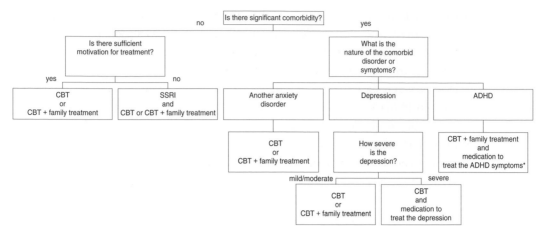

*Note: There have been some reports of childrewn with comorbid ADHD and anxiety disorders developing tics with psychostimulant medication. These tics may or may not remit with discontinuation of the medication treatment.

Fig. 5.1.   Decision tree for determining first line of treatment for youth with anxiety disorders.

than symptoms are considered. Furthermore, when a primary disorder remits, secondary problems often come to the fore. Thus, combining treatments is often more common as treatment progresses and the limits of initial treatment become apparent.

The treatment refractory patient

When a patient has had two trials of different medications, and, where appropriate, combinations of medications as well as optimal psychosocial treatment, and where these trials are adequate in dose and duration and the patient still shows little or no improvement, it is justifiable to label the patient as treatment resistant. In this situation, newer treatments, treatments with a lower probability of success and riskier combinations of treatment all seem warranted.

Maintenance treatment

Finally, when a patient is a responder, it is critical from a personal and public health perspective to know how long to continue treatment at what dose and visit schedule before trying, if appropriate, to discontinue treatment. If discontinuation is desirable, and it may not be in the face of persisting symptoms or previous relapses, then the optimal schedule for discontinuing medications vs. psychosocial treatment, given that these two modalities may show differences in durability of benefit, must be considered.

Most of the time, the extant treatment literature and, typically, unsystematic reviews of the treatment literature, do not provide much guidance once past the choice of initial unimodal interventions. This is especially true for treatment reviews that focus on either medication or psychosocial interventions alone and hence cannot address issues associated with combining treatments. Because this leaves out a significant number of patients for whom combined treatment is appropriate if not *de rigueur* (e.g. partial responders to initial treatment, those who have failed to respond to several treatments, and/or those who require a combination of treatments because of co-morbidity), typical unsystematic treatment reviews are of less use in clinical practice.

On being multidisciplinary

Although cognitive–behavioural and pharmacological treatment strategies for anxious children combine readily, clinical psychology and psychiatry are often at odds over stakeholder issues. We believe that it is not possible to practise competent and ethical psychopharmacology without the availability of evidence-based psychosocial interventions. Similarly, it is not possible to practise competent and ethical psychotherapy without the availability of empirically supported psychopharmacology. Physicians (who typically write prescriptions) and psychologists (who, for the most part, have developed and typically implement CBT) must join hands in the care of individual patients if for no other reason than that the complexity of modern mental health care is beyond the capacity of any one individual to master. Without this commitment to multidisciplinary practice, we short change our patients.

Outcome

A growing body of literature documents the outcomes for both treated and untreated youth with anxiety disorders. A review of the empirical literature suggests the conclusions outlined below.

- Without treatment these disorders are persistent and they result in academic, social and emotional complications for the youths who evince them.
- Recent advances suggest that CBT and the SSRIs are the most promising treatment options
- With CBT, approximately two-thirds to three-quarters of children will experience a remission of the anxiety disorder. Most will experience some reduction in symptoms.
- The effects of CBT appear to continue after the active treatment phase is terminated and most children whose symptoms remit after treatment will continue to be diagnosis free for at least 1 year post-treatment. Additionally, a sizeable portion of those children who experienced symptom relief but not total remission at the end of treatment will continue to make improvements post-treatment.
- Adding a parent or family component to CBT for anxious children can increase the success of treatment. Some evidence suggests that approximately 85 per cent of children receiving this type of treatment will be diagnosis free at the end of treatment and that this number grows even after the active phase of treatment has been discontinued.

- Although we have less information about the use of medications with anxious children, it appears that about three-quarters of children treated with SSRIs will also experience remission of the disorder. However, it is also true that children with anxiety disorders seem to experience a sizeable placebo effect in response to medication treatment.
- The long-term maintenance of medication treatment is unknown at this time. We also know little about combined treatments in children at this time. Speculation based on adult studies, however, suggests that caution should be exercised when combining CBT and medication treatments, in that long-term outcome may be compromised.
- Finally, it will be imperative that we examine and treat these disorders from a multidisciplinary perspective if we are to make significant and lasting advances.

SUGGESTED READING

American Academy of Child and Adolescent Psychiatry. Practice parameters for the assessment of children and adolescents with anxiety disorders. *Journal of the American Academy of Child and Adolescent Psychiatry* **36** (1997), 69–84.

G. A. Bernstein, C. M. Borchardt & A. R. Perwein, Anxiety disorders in children and adolescents: a review of the past 10 years. *Journal of the American Academy of Child and Adolescent Psychiatry* **35** (1996), 1110–19.

B. Birmaher, D. A. Axelson, K. Monk *et al.*, Fluoxetine for the treatment of childhood anxiety disorders. *Journal of the American Academy of Child and Adolescent Psychiatry* **42** (2003), 415–23.

D. L. Chambless & T. H. Ollendick, Empirically supported psychological interventions: controversies and evidence. *Annual Review of Psychology* **52** (2001), 685–716.

A. E. Grills & T. H. Ollendick, Multiple informant agreement and the Anxiety Disorders Interview Schedule of Parents and Children. *Journal of the American Academy of Child and Adolescent Psychiatry* **42** (2003), 30–40.

N. J. King, B. J. Tonge, D. Heyne *et al.*, Cognitive–behavioral treatment of school refusing children: a controlled evaluation. *Journal of the American Academy of Child and Adolescent Psychiatry* **37** (1998), 395–403.

C. G. Last, C. Hansen & N. Franco, Anxious children in adulthood: a prospective study of adjustment. *Journal of the American Academy of Child and Adolescent Psychiatry* **36** (1997), 645–52.

S. G. Mattis & T. H. Ollendick, *Panic Disorder and Anxiety in Adolescence*. (Oxford: British Psychological Society, 2002).

P. Muris, H. Merckelbach, T. H. Ollendick, N. J. King & N. Bogie, Three traditional and three new childhood anxiety questionnaires: their reliability and validity in a normal adolescent sample. *Behaviour Research and Therapy* **40** (2002), 753–72.

T. H. Ollendick & J. A. Cerny, *Clinical Behavior Therapy with Children.* (New York: Plenum Press, 1981).

T. H. Ollendick & D. R. Hirshfeld-Becker, The developmental psychopathology of social anxiety disorder. *Biological Psychiatry* **51** (2002), 44–58.

T. H. Ollendick & J. S. March (eds.), *Phobic and Anxiety Disorders: A Clinician's Guide to Effective Psychosocial and Pharmacological Interventions.* (New York: Oxford University Press, 2003).

T. H. Ollendick, A. E. Grills & N. J. King, Applying developmental theory to the assessment and treatment of childhood disorders: Does it make a difference? *Clinical Psychology and Psychotherapy* **8** (2001), 304–15.

T. H. Ollendick, N. J. King & P. Muris, Fears and phobias in children: phenomenology, epidemiology, and aetiology. *Child and Adolescent Mental Health* **7** (2002), 98–106.

P. M. J. Prins & T. H. Ollendick, Cognitive change and enhanced coping: missing mediational links in cognitive behavior therapy with anxiety-disordered children. *Clinical Child and Family Psychology Review* **6** (2003), 87–105.

M. A. Rynn, A. L. Siqueland & K. Rickels, Placebo-controlled trial of sertraline in the treatment of children with GAD. *American Journal of Psychiatry* **158** (2001), 2008–14.

RUPP Anxiety Study Group. Fluvoxamine for the treatment of anxiety disorders in children and adolescents. *New England Journal of Medicine* **344** (2001), 1279–85.

L. D. Seligman & T. H. Ollendick, Anxiety disorders. In H. C. Steinhauser & F. Verhulst (eds.), *Risks and Outcomes in Developmental Psychopathology.* (New York: Oxford University Press, 1999), pp. 103–20.

L. D. Seligman & T. H. Ollendick, Co-morbidity of anxiety and depression in children and adolescents: an integrative review. *Clinical Child and Family Psychology Review* **1** (1998), 125–44.

Appendix 5.1. Self-rating questionnaire (The Fear Survey Schedule for Children – Revised, FSSC-R)

© Thomas H. Ollendick

B. Name:_____ Age: ____ Date: _____

Directions: A number of statements which boys and girls use to describe the fears they have are given below. Read each carefully and put an **X** in the box in front of the words that best describe your fear. There are no right or wrong answers. Remember, find the words which best describe how much fear you have.

1. Giving an oral report	☐ None	☐ Some	☐ A lot
2. Riding in the car or bus	☐ None	☐ Some	☐ A lot
3. Getting punished by mother	☐ None	☐ Some	☐ A lot

  4. Lizards . . . . ☐ None   ☐ Some   ☐ A lot

  5. Looking foolish. . . . . ☐ None   ☐ Some   ☐ A lot

  6. Ghosts or spooky things . . . . ☐ None   ☐ Some   ☐ A lot

  7. Sharp objects. . . . . ☐ None   ☐ Some   ☐ A lot

  8. Having to go to the hospital. . . . . ☐ None   ☐ Some   ☐ A lot

  9. Death or dead people . . . . ☐ None   ☐ Some   ☐ A lot

 10. Getting lost in a strange place . . . . ☐ None   ☐ Some   ☐ A lot

 11. Snakes. . . . . ☐ None   ☐ Some   ☐ A lot

 12. Talking on the telephone . . . . ☐ None   ☐ Some   ☐ A lot

 13. Roller coaster or carnival rides . . . . ☐ None   ☐ Some   ☐ A lot

 14. Getting sick at school . . . . ☐ None   ☐ Some   ☐ A lot

 15. Being sent to the principal . . . . ☐ None   ☐ Some   ☐ A lot

 16. Riding on the train . . . . ☐ None   ☐ Some   ☐ A lot

 17. Being left at home with a sitter . . . . ☐ None   ☐ Some   ☐ A lot

 18. Bears or wolves . . . . ☐ None   ☐ Some   ☐ A lot

 19. Meeting someone for the first time . . . . ☐ None   ☐ Some   ☐ A lot

 20. Bombing attacks – being invaded . . . . ☐ None   ☐ Some   ☐ A lot

 21. Getting a shot from the nurse or doctor . . . . . ☐ None   ☐ Some   ☐ A lot

 22. Going to the dentist . . . . ☐ None   ☐ Some   ☐ A lot

 23. High places like mountains . . . . ☐ None   ☐ Some   ☐ A lot

 24. Being teased. . . . . ☐ None   ☐ Some   ☐ A lot

 25. Spiders . . . . ☐ None   ☐ Some   ☐ A lot

 26. A burglar breaking into our house . . . . ☐ None   ☐ Some   ☐ A lot

 27. Flying in an airplane . . . . ☐ None   ☐ Some   ☐ A lot

 28. Being called on by the teacher . . . . ☐ None   ☐ Some   ☐ A lot

 29. Getting poor grades. . . . . ☐ None   ☐ Some   ☐ A lot

30. Bats or birds .... ☐ None   ☐ Some   ☐ A lot

31. My parents criticizing me................. ☐ None   ☐ Some   ☐ A lot

32. Guns .... ☐ None   ☐ Some   ☐ A lot

33. Being in a fight .... ☐ None   ⊔ Some   ☐ A lot

34. Fire – getting burned..................... ☐ None   ☐ Some   ☐ A lot

35. Getting a cut or injury .... ☐ None   ☐ Some   ☐ A lot

36. Being in a big crowd .... ☐ None   ☐ Some   ☐ A lot

37. Thunderstorms.......................... ☐ None   ☐ Some   ☐ A lot

38. Having to eat some food I don't like .... ☐ None   ☐ Some   ☐ A lot

39. Cats...................................... ☐ None   ☐ Some   ☐ A lot

40. Failing a test .... ☐ None   ☐ Some   ☐ A lot

41. Being hit by a car or truck .... ☐ None   ☐ Some   ☐ A lot

42. Having to go to school .... ☐ None   ☐ Some   ☐ A lot

43. Playing rough games during recess .... ☐ None   ☐ Some   ☐ A lot

44. Having my parents argue .... ☐ None   ☐ Some   ☐ A lot

45. Dark rooms or closets.................... ☐ None   ☐ Some   ☐ A lot

46. Having to put on a recital................. ☐ None   ☐ Some   ☐ A lot

47. Ants or beetles .... ☐ None   ☐ Some   ☐ A lot

48. Being criticized by others................. ☐ None   ☐ Some   ☐ A lot

49. Strange looking people .... ☐ None   ☐ Some   ☐ A lot

50. The sight of blood .... ☐ None   ☐ Some   ☐ A lot

51. Going to the doctor .... ☐ None   ☐ Some   ☐ A lot

52. Strange or mean looking dogs.............. ☐ None   ☐ Some   ☐ A lot

53. Cemeteries.............................. ☐ None   ☐ Some   ☐ A lot

54. Getting a report card..................... ☐ None   ☐ Some   ☐ A lot

55. Getting a haircut .... ☐ None   ☐ Some   ☐ A lot

56. Deep water or the ocean . . . . □ None   □ Some   □ A lot

57. Nightmares . . . . □ None   □ Some   □ A lot

58. Falling from high places . . . . □ None   □ Some   □ A lot

59. Getting a shock from electricity . . . . □ None   □ Some   □ A lot

60. Going to bed in the dark . . . . □ None   □ Some   □ A lot

61. Getting car sick . . . . □ None   □ Some   □ A lot

62. Being alone . . . . □ None   □ Some   □ A lot

63. Having to wear clothes different from others.   □ None   □ Some   □ A lot

64. Getting punished by my father . . . . □ None   □ Some   □ A lot

65. Having to stay after school . . . . □ None   □ Some   □ A lot

66. Making mistakes . . . . □ None   □ Some   □ A lot

67. Mystery movies . . . . □ None   □ Some   □ A lot

68. Loud sirens . . . . □ None   □ Some   □ A lot

69. Doing something new . . . . □ None   □ Some   □ A lot

70. Germs or getting a serious illness . . . . □ None   □ Some   □ A lot

71. Closed spaces . . . . □ None   □ Some   □ A lot

72. Earthquakes . . . . □ None   □ Some   □ A lot

73. Terrorists . . . . □ None   □ Some   □ A lot

74. Elevators . . . . □ None   □ Some   □ A lot

75. Dark places . . . . □ None   □ Some   □ A lot

76. Not being able to breathe . . . . □ None   □ Some   □ A lot

77. Getting a bee sting . . . . □ None   □ Some   □ A lot

78. Worms or snails . . . . □ None   □ Some   □ A lot

79. Rats or mice . . . . □ None   □ Some   □ A lot

80. Taking a test . . . . □ None   □ Some   □ A lot

Appendix 5.2. The Childhood Anxiety Sensitivity Index

(Silverman, Fleisig, Rabian & Peterson, 1991)

Directions: A number of statements which boys and girls use to describe themselves are given below. Read each statement carefully and put an 'X' in the blank in front of the words that describe you. There are no right or wrong answers. Remember, find the words that best describe you.

1. I don't want other people to know when I feel afraid. __None __Some __A lot

2. When I cannot keep my mind on my schoolwork I worry that I might be going crazy. __None __Some __A lot

3. It scares me when I feel 'shaky'. __None __Some __A lot

4. It scares me when I feel like I am going to faint. __None __Some __A lot

5. It is important for me to stay in control of my feelings. __None __Some __A lot

6. It scares me when my heart beats fast. __None __Some __A lot

7. It embarrasses me when my stomach growls (makes noise). __None __Some __A lot

8. It scares me when I feel like I am going to throw up. __None __Some __A lot

9. When I notice that my heart is beating fast, I worry that there might be something wrong with me. __None __Some __A lot

10. It scares me when I have trouble getting my breath. __None __Some __A lot

11. When my stomach hurts, I worry that I might be really sick __None __Some __A lot

12. It scares me when I can't keep my mind on my schoolwork. __None __Some __A lot

13. Other kids can tell when I feel shaky. __None __Some __A lot

14. Unusual feelings in my body scare me. __None __Some __A lot

15. When I am afraid, I worry that I might be crazy.   __None __Some __A lot

16. It scares me when I feel nervous.   __None __Some __A lot

17. I don't like to let my feelings show.   __None __Some __A lot

18. Funny feelings in my body scare me.   __None __Some __A lot

Appendix 5.3. A relaxation training script for children (Ollendick, 1978)

Hands and arms

Make a fist with your left hand. Squeeze it hard. Feel the tightness in your hand and arm as you squeeze. Now let your hand go and relax. See how much better your hand and arm feel when they are relaxed. Once again, make a fist with your left hand and squeeze hard. Good. Now relax and let your hand go. (Repeat the process for the right hand and arm.)

Arms and shoulders

Stretch your arms out in front of you. Raise them high up over your head. Way back. Feel the pull in your shoulders. Stretch higher. Now just let your arms drop back to your side. Okay, let's stretch again. Stretch your arms out in front of you. Raise them over your head. Pull them back, way back. Pull hard. Now let them drop quickly. Good. Notice how your shoulders feel more relaxed. This time let's have a great big stretch. Try to touch the ceiling. Stretch your arms way out in front of you. Raise them way up high over your head. Push them way, way back. Notice the tension and pull in your arms and shoulders. Hold tight now. Great. Let them drop very quickly and feel how good it is to be relaxed. It feels good and warm and lazy.

Shoulders and neck

Try to pull your shoulders up to your ears and push your head down into your shoulders. Hold in tight. Okay, now relax and feel the warmth. Again, pull your shoulders up to your ears and push your head down into your shoulders. Do it tightly. Okay, you can relax now. Bring your head out and let your shoulders relax. Notice how much better it feels to be relaxed than to be all tight. One more time now. Push your head down and your shoulders way up to your ears. Hold it. Feel the tenseness in your neck and shoulders. Okay. You can relax now and feel comfortable. You feel good.

Jaw

Put your teeth together real hard. Let your neck muscles help you. Now relax. Just let your jaw hang loose. Notice how good it feels just to let your jaw drop. Okay, bite down again hard. That's good. Now relax again. Just let your jaw drop. It feels so good just to let go. Okay, one more time. Bite down. Hard as you can. Harder. Oh, you're really working hard. Good. Now relax. Try to relax your whole body. Let yourself go as loose as you can.

Face and nose

Wrinkle up your nose. Make as many wrinkles in your nose as you can. Scrunch your nose up real hard. Good. Now you can relax your nose. Now wrinkle up your nose again. Wrinkle it up hard. Hold it just as tight as you can. Okay. You can relax your face. Notice that when you scrunch up your nose that your cheeks and your mouth and your forehead all help you and they get tight, too. So when you relax your nose, your whole face relaxes too, and that feels good. Now make lots of wrinkles on your forehead. Hold it tight now. Okay, you can let go. Now you can just relax. Let your face go smooth. No wrinkles anywhere. Your face feels nice and smooth and relaxed.

Stomach

Now tighten up your stomach muscles real tight. Make your stomach real hard. Don't move. Hold it. You can relax now. Let your stomach go soft. Let it be as relaxed as you can. That feels so much better. Okay, again. Tighten your stomach real hard. Good. You can relax now. Kind of settle down, get comfortable, and relax. Notice the difference between a tight stomach and a relaxed one. That's how we want it to feel. Nice and loose and relaxed. Okay. Once more. Tighten up. Tighten hard. Good. Now you can relax completely. You can feel nice and relaxed.

This time, try to pull your stomach in. Try to squeeze it against your backbone. Try to be as skinny as you can. Now relax. You don't have to be skinny now. Just relax and feel your stomach being warm and loose. Okay, squeeze in your stomach again. Make it touch your backbone. Get it real small and tight. Get as skinny as you can. Hold tight now. You can relax now. Settle back and let your stomach come back out where it belongs. You can really feel good now. You've done fine.

Legs and feet

Push your toes down on the floor real hard. You'll probably need your legs to help you push. Push down, spread your toes apart. Now relax your feet. Let your toes go loose and feel how nice that is. It feels good to be relaxed. Okay. Now push your toes down. Let your leg muscles help you push your feet down. Push your feet. Hard. Okay. Relax your feet, relax your legs, relax your toes. It feels so good to be relaxed. No tenseness anywhere. You feel kind of warm and tingly.

Source: Ollendick, T. H. & Cerny, J. A. (1981). *Clinical Behavior Therapy with Children.* New York: Plenum Press.

6

Obsessive-compulsive disorders

Per Hove Thomsen

Department of Child and Adolescent Psychiatry, University Hospital Aarhus, Denmark

Introduction

Research in children and adolescents over the past 20–30 years has documented that OCD (obsessive-compulsive disorder) is considerably more common than believed previously. The need for treatment of this, in many cases rather disabling disorder, has been recognized. The availability of treatment has increased immensely, and a number of studies have documented the role of psychopharmacological treatment and to a lesser extent cognitive behavioural treatment.

Definition and classification

Many children experience ritualistic behaviour during certain phases of their normal development as shown in Table 6.1. This ritualistic behaviour, however, is characterized as being non-disabling and non-distressing to the child. However, this normal ritualistic behaviour seems to help the child in structuring daily life, to perform controlling behaviour and to develop reasonable habits.

OCD is defined by the presence of obsessions and/or compulsions, a definition which applies to both children and adults. The main characteristics of obsessions are shown in Table 6.2. Obsessions are recurrent, persistent ideas, thoughts, images or impulses, which are egodystonic and regarded by the child as futile or repugnant. Egodystonic means that the child recognizes the obsessions as thoughts alien to his or her conscience. Compulsions are repetitive and seemingly purposeful actions which are performed in accordance with certain rules or in a stereotyped fashion. The obsessions and compulsions must be a significant source of distress to the child or they must interfere with social or role functioning.

Diagnostic criteria according to ICD-10 and DSM-IV are shown in Table 6.3. According to DSM-IV the principle of egodystonic thoughts is not applicable to all

A Clinician's Handbook of Child and Adolescent Psychiatry, ed. Christopher Gillberg,
Richard Harrington and Hans-Christoph Steinhausen. Published by Cambridge University Press.
© Cambridge University Press 2005.

Table 6.1. Rituals and superstition in normal children

Bed rituals	Small children
Avoiding stepping on cracks	Younger children
Control/checking	Younger and older children (mild form)
Counting/lucky numbers	Older children
Touching	Older children (when playing) – not common
Washing/showering	Preschool children (mild), seldom in teenagers (unless OCD)
Fear of dirt and contamination	Younger children and older children (only in mild forms)

Table 6.2. What characterizes an obsession?

Recognized as part of own thoughts or urges (not transferred from the outside)
Recurrent
Unpleasant
Recognized as unreasonable
Distressful and affects social functioning

children. In DSM-IV the subcategory OCD with poor insight has been introduced. This subgroup of OCD-patients is characterized by having constantly poor insight in which OCD-patients are unable to rationalize and detach themselves from their symptoms. In many children the poor insight category may well apply, as children are known to have poorer insight regarding their symptoms as they are also usually less resistant to obsessions. In ICD-10, the only subgroups are whether obsessions or compulsions dominate.

Epidemiology

Prevalence rates

Transient, mild obsessive and compulsive behaviours are not rare in children and adolescents. OCD, defined as described above, affects 0.8–1.5 per cent of the paediatric and adolescent population. Table 6.4 presents recent epidemiological studies, all using DSM-diagnostic criteria for case definition.

Incidence rates

OCD onset is found frequently in childhood or during adolescence. Newer studies indicate that between 50 and 80 per cent of adult OCD-patients have experienced symptoms before the age of 18 years. In children with OCD the ratio of males to females is normally 2:1.

Table 6.3. ICD-10 and DSM-IV criteria for OCD[1]

A. Either obsessions or compulsions:

Obsessions as defined by (1), (2), (3), and (4):

(1) recurrent and persistent thoughts, impulses or images that are experienced, at some time during the disturbance, as intrusive and inappropriate and that cause marked anxiety or distress;

(2) the thoughts, impulses or images are not simply excessive worries about real-life problems;

(3) the person attempts to ignore or suppress such thoughts, impulses or images, or to neutralize them with some other thought or action;

(4) the person recognizes that the obsessional thoughts, impulses or images are a product of his or her own mind (not imposed from without as in thought insertion).

Compulsions as defined by (1) and (2):

1. repetitive behaviours (e.g. hand washing, ordering, checking) or mental acts (e.g. praying, counting, repeating words silently) that the person feels driven to perform in response to an obsession, or according to rules that must be applied rigidly;

2. the behaviours or mental acts are aimed at preventing or reducing distress or preventing some dreaded event or situation; however, these behaviours or mental acts either are not connected in a realistic way with what they are designed to neutralize or prevent or are clearly excessive.

A. At some point during the course of the disorder, the person has recognized that the obsessions or compulsions are excessive or unreasonable. *Note*: This does not apply to children.

B. The obsessions or compulsions cause marked distress, are time consuming (take more than one hour a day), or significantly interfere with the person's normal routine, occupation (or academic) function, or usual social activities or relationships.

C. If another Axis I disorder is present, the content of the obsession or compulsion is not restricted to it (e.g. preoccupation with food in the presence of an eating disorder, hair pulling in the presence of trichotillomania, concern with appearance in the presence of body dysmorphic disorder; preoccupation with drugs in the presence of a substance use disorder; preoccupation with having a serious illness in the presence of hypochondriasis; preoccupation with sexual urges or fantasies in the presence of a paraphilia; or guilty rumination in the presence of major depressive disorder).

D. The disturbances are not due to the direct physiological effects of a substance (e.g. a drug of abuse, a medication) or a general medical condition.

Specify if:

With poor insight: if, for most of the time during the current episode, the person does not recognize that the obsessions and compulsions are excessive or unreasonable.

---

[1] The ICD-10 criteria are identical. However, ICD-10 does not include the poor insight subtype
Source: The Diagnostic and Statistical Manual of Mental Disorders, Fourth Edition.
Copyright 1994 American Psychiatric Association, pp. 422–3.

Table 6.4. Prevalence of OCD in children and adolescents. Community studies with structured clinical interviews

Author	Country	n(age)	Prevalence (%)
Douglass, H. M., Moffitt, E. H., Dar, R., McGee, R. & Silva, P. (1995). Obsessive-compulsive disorder in a birth cohort of 18-year-olds: prevalence and predictors. *J. Am. Acad. Child Adolesc. Psychiatry*, **34** (11), 1424–31.	New Zealand	930 (18)	4.0
Esser, G., Scmidt, M. H. & Woerner, W. (1990). Epidemiology and course of psychiatric disorders in school-age children – results of a longitudinal study. *J. Child Psychol. Psychiatry*, **31** (2), 243–63.	Germany	356 (8–13)	2.8–4.6 (8 yr olds)[a]
Flament, M., Whitaker, A., Rapoport, J. L. *et al.* (1988). Obsessive compulsive disorder in adolescence: an epidemiological study. *J. Am. Acad. Child Adolesc. Psychiatry*, **27** (6), 764–71.	USA	5108 (14–18)	1.0
Reinherz, H. Z., Giaconia, R. M., Lefkowitz, E. S., Pakiz, B. & Frost, A. K. (1993). Prevalence of psychiatric disorder in a community population of older adolescents. *J. Am. Acad. Child Adolesc. Psychiatry*, **32** (2), 369–77.	USA	386 (18)	1.3
Thomsen, P. H. (1993). Obsessive-compulsive disorder in children and adolescents. Self-reported obsessive-compulsive behaviour in pupils in Denmark. *Acta Psychiatr. Scand.*, **88**, 212–17.	Denmark	1032 (11–17)	4.1[a]
Valleni-Basile, L. A., Garrison, C. Z., Jackson, K. L. *et al.* (1994). Frequency of obsessive-compulsive disorder in a community sample of young adolescents. *J. Am. Acad. Child Adolesc. Psychiatry*, **33** (6), 782–91.	USA	3283 (12–15)	3.0
Zohar, A. H., Ratzosin, G., Pauls, D. L. *et al.* (1992). An epidemiological study of obsessive-compulsive disorder and related disorders in Israeli adolescents. *J. Am. Acad. Child Adolesc. Psychiatry*, **31**, 1057–61.	Israel	562 (16–17)	1.8[b]–3.6[c]

Diagnostic criteria are DSM-III or DSM-III-R.
a: obsessive-compulsive symptoms.
b: excluding pure obsessional.
c: all with obsessions and/or compulsions.

Boys with OCD may experience more severe manifestations of OCD in childhood or they may have more co-morbid illnesses forcing the child to referral. Boys may also have a higher prevalence of neurological impairments. On the other hand, the clinical picture and the severity appears to be identical in males and females.

Implications for clinical practice

For many children and adolescents, OCD takes a chronic course. Only a few follow-up studies have been conducted in child and adolescent populations with OCD; however, there are strong indications that OCD affects social life, quality of life and that many OCD-patients suffer from a waxing and waning course with partial remission or constantly distressing obsessive-compulsive symptoms throughout a lifelong perspective.

Clinical picture

The most common OCD symptoms seen in affected children and adolescents are anxiety regarding dirt and contamination and exaggerated washing rituals or checking behaviour. The most common OCD symptoms in paediatric populations of OCD patients are presented in Table 6.5.

Another very common obsession is fear of harming oneself or another person. Quite a number of patients have obsessions regarding illness and death. Some children have a totally irrational fear of contracting AIDS, being infected with salmonella or getting cancer. In spite of these children's insight and sensible distance towards their symptoms, they are very often totally dominated by obsessions of illness and death. Many children, therefore, exhibit avoidant behaviour in which they increasingly isolate themselves and avoid any situation where such dangerous thoughts about illness or death might occur.

Some children have repeating rituals, i.e. they have to repeat daily routines or specific actions endlessly. Obsessions and compulsions on symmetry indicates that every action done with the right hand has to be repeated by the left, etc. Some children are not able to describe any specific obsessions, but merely experience 'just right' perceptions in which they feel they can relax after having done the compulsions. Some children exclusively have mental rituals. These compulsions are done within the mind of the child, such as counting, calculating specific numbers, thinking about and memorizing specific words or names of people.

There seems to be a great deal of overlap between symptoms and between different groups of obsessions and compulsions. No specific correlation has been shown between types of obsessive-compulsive symptoms and age or sex, neither in the adult nor in the paediatric population. In the long-term perspective obsessive-compulsive symptoms seem to change over time.

Table 6.5. Most common OCD symptoms

Obsessions	Compulsions
Concern with dirt, germs	Hand washing, showering, grooming
Something terrible happening	Repeating
Symmetry, order	Checking
Scrupulousness (religious)	Writing, moving, speaking
Concern with bodily secretions	Removing contact with contaminants
Lucky/unlucky numbers	Touching
Forbidden, aggressive, sexual thoughts	Counting
Fear might harm others/self	Ordering/arranging
Concern with household items	Preventing harm to self or others
Nonsense sounds, words or music	Hoarding/collecting
	Cleaning objects

Differential diagnoses and co-morbidity

Various disorders have to be considered for differential diagnoses with some occurring also as a co-morbid condition. Specifically Tourette syndrome, schizophrenia, eating disorder, pervasive developmental disorder, depressive symptoms and anxiety disorder have to be considered.

- Obsessions and compulsions as part of OCD must be differentiated towards elaborated tics as part of the Tourette syndrome. Obsessions are egodystonic and are experienced as invading, senseless and distressful. In Tourette syndrome tics are usually not experienced as invading and on the contrary they are often followed by a pleasant feeling of relaxation. Many patients with Tourette syndrome also fulfil the criteria for OCD. In these patients the most common obsessions and compulsions are regarding symmetry, spitting, staring and touching. Family studies suggest genetic relations between OCD and Tourette syndrome.

- In schizophrenia the patients suffer from delusions and hallucinations. Delusions are not experienced as egodystonic; on the contrary they are ego-syntonic. However, during recent years researchers and clinicians have acknowledged increasingly that a high number of patients with schizophrenia also suffer from OCD.

- Eating disorders are characterized by a distorted body image and a fear of gaining weight. In anorexia nervosa, for instance, the thought about gaining weight and the distortion of body image is ego-syntonic and not an ego-alien obsession. However, in many patients with eating disorders OCD is present and several studies indicate a relation between eating disorders and OCD.

- Pervasive developmental disorders are characterized by disturbance of social interaction, ritualized and extremely habitual behaviour and particular areas of interests. In clinical practice it is usually not difficult to differ OCD from Asperger's syndrome. In some patients with Asperger's syndrome however, obsessions may be present and should be treated as such.

- Depressive symptoms are often seen in OCD and several long-term studies indicate that more than half of adult OCD patients will at some point fulfil the criteria for depression.
- Anxiety disorders, such as separation anxiety and social phobia, are seen rather frequently as co-morbid disorders to OCD.

Assessment

OCD is a psychiatric disorder in which no blood test or other objective examination can be performed in order to diagnose. Pure OCD is usually easy to diagnose but very often co-morbid conditions are present and sometimes social consequences of the disorder may complicate the diagnostic procedure. However, a thorough diagnostic procedure is necessary to fully understand the extent and severity of the OCD symptoms and thereby the whole situation of the child. Further, a thorough and detailed diagnostic procedure is necessary for initiating treatment with cognitive behavioural therapy or medication.

First of all, it is essential to distinguish between obsessive-compulsive symptoms as an expression of OCD and temporary, light rituals as part of normal development. It is important to get a picture of how much symptoms dominate the daily life of the child, how distressing they are to the child, and also how symptoms seem to affect the whole family situation. The following will be necessary to include in the assessment procedure: Disposition, assessment of the family pattern and family climate (in order to detect which factors might possibly maintain symptoms). The developmental history, the time of onset of OCD, and the way in which the obsessive-compulsive symptoms were recognized by parents, the presence of other psychiatric disorders (especially depression, eating disorder or Tourette syndrome), psychosocial functioning (in school and at home), somatic disorders (especially infectious diseases (see description of PANDAS) and description of critical life events (which might be relevant for the onset of OCD).

Diagnostic instruments

The screening most commonly used and well estimated for obsessive-compulsive symptoms and indicator of severity is the Yale–Brown Obsessive Compulsive Scale, which also exists in a children's version (CY-BOCS). In this interview both obsessions and compulsions are covered. The degree of interference, distress, resistance towards symptoms and control over symptoms are measured. Furthermore, aspects of insight in symptomatology, avoidant behaviour, indecisiveness, the feeling of responsibility and obsessive slowness and pathological doubt are included in this fine instrument. A total score of 10–18 indicates mild OCD, which might be distressful but does not cause dysfunction. A total score between 19 and 29 indicates moderate OCD causing both distress and social dysfunction. A total score above 30 indicates severe OCD with clear dysfunction and distress.

Advantages and disadvantages

The CY-BOCS has quite a high reliability, a partially documented validity, the measurement of severity is not dependent on the number of obsessive symptoms and the instrument is very good at measuring changes (such as treatment response); however, the instrument demands knowledge and understanding of OCD by the clinician, and the major disadvantage seems to be the simplified total score. Patients with severe obsessions but without compulsions, for instance, will not score as high as patients with moderate symptoms with both obsessions and compulsions. This gives a somewhat skewed picture of the severity of the patient's disease.

Another instrument is the Leyton Obsessional Inventory. This instrument was originally designed for measuring obsessive traits in house mothers and consisted of 69 questions. An 11-item short version has been developed for children and adolescents and is included in the appendix.

Advantages and disadvantages

The Leyton Obsessional Inventory has been used relatively frequently in epidemiological studies. It detects both symptoms and traits, resistance against symptoms and the degree of interference of the symptoms. However, no studies of reliability or validity have been performed. The total score seems to be not clinically relevant. The instrument is not specifically designed for OCD patients, and the instrument is not good at measuring changes as a result of treatment.

Aetiology

Multiple aetiological theories for OCD have been suggested, including neuropsychiatric, immunological, aetiological, psychodynamic and behavioural pathways.

- Evidence from neuropsychological studies, family genetic studies, and neuroimaging strongly suggest a neurobiological cause of OCD. Pharmacological and biochemical challenge studies suggest that abnormalities in serotonergic activity in the brain are related to at least a significant proportion of OCD cases. Position erission tomography (PET) scans have shown increased glucose metabolism in orbito-frontal and pre-frontal cortex, right caudate nucleus in adults as well as children with OCD. A successful treatment with either behavioural therapy or SSRI medication has led to a normalization of these deviations in frontal and basal ganglia glucose metabolism.

- A subtype of early onset OCD has been suggested: PANDAS (paediatric autoimmune psychiatric disorder associated with streptococcal infections). This subtype of OCD describes the presence of OCD following infection with group-A beta-hemolytic streptococcus leading to an autoimmune response to the infection. The symptoms have been explained to be caused by the development of nuclear antibodies against nucleus caudatus in the basal ganglia. The PANDAS-picture is characterized by the following: presence of OCD or tics, onset of OCD-symptoms before puberty, sudden onset and a typically saw tooth course with sudden changes simultaneously with exacerbation of symptoms and neurologic abnormalities and simultaneously infections with hemolytic streptococcus. This subtype of OCD has not yet led to any established treatment algorithms relevant to this group of patients. From a research point of view, however, the findings are very interesting and further stress the involvement of nucleus caudatus in the pathogenesis of OCD.
- Family studies and a few twin studies demonstrate that OCD is a heritable disorder where as many as 50 per cent of paediatric OCD cases may be familial.

Treatment

General treatment principles

Before a treatment is started, a thorough evaluation of the child must be undertaken. In mild cases of OCD, the school psychologist or a general practitioner may help the child in controlling and suppressing the OCD symptoms. In more severe cases, however, referral to specialist treatment is warranted.

Treatment algorithms

The first, and very important, part of a treatment programme is psychoeducation. Information about aetiology, treatment methods and their efficacy is provided to the child or adolescent, to the parents and siblings. A number of parents may be annoyed that their child is not capable of 'pulling itself together' and suppress the more dominant obsessive-compulsive symptoms. On the other hand, many parents are, naturally, worried about their child's condition and they may also feel guilt that they have done something wrong in their education of the child. Therefore, information and counselling is very important.

During this phase of treatment one must also consider whether the teachers in school, the mates of the child and other family members should be told about the child's condition. Many children with OCD are very secretive as to the symptoms and find it very embarrassing to reveal them. Thus, it is very important to include the child in these decisions. As a second step it should be considered what kind of support is needed for the child in school, in its spare time and at home. For some children with severe OCD it may be helpful to lower the demands regarding school work etc. for a period of time.

As a general principle the following guidelines can be used when planning an OCD treatment programme.

- Assess degree of insight into OC-symptoms and treatment motivation.
- Assess co-morbid symptoms such as depression, anxiety, drug abuse, tics or Tourette syndrome. If the latter is present, antipsychotic medication may be helpful in addition to SSRI and CBT.
- Assess OCD symptoms thoroughly (with Yale-Brown Obsessive Compulsive Scale, Children's version (CY-BOCS), symptom check list).
- Assess severity of OCD (with CY-BOCS).
- Inform child and family about OCD and treatment procedure. Distribute literature and brochures on OCD.
- Assess need for CBT (with exposure and prevention), maybe combined with SSRI-treatment.
- Assess efficacy of 4–6 CBT-sessions and consider SSRI-treatment.
- Initiate medication. A trial should be performed for at least 10–12 weeks with at least 6 weeks on adequate dose (usual or maximum dose).
- In case of poor response reassess motivation and compliance to both the CBT and medication. Include support from parents or others.
- In case of consistent poor or non-response consider augmentative medication.

The treatment tree shown in Fig. 6.1 may be a useful guidance.

Cognitive behavioural therapy

The next step in the treatment programme would be application of psychotherapy based on cognitive behavioural principles.

During the behavioural therapy focus is upon change of behavioural patterns. The main approach is exposure and prevention therapy (exposure: The child is exposed to the stimulus that increases anxiety and releases a compulsive behaviour; prevention: The usual compulsive act is prevented and the child is helped to overcome the anxiety without performing compulsive or avoiding behaviour). In the cognitive therapy the main focus is upon changing the cognitive distortions (e.g. If I don't wash my hands 100 times, I will catch AIDS). These cognitive distortions are supposed to create the compulsive behaviour.

Much of this cognitive behavioural therapy (CBT) is based on home tasks. In small children the primary approach is behavioural, whereas cognitive aspects should be included with increasing age as shown in Fig. 6.2. Parents play a very important role in performing the CBT and in maintaining compliance to the therapy.

Choose <u>initial</u> treatment based on severity and age

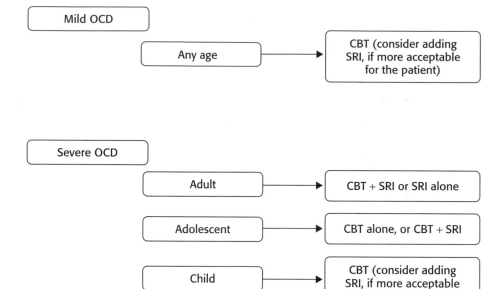

Insufficient efficacy:

If initial treatment was:

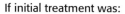

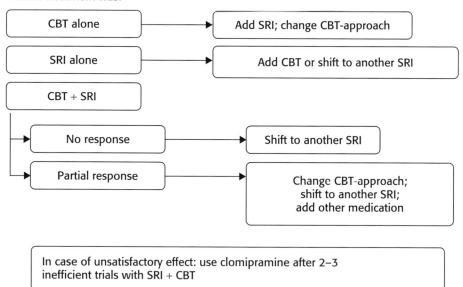

Fig. 6.1.   'Treatment tree'.

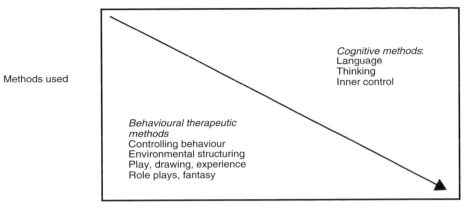

Fig. 6.2.   CBT components by age.

The cognitive behavioural therapy of the obsessive-compulsive symptoms in children and adolescents should always be individually organized. The obsessive-compulsive symptoms, as described previously, seem rather homogenous according to form and content, but choice of speed of therapy, in which order things should be done, and which specific methods seem to be optimal, must be dependent on the individual child. The treatment is structured with a combination of sessions with the child, therapist (and parents) and home tasks. During sessions the child's work with home tasks is discussed and new tasks are formulated. Parents should be involved partly in these sessions and should be informed of the home tasks and how they can support the child's duties at home. Table 6.6 describes how a treatment programme can be structured, session by session.

In order to increase compliance and to engage the child in the therapeutic programme, the initial sessions should be rather intense without too long intervals in between. Many children will benefit from – in between sessions – telephone talks or communication via email. The individual session should have a set structure and content, which could be as shown in Table 6.7.

Registration of obsessive-compulsive symptoms is an important element of CBT. The CY-BOCS detects different kinds of obsessive and compulsive symptoms and rates also severity, distress, resistance and insight into OCD symptoms. Using this instrument would help the therapist and the child to keep on track and to measure changes throughout the therapy. Examples of symptom registration are presented in Table 6.8.

Based on the symptom registration, a hierarchy of the symptoms is created. Based on this hierarchy, the exposure and prevention therapy (ERP) can be planned. The ERP can be imaginary or in vivo. When choosing items from the hierarchy of symptoms for ERP, it is important to have the opinion of the child/adolescent,

Table 6.6. Treatment model

Sessions	Contents

1. session	Psychoeducation
	    Actual knowledge on OCD
	    Rationale behind CBT

2.–5. session	Registration of symptoms Stimulus hierarchy Exposure and response prevention (ERP)
6.–14. session	ERP + cognitive therapy/training
15.–16. session	Repetition of learnt strategies and psychoeducation concerning maintenance, generalization and relapse prevention
Few sessions	Repetition of strategies, etc.

Table 6.7. Structure in the treatment session

A. Contact
B. Review, since last
C. What problems do you want to work with? Itinerary
D. Home work from last session, go through and work with
E. Today's subject(s) – guided analysis and work, identifying themes
F. Choice of new home work, ERP
G. Summary of session and new home task(s)
H. Information and summary with parents

and the therapist must make sure that the ERP concentrates on items that are of high relevance to the OCD patient, and, on the other hand, is not too difficult (because of high level of anxiety). During therapy the therapist must consider and be aware of avoiding behaviour in which the child avoids confrontation with the feared stimulus.

Treatment of obsessions and mental rituals

In cases with obsessions and mental rituals the exposure could be organized as one to two daily periods of worry, in which the child devotes himself to an obsession, and during the rest of the day tries to resist the thoughts. The child is encouraged to postpone the obsessions to these times of worry. Other children may benefit from ERP based on sound recordings. The child writes down obsessions or mental rituals and during therapy session dictates these to a tape recorder, which the child must listen to repeatedly at home, up to for instance 30–45 minutes every day. The

Table 6.8. Example of use of symptom hierarchy and anxiety barometer in a treatment course

	Level of anxiety (range: 0–10; 10 is most severe anxiety)				
Session no.	1	2	3	4	5
1 Writing on computer	5	3	1	1	0
2 Cleansing spoons before use at home	1	1	0	0	0
3 Eating at friend's house	10	10	7	7	6
4 Eating in restaurant	7	1	1	0	0
5 Touching objects	5–10	4–7	3–5	0	0
6 Drinking from opened milk carton	5–6	1–3	0	0	0

Table 6.9. Techniques to break OCD rituals

Methods	Description	Example
Postpone the ritual	Decide on postponing ritual until it fades away	Postpone washing ritual 1 hour
Shorten the ritual	Perform the ritual, but for shorter and shorter time, until it no longer feels necessary	Wash for 10 min instead of 15 min
Change the ritual	Change some of the ritual in a way that breaks the OCD-rule	Do not wash fingers consecutively
Perform the ritual	Instead of rushing through the ritual to get it over with, do it slowly and carefully with your attention on the detail in the ritual	Wash each finger one time carefully instead of washing hands over and over

goal of treatment is to break down OCD rituals. Table 6.9 shows some techniques to break OCD rituals.

Psychopharmacological treatment

A variety of medications has been used in the treatment of adult OCD patients. The treatment has involved the use of antidepressants and has emerged from the hypothesis that a dysregulation of the serotonin neurotransmitter system may be responsible for OCD. Looking upon the psychopharmacological approach, the first choice would be an antidepressant agent with serotonergic efficacy. Clomipramine is the most extensively studied of the antidepressants in child and adolescent cases. Double-blind, placebo-controlled, cross-over and parallel studies have found that

Table 6.10. Usual start dose and end dose and maximum dose are given below

Drug	Usual start dose (mg)	Usual end dose (mg)	Usual maximum dose (mg)
Citalopram	10 (in small children 5)	40–60	60
Fluoxetine	10	40–60	80
Fluvoxamine	25	200	250
Paroxetine	10	40–50	60
Sertraline	25	100–125	200

clomipramine is significantly superior to placebo. Clomipramine, however, can, as a tricyclic antidepressant, cause tachycardia and prolongation of ECG intervals.

Large systematic trials of SSRI's in adult OCD patients have documented their efficacy. Randomized controlled trials now exist for paediatric OCD for fluoxetine, fluvoxamine and sertraline, and open label trials have shown efficacy for citalopram. One study on a paediatric population shows that sertraline has the same pharmacokinetics and dynamics as seen in adult patients, and tolerability has been documented. The side effects most commonly described include nausea, headache, tremor, gastrointestinal complaints, insomnia and – in some children – disinhibition, agitation or even hypomania at higher doses of SSRI.

In the majority of cases significant to moderate improvement can be observed after several weeks on SSRI. In most cases, an improvement rate of 20–50 per cent is reported following medication. It is thus recommended that medication is combined with CBT in order to obtain results that are more permanent.

Effective doses

So far, the optimal dose has not been described for children and adolescents with OCD. A low dose is recommended initially followed by a gradual increase in order to avoid side effects and to monitor efficacy. During the first approximately 10 days of treatment some children might complain from a deterioration of their obsessive-compulsive symptoms or may seem agitated. It is crucial that, during this phase of treatment, the child or adolescent is encouraged to continue medication, temporarily a lower dose might be needed, as these side effects seem to disappear after a few days. It should be stressed that these doses are only intended as a guide and the optimal therapeutic doses are still not determined. Table 6.10 provides information on recommended doses.

Duration of treatment

It is difficult exactly to determine how long the medication should be continued. Many OCD patients, adults as well as children, show a relapse of OCD symptoms when treatment is discontinued. On the other hand, some long-term studies show that children and adolescents with OCD will not have chronic OCD symptoms. It is therefore, recommended to try discontinuation of medication after $1\frac{1}{2}$–2 years effective treatment.

Discontinuation

Discontinuation is recommended after $1\frac{1}{2}$–2 years of effective treatment. In some OCD patients deterioration in obsessive-compulsive symptoms may be seen following the discontinuation. Some studies suggest that concurrent CBT may reduce this deterioration. Discontinuation of psychopharmacological treatment is recommended to be slow, partly in order to avoid withdrawal symptoms but mainly for psychological reasons. It is recommended that discontinuation is done by reducing by 25 per cent every second month and that discontinuation is done in the absence of stressful life events or turmoil in the child's life.

Compliance

Some children and adolescents may be reluctant to take the medication in case this becomes entangled with an OCD ritual, or if side effects are too prominent. Some children with OCD may even experience the obsession that medication is contaminated. In these cases it is important to note that medication alone is rarely as effective as medication combined with behavioural therapy.

The treatment of non- or poor-responders

In case the child does not respond to the recommended combination of CBT and SSRI, one must examine the possible factors to explain this lack of efficacy. When compliance is OK, one should try shifting to another SSRI as some patients may not respond as well to one particular SSRI as others do. However, this shift should not be made before a trial of at least 12 weeks of treatment.

Augmenting strategies

There are only a few descriptions of augmenting strategies in the child and adolescent population. Risperidone has been described and has proved superior to placebo in controlled studies in adults, but no other studies have so far proved superior to a placebo. This agent can be used with co-morbid tics, in subgroups with poor insight in obsessive-compulsive symptoms, and in adolescents with co-morbid disorder of borderline personality disorder. In cases with much anxiety, buspirone can be tried; however, only one report has suggested it to be effective in adolescents with severe OCD and anxiety.

Outcome

For many children and adolescents with OCD, the disorder takes a chronic course. There still are a limited number of long-term studies that illustrate the course of disorder from childhood to adult age. However, studies from the USA, Denmark, Germany and India seem very consistent that more than half of the patients will still suffer from OCD as adults. The longest study on the course of OCD was performed in Sweden. With the total follow-up time of 47 years, the researchers concluded that 83 per cent of the patients were better (reduction of obsessions and compulsions) of whom 20 per cent were completely well. Twenty-eight per cent had obsessive-compulsive symptoms on a subclinical level.

From most of the studies it is concluded that early age of onset and the presence of both obsessions and compulsions compromise the social function, and that co-morbid disorders such as Tourette syndrome predict negative outcome. It must be borne in mind that most of the studies referred to here were conducted in a time when treatment options were not optimal because access to cognitive behavioural therapy and medication was very limited.

SUGGESTED READING

J. Alderman, R. Wolkow, M. Chung & H. F. Johnston, Sertraline treatment of children and adolescents with obsessive-compulsive disorder: pharmacokinetics, tolerability, and efficacy. *Journal of the American Academy of Child and Adolescent Psychiatry*, **37** (1998), 386–94.

L. Barr, W. K. Goodman, L. H. Price, C. J. McDougle & D. S. Charney, The serotonin hypothesis of obsessive-compulsive disorder: Implications of pharmacologic challenge studies. *Journal of Clinical Psychiatry*, **53** (1992), 17–28.

E. H. Cook, K. D. Wagner, J. S. March *et al.*, Long-term sertraline treatment of children and adolescents with obsessive-compulsive disorder. *Journal of the American Academy of Child and Adolescent Psychiatry*, **40** (10) (2001), 1175–81.

E. J. Berg, J. L. Rapoport & M. Flament, The Leyton Obsessional Inventory-Child Version. *Journal of the American Academy of Child Psychiatry*, **25** (1986), 84–91.

J. Cooper, The Leyton Obsessional Inventory. *Psychological Medicine*, **1** (1970), 48–64.

J. DeVeaugh-Geiss, G. Moroz, J. Biederman *et al.*, Clomipramine hydrochloride in childhood and adolescent obsessive-compulsive disorder – a multicenter trial. *Journal of the American Academy of Child and Adolescent Psychiatry*, **31** (1992), 45–9.

M. Flament, A. Whitaker, J. L. Rapoport *et al.*, Obsessive compulsive disorder in adolescence: an epidemiological study. *Journal of the American Academy of Child and Adolescent Psychiatry*, **27** (6) (1988), 764–71.

H. L. Leonard, S. E. Swedo, M. Lenane *et al.*, A two to seven year follow-up study of 54 obsessive compulsive children and adolescents. *Archives of General Psychiatry*, **50** (1993), 429–39.

J. S. March, J. Biederman, R. Wolkow *et al.*, Sertraline in children and adolescents with obsessive-compulsive disorder: a multicenter randomized controlled trial. *Journal of the American Medical Association*, **280** (20) (1998), 1752–6.

J. S. March & H. L. Leonard Obsessive-compulsive disorder in children and adolescents: a review of the past 10 years. *Journal of the American Academy of Child and Adolescent Psychiatry*, **35** (1996), 1265–73.

J. S. March & K. Mulle, *OCD in Children and Adolescents. A Cognitive-Behavioral Treatment Manual.* (The Guilford Press, New York: The Guilford Press, 1998).

J. S. March, K. Mulle & B. Herbel, Behavioral psychotherapy for children and adolescents with obsessive-compulsive disorder: an open trial of a new protocol-driven treatment package. *Journal of the American Medical Association*, **33** (3) (1994), 333–41.

J. L. Rapoport, *The Boy Who Couldn't Stop Washing.* (New York: Penguin Books, 1991).

M. Riddle, J. Claghorn, G. Gaffney *et al.*, A controlled trial of fluvoxamine for obsessive-compulsive disorder in children and adolescents. *Psychopharmacology Bulletin*, **32** (3) (1996), 399.

M. A. Riddle, M. Scahill, R. A. King *et al.*, Double-blind, crossover trial of fluoxetine and placebo in children and adolescents with obsessive-compulsive disorder. *Journal of the American Academy of Child and Adolescent Psychiatry*, **31** (1992), 1062–9.

M. A. Riddle, E. A. Reeve, J. A. Yaryura-Tobias *et al.*, Fluvoxamine for children and adolescents with obsessive-compulsive disorder: a randomized, controlled, multicenter trial. *Journal of the American Academy of Child and Adolescent Psychiatry*, **40** (2) (2001), 222–9.

G. Skoog & I. Skoog, A 40-year follow-up of patients with obsessive-compulsive disorder. *Archives of General Psychiatry*, **56** (1999), 121–7.

P. H. Thomsen, Children and adolescents with obsessive-compulsive disorder. A 6–22 year follow-up study. Clinical descriptions of the course and continuity of obsessive compulsive symptomatology. *European Child and Adolescent Psychiatry*, **3** (1994), 82–96.

P. H. Thomsen, *From thoughts to obsessions – children and adolescents with obsessive-compulsive disorder.* (London: Jessica Kingsley Publications, 1998).

P. Thomsen & J. Leckman, Obsessive-compulsive disorder and the Anxiety Spectrum in Children. *CNS Spectrums*, **5** (6, suppl. 4, 2000), 18–23.

P. H. Thomsen & H. U. Mikkelsen, The addition of buspirone to SSRI in the treatment of adolescent obsessive-compulsive disorder. A study of six cases. *European Child and Adolescent Psychiatry*, **8** (1998), 143–8.

P. H. Thomsen, C. Ebbesen & C. Persson, Long-term experience with citalopram in the treatment of adolescent OCD, *Journal of the American Academy of Child And Adolescent Psychiatry*, **40** (8) (2001), 895–902.

Appendix 6.1. Short Leyton Obsessional Inventory-Child Version (SLOI-CV)

Bamber *et al.* (2002) This form is about how you might have been feeling or acting recently. For each item please tick the box that best describes how often you have felt or acted in this way *over the past 2 weeks*. If a sentence was true about you *all the time* over the past 2 weeks, tick 'Always'. If it was true *most of the time*, tick 'Mostly'. If it was only *sometimes* true, tick 'Sometimes'. If you *never* felt like that over the past 2 weeks, tick 'Never'.

	Always	Mostly	Sometimes	Never
1. I felt I had to do things in a certain way, like counting or saying special words, to stop something bad from happening.				
2. I had trouble finishing my homework or other jobs because I had to do things over and over again.				
3. I hated dirt and dirty things.				
4. I had a special number that I counted up to, or I felt I had to do things just that number of times.				
5. I often felt guilty or bad about things I had done even though no one else thought I had done anything wrong.				
6. I worried about being clean enough.				
7. I moved or talked in a special way to avoid bad luck.				
8. I worried a lot if I did something not exactly the way I liked.				
9. I was fussy about keeping my hands clean.				
10. I had special numbers or words that I said because I hoped they kept bad luck or bad things away.				
11. I kept on thinking about things that I had done because I wasn't sure that they were the right things to do.				

7

Adjustment disorders

Peter Hill

Department of Psychological Medicine, Great Ormond Street Hospital for Children, London, UK

Introduction

The concept of adjustment disorder (or a group of adjustment disorders) has a long history, though what is actually meant by the term has changed over time. Originally, as 'adjustment reaction', it was one of a very few disorder categories included in major psychiatric classification schemes specifically for use in children and adolescents. In DSM-I, for instance, adjustment reaction and childhood schizophrenia were the only two categories of childhood psychiatric disorder. The intention was to indicate that some instances of disordered behaviour or emotions arose specifically because of an identified stressor rather than, say, a process of mental illness. The source of stress was originally thought of as including both external events (such as bereavement) or an internal developmental process, which might require significant adaptation of mental functioning (such as maturational changes during adolescence). There was an implicit idea that adjustment to adversity or intrapsychic conflict could be either adaptive or maladaptive. If it was maladaptive, then personal dysfunction was to be seen as a psychiatric condition.

Historically, the most widespread way of understanding a psychological response to adversity or conflict was initially through psychoanalytic theory and a concept of trauma or intrapsychic conflict secondary to external events or developmental challenges. Subsequently, the development of a model of social influences led to a rather different way of thinking which emphasized processes rather more than events. A sophisticated approach developed, which emphasized interplay between events, processes, vulnerability and coping, and could be understood as interactive and systemic rather than relying on linear causality. It became harder to maintain a simple idea of a single stressor causing a reaction which could be sufficiently unfortunate for the young person to develop a psychiatric condition. Factors in the child or the environment modified the impact of events. Adverse circumstances

A Clinician's Handbook of Child and Adolescent Psychiatry, ed. Christopher Gillberg,
Richard Harrington and Hans-Christoph Steinhausen. Published by Cambridge University Press.
© Cambridge University Press 2005.

might only have an effect when vulnerability factors in the child were present or when other potentiating adversities in the environment existed, or because the child's attempts to cope evoked further difficulties. Interaction rather than reaction became the issue when causality was considered.

Furthermore, it became clear that adverse circumstances, acute or chronic, could be implicated in the causation of a whole range of disorders so the question arose as to whether there was any point in retaining a separate adjustment disorder concept.

During the middle years of the last century, this realization that aetiology of psychiatric disorders was complex paralleled a general reluctance to apply adult-type categorical psychiatric diagnoses to children, together with a belief that maladaptive reactions to adversity in childhood were generally mild, brief and easily related to identifiable stressors. In the 1960s and 1970s, the most popular diagnoses in American child psychiatry were 'adjustment reaction' and 'transient situational disturbance'. Yet in the same era, and subsequently, various articles appeared that were critical of either the concept of adjustment reaction/disorder or of its application in practice. Vagueness and an over-inclusive approach were the main criticisms applied to the concept.

Furthermore, although there are operational definitions in both ICD and DSM, it seems, from surveys, that psychiatrists and psychologists do not consistently adhere to these in practice. The newer term adjustment disorder continues to be popular with a number of psychiatrists, partly because of enduring prejudices similar to the above, partly because it is seen as less stigmatizing than what has come to be known as a 'major category' psychiatric disorder. It is generally thought, for instance, to be less likely to affect an individual's future life insurance premium.

In parallel with this, the fact that impairment does not always correlate with severity or number of symptoms means that psychiatrists can find themselves treating children who are distressed or functionally impaired but do not meet criteria for major category disorders. Some clinicians refer to the clinical conditions of such children as adjustment disorders even though there is no obvious stressor, perhaps because the low symptom count suggests low severity in spite of impairment or distress. Although this is technically incorrect, there does seem to be a need to find a way of recognizing these children's problems and justifying treatment even though no diagnostic label may be applicable.

Definition and classification

Adjustment disorders are, in ICD-10-DCR (the diagnostic criteria for research version of ICD-10):

states of subjective distress and emotional disturbance, usually interfering with social functioning and performance, arising in the period of adaptation to a significant life change or a stressful life event . . . the condition would not have arisen without the stressor.

Uniquely, there is no specific set of clinical phenomena that define adjustment disorders; it is the relation to a defined stressor and the duration that set them apart from other conditions.

The stressor is non-catastrophic (cf. post-traumatic stress disorder) and symptoms must develop within 1 month of exposure to it (usually 1 month but up to 3 months in the ordinary descriptive version of ICD-10). Normal grief following bereavement is not included.

Duration of symptoms should not exceed 6 months except in the case of prolonged depressive reaction (see below) in which case they may last up to 2 years. Mild depressive reaction does not exceed 1 month.

DSM-IV-TR diagnostic criteria are essentially similar but 3 months may elapse between stressor and onset and the subtyping of depressive reactions is not included, all adjustment disorders having to be re-classified as major category diagnoses after six months.

The stressor can be coded with a Z code from ICD-10 (see Box 7.1.). This is by no means a complete list of potential stressors (omitting a number to do with physical health or school events) but is included for illustration.

Box 7.1. Selected Z codes from ICD-10 (problems related to negative life events in childhood)

Z61.0 Loss of love relationship in childhood

Z61.1 Removal from home in childhood

Z61.2 Altered pattern of family relationships in childhood

Z61.3 Events resulting in loss of self-esteem in childhood

Z61.4 Problems related to alleged sexual abuse of child by person within primary support group

Z61.5 Problems related to alleged sexual abuse of child by person outside primary support group

Z61.6 Problems related to alleged physical abuse of child

Z61.7 Personal frightening experience in childhood

Z61.8 Other negative life events in childhood

As far as clinical symptoms are concerned, the text of ICD-10 states:

The manifestations vary and include depressed mood, anxiety or worry (or a mixture of these), a feeling of inability to cope, plan ahead or continue in the present situation . . . . . . conduct disorders may be an associated feature, particularly in adolescents . . .

The category F43.2 in ICD-10 is subcategorized according to symptom pattern, e.g. depressive, other emotions, conduct or various combinations of these, which means that it is a plural category of adjustment disorders (Box 7.2).

Box 7.2. Subtypes of ICD-10 adjustment disorder

F43.2 Adjustment Disorders
F43.20 Brief depressive reaction (under one month)
F43.21 Prolonged depressive reaction (up to two years)
F43.22 Mixed anxiety and depressive reaction
F43.23 With predominant disturbance of other emotions (including tension, anger, regressive behaviour)
F43.24 With predominant disturbance of conduct

In ICD-10 it is implied that a re-diagnosis is needed if symptoms persist longer than specified time criteria. This is explicit in DSM-IV. Similarly, DSM-IV states that the condition can only be regarded as an adjustment disorder if it does not fulfil symptom criteria for a major category disorder (a psychiatric disorder on axis I that is not an adjustment disorder). This is less clearly stated in ICD-10 but implicit in some of the coding instructions. It is also the case that a condition can only be regarded as an adjustment disorder for a limited amount of time for so long (6 months for most subcategories in ICD-10-DCR) and, once this time period has been exceeded, the condition should be reclassified as a major category disorder. Nevertheless, adjustment disorder (the collective term for different adjustment disorders defined by predominant symptomatology) is on the same axis as so-called major category disorders.

This probably indicates a logical fault in the major classification systems. Yet there does seem to be an enduring need to recognize that children (a term which in this chapter includes adolescents) can react maladaptively or with disproportionate distress to adversity in a way that is mild or time limited. Similarly, some children have impaired functioning or substantial suffering yet have insufficient symptoms or signs for their clinical condition to qualify as a major category psychiatric disorder. It is possible that moving such mild or time-limited conditions to a separate axis (such as a V code) or, for each disorder, including the possibility of a code indicating that the form is mild, brief (and possibly reactive), would solve the problem.

Nevertheless, as things stand one can take the two major psychiatric classification schemes together and distil the core components of the concept as set out in Box 7.3.

Box 7.3. Core components of adjustment disorder

1. Distress or disturbance of functioning that is beyond the normal range for age and culture
2. Psychopathology that is less severe or extensive than expected in a major category axis 1 disorder
3. An identifiable stressor, usually an event or onset of change in personal circumstances occurring within a few months prior to the onset of the disorder
4. Relatively short duration – about 6 months in most cases
5. Not
   a. a normal bereavement reaction
   b. an exacerbation of pre-existing psychopathology
   c. an acute stress reaction
   d. post-traumatic stress disorder

Another way of expressing this is to say that adjustment disorder is a mild, short-lived and psychopathologically non-specific reaction to an adversity. Although it is obviously sensible to adhere to the diagnostic criteria in ICD or DSM, evidence from prospective studies suggests that the time constraints in these schemes may be too restrictive. Evidence from such work indicates that not all children who develop an abnormal state of mind following a defined stressor will do so within 3 months. Similarly, an appreciable minority will continue to have symptoms beyond 6 months though persistence beyond 9 months is probably rare. No evidence from childhood studies supports the idea that depressive reactions run a more protracted course than other presentations where there is a circumscribed, acute precipitating event.

To what extent one should regard disturbed mood or behaviour secondary to persisting adversity as an adjustment disorder is not addressed by classification manuals but since this is well known to be a causal factor in a range of major category disorders it would not seem necessary. When there is continuing stress, some psychiatrists ignore diagnostic guidelines and use the term 'adjustment disorder' to indicate a reaction with a milder psychopathological picture than a major category condition. This is not obviously the same sort of thing as a circumscribed reaction to acute adversity and the practice is best avoided.

A protracted reaction to a stressor, even an acute one, may indicate that the parents are also affected and their reactions complicate the child's adjustment. In such instances, the child may be faced with further adversity in the form of parental psychopathology so that perpetuating factors become more significant than precipitating ones.

Epidemiology

It is hard to find good data from which to generate point prevalence rates. Two studies, in Finland and Puerto Rico have used reasonably modern definitions and total populations, and come up with point prevalence rates for school-age children of 3–4 per cent. The prevalence among clinical populations is not surprisingly higher – about 6–7 per cent in out- or day-patient clinics.

In whole populations there is little to suggest one sex as being more likely than the other to develop an adjustment disorder. In clinical practice, however, the tendency for psychiatrists to use adjustment disorder as a diagnosis associated with deliberate self-harm means that more girls and more adolescents will receive the diagnosis.

Clinical picture

There is no pattern of signs and symptoms that characterize adjustment disorder in general, though sub-types can be recognized according to diagnostic subcategories (Box 7.2). Thus depressive symptoms, conduct problems and a variety of symptoms expressing tension, anger, anxiety and behavioural manifestations of these (such as regression or clinging to an attachment figure) would be expected as indicated by the sub-classification framework. In addition, other behaviours such as self-isolation, spurning the attempts of others to communicate or sympathize, general uncommunicativeness, avoiding certain situations, apparent preoccupation, disrupted sleep or appetite and irritability may be noted by parents or teachers.

However, if one follows a group of children exposed to a defined stressor (as has been done with newly diagnosed diabetes) or examines DSM-IV field trials, then depression is the commonest picture, followed by mixed depression and anxiety.

Aetiology

Research on stress and coping usually uses a typology of stressors.

- Normative/generic, experienced by all children during development (e.g. separation from parents in order to attend school, examinations). Within this group the term 'transitions' is sometimes used to indicate stress secondary to universal experiences in development such as pubertal body changes.
- Non-normative, specific to an individual child, such as bereavement, bullying or parental discord. Sometimes referred to as 'turning points'.
- 'Daily hassles', minor but cumulative. Classically, these are irritating, frustrating, distressing demands arising during everyday life at home, with peers or at school. Clearly there is a long list of possible everyday hassles but irritable demands from parents, hostile responses from a sibling, ignoring by a favoured friend,

criticism by a teacher and practical difficulties with transport or money would be typical.

Clearly, the concept of adjustment disorder implicates the first two types rather than the third, though extensive daily hassles may provide a vulnerability exaggerating the impact of an acute normative or non-normative event from which the timing requirements of the diagnostic criteria are taken.

Generally, the impact of experiences is understood to be a function of their:

- number
- timing
- synchronicity.

In addition to which there are a number of event parameters:

- unpredictability (no opportunity for anticipatory coping)
- previous exposure (sensitizing or steeling)
- subjective appraisal by the child.

Following which the style of coping may be

- emotion focused
- engagement vs. avoidance
- problem solving
- cognitive reframing.

The manner of coping can itself complicate the situation. For instance, protracted avoidance will not allow problem-solving to be brought into play which may result in prolongation of the adjustment reaction so that coping becomes maladaptive.

In clinical practice speaking there are acute stressors, which commonly present with adverse psychological sequelae: parental illness or death, intra-familial crises, personal ill-health or injury, moves of house or school, examinations, crises in peer relations, or brushes with the law. However, these are no different from those associated with major category psychiatric disorder and there are none that are specific to adjustment disorder. It is important to note that colloquial myth can be misleading. For instance, there are no grounds for thinking that normal adolescent development is inherently more stressful than developmental challenges in young adult life and most adolescents are mentally healthy. Myth can also obscure the fact that some children profit from mild adversities. For instance, the birth of a younger sibling, for instance, more commonly results in greater independence in self-care than it causes a regression in behaviour.

Assessment

A normal history from both child and parents is obviously needed. There should be particular emphasis on the following.

Demonstrating a link between a putative stressor and current psychopathology

Consider:

– temporal proximity
– form of psychopathological reaction
– content of psychopathological reaction.

In part this will depend upon timing; the appearance of new psychopathology follows an identified stressor. But it is also important to relate the form and content of a psychological reaction to the nature of the adversity, especially from the child's point of view, demonstrating a semantic link. Essentially a *verstehende* concept is required, in other words that, by empathizing with the child, it is possible to understand how stress and reaction are linked. However, it has to be said that the association between type of life event and type of disorder is weak.

It should also be possible to say that the condition would not have arisen without the stressor. Yet an acute adversity may have been merely the last straw to break the camel's back. Single life events occurring in isolation are not usually pathogenic and a potentiation by chronic stressors or vulnerabilities is more likely.

Understanding the subjective evaluation of the stressor from the child's point of view

A core issue in stress and coping research has been the realization that the subjective evaluation of the life event is crucial. Two themes emerge from coping research as important:

– perceived threat including whether support (e.g. from parents) is readily available
– perceived lack of control (helplessness).

Previous exposure to similar events or experiences is highly relevant. Successful management of a previous similar adversity can result in cognitive or practical mastery – so-called steeling. Conversely, a bruising earlier experience can result in sensitization so that the impact of a current experience is magnified.

Examining parental attitudes and psychopathology, especially those that have arisen from the same acute adversity

Many adverse events affecting children also affect one or both parents or siblings. Their reaction can modify the impact of the event or choice of coping strategy. Avoidant behaviour by the parent conveys a message to the child that the event is seriously threatening, refusal to discuss an event (hoping the child will then forget it) may not allow the child to mentally process the experience, irritability in the parent's interactions with the child causes insecure unhappiness and so on.

Understanding what coping strategies the child and family have used in the past

There is the possibility that coping methods used in the past may no longer be age-appropriate for the child. By and large, an authoritative parenting style allows for a greater feeling of competence and control in the child. Children from families that encourage independence and the open expression of feelings are more likely to use family and social resources actively rather than withdrawing. A predominant use of active coping is likely to result in the child feeling more in control of adverse events, diminishing their perceived threat.

Noting what coping strategies are currently being employed by child and family

There is rather little information available from formal studies as to what is normal coping. Younger children are more likely to use emotion-focused strategies with predominant use of attachment relationships or practical help from adults in terms of problem-solving. In middle childhood, children learn functional strategies: active problem-solving, seeking advice or information, using social support. Adolescents are more adept at using people outside their family such as friends or teachers. Although functional strategies are the most widely used by teenagers, the ability to use emotion-focussed coping on one's own increases with age so that by mid-adolescence young people normally have quite a good range of coping skills though thinking of several possible courses of action rather than just one remains a problem for many.

Dysfunctional coping is defined in its own terms as something which does not help or makes matters worse. Social withdrawal, wishful thinking, avoidance of engagement with the problem all are likely to prove maladaptive if used to excess, though each may prove useful in the short term.

There are some gender differences. Boys are more likely to rely on problem-solving but girls preferentially use social support. This means that girls who employ avoidant strategies are doubly disadvantaged since this cuts them off from a coping resource, something very evident in depressive reactions when social withdrawal is common.

The importance of individual interviews with child and parent(s)

Key diagnostic issues such as the timing of the stressful event and onset of subjective symptoms need information that may only be available from the child. Much the same applies to stress that the parents have caused themselves – such as child abuse. Children are often secretive about some extra-familial stressors such as bullying or extra-familial abuse.

The subjective evaluation of the event is something about which information from the child is crucial. Yet children may not be open about this in their parent's hearing. Not all children will voice worries such as the possibility of parental death when the parent is present in the room. Nor will they necessarily talk openly about 'childish' ways of coping such as magical rituals.

In parallel with these issues, parents may be unwilling to disclose their mental state fully or discuss their own appraisal of the event in the presence of their child. Similarly there may be adult evaluations of risk that they do not wish to discuss openly.

Having made this point, there is obvious advantage in conducting part of the assessment with parents and child jointly present so that attachment interactions can be observed or discrepancies in the factual account of events examined. In such a setting, siblings may usefully be included so some flexibility and sensitivity is clearly needed when deciding to do so.

Taking chronic adversities and individual strengths/vulnerabilities into account

The impact of the event or change in circumstances in question can only be evaluated when it is known what the background is. The general state of family relationships, particularly attachment relationships, is most important. Peer relations become increasingly important with adolescence. Previous adverse experiences including the amount of daily hassles are clearly relevant. Constitutional vulnerability factors (intelligence, temperament, physical illness) should not be neglected.

Taking a measure of current functioning

Functional impairment is not an absolute entity and can be measured by various instruments. The Children's Global Assessment Scale (C-GAS) has the advantage that it can be discussed with the family and scores on this can be compared with clinic populations. The disadvantage, as with most impairment scales is that an overall score may conceal the fact that a child may be functioning reasonably well in some areas and poorly in others.

Alternatively a pre- and post-event comparison may be the better indicator of what this child and family expect normal functioning to be – something which may require re-appraisal.

Differential diagnosis

This is a technical exercise. The acute stress reaction is typically a state of mute, disorientated bewilderment with high autonomic arousal lasting a few hours or days after a severe life-threatening experience such as a road traffic accident. Post-traumatic stress disorder (PTSD) (see Chapter 8) is a pattern of more protracted symptoms involving memory dysfunction, anxious arousal and behavioural avoidance which follows a highly stressful, catastrophic, abnormal experience. In a number of cases of post-traumatic reaction in childhood the full criteria for PTSD are not met and a diagnosis of adjustment disorder is queried. Technically, the experience from which an adjustment disorder arises should not be as overwhelming or extreme as one which produces PTSD but in practice, psychiatrists seem often to use adjustment disorder as a diagnosis in such situations.

A range of psychological reactions to stress can be observed and it is correct to make a major category axis 1 diagnosis if criteria for one are fulfilled in spite of the obvious precipitation by an event. In the present classification schemes there is a problem with how best to diagnose partial syndromes which persist more than six months, beyond the time criteria for non-depressive adjustment disorders.

Assessment has to be a continuing process since the initial diagnosis of an adjustment disorder seems to increase the likelihood of developing a major category diagnosis, especially depressive disorder, subsequently.

Treatment

It is rather unlikely that many children with adjustment disorders will be detected, referred to a specialist mental health service and treated to completion within a 6-month period so it is not surprising that there are no good scientific trials of treatment. Consequently, it is not possible to create a strong evidence base for treatment efficacy. Given the range of symptoms possible, it is inevitable that treatment has to proceed on first principles.

Clearly the stressor should be removed or the child removed from the stressful situation if at all possible. If this is impossible then psychological support is provided to child and family by the therapist. In outline, this includes:
– open acknowledgement of suffering and impaired functioning, re-framing problematic behaviours as understandable responses (where appropriate)
– empathizing with distress and providing a vocabulary of emotional terms so that emotions can be discussed and differentiated
– appraisal of the power and quality of the stressor, correcting misperceptions and misunderstandings
– discussion of ways of coping and their strengths and weaknesses; ensuring that basic techniques such as self-distraction, activity scheduling and relaxation are present
– encouragement to select and pursue optimal coping strategies with praise and other social reinforcement used to maintain these.

In parallel with this, the family's inherent strengths are used in order to provide emotional support for the child. This usually involves a therapist recognizing and promoting attachment relationships which are the basic framework for anxiety reduction and empowerment for the child. In the time-frame which adjustment disorders are recognized, long-term work is unlikely and personal support from a therapist is not likely to be more effective than from parents. This means that working through parents becomes the usual approach. A possible exception to this

is in a bitter divorce when the parents are mutually so hostile that the child's family relationships become polarized and a therapist from outside the situation is best place to provide support.

In carrying out work through parents, the components of support, identified above, provide a general framework. This can be developed by a therapist so that parents and possibly siblings of a child or adolescent with an adjustment disorder can take over some of the supportive activities. Such an approach derives from social problem-solving work within cognitive-behavioural treatments as well as from observational studies of healthy families. Family members are encouraged to
- name the situation or predicament following the event in question
- acknowledge and empathize with the child's distress
- discuss ways out of the situation with the child
- help the child select one and encourage its implementation
- review progress and adapt if necessary.

In general, the principle that an authoritative style of parenting facilitates coping means that parents should be seen to be in control whilst remaining receptive to the child's view and being emotionally supportive. There is no evidence to support parental indulgence of bad behaviour in a child with an adjustment disorder characterized by poor conduct. Therefore, a therapist may need to ensure the preservation of justifiable parental authority alongside parental sympathy and support.

Given that many adjustment disorders seem to include a depressive component, it is rational to use methods found to be useful in the treatment of depression in the young. Mild depressive reactions in older children and adolescents will respond to a psycho-educational and cognitive approach and it seems likely that this approach will also help with mild pathological anxiety. Key components identified in studies of cognitive behavioural interventions and interpersonal psychotherapy include many of those listed in the section on emotional support above, adding tuition in self-evaluation, self-reinforcement and cognitive restructuring.

It is unlikely that psychopharmacological interventions will have much of a role to play in the absence of a major category diagnosis. Clinical anecdote suggests that some school-age children with sleep onset difficulties may be helped by melatonin 1–6 mg at night for a few weeks but there is no systematic evidence to support this. Although unfashionable, short-term benzodiazepines seem helpful for markedly anxious adolescents when the prescriber is confident that the stressor is self-limiting or has passed.

Outcome

By definition, adjustment disorder according to the standard classification schemes has a good prognosis since, as currently defined, it cannot last longer than the specified time periods. When there is a specific time-limited stressor, most cases seem to resolve within 6–9 months. However, not all will and the existence of an adjustment disorder increases, perhaps by threefold, the chance of a major category diagnosis subsequently developing. It has not yet been shown how to predict which cases will follow this course though there is evidence that the co-existence of parental psychopathology is an adverse influence.

Presumably the general rules of vulnerability and resilience apply as far as the characteristics of the individual child go. These cannot be taken in isolation from the likelihood of the stressor re-occurring, the possibility of the child's adjustment compounding or maintaining the problem, and the quality of family, peer group and indeed professional support.

SUGGESTED READING

General, critical overview

P. Hill, Adjustment disorders. Chap 31 in Rutter, M. & Taylor, E. (eds.), *Child and Adolescent Psychiatry*. 4th edn. (Oxford: Blackwell Scientific Publications, 2002).

Epidemiology

F. Almqvist, K. Puura, K. Kumpulainen *et al.*, Psychiatric disorders in 8–9 year-old children based on a diagnostic interview with the parents. *European Child and Adolescent Psychiatry*, **8** (1999) suppl. 4, 17–28.

A. Angold, E. J. Costello, E. M. Z. Farmer, B. J. Burns & A. Erkanli, Impaired but undiagnosed. *Journal of the American Academy of Child and Adolescent Psychiatry*, **38** (1999), 129–37.

Impact of life events

S. Sandberg & M. Rutter, The role of acute life stresses. Chap 17 in Rutter, M. & Taylor, E. (eds.) *Child and Adolescent Psychiatry*. 4th edn. (Oxford: Blackwell Scientific Publications, 2002).

Coping

E. Frydenberg, *Adolescent Coping: Theoretical and Research Perspectives.* (London: Routledge, 1997).

I. Seiffge-Kranke, *Stress, Coping and Relationships in Adolescence.* (Hove, UK: Lawrence Erlbaum Associates, 1995).

Valuable empirical studies

M. Kovacs, C. Gatsonis, M. Pollock & P. L. Parrone, A controlled prospective study of DSM-III adjustment disorder in childhood: short-term prognosis and long-term predictive validity. *Archives of General Psychiatry*, **51** (1994), 535–41.

M. Kovacs, V. Ho & M. H. Pollock, Criterion and predictive validity of the diagnosis of adjustment disorder: a prospective study of youths with new-onset insulin-dependent diabetes mellitus. *American Journal of Psychiatry*, **152** (1995), 523–8.

Children's Global Assessment Scale

D. Shaffer, M. S. Gould, J. Brasic, *et al.*, A Children's Global Assessment Scale (CGAS) *Archives of General Psychiatry*, **40** (1983), 1228–31.

8

Post-traumatic stress disorder

Paul Stallard

Department of Child and Family Psychiatry, Royal Hospital Bath, UK

Introduction

It has only been in the last 20 years that researchers have systematically investigated the psychological effects of trauma on children. Early studies of children's reactions to traumatic events did not use a consistent format to report symptoms and relied upon general assessments of global behaviours typically completed by parents or teachers. Adults tend to underestimate the severity of the psychological effects experienced by their children with global measure of behaviour being insensitive to the specific changes in cognitions or emotions associated with traumatic reactions. Interviews undertaken with children using assessments sensitive to the core features of post-traumatic stress disorder (PTSD), namely trauma re-experiencing, avoidance and arousal, reveal that children are significantly affected by traumatic events.

Since the mid-1980s considerable knowledge about PTSD in children exposed to single and multiple traumas has accrued. Children have been found to experience PTSD following a range of traumatic events including natural disasters such as flooding, fires, lightening strikes, hurricanes, landslides and earthquakes. PTSD following a range of human-made traumas such as wars, kidnapping, bombings, sniper attacks, abuse and hostage taking has also been documented as well as following transportation accidents such as shipping disasters and coach accidents. Finally post-traumatic stress disorder arising from more common everyday traumatic events such as road traffic accidents, acute physical injury and chronic illness has also been reported.

Definition and classification

PTSD is defined as an anxiety disorder associated with a traumatic event in which the trauma is repetitively re-experienced. In addition to re-experiencing, symptoms

A Clinician's Handbook of Child and Adolescent Psychiatry, ed. Christopher Gillberg,
Richard Harrington and Hans-Christoph Steinhausen. Published by Cambridge University Press.
© Cambridge University Press 2005.

Table 8.1. ICD-10 Diagnostic guidelines for post-traumatic stress disorder

This disorder should not generally be diagnosed unless there is evidence that it arose within 6 months of a traumatic event of exceptional severity. A 'probable' diagnosis might still be possible if the delay between the event and the onset was longer than 6 months, provided that the clinical manifestations are typical and no alternative identification of the disorder (e.g. as an anxiety or obsessive-compulsive disorder or depressive episode) is plausible. In addition to evidence of trauma, there must be a repetitive, intrusive recollection or re-enactment of the event in memories, daytime imagery or dreams. Conspicuous emotional detachment, numbing of feeling and avoidance of stimuli that might arouse recollection of the trauma are often present but are not essential for diagnosis. The autonomic disturbances, mood disorder and behavioural abnormalities all contribute to the diagnosis but are not of prime importance.

The late chronic sequelae of devastating stress, i.e. those that manifest decades after the stressful experience, should be classified under F62.0.

Includes: traumatic neurosis.

Reprinted with permission from the *International Classification of Diseases*, 10th edn. © 1993, World Health Organization.

of trauma avoidance and increased arousal are often present although the classification systems differ regarding whether their presence is required to fulfil diagnostic criteria.

ICD-10

PTSD was not included as a specific diagnosis until the latest edition of the *International Classification of Diseases* (ICD-10). This saw the introduction of a new category, 'reaction to severe stress, and adjustment disorders (F43)' which, in addition to the diagnoses of PTSD, includes acute stress reactions and adjustment disorders. The diagnostic criteria for these disorders relate to all age groups, including children, although how specific symptoms manifest themselves within the younger age group is not specified (Table 8.1).

The diagnostic criteria require the identification of a specific threatening event that is associated with the onset of the disorder. The traumatic event is defined as 'exceptionally threatening or catastrophic in nature, which is likely to cause pervasive distress in almost anyone (e.g. natural or human-made disaster, combat, serious accident, witnessing the violent death of others or being a victim of torture, terrorism, rape or other crime)'. The symptoms arising from the stressful event should occur within 6 months of the trauma for the diagnosis to be made.

The core diagnostic symptoms are based upon evidence of trauma re-experiencing as manifest by repetitive intrusive thoughts and images, trauma 'flashbacks' or dreams. These typically occur within the context of emotional changes such as persistent numbness, emotional blunting and detachment from other people, unresponsivness to surroundings, anhedonia and avoidance of activities and situations reminiscent of the trauma. Commonly there is fear and avoidance of cues that trigger memories of the trauma. Rarely there may be dramatic, acute bursts of fear, panic or aggression, triggered by stimuli arousing a sudden recollection and/or re-enactment of the trauma or of the original reaction to it.

Increased physiological arousal is common as manifest by autonomic hyperarousal with hypervigilance, an enhanced startle reaction, and insomnia. Associated anxiety and depression are common, suicidal ideation is not infrequent and excessive use of alcohol or drugs may be a complicating factor.

The cardinal diagnostic criteria for ICD-10 are therefore twofold. Diagnosis requires evidence of exposure to a stressful event, which is then remembered persistently or relived. The other symptoms are identified as commonly present rather than required and as such it is often easier for trauma victims to satisfy these diagnostic criteria, rather than the more specific criteria of DSM-IV.

DSM-IV

PTSD was first recognized as a psychiatric diagnosis in the *Diagnostic and Statistical Manual of the American Psychiatric Association* in 1980 and is currently defined within the anxiety disorders section (309.81). The latest edition, DSM-IV, incorporates two significant developments. First, it attempts to define more clearly what constitutes a traumatic event and secondly describe how symptoms may manifest themselves in children (Table 8.2).

As with ICD-10, the gateway to the diagnosis is through exposure to a traumatic event. However DSM-IV recognizes the importance of both the objective severity of the event as well as the individual's subjective appraisal of it. This goes some way to addressing the finding that children exposed to the same traumatic event may react very differently.

The previous DSM-111-R definition of a traumatic event as 'an event that is outside the range of usual human experience' has been replaced with dual criteria requiring both exposure to a traumatic event and the person's reaction involving 'fear, helplessness or horror'. This revision acknowledges that some traumatic events that result in PTSD in children (e.g. abuse, road traffic accidents) are not rare. The guidelines specify that in children fear, helplessness or horror may be expressed by disorganized or agitated behaviour. The nature of the traumatic event has also been widened to include 'actual or threatened death or serious injury, or a threat to the physical integrity of self or others'. Greater emphasis is therefore placed upon how the individual appraises the event rather than its objective severity.

In addition to exposure to a traumatic event (criteria A), DSM-IV requires evidence of persistent symptoms in the three core areas of trauma re-experiencing (criteria B), avoidance (criteria C) and increased arousal (criteria D). In order to

Table 8.2. DSM-IV Criteria for PTSD

A. The person has been exposed to a traumatic event in which both of the following were present:
  (1) The person experienced, witnessed, or was confronted with an event or events that involved actual or threatened death or serious injury, or a threat to the physical integrity of self or others,
  (2) The person's response involved fear, helplessness or horror. *Note:* In children, this may be expressed instead by disorganized or agitated behaviour.

B. The traumatic event is re-experienced persistently in one (or more) of the following ways:
  (1) Recurrent and intrusive distressing recollections of the event, including images, thoughts or perceptions. *Note:* In young children, repetitive play may occur in which themes or aspects of the trauma are expressed.
  (2) Recurrent distressing dreams of the event. *Note:* In children, there may be frightening dreams without recognizable content.
  (3) Acting or feeling as if the traumatic event were recurring (includes a sense of reliving the experience, illusions, hallucinations and dissociative flashback episodes, including those that occur on awakening or when intoxicated) *Note:* In young children, trauma specific re-enactment may occur.
  (4) Intense physiological distress at exposure to internal or external cues that symbolize or resemble an aspect of the traumatic event.
  (5) Physiological reactivity on exposure to internal or external cues that symbolize or resemble an aspect of the traumatic event.

C. Persistent avoidance of stimuli associated with the trauma and numbing of general responsiveness (not present before the trauma), as indicated by three (or more) of the following:
  (1) Efforts to avoid thoughts, feelings, or conversations associated with the trauma.
  (2) Efforts to avoid activities, places, or people that arouse recollections of the trauma.
  (3) Inability to recall an important aspect of the trauma.
  (4) Markedly diminished interest or participation in significant activities.
  (5) Feelings of detachment or estrangement from others.
  (6) Restricted range of affect (e.g. unable to have loving feelings).
  (7) Sense of foreshortened future (e.g. does not expect to have a career, marriage, children, or a normal lifespan).

D. Persistent symptoms of increased arousal (not present before the trauma) as indicated by two (or more) of the following:
  (1) Difficulty falling or staying asleep.
  (2) Irritability or outbursts of anger.
  (3) Difficulty concentrating.
  (4) Hypervigilance.
  (5) Exaggerated startle response.

Table 8.2. (*cont.*)

E. Duration of the disturbance (symptoms in criteria B, C, and D) is more than one month.

F. The disturbance causes clinically significant distress or impairment in social, occupational, or other important areas of functioning.

Specify if:
Acute: if duration of symptoms is less than 3 months.
Chronic: if duration of symptoms is 3 months or more.

Specify if:
With delayed onset: if onset of symptoms is at least 6 months after the stressor.

Reprinted with permission from the *Diagnostic Manual of Mental Disorders*, 4th edn. © 1994, American Psychiatric Association.

fulfil diagnostic criteria, the child must meet one or more of the specified five re-experiencing symptoms, three or more of the seven avoidance and numbing symptoms and two or more of the five-arousal symptoms. Attempts have been made to define how re-experiencing may occur in children noting that this may be expressed through repetitive play, frightening dreams and through trauma re-enactment. In terms of avoidance, the difficulty of children reporting a diminished interest in significant activities or a constriction of affect is noted and the need to evaluate these symptoms by observations from parents, teachers and others suggested. Similarly, it is suggested that a foreshortened future may be evidenced by the belief that life will be too short to include becoming an adult. Finally, in terms of arousal, DSM-IV notes that children may also exhibit various physical symptoms, such as stomach aches and headaches.

These symptoms have to be present for more than 1 month (criteria E) and cause clinically significant distress or impairment in social, occupational, or other important areas of functioning (criteria F). For children this would include school.

Finally, specifiers can be used to categorize PTSD according to duration and onset. For acute PTSD, symptoms will have been present for between 1 and 3 months with chronic PTSD referring to symptoms being present for longer than 3 months, Finally, delayed onset can be specified if symptoms occur within 6 months of the traumatic event.

Clinical applicability

Both ICD-10 and DSM-IV were developed for adults thereby raising questions regarding whether these criteria are developmentally sensitive to the signs and symptoms of trauma in children. The evidence to date would suggest that PTSD is manifest in a similar manner, with children displaying many of the same PTSD symptoms as adults. However, as noted in DSM-IV, the manner in which children will, for example, re-enact their trauma may be different to the way this is expressed by adults. Repetitive drawing and play whereby aspects of the trauma are acted out is more often observed in young children whilst avoidance symptoms, such as emotional numbing or a sense of a foreshortened future are observed less frequently.

Although children and adults demonstrate comparable reactions, PTSD will be manifest differently across different stages of childhood. Pre-school children demonstrate more circumscribed symptoms displaying fewer re-experiencing symptoms and little avoidance. This has led some researchers to identify an alternative set of criteria that describe trauma reactions in very young children (Table 8.3).

Based upon a series of observations of traumatized pre-school children a set of criteria that include more behavioural symptoms such as play re-enactment, separation anxiety, the development of new fears and aggression have been proposed. The criteria are based upon DSM-IV and under Criterion A, only require young children to have experienced a traumatic event with evidence of a subjective appraisal suggesting fear, helplessness or horror being dropped. Evidence of only one item from each of the re-experiencing (Criterion B), numbing of responsiveness/avoidance (Criterion C) and increased arousal (criterion D) categories is required. A new cluster of symptoms (criterion E) relating to new fears and aggression has been introduced for which one item is required. The disturbance has to last longer than 1 month with the DSM-IV requirement of causing significant impairment being omitted. In a subsequent study, Scheeringa et al. (2001) found that children under 4 years of age displayed significantly more of the alternative criteria for PTSD than the DSM-IV criteria.

Finally, while there is a need to ensure that diagnostic criteria are developmentally appropriate, a second issue focuses upon the number of symptoms in each PTSD category that are required to make a diagnosis in children. This highlights the question of whether children who do not meet full diagnostic criteria are in someway different from those who fulfil partial criteria (i.e. present with a number of symptoms but do not meet the number specified by DSM-IV). Recent research has demonstrated that children fulfilling requirements for two of the three PTSD symptom clusters (i.e. re-experiencing, numbing/avoidance and arousal) were not significantly different from those meeting all three-cluster criteria in terms of impairment or distress. Thus, while PTSD provides a structured way of assessing trauma reactions, interventions need to be provided on the basis of clinical need rather than on fulfilment of diagnostic criteria.

In summary, clinicians need to assess both the presence of particular symptoms and also the degree of distress or impairment they cause the child. Distress may take the form of strong emotional reactions such as anxiety, depression and angry outbursts. Various aspects of the child's life could be impaired including family relationships, friendships, social life, their ability to participate in recreational/social

Table 8.3. Criteria for post-traumatic stress disorder in infancy and early childhood. (Scheeringa, Zeanah, Drell & Larrieu 1995)

A. The person has been exposed to a traumatic event in which both of the following were present:
   (1) The person experienced, witnessed, or was confronted with an event or events that involved actual or threatened death or serious injury, or a threat to the physical integrity of self or others.

B. Re-experiencing: One item needed:
   (1) Post-traumatic play: compulsive repetitive, represents part of the trauma, fails to relieve anxiety and is less elaborate and imaginative than unusual play.
   (2) Play reenactment: represents part of the trauma but lacks the monotonous repetition and other characteristics of post-traumatic play.
   (3) Recurrent recollections of the traumatic event other than what is revealed in play, and which is not necessarily distressing.
   (4) Nightmares: may have obvious links to the trauma or be of increased frequency with unknown content.
   (5) Episodes with objective features of a flashback or dissociation.
   (6) Distress at exposure to reminders of the event.

C. Numbing of responsiveness. One item needed:
   (1) Constriction of play. Child may have constrictions of play and still have post-traumatic play or play re-enactment.
   (2) Socially more withdrawn.
   (3) Restricted range of effect.
   (4) Loss of acquired developmental skills, especially language regression and loss of toilet training.

D. Increased arousal. One item needed:
   (1) Night terrors.
   (2) Difficulty going to sleep which is not related to being afraid of having nightmares or fear of the dark.
   (3) Night-waking not related to nightmares or night terrors.
   (4) Decreased concentration: marked decrease in concentration or attention span compared to before the trauma.
   (5) Hypervigilance.
   (6) Exaggerated startle response.

E. New fears and aggression: One item needed:
   (1) New aggression.
   (2) New separation anxiety.
   (3) Fear of toileting alone.
   (4) Fear of the dark.
   (5) Any other new fears of things or situations not obviously related to the trauma.

F. Duration of disturbance greater than 1 month.

activities, school/work attendance and performance. On a few occasions, children may present with a number of symptoms consistent with a diagnosis of PTSD but these may not cause significant impairment or affect the child's everyday life or functioning adversely. Similarly, failure to meet diagnostic criteria does not imply that a child has not been affected significantly by their trauma and does not require treatment. Good practice would suggest that children with clinically significant post-traumatic reactions that cause significant distress or impairment, regardless of whether or not they meet full diagnostic criteria for PTSD should be offered treatment.

Epidemiology

Prevalence and incidence rates

Estimated lifetime prevalence rates of PTSD in the general population range from 1–14 per cent. For children and adolescents under the age of 18 studies suggest that 6–8 per cent will meet diagnostic criteria for lifetime PTSD. Within specific trauma populations, rates are considerably higher and typically evidence of PTSD is found when symptoms are sought. In terms of human-made disasters, 77 per cent of children involved in a school playground sniper shooting were found to have moderate to severe PTSD when assessed 1 month later. Almost half of Cambodian children exposed to war met criteria for PTSD when assessed up to 4 years later. Natural disasters such as earthquakes have found up to 92 per cent of children to present with severe or very severe post traumatic stress reactions 18 months after the quake. In terms of transportation accidents, half of the children involved in the sinking of the cruise ship *Jupiter* developed PTSD at some stage during the 5–8 year follow-up period. PTSD has also been found in children involved in the everyday trauma of road traffic accidents (RTAs). Up to one-third of child RTA survivors have been found to fulfil the diagnostic criteria for PTSD 6 weeks after their accident. Finally, a meta-analysis of 34 studies involving over 2500 children who had been exposed to various traumatic events found 36 per cent met criteria for PTSD. Rates of diagnosed PTSD did not differ significantly across developmental levels.

The evidence therefore suggests that PTSD is a common reaction in children exposed to traumas. A range of factors including the diagnostic criteria used (ICD vs DSM); method of assessment (diagnostic interview vs questionnaires) source of information (adult vs child) methodological variables (time assessed) and whether lifetime or current status is being determined will contribute to the variation in reported prevalence rates.

Sex ratios

Although the results are not consistent, there is growing evidence to indicate that girls are more at risk of developing PTSD than boys. Whether this reflects true differences in experienced symptoms or a greater frequency of internalizing as opposed to externalizing symptoms in girls or an increased willingness for girls to report them is unclear.

Clinical implications

These results suggest that a wide variety of traumatic events can result in PTSD. Although a number of children involved in traumatic events will not experience significant trauma reactions, a significant number of children will develop PTSD. Girls are more likely to develop PTSD.

Clinical picture

Main features and symptoms

Immediately following a traumatic event, a child may appear frightened and scared. They may cry, shake, become clingy and want to spend time with their main carer. Alternatively, they may appear quiet and withdrawn or dazed as if in a state of shock. The symptoms typically occur within a few minutes of the trauma and tend to subside once the stressor has been removed. Acute stress reactions such as these are common. These reactions typically are transient in nature with symptoms tending to reduce in severity and frequency within a few hours becoming almost minimal after 3 days. For some children, however, their symptoms persist, and develop into the more chronic condition of PTSD.

A cardinal feature of PTSD in both diagnostic systems is trauma re-experiencing whereby frequent, vivid trauma related thoughts are often recalled. Children may describe detailed intrusive memories, thoughts and images of the traumatic event, particularly at those times when they are unoccupied or trying to sleep. These thoughts break though into consciousness without any effort and 'just seem to happen'. They can occur several times each day and are often accompanied by increased levels of arousal and intense feelings of panic.

A smaller number of children report more intense and distressing trauma images in the form of flashbacks where they feel as if the traumatic event is recurring. These are more common with older children, as younger children tend to re-experience the trauma through play and drawing. During a flashback, the child may report a brief period when they feel disassociated and disengaged from what is happening as they visualize vividly and re-experience the trauma intensely.

Intrusive thoughts and flashbacks can be triggered by a variety of stimuli associated with the trauma including physical sensations, noises, smells and visual cues. Re-experiencing symptoms often prove intensely distressing and episodes of regular tearfulness and uncontrollable crying are often reported. In many cases accident cues trigger a range of acute physiological anxiety symptoms such as palpitations, difficulty breathing, clammy and sweaty hands, feelings of nausea and light headedness. Emotional changes are common and children often report feeling angry, irritable and intolerant and in some cases become aggressive. These feelings may be associated with thoughts of self-blame or responsibility for the trauma, survivor guilt at for example escaping with comparatively less severe injuries, or for the way the child acted during the trauma.

At night-time recurrent distressing dreams may be reported especially during the first few weeks after the trauma. Difficulty sleeping, early morning waking, fears of the dark and nightmares are common, particularly in younger children. In some instances the content of the dream/nightmares will be related to the trauma whereas younger children may report frightening dreams without any recognizable trauma related content. Separation anxiety may be reported where the child is reluctant to leave their parents, clinging to them during the daytime and sometimes sleeping with them at night. With younger children, a loss of previously acquired skills, particularly toileting problems may be noted. These tend to be more common in the period immediately after the trauma. Parents may not necessarily attribute these behaviour changes to the trauma but may instead perceive their child to be willful, defiant and problematic.

Avoidance whereby children and young people avoid talking or thinking about the trauma or activities, places or people associated with the traumatic event is common. Significant changes in social life and relationships may be noted with previously enjoyable activities stopping, friendship patterns changing and family relationships being effected. Children may find it difficult to talk with their parents about the trauma, particularly if they were involved or in some way responsible for what occurred. Parents may also avoid initiating conversations about the trauma, wishing to protect their children from further upset. This can lead to a conspiracy of silence, where the trauma is not talked about, leading the parents to underestimate the effects of the trauma upon the child. Similarly, friendship patterns change as children complain that their friends do not understand the significance or impact of the trauma upon them. Children may describe a sense of estrangement/alienation, as they talk about feeling different and distant from their friends.

Cognitive changes such as difficulty concentrating may be reported, particularly at school, where the child may seem more distractable and less able to focus upon their work or listen to instructions. Younger children may present with similar symptoms and appear restless and unable to sustain any play for more than a brief period. Memory problems in terms of increased difficulty mastering new skills or remembering and recalling previously learned material may be noted. Educational attainments may decline and teachers may attribute this to a conscious lack of interest or effort on the part of the child rather than a possible consequence of the trauma.

Children may become hyper-vigilant, appearing more alert and aware of possible danger feeling themselves to be more vulnerable and susceptible to further trauma.

Previously held assumptions about the future may be shattered as life is re-appraised as more uncertain. Children may appear increasingly worried and preoccupied that something bad will happen when they get older. Planning for the future may become more difficult as longer-term plans are suspended and replaced by a shorter-term perspective in which each day is taken as it occurs. For others, the trauma may provide a more positive opportunity to reappraise life and re-prioritize values and goals.

Differential diagnosis and co-morbidity

The diagnostic criteria for PTSD require exposure to a stressor of an extreme nature. This is in contrast to an adjustment disorder where the stressor can be of any severity. In situations where a PTSD symptom pattern occurs in response to a non-extreme stressor (e.g. birth of sibling, house move, change of school) or where the response to an extreme stressor does not meet criteria for PTSD, an adjustment disorder diagnosis may be appropriate.

An acute stress disorder (ASD) is distinguished from PTSD because the symptom pattern must both occur and resolve within 4 weeks of the traumatic event. If symptoms persist for more than 1 month and meet criteria for PTSD, the diagnosis is changed from ASD to PTSD.

The repetitive re-experiencing symptoms of PTSD in terms of intrusive thoughts, images and flashbacks need to be distinguished from those that occur in obsessive-compulsive disorder (OCD). In OCD recurrent thoughts typically are not related, or confined to, an experienced traumatic event.

If avoidance, numbing and symptoms of increased arousal were present before the traumatic event, then a diagnosis of PTSD may not be appropriate. Where the trauma clearly did not precede the onset of symptoms, other diagnosis, such as depression or anxiety disorder may need to be considered. However, assessment needs to be thorough in order to ascertain whether the identified trauma is a single event or part of a series of traumas as may occur with child abuse or domestic violence. Careful assessment may reveal that the onset of symptoms coincided with an earlier or previous traumatic event.

Co-morbid conditions are common. In particular depression, generalized anxiety, specific phobias, and with adolescents, alcohol and drug abuse should be considered. There is considerable symptom overlap between mood and anxiety disorders and PTSD where increased arousal and emotional numbing form two of the core diagnostic features of PTSD. If the symptom pattern fulfils criteria for PTSD and also for other disorders, then these diagnoses should be provided in addition to PTSD. Co-morbidity is important to assess as its presence may indicate more chronic PTSD.

Diagnostic instruments

A range of diagnostic assessments based largely upon DSM criteria have been developed for use with children. These are either interviewer-led semi-structured interviews or self/parent completed assessments of PTSD symptoms. Instruments are summarized in full in the American Association of Child and Adolescent Psychiatry Practice Parameters. The report concludes that, although there are several instruments available to assess PTSD-related symptoms, none is optimal and no single instrument is accepted as a 'gold standard' for diagnostic or monitoring purposes.

A more limited summary of key instruments is produced in Table 8.4.

- The psychometric properties of none of the semi-structured interviews has been extensively evaluated and none of the existing parent or self-completed measures is optimal.
- The most extensively used assessment is the Children's Post-Traumatic Stress Reaction Index (CPTS-RI). This is a 20-item self-report scale that can also be used as a semi-structured interview. The index has good internal consistency and correlates well with clinical diagnosis.
- The Children's Post-traumatic Stress Disorder Inventory is a self-report measure that covers all DSM-IV diagnostic symptoms. This is a self-report measure providing information in five areas of exposure, re-experiencing, avoidance, hyperarousal and degree of distress. The inventory has high inter-rater and test–retest reliability, is sensitive, and correlates well with clinical diagnosis.
- The Impact of Events Scale has been used widely with adults to assess the degree of subjective distress arising from a specific traumatic event. A number of items in the original scale were misinterpreted by younger children, resulting in the scale being adapted for use with this age group. An 8-item version, containing intrusion and avoidance items and a 13-item version which includes additional arousal items has been developed and can be used with children as young as 8 years of age. The psychometric properties of the self-completed questionnaire are good with a total score of 17 on the 8-item version being used to identify children with possible PTSD.
- In addition to PTSD, attention should be paid to the assessment of other comorbid conditions, particularly depression and generalized anxiety. The Birleson Depression Inventory is an 18-item self-completed scale. A cut-off of 15 has been found to differentiate depressed and non-depressed children aged 7–18. The Revised Children's Manifest Anxiety Scale is a 37-item self-completed questionnaire that can be used with children aged 6–19. An overall cut-off of 19 is suggested in order to identify children experiencing clinically significant levels of anxiety.

In summary, structured diagnostic interviews and assessments provide clinicians with a useful way of systematically assessing the core features of PTSD. In clinical practice these should be used to complement a fuller and more comprehensive

Table 8.4. Semi-structured interviews and self/parent report scales for the assessment of PTSD and PTSD symptoms

Measure	Author	Source
Semi-structured interviews for assessing PTSD		
Clinician-Administered PTSD Scale for Children and Adolescents, DSM-IV version	Nader, K. O. *et al.* (1997)	National Centre for PTSD, Department of Psychiatry, Los Angeles.
Childhood PTSD Interview-Child Form	Fletcher, K. (1997).	*Trauma Assessments: A Clinician's Guide.* Carlson, E. (Ed), New York, Guilford Press.
Schedule for Affective Disorders and Schizophrenia for School-Age Children – Present and Lifetime version, PTSD scale	Kaufman J. *et al.* (1997)	*Journal of the American Academy of Child and Adolescent Psychiatry*, **36**, 980–8.
Questionnaires/Scales assessing PTSD symptoms		
Children's PTSD Reaction Index	Fredrick, C. J. (1985)	*Post-traumatic Stress Disorder in Children.* Eth, S & Pynoos, R. S. (Eds). American Psychiatric Press.
Children's PTSD Inventory	Saigh, P. (1989)	*International Journal of Special Education*, **4**, 75–84.
Post-traumatic Symptom Inventory for Children	Eisen, M. (1997)	*Trauma Assessments: A Clinician's Guide.* Carlson, E. (Ed), New York, Guilford Press.
Questionnaires measuring specific PTSD symptoms and associated conditions		
Children's Impact of Event Scale (IES).	Yule, W. (1997)	*Child Psychology Portfolio.* I. Sclare (ed). Windsor: NFER-Nelson.
The Birleson Depression Scale	Birleson, P. (1981)	*Child Psychology Portfolio.* I. Sclare (ed). Windsor: NFER-Nelson.
The Fear Survey Schedule for Children – Revised (FSSC-R)	Nakamaure, C. Y. (1968) revised by Ollendick, T. H. & Yule, W. (1983)	*Child Psychology Portfolio.* I. Sclare (ed). Windsor: NFER-Nelson.
Spence Children's Anxiety Scale (SCAS)	Spence, S. H. (1997).	*Child Psychology Portfolio.* I. Sclare (ed). Windsor: NFER-Nelson.
Revised Measure of Children's Manifest Anxiety	Reynolds, C. R. & Richmond, B. O. (1978)	*Journal of Abnormal Child Psychology*, **8**, 271–80

assessment. As described below, the assessment should start with open questions encouraging the child to describe their trauma and any subsequent cognitive, emotional and behavioural changes. More structured assessments should be used after this discussion in order to complement and substantiate the information obtained during interview.

Assessment

The assessment of PTSD requires direct interviews with both the child and their parents/carers. It is important to remember that parents may fail to recognize or under-report PTSD symptoms or to minimize their child's distress. It is therefore essential that time is spent separately with the child and their carers. However, often clinicians do not ask the child directly about the traumatic event. Clinicians may want to protect the child or minimize future distress and avoid a potentially distressing or upsetting conversation about the trauma. On other occasions, concerns about contaminating or biasing a child's account of a trauma and possible testimony in court (e.g. child abuse) have been used as the rationale for professional avoidance. Indications that the child appears to be coping may be interpreted incorrectly as evidence that the trauma does not need to be revisited. At other times, the clinician's own anxiety and distress about discussing potentially upsetting events acts as a barrier that prevents and limits any open dialogue. At these times it is likely that possible symptoms of PTSD will remain undetected. The overriding clinical view is that, if children are not directly asked about their trauma, they are less likely to report symptoms of PTSD.

Children

The interview with the child provides an opportunity to hear directly from them their account of the traumatic event and how they feel they have been affected. In view of the above comments, it is important to recognize that in many cases the child will not have previously talked about their trauma in any detail. The clinician needs to be sensitive to this issue and receptive to any distress the child may demonstrate.

- Children should be asked directly and sensitively about the traumatic event. Initially, the children should be encouraged to provide their own account and this can be done either verbally or through the drawing of a picture. A series of prompts should then be used to build up a detailed picture of the trauma.
- The trauma should be tracked through in time with prompts being used to help the child describe events before, during and immediately after the traumatic event. The prompts can be descriptive (e.g. what happened after you fell down), or concerned with eliciting feelings (how did you feel when you saw that happen?) or thoughts (what did you think was going to happen to you?).

- Once the trauma has been described the assessment should focus upon detailing the behavioural and emotional changes that have occurred following the trauma. These need to be tracked in time so the child may, for example, be prompted to recall how they were on the first night after the event, when they returned to school and how they are now.
- The symptoms volunteered should be clearly specified and simple visual rating scales used to quantify relevant dimensions such as frequency, severity, or degree of distress or impairment caused. Depending upon the child's age and developmental level, self-report assessments can complement interview information.
- The onset of the symptoms should be checked and the relationship to the trauma ascertained.
- The clinician should then assess directly whether the child has experienced other symptoms described in the diagnostic classification systems and to detail their onset and severity.
- Evidence of other co-morbid conditions including depression, generalized anxiety disorders, specific phobias, substance alcohol abuse and self-injurious behaviour should be explored.
- Finally, the child's thoughts about the trauma, why it occurred, how they reacted, its effect upon the future should be checked. Issues such as possible guilt (e.g. at surviving or receiving only minor injuries), responsibility and blame (for what occurred), thoughts of death or serious injury and feelings of being different from others should be checked.

Younger children are more likely to experience difficulty with verbal assessments and, at these times, developmentally more appropriate methods should be used. An interview format has been described and used with younger children (aged 3 and older) shortly after witnessing violent traumatic events. This format is helpful for encouraging children to talk about the traumatic event although further questioning is required, either from the child, their carer, or both, in order to specify any changes in behaviour that have occurred.

- The interview starts by informing the child that the therapist has met many children whom have 'gone through what you have gone through'.
- The young person is encouraged to draw a picture about anything they like as long as they can tell a story about it. Young children will find this helpful and usually are able to provide more detailed verbal accounts of traumatic events if they talk whilst drawing.
- The facilitator probes the child's drawing and story, identifies possible traumatic references, which are then explored and built upon during the second stage of the interview.
- Within a supportive holding relationship, the child is encouraged to describe what happened as the traumatic event is systematically reconstructed. The

factual content is discussed in detail, accompanying sensory experiences described, and the worst moment for the child explored. Common feelings and emotional reactions including guilt, accountability and anger are discussed.

- The interview is then closed by the facilitator reviewing and summarizing the session. Children are reassured that feelings of helplessness and fear are common, alerted to the possible future course of their reactions and invited to contact the facilitator if they wish to talk again.
- The interview is used as a way of screening the child to identify whether any further professional intervention is required.

Parents/carers

The interview with the parents/carers provides an opportunity to place the trauma and child's subsequent reaction and symptoms within a wider context.

- A developmental history looking at the child's general development, educational ability, temperament and history of previous medical and psychological problems should be obtained. This will help to determine whether symptoms were present before, or arose as a result of the trauma.
- The family and social context should be discussed with relationships between key family members identified, friendship patterns established, relationship difficulties noted and the child's areas of interest and social activities established. Marital difficulties and previous or current mental health problems in the child's carers should be checked. In addition, the presence of other recent or on-going stressors should be explored.
- The parent/carer's account of the trauma and their views regarding its impact upon the child, (and themselves if involved) should be determined.
- Behaviour and emotional changes that have occurred following the trauma, both immediately after and currently should be assessed. The assessor should be aware of developmental variations in the presentation of PTSD symptoms, particularly with pre-school children where parents may construe significant behaviour changes (toileting accidents, refusal to go to bed on their own) as willful naughtiness rather than trauma related.
- The presence of any co-morbid conditions should be explored and in particular symptoms of depression and generalized anxiety.
- Finally, the clinician should establish what help has been provided for the child and what strategies the family has found effective in reducing their child's distress.

Aetiology

Comparatively little is known about risk and protective factors that affect the onset and long-term course of PTSD in children and young people. The evidence currently available points to the importance of child characteristics, family factors and disaster-related variables.

Child characteristics

- As highlighted earlier, gender appears important with girls tending to be more vulnerable to the development of PTSD than boys. Girls tend to demonstrate more internalizing symptoms whereas boys are more likely to exhibit more externalizing symptoms.
- Children of all ages are affected by traumatic events although there is continuing debate as to whether younger children are at a greater or lesser risk of developing PTSD. Little is known about possible changes in cognitive development that may affect understanding and beliefs about how the trauma is appraised.
- The child's response may be affected by prior life events or pre-existing problems that increase the risk of them developing PTSD symptomatology. Previous psychological problems tend to increase the child's vulnerability to PTSD, whereas higher educational attainment tends to be a protective factor.

Family factors

- The relationship between child and parent symptomatology is not entirely consistent, although on balance it would appear that parental and child adjustment are related. Higher rates of PTSD have been found in children whose parents have themselves experienced strong emotional distress and are less able to help their children.
- Alternatively, social support either from parents, friends or professionals in which the child is encouraged and helped to discuss, understand and come to terms with the trauma appears protective. Children who have such a supportive environment tend to present with fewer symptoms and appear to recover more quickly.

Trauma-related variables

- Level of exposure to the trauma is an important factor. Children who have higher or more severe levels of exposure to traumatic events generally have been found to have higher rates of PTSD symptoms.
- There is some evidence that incurring a physical injury can adversely affect adjustment.
- The child's appraisal of the event is an important factor and goes some way to explaining why objectively minor traumas can result in PTSD. Those children who perceive traumatic events as life threatening are more likely to develop PTSD.

Treatment

Clinical management and setting

The treatment of PTSD is usually undertaken in community settings. In-patient admission is typically not required unless the child presents with a severe co-morbid condition (e.g. depression) that may benefit from in- or day-patient treatment. A variety of modalities can be used including individual, family and group interventions, which can be delivered at various times following the trauma.

There is comparatively little well-controlled research examining the effectiveness of interventions for the treatment of child PTSD. Research with children has to date largely focused upon documenting symptoms and on the course of the disorder rather than evaluating the efficacy of interventions.

Consensus amongst child trauma experts would suggest that interventions should include:

- a direct discussion about the traumatic event
- identification and correction of inaccurate cognitions and attributions about the trauma
- anxiety management
- the involvement of parents in treatment.

Psychological interventions – crisis interventions

The period immediately following a traumatic event is often very emotional, characterized by high rates of anxiety and uncertainty. Children will have many needs during the immediate post-trauma stage, with the most pressing being the need to be re-united with their carers. It is only once the child's sense of safety has been re-established that psychological interventions should be considered.

Crisis or impact phase interventions, typically delivered within 72 hours of the trauma, are concerned primarily with preventing or ameliorating the possible psychological distress arising from the traumatic event. Often, these are provided to everyone involved in the trauma regardless of symptomatology or diagnosis. At this stage children will not be suffering from PTSD but, if assessed, may meet diagnostic criteria for an acute stress disorder.

Psychological debriefing

Psychological debriefing, sometimes known as critical incident stress debriefing, has become an integral part of front-line interventions for adult victims and helpers involved in major traumas. Debriefing has a compelling and widespread appeal as an acceptable, moral, ethical, humane and immediate way of providing psychological help to those involved in traumatic events. Although widely used with adults, there is considerable debate as to whether debriefing is effective in preventing or minimizing subsequent psychological distress. The recent guideline from the National Institute of Clinical Excellence (NICE) on the management of PTSD (2005) concludes that the systematic provision of single session debriefing interventions should not be routinely provided. Although all but one of the studies reviewed were conducted with adults, the results of the trial with children do not support the widespread use of single session debriefing. When re-assessed 8 months post-trauma, the psychological functioning of children and young people involved in road traffic accidents who received debriefing was not significantly better or worse than those who did not.

Psychological interventions – cognitive behaviour therapy (CBT)

CBT has been successfully used in the treatment of PTSD and tends to address the cardinal features of the condition, namely trauma re-experiencing (cognitive element), avoidance (behavioural element) and increased arousal (emotional element). CBT is based upon the underlying assumption that affect and behaviour are largely a product of cognitions. CBT aims to ameliorate and/or reduce psychological distress and maladaptive behaviour by focusing upon altering cognitive processes.

CBT can be used with children aged over 7 years of age, although it is important to ensure that the intervention and techniques are adapted so that they do not exceed the child's cognitive or emotional capabilities. With younger children there may be a greater emphasis upon behavioural techniques. The cognitive element may be less sophisticated, relying more upon specific, concrete cognitive techniques such as developing positive self-talk. Adolescents will typically be able to work with higher order, more abstract and complex cognitive tasks such as identifying dysfunctional assumptions, evaluating evidence for and against beliefs and cognitive restructuring.

CBT for children with PTSD is often delivered within 6–12 sessions and typically involves the following treatment elements.

- Psychoeducation is required to provide both the treatment rationale and an understanding for both the child and their parents/carers as to the possible reactions and symptoms that might follow a traumatic event. The child's symptoms are placed within the context of a typical response to an abnormal event. The relationship between cognitions, emotions and behaviour is explained and a formulation of the child's presenting difficulties provided. Goal setting occurs whereby the child, their parents and the therapist mutually agree the targets of the intervention and the overall goals that are to be achieved. Quantification is helpful with measurable targets such as reducing intrusive thoughts to once per week or travelling to school on the bus, ensuring that progress can be carefully monitored and reviewed.

- Anxiety management is the vehicle whereby the arousal symptoms of PTSD are addressed. Typically, this involves emotional education whereby the child is helped to identify and label their emotions and the physiological symptoms associated with anxiety. Thoughts associated with anxious feelings are identified and alternative coping self-talk (i.e. non-anxiety producing) developed and practised. Specific relaxation skills such as relaxing imagery, controlled breathing and progressive muscular relaxation may be taught in order to provide the child with ways in which anxious feelings can be controlled and reduced. The use of objective scales to monitor the intensity of subjective feelings of anxiety is encouraged. These are often referred to as subjective units of distress (SUDS) and consist of a 0–10 point scale (0 = no distress at all; 10 = the most upset I have ever been).

- Avoidance is addressed through the process of exposure designed to help the child face and overcome their traumatic experience and the consequences that may arise. The child is helped to develop a hierarchy of feared/avoided situations, which are arranged in order of increasing difficulty. Exposure can occur both imaginal or in vivo (real life). Starting with the least distressing event, once relaxed, the child is encouraged to master and successfully confront the feared event. The child will be encouraged to use coping self-talk to help them cope. The child and their parents/carers should reinforce and reward any success, no matter how small. The child systematically works their way through the hierarchy until the feared events and situations have been confronted and overcome.

- The cognitive element of the intervention aims to develop an understanding of the way the child appraises the trauma and to challenge and restructure distorted or biased cognitions. Once relaxed, the child is encouraged to build up a comprehensive picture of the traumatic event with the therapist paying particular attention to those parts of the child's account that are lacking in detail or poorly remembered. At various times the child's distress can be checked by asking them to rate their SUDS. If levels of anxiety are high, the child should be encouraged to stop, relax and regain control of their anxiety before continuing. Care should be taken to pace the intervention appropriately and to ensure that the child does not experience undue anxiety. Beliefs and cognitions about the trauma will emerge and these should be discussed, checked and re-appraised. Important cognitions may focus around issues of blame (feeling responsible for what occurred or being unable to prevent it), survivor guilt (why they were perhaps less effected/injured than others), life threat (thinking that they would die during the trauma), a perception of continuing current threat (increased vulnerability to on-going and future harm) and impact (devastating and shattering event). The process of discussion will help the child to normalize some of their cognitions and allows others to be re-appraised and restructured.

- Finally, the intervention may involve programmes designed to address specific problems such as night-time difficulties or school refusal. Typically these are addressed in a positive way whereby the child's appropriate behaviour is reinforced and rewarded with inappropriate behaviour receiving minimal reinforcement.

A few randomized-controlled trials evaluating the effectiveness of CBT in treating PTSD have been undertaken. Most have focused upon abuse as the traumatic event with the studies consistently indicating that CBT results in reductions in PTSD symptomatology. Further support for the efficacy of CBT comes from uncontrolled studies. However, the results do not yet indicate consistently whether CBT is superior to, or results in additional gains, over and above other forms of active treatment.

Psychological interventions – eye movement desensitization (EMDR)

Recent interest in the use of eye movement desensitization and reprocessing has indicated that substantial reductions in traumatic images may occur when used with children. EMDR is based on the premise that PTSD is a result of inadequate processing of trauma-related information. EMDR combines elements of a behavioural and client-centred approach to free traumatic images and memories in order to allow them to be processed, thereby reducing their potency. Specialist training is required to undertake EMDR and the process involves the following.

- The most distressing aspect of the trauma is identified. This could be a specific image, physical sensation, thought or belief.
- The child is then encouraged to concentrate on this emotionally disturbing material whilst simultaneously focusing upon an external stimulus. This is achieved most commonly by asking the child to track the movement of the therapist's finger, which is moved from side to side across the child's visual field. The traumatic event is held in the child's memory but is not discussed as the child rapidly moves their eyes from side to side.
- After approximately 30 seconds the child is asked whether anything happened and whether a particular image, thought, emotion or physical sensation occurred.
- If a dominant aspect of the trauma emerges, the child is asked to concentrate on this as the process is repeated. Thus if the child reports that they have become more angry, they will be asked to focus upon this anger.

• The process is repeated until the memory produces less distress.

Evidence from small-scale uncontrolled case studies is beginning to accumulate to suggest that EMDR may be effective in the treatment of childhood PTSD. Large-scale, methodologically sound, randomized-controlled treatment trials have not yet been undertaken.

The involvement of parents

Consideration needs to be given to the role of parents in interventions with children with PTSD. There is a general consensus that the involvement of parents/carers in treatment is important for resolving symptoms of PTSD. Parents have important roles in providing their child with post-trauma support and in encouraging the use of appropriate coping strategies. There is evidence to suggest that parental emotional reaction to the trauma and parental support of the child are important mediators of the child's PTSD. The parent's own distress may therefore need to be addressed as it may have an impact upon the maintenance of the child's problems. Parents will require education about the nature and possible course of PTSD symptoms in order to allow them to put their child's behaviour in context. This may help them to be more aware of, and responsive to, their child's emotional needs. Similarly, with young children parental involvement is important and will help the child to feel safe and comforted during clinical sessions.

At other times parents/carers may not be best placed to participate in the child's treatment programme, particularly if they were involved or responsible for what had occurred. Parents/carers may themselves be severely traumatized, being pre-occupied with their own problems and thus unable to help their child. Similarly, some parents may find their child's trauma particularly distressing and the child's concern about upsetting their parent may inhibit open discussion of important cognitions and events.

These factors need to be assessed and a decision made as to how to involve the parent in the intervention. Parents could have a very limited role participating in parallel psycho-educational sessions. They could be involved as co-therapists, attending all treatment sessions and prompting and reinforcing the practising of skills and attainment of goals outside of treatment sessions. Alternatively, the parents themselves could also be the subject of direct intervention, learning ways of addressing their own problems.

Pharmacotherapy

There is an absence of methodologically sound research evaluating the effectiveness of pharmacotherapy in the treatment of PTSD in children. The suggestion that PTSD symptoms may be due to excessive activity of the central adrenergic system has led some to explore whether adrenergic blocking agents such as propanolol and clonidine may be helpful. Recent practice guidelines for the assessment and treatment of children and adolescents with PTSD published by the American Psychiatric Association identifies that carbamazepine, propranolol, clonidine and guanfacine have been reported to ameliorate PTSD symptoms. The report, however, highlights that none of the studies reported used a control group or allocated children randomly to treatment conditions. The guidelines further note that, although antidepressants have been suggested to help some children with PTSD, particularly those with predominantly depressive or anxiety panic symptoms, there are no empirical studies of antidepressants for PTSD in children.

The report concludes that the present state of knowledge is not adequate to support the use of any particular medication to treat PTSD in children specifically.

Group vs. individual therapy

Empirical evidence comparing the efficacy of group vs individual therapy in the treatment of PTSD is lacking. The practice parameters of the American Academy of Child and Adolescent Psychiatry suggest that the treatment modality (individual, group, family) is less important than the content of the intervention, which should focus upon and treat the child's specific symptoms.

Monitoring and evaluation of treatment

Good practice requires that the purpose and nature of the intervention be fully explained to the child in a developmentally appropriate manner. The child and their parents/carers should be fully informed and consent to the indicated intervention. Targets should be agreed mutually, monitored and reviewed regularly in order to evaluate progress. Measures should be put in place to quantify the child's possible distress during clinical sessions. If high levels are reported, the clinical session should continue until any significant distress has been reduced to a more tolerable level.

Problematic issues

Exposure is a core element in the treatment of PTSD. In order for exposure to be effective, the child needs to experience and overcome high levels of arousal. If exposure is not sufficiently long, habituation will not occur and the emotional distress will not reduce. Treatment sessions therefore should be sufficiently long to allow the traumatic memory to be overcome, mastered and integrated rather than simply rehearsed. Treatment sessions should end with the child feeling relaxed and in control.

Outcome

Unfortunately, comparatively little is known about the long-term course of PTSD in children. Recent results from a longitudinal follow-up study of children involved in the cruise ship *Jupiter* sinking indicate the following.

- That delayed onset of PTSD (i.e. occurring later than 6 months after the trauma) is unusual. If children are going to develop trauma reactions, most will present with persistent and significant symptoms within 6 months of the event.
- Of those children who develop PTSD, between one-third and a half will recover within 1 year of onset.
- Approximately one-third of those who develop PTSD will go on to develop chronic symptoms lasting in excess of 5 years.

In summary, the data available would suggest that, although PTSD symptoms will remit in a number of children over time, a substantial proportion will continue to be significantly affected for long periods of time.

SUGGESTED READING

American Academy of Child and Adolescent Psychiatry, Practice parameters for the assessment and treatment of children and adolescents with post-traumatic stress disorder. *Journal of the American Academy of Child and Adolescent Psychiatry*, **37**, 10 Suppl. (1998).

A. Dyregrov, Grief in Children: A Handbook for Adults. (London: Jessica Kingsley, 1991).

K. E. Fletcher, Childhood posttraumatic stress disorder. In E. J. Mash & R. Barkley (eds). *Child Psychopathology.* (New York: Guilford Press, 1996)

S. Joeseph, R. Williams & W. Yule, *Understanding Post-traumatic Stress: A Psychological Perspective on PTSD and Treatment.* (Chichester: Wiley, 1997)

S. Perrin, P. Smith & W. Yule, Practitioner review: the assessment and treatment of post-traumatic stress disorder in children and adolescent. *Journal of Child Psychology and Psychiatry*, **41** (3) (2000), 277–89.

Post Traumatic Stress Disorder (PTSD): the management of PTSD in adults and children in primary and secondary care (2005). National Institute of Clinical Excellence www.nice.org.uk.

R. S. Pynoos & S. Eth, Witness to violence: the child interview. *Journal of the American Academy of Child Psychiatry*, **25** (1986), 306–19.

K. Salmon & R. A. Bryant, Posttraumatic stress disorder in children: the influence of developmental factors. *Clinical Psychology Review*, **22** (2002), 163–88.

M. S. Scheeringa, C. D. Peebles, C. A. Cook & C. H. Zeanah, Towards establishing procedural, criterion, and discriminative validity for PTSD in early childhood. *Journal of the American Academy of Child and Adolescent Psychiatry*, **40** (1) (2001), 52–60.

O. Udwin, S. Boyle, W. Yule, D. Bolton & D. O'Ryan, Risk factors for long-term psychological effects of a disaster experienced in adolescence: predictors of post traumatic stress disorder. *Journal of Child Psychology and Psychiatry*, **41** (8) (2001), 969–79.

W. Yule, D. Bolton, O. Udwin, S. Boyle, D. O'Ryan & J. Nurrish, The long-term psychological effects of a disaster experienced in adolescence: 1: The incidence and course of PTSD. *Journal of Child Psychology and Psychiatry*, **41** (4) (2000), 503–11.

9

Functional somatic symptoms and somatoform disorders in children

M. Elena Garralda

Child and Adolescent Psychiatry, Imperial College London, St Mary's Campus, London, UK

Introduction

Somatoform disorders differ from other psychiatric disorders in two main respects: first through the fact that presenting complaints are physical as opposed to psychological in nature; secondly because parents and children usually attribute these symptoms to physical illness in spite of the lack of medical evidence, including examination and physical investigations. As a result somatoform disorder tends to present to psychiatrists only after repeated paediatric or other specialist investigations have taken place, and the referral may be accepted only reluctantly by a number of families who are sceptical about the usefulness of a psychiatric assessment, even sometimes hostile to this. This calls for special expertise at the child psychiatry clinic in assessment and management.

A crucial feature of somatoform disorders is the presence of somatization or the manifestation of distress through somatic symptoms, a tendency to experience and communicate somatic distress and symptoms unaccounted for by pathological findings, to attribute them to physical illness and to seek medical help. Functional or unexplained physical symptoms (ie those without an established organic substrate) are common in the general population but do not necessarily lead to impairment, nor are they always an expression of distress or linked to illness beliefs and medical help seeking. However, the associations of unexplained recurrent physical symptoms in the child and adolescent general population have a great deal in common with those of somatoform disorders, and unexplained physical symptoms will also be considered in this chapter alongside these disorders.

There are several categories of psychiatric disorders where physical symptoms are a key or presenting feature. They include mental factors influencing the development of physical pathology or psychophysiological processes (for example, asthma, ulcerative colitis). Physical symptoms may also be the main feature of

A Clinician's Handbook of Child and Adolescent Psychiatry, ed. Christopher Gillberg,
Richard Harrington and Hans-Christoph Steinhausen. Published by Cambridge University Press.
© Cambridge University Press 2005.

well-recognized psychiatric or developmental conditions (for example, eating and sleeping disorders, bedwetting, abnormal movement disorders). These are discussed elsewhere in this book. This chapter will focus on somatoform disorders, where somatic symptoms are seen primarily as manifestations of psychic distress or difficulty, as masquerading mental factors which are assumed to have major aetiological significance.

Definition and classification

Somatoform disorders are described comparably in both ICD-10 and DSM-IV classification systems as those where:
- physical symptoms suggest an underlying medical condition; however, no medical disease, substance misuse or another mental disorder can be found to account for the degree of functional disability or distress
- the symptom production is not under conscious control.

These diagnostic criteria were established for adults and by extrapolation are applied to children. It is probably more difficult to assess the degree of conscious control in childhood.

Somatoform disorders include a number of sub-categories, including:
- somatization disorder
- pain disorder
- conversion (dissociative) disorder
- undifferentiated somatoform disorder
- hypochondriasis.

ICD-10 includes under neurotic disorders neurasthenia, with chronic fatigue as the defining symptom and now more commonly referred to as chronic fatigue syndrome.

Not all of the above are described consistently in children and adolescents. This chapter will cover predominantly those that are, namely pain, conversion and dissociative disorders though some mention will also be made of somatization disorder. Chronic fatigue syndrome will also be considered.

The main criteria according to ICD-10 and DSM-IV are given in Appendix 9.1.

Epidemiology

Prevalence rates

General population

Much more is known about the general population epidemiology of symptoms likely to be functional or unexplained than that of somatoform disorder categories. Surveys across different countries have found that about one in four children complain of at least one of a set of somatic symptoms weekly or every other week.

Symptoms are generally more common in girls than in boys, headaches and tiredness being especially frequent.

As for recurrent and troubling somatic symptoms, studies converge in finding that 2–10 per cent of children and adolescents in the general population have recurrent aches and pains, most likely to be unexplained, and 5–10 per cent report distressing symptoms or are regarded by their parents as 'sickly'. Rates vary according to problem definition and it is common for several symptoms to coexist in the same child.

Over the years, recurrent abdominal pains have attracted most attention. Apley's classic study of school children found that around 10 per cent (12 per cent of girls and 9 per cent of boys) of children in the general population had at least three bouts of pain defined as severe enough to affect activities over a 3-month period. Similar rates of recurrent abdominal pains were documented amongst medical out-patient clinics.

The recent German Early Developmental Stages of Psychopathology project in adolescence and young adulthood has documented the prevalence of somatoform disorders amongst 3021 14–24-year-old representative adolescents and young people. It has used research clinical interviews, and ascertained clinical significance and impairment, lack of explanatory medical conditions or substance use (though not of explanatory psychiatric disorders). The main findings are outlined here.

- More than 12 per cent of the population suffered during their lifetime (12-month prevalence of 7.2%) from at least one of the somatoform disorders (i.e. somatization, pain, conversion and hypochondriasis disorders; dissociative disorder not otherwise specified or NOS, abridged somatization disorder or SS14,6 (a disorder requiring fewer symptom types than somatization disorder: four for males and six for females), undifferentiated somatoform/dissociative syndrome or USDS.
- Whereas the less specific disorders were present more frequently, the most prevalent specific disorders were somatoform pain disorder (lifetime 1.7%, 12-month 0.9%) and conversion disorder (0.4% and 0.2%, respectively). Only one case fulfilled diagnostic criteria for hypochondriasis and none for somatization disorder.
- Disorders were linked generally to low socio-economic status, except for pain disorder which was associated to higher (university) education.

Chronic fatigue syndrome was not included in this study but population rates of 2 per cent 'chronic fatigue syndrome-like' syndromes assessed from questionnaire information are reported in 5–17-year olds in the USA, with indications of particularly higher rates in Latino subjects. In children with severe chronic fatigue disorders assessed in tertiary paediatric units, a predominance of high socio-economic backgrounds and white ethnicity is reported.

Paediatric clinics

About 10 per cent of children attending general practice or paediatric clinics are reported as having medically unexplained medical symptoms. When a broader psychosomatic concept is used (i.e. children presenting with any kind of physical presentations, where doctors identify associated or contributing psychological factors, for example, stress-exacerbating asthma) psychosomatic problems are seen in between a quarter to nearly half the children consulting.

Most of what we know in this area refers to school children and adolescents. However, unexplained somatic symptoms are seen almost as frequently in early childhood or nursery children, with frequent complaining of abdominal pains in nearly one in ten, tiredness and leg pains being less common and fewer complaining of headaches.

Sex and age ratios

Adolescent girls in the general population report more physical symptoms than boys and parents describe more girls than boys as suffering from a variety of physical symptoms or being sickly. Similarly, somatoform disorders are also more common in adolescent girls, as girls are over-represented amongst cases of conversion disorder and chronic fatigue syndrome seen in paediatric and psychiatric clinics.

Interesting trends emerged from the German epidemiological survey of older adolescents and young adults as follows.

• Most pain and undifferentiated disorders had started in childhood or early adolescence.

• Conversion and dissociative disorders started later (median age of onset at 16 years).

• For females, pain disorder showed the steepest age of onset increase between 11 and 19 years of age, whereas all men had onset of pain disorder by 13 years of age.

Amongst patients consulting general paediatricians, unexplained physical symptoms are more common in older than in preschool children. There are indications that abdominal symptoms increase gradually from 3 to 9 years of age and then decrease steadily up to adolescence. The converse is likely to be true of headaches, which appear considerably less common in pre-school than in older children and adolescents.

Implications for clinical practice

It is important for parents consulting for unexplained medical symptoms in their children to be made aware of the high frequency of these symptoms in the population and amongst children attending paediatric clinics. Information of this kind may provide a helpful perspective for their anxieties about a possible medical aetiology. Knowledge about the frequency of unexplained somatic symptoms and possible somatization amongst children attending paediatricians and family doctors also helps provide a context for the planning of paediatric and child psychiatric paediatric liaison services.

Clinical picture

Factors which raise suspicion that psychological factors are playing a part in somatic presentations include:

- the presence of a time relationship between a likely stress and physical symptoms
- severity of handicap from the symptom out of keeping with the established pathophysiology
- concurrent psychiatric disorder.

Main features and symptoms

Headaches commonly present as migraine and tension headaches. In migraine – which is regarded as a neurological disorder – the headache is periodic, severe and unilateral, accompanied by a visual aura, nausea, vomiting and a family history of migraine. Tension headaches are described as non-paroxysmal, frequent, bilateral and often frontal, like 'a band or heavy weight or fullness', with associated dizziness. In practice, the differentiation between the two types is often not clear-cut and both may co-exist in the same patient.

Except for headaches, more is known about recurrent unexplained stomach aches or recurrent abdominal pains (RAP) leading to medical help-seeking than about other physical symptoms, though it is common for multiple symptoms to co-exist, whatever the most prominent or presenting complaint. Typically abdominal pains will have a diffuse or peri-umbilical distribution, be intense and cause distress to the child. The pain is often worse during the day and may not keep the child awake at night. It may be more noticeable on Monday mornings and less bothersome during holidays. Medication tends to be of little use. Although onset may follow an episode of diarrhoea and vomiting, or the pain may be associated with constipation, marked abnormalities of bowel habit are not often seen. Children may look pale and quite unwell and this reinforces parental worries about physical pathology.

Abdominal pains and headaches form part of ICD-10s persistent somatoform pain disorder when the pain is persistent, severe and distressing, when it occurs in association with emotional conflict or psychosocial problems that are sufficient to allow the conclusion that they may have an aetiological influence.

In dissociative (conversion) disorders there is a partial or complete loss of bodily sensations or movements. Most children present with disturbances of motor function such as weakness of legs and bizarre gait, but they can also show total incapacitation. Symptoms are often brought on by a particularly traumatic event and they tend to remit after a few weeks or months. Visual symptoms can be reported, with loss of or restricted vision, though as with recurrent backache and stiffness, by the time they present to specialist services they can be a warning sign of underlying neurological disorder. As well as conversion blindness, mutism or inability to produce vocal sounds may be a presenting or associated feature. Children may communicate different levels of distress about their symptoms but the concept of 'belle indifference' is probably not particularly helpful with young patients.

Pseudoseizures are seen in western countries but may be specially common in some specific cultures. In a recent study from Turkey of predominantly girls presenting to a tertiary child psychiatry unit with conversion, most had pseudoseizures. They tended to come from middle-class nuclear families and virtually all reported precipitant events – either relationship problems or medical illness in the family. The mean time to diagnosis was long (1 year), and the average age at symptom onset 12 years.

In chronic fatigue syndrome (or neurasthenia) the main complaint is increased fatigue after mental or physical effort. Unlike post-infectious tiredness or medically related fatigue, which tend to be either short-lived or dependent on concurrent medical disease, fatigue is chronic and medically unexplained. It is associated with decrease in occupational performance or coping efficiency in daily tasks. There is difficulty in concentrating and dizziness, physical fatigability with physical weakness and exhaustion after only minimal effort, muscular aches and pains, tension headaches, sleeping problems and worry about decreasing mental and bodily wellbeing. Whilst there is little supporting evidence for a medical substrate to this disorder, high levels of associated psychopathology have been reported consistently in severely affected cases, mostly from the adult literature. In spite of this, it is common for parents and patient support groups to ascribe the condition to neurological pathology as implied in the term ME (for myalgic encephalomyelitis), preferred by patient support groups.

Marked functional impairment unexplained by any associated physical or psychiatric pathology is a key feature of somatoform disorders as seen in specialist clinics. This may be specially marked and prolonged in chronic fatigue syndrome. For example, a follow-up study of children attending tertiary paediatric clinic has documented long mean duration of illness to recovery (38 months) and marked functional impairment. Two-thirds of the children had had prolonged periods of bed rest and had stopped school attendance altogether, with a mean of time out of school of three school terms. This was accompanied by marked reduction of social and everyday activities. This degree of impairment is not seen in other paediatric or psychiatric disorders and can be regarded as central to the syndrome.

The association with functional impairment – though less strong than in tertiary referred children – is seen across the age and severity range of recurrent somatic symptoms in children. Young nursery children in the general population with frequent somatic symptoms are significantly more likely than children without symptoms to have associated behavioural and emotional problems, to be kept out of nursery and to attend paediatric services. Similar associations are seen amongst children with unexplained physical symptoms attending general paediatric clinics. This suggests that a somatization pattern of psychological difficulty expressed through somatic symptoms and leading to paediatric help seeking and impairment of everyday activity starts early in childhood. In some children it may be the forerunner of somatoform disorders which tend to become expressed in later childhood or adolescence.

Attendance to many different specialist clinics is also common in these cases. In the above study of children with chronic fatigue syndrome attending tertiary paediatric clinics, subjects had seen a mean of close to seven professionals about their condition (range of 2 to 22). Excessive medical investigations may contribute to the maintenance of the disorder by undermining parents' confidence and delaying appropriate management.

Differential psychiatric diagnosis of medically unexplained physical symptoms

Physical symptoms are found commonly in children and adolescents with psychiatric disorders and are, in fact, key features of emotional disorders. The following psychiatric disorders should be considered specially in differential psychiatric diagnosis:

- school phobia and refusal, where the key features are marked fear and avoidance of school; although children with somatoform disorders avoid school, the reasons given are typically inability to function because of the physical symptoms, worry about the symptoms getting worse, and concern about how to explain their disorder to others
- anorexia nervosa, with deliberate weight loss and an intrusive dread of fatness
- depressive disorder, with consistent and persistent lowering of mood and associated cognitive and behavioural changes
- anxiety disorders, with prominent, prolonged and persistent feelings of anxiety, worry and restlessness
- elective mutism, with marked, emotionally determined selectivity in speaking, so that the child demonstrates verbal competence in some situations only
- factitious illness (also called Munchausen by proxy), where physical symptoms or signs in the child are fabricated deliberately or induced, nearly always by the mother.

An example of functional somatic symptoms likely to be an expression of an anxiety disorder was an epidemic of fainting, dizziness and fears of possession in adolescents and young adults (mostly female) who were residents in a Bhutanese refugee camp in Nepal. Detailed examination of the accompanying symptoms (for example, hyperventilation, fearfulness, palpitations and trembling) led the authors to conclude that these may have been an expression of acute anxiety states.

Differential diagnosis can be particularly complex in cases where biologically and psychologically determined symptoms co-exist. For example pseudoseizures may be present alongside epileptic seizures or fainting episodes and mimic them.

Research diagnostic criteria for syndromes such as chronic fatigue syndrome make the presence of primary mental disorders such as psychotic states or anorexia nervosa exclusion criteria. However, it is possible and, indeed, common for somatoform to co-exist with other psychiatric disorders. The somatoform disorder is regarded as primary as opposed to a direct expression of an emotional disorder, when physical symptoms are more prominent than emotional or behavioural features, when they are the main cause of functional impairment, when there is an unwarranted belief in an underlying medical disorder and repeated medical help seeking.

Psychiatric co-morbidity

Psychiatric symptoms and co-morbidity are reported commonly in children with functional symptoms or somatoform disorders. The strongest associations are with anxiety and depressive disorders.

In a general population sample of USA school children and adolescents, one in five girls with stomach aches had co-morbid anxiety disorders, a comparable one in five children with musculo-skeletal pains had depressive disorders (compared with only 2 or 3 per cent in children without pains). In addition, 7 per cent of the boys with musculo-skeletal pains had co-morbid oppositional defiant or attention deficit hyperactivity disorder (compared with 2 per cent of those without these physical symptoms). Associations with attention deficits, adjustment disorders and other problems such as dependency, feeding and elimination disorders may be specially common in young preschool children.

Amongst children attending services a third to a half may be expected to have psychiatric co-morbidity at the time of assessment, but 12-month prevalence can be as much as three-quarters in some severely affected children with chronic fatigue syndrome. In some cases psychiatric disorders will precede the development of the handicapping functional somatic symptoms, but it seems more common for the latter to develop in the course of the somatoform disorder.

Different rates of psychiatric co-morbidity have been reported for specific somatoform disorders. For example, in the German adolescent epidemiology study, psychiatric co-morbidity was present in 80 per cent of subjects with modified somatization disorder. Conversion and dissociative disorders were associated strongly with eating disorders, and pain disorders with major depression, panic disorder and post-traumatic stress disorder. Pain disorder was usually reported as temporally or sequentially primary to psychiatric disorders, but conversion and dissociative disorder followed frequently on other psychopathology.

The strongest current impairment was seen in conversion disorder and in modified somatoform disorders, degree of impairment increasing with more co-morbid psychopathology. However, somatoform disorders were associated with impairment in childhood (ie missing school, seeing doctors, seeking professional help for mental problems) even after controlling for psychiatric disorders.

The high levels of co-morbid psychopathology underscore the importance of carrying out a careful psychiatric assessment of children with somatoform disorders, to make sure that psychopathology is attended to and managed adequately.

Diagnostic instruments

Instruments to measure physical symptoms and associated functional impairment, symptom diaries and severity ratings may all be helpful during assessment and for monitoring progress. References on specific instruments are given alongside suggested reading, and the Child Symptom Inventory, Functional Disability Index, fatigue scale and a sample symptom diary are given in Appendix 9.2.

The Child Somatization Inventory (CSI) measures 35 symptoms and their severity if present in the 2 weeks prior to assessment. Total number and severity symptom scores are derived. A somatization score identifies somatization disorder-related symptoms of marked severity. The linked Functional Disability Index (FDI) is a 14-item questionnaire of documented validity, stability and sensitivity to change. It scores the presence and severity of functional disability in areas such as walking, travelling, daily chores, social and leisure activities, sleeping and eating.

It is helpful to complement the above with specific symptom scales. The fatigue self-report scale lists features of both physical and mental fatigue; it has acceptable reliability and a cut-off of 3 is associated with clinically relevant fatigue symptoms from research interviews. It is easy to use with young people.

Symptoms diaries using Likert scales (often 0–10) to assess the severity of the key symptoms are helpful to map frequency, severity and contingencies of symptoms and to document changes with treatment over time. Symptom improvement may be ascertained through these before patients have experienced subjective relief: visualization of improved scores may help maintain therapeutic optimism and motivation. For all children, an essential measure of functional impairment is precise information about school attendance.

Also useful are scales to measure changes in symptom of anxiety, fears and depression and general behavioural scales as described in relevant chapters in this book.

Assessment

The family doctor or general practitioner will be the first port of call for most children. Some may already be well known to the doctor because of comparatively frequent family ill health and consulting. Nursery children with unexplained somatic symptoms consult their family doctor more than other children, and those with chronic fatigue syndrome tend to have a pre-morbid history of an excess of upper respiratory or infectious illnesses leading to school absence. Usual assessment and investigations by the family doctor will often relieve concerns sufficiently for the child to improve and to ensure an adequate level of functioning.

Children and families with frequent symptoms and high anxiety levels may be expected to be referred to a general or specialist paediatric or medical service for further assessment and investigations. Given the frequent psychiatric co-morbidity, the excess of life stresses, personality vulnerabilities and family illness and distress discussed below under aetiology, systematic psychiatric history taking and mental state examination as well as exploration of a psychosocial contribution are highly relevant at this stage.

Few children are likely to be referred to child psychiatrists and referral needs to be handled carefully. Many children and families fear that a referral means that the child's symptoms are not being taken seriously, that they are assumed to be 'all in the mind' and therefore somehow unreal, purely an expression of psychopathology or of parental anxiety. Even after referral, some families will remain highly anxious and sometimes even 'hopeful' that an underlying physical disorder will become manifest. It is therefore appropriate for the psychiatric assessment to include medically informed history-taking, acknowledgement of what medical disorders have been excluded and of possible physiological explanations for symptoms.

Psychiatric assessment needs to include a detailed psychiatric history, mental state of the child and assessment of family function. Psychometry can be helpful when the child has a history of putting him or herself under academic pressure and where there is a possible mismatch between the child's achievements, capability and expectations. As already mentioned, a detailed history of school attendance is essential.

Aetiology

Precipitants and stress

It is not uncommon for somatoform disorders to be brought about or precipitated by physical problems and medical treatments, for example severe abdominal pains may start after an acute gastrointestinal infection. Pseudoseizures may follow episodes of fainting or epileptic seizures. An injury and treatment with immobilization may precede loss of sensation or motility in a limb. A 'flu'-type, glandular fever or other infectious illness often brings on chronic fatigue syndrome. It may be expected that, in some families, this will influence or bias physical aetiological beliefs. Whereas most cases of 'flu'-type illness will recover normally within a couple of weeks, recovery from glandular fever can take longer. However, only a small proportion of those affected will have prominent fatigue syndrome 6 months later.

Psychosocial stress and events are also linked to the onset and maintenance of somatoform disorders and for a number of children the somatic symptoms may represent a psychiatric adjustment reaction. Stresses need not be isolated, uncommon or specially threatening. Children with unexplained medical symptoms present as specially sensitive to daily hassles such as harsh comments on school work, or ups and downs in peer relationships, and are likely to report close links between these stresses and somatic symptoms. The combination of the stress of moving to secondary school with a flu-type illness in the autumn term may trigger a chronic fatigue state. Pre-schoolers with frequent somatic symptoms experience an excess of common life events – such as birth of a sibling – compared with children without symptoms.

The effect of life stresses on children with recurrent functional symptoms or somatoform disorders is likely to be mediated by problems in social competence or personality difficulty in the child, and by high levels of physical symptoms in their parents.

Personality features

Personality factors have long been recognized as of relevance for functional symptoms in children. Clinicians consistently have described them as conscientious, sensitive, insecure and anxious. More recently the use of research personality instruments has led to identification of an excess of personality problems in children with severe forms of chronic fatigue syndrome. Traits indicative of conscientiousness, vulnerability, worthlessness and emotional lability would appear to be particularly common amongst them. If very marked, these traits would make it specially difficult for children to adapt emotionally and behaviourally to the vicissitudes of everyday life. They may lead to children putting themselves under pressure to work and succeed in school, or to be specially sensitive to social interactions.

Illness beliefs

Family beliefs about a medical causation for the child's symptoms can militate against efforts towards rehabilitation and recovery. They can be an expression of a persistent and generalized tendency to believe in physical explanations for symptoms in the absence of medical evidence and reassurance to the contrary. Children with chronic fatigue syndrome tend to underestimate normative adolescent fatigue levels and feel specially frustrated by fatigue that other young people might not regard as abnormal.

Family factors

The combination of high levels of maternal distress and family health problems seems characteristic. A history of health problems in other family members is common, and there may be shared illness features with the unexplained symptoms in children. More families of children with severe chronic fatigue syndrome report an excess of comparable disorders in parents or siblings, and children with somatoform pain disorders tend to have relatives with other unexplained symptoms. Mothers of young children with recurrent physical symptoms are likely to perceive their own health as poor and be frequent attendees to their family doctor. There is some evidence that children with unexplained medical symptoms report more possible family illness models (i.e. instances of similar physical problems in the family) than those with established organic disorders, perhaps reflecting both the presence of symptoms and a special focus or attention to them by the child. It is assumed that this may contribute to the child's symptoms through the behavioural learning mechanism of modelling. There is moreover evidence that the presence of parental ill-health is associated with the continuation of the children's unexplained or recurrent symptoms during childhood and into adulthood.

High levels of parental mental distress are characteristic. This distress is often focused on the child's symptoms and may be striking to clinicians through its intensity and emotional over involvement. This involvement may contribute to the continuation of symptoms, by anxiously sensitizing the child and family and focusing their attention on physical symptoms and by militating against the use of coping mechanisms such as distraction. Parents of children with unexplained medical symptoms report more behaviours likely to reinforce child illness behaviour than those of children with other paediatric disorders, they are likely to respond to them with comparatively less anger, disappointment and punishment.

Unexplained medical symptoms and associated functional impairment may have profound effects on the family, everyday life revolving on the child's health, with a decrease in leisure activities and an increase in interpersonal tension. Parents often feel stressed and uncertain in their search for the right balance between encouraging active positive coping in children and pampering them, given their poor physical health. Long illness episodes can result in sustained changes in family function and these can be slow to shift during rehabilitation treatment.

Educational concerns and social factors

Concerns about school, often over educational performance but also over interactions with teachers and specially with peers are very common. At times bullying may be involved. Once children stop school attendance, they can become acutely anxious when the issue of return to school is approached. They do not see themselves as wishing to avoid attendance per se. The concerns usually involve a sense of inability to perform educationally because of their symptoms and about school attendance making them worse. Children are often acutely sensitive about assumptions by others that they are using their health to avoid unpleasant aspects of school attendance and feel misunderstood, embarrassed and angry about this.

Wider social factors may be relevant. For example, particularly high rates of pseudo-seizures have been reported in some Turkish clinical samples when compared with those from western countries.

Treatment

The assessment and planning of treatment, once explanatory physical or psychiatric disorders have been excluded, should involve a special effort to engage families. The following may be useful in assessment.

- Fully discuss physical concerns preoccupying the family and physical tests carried out
- Address physiological mechanisms contributing to symptoms when understood (i.e. muscle pains as a consequence of immobilization and abnormal gait; excessive rest may alter sleep)
- Avoid questioning the child's truthfulness regarding the symptom: attribution of symptoms such as 'all in the mind' is particularly unhelpful
- The significance of the 'belle indifference' is questionable
- It is important not to communicate a sense of embarrassment regarding the diagnosis of somatoform disorder or of other psychiatric disorders
- Families and children are more likely to accept stress and psychological factors contributing to the maintenance of the condition than to its cause
- Move from the physical to the psychological at a pace the family can cope with
- The essence of treatment is the development of strategies to help the child and family cope with the symptoms and reduce the associated functional impairment
- Emphasize that response to treatment may be slow but that most children can recover
- Liaison with school is usually required, specially so in the presence of dramatic, episodic symptoms such as pseudo-seizures
- The use of placebo, sham interventions or excessive reassurance is seldom helpful.

Clinical management and treatment setting

Clinical management thus starts with assessment by the family practitioner or paediatrician. When the problem fails to respond to paediatric assessment and advice, it is best managed within a psychosocial perspective. The severity of the problem and the extent of parental concerns about underlying medical illness will help determine whether psychiatric referral is indicated. This is specially appropriate:

- for diagnostic purposes, when there is uncertainty about the relevance of psychological factors
- when there is associated psychiatric disorder
- when the child fails to respond to standard paediatric treatment
- when major family problems affect the resolution of the symptoms.

It is essential that referring doctors to child psychiatry make a careful assessment of family attitudes towards psychiatric and other psychosocial problems and are able to discuss these with families in a productive way.

Psychological interventions

Treatment should aim to develop a partnership with child and families and – for cases with definite stress about school performance and school attendance problems – a co-ordinated approach with teachers. Co-ordination with other therapists involved, to ensure that everyone is working effectively towards similar goals, is crucial when several professionals are involved.

A specific treatment programme will contain certain features in common whether delivered by family doctors, paediatricians or psychiatrists. The intensity of contact required will vary depending on severity. Cases seen by psychiatric liaison teams typically will involve at early stages weekly or 2-weekly therapy sessions to help identify and review goals.

Treatment features are likely to involve a rehabilitative approach which aims to:

- emphasize the central role in treatment of reducing disability
- develop an active, problem-focused attitude to coping
- ascertain precise daily variations in severity of symptom and associated impairment (diaries help)
- develop special techniques to deal with individual symptoms (i.e. distraction techniques, rest periods, relaxation for headaches, analgesics as appropriate, physical exercises for muscular dysfunction; examination of contingencies and practical management of pseudoseizures)
- attend to dietary habits and sleep which may have become altered
- acknowledge and address as appropriate concerns by child and family that a rehabilitation programme might make the symptoms worse
- impose modest initial goals to increase normalization of daily activities
- gradually increase daily activities (including school work and attendance), change being set at achievable, consistent, agreed levels
- explore child expectations on ultimate goals (i.e. on usual well-being or fatigue levels) as these may be unrealistically high

- manage. underlying anxieties
- treat. associated emotional disorders
- family work
- gradually shift the burden of responsibility for therapeutic success from the clinician to the parent and patient.

School

It is important to look at ways of reducing any existing school-related stresses and conflicting expectations in discussion with parents and teachers. This may involve missing certain lessons or strategies to help the child cope with the symptom within school. The exact management of pseudoseizures needs to be made explicit and should include consideration of ways of reducing their dramatic impact within the school setting. In very incapacitated children a period out of school, or working with a home tutor or in a small home tuition centre may be indicated. Rehabilitation into school will usually involve gradual and partial re-introduction. For vulnerable children a school for 'delicate' children may be required. Some children benefit from admission to a paediatric unit with psychiatric input or to a psychiatric unit with educational provision.

Family work

Family work is essential in all cases. The aim is to facilitate the parents' engagement in treatment, by discussing on-going parental concerns about the nature of the condition. Parents will be central to planning a treatment programme that helps the child develop distracting and other coping mechanisms, and to understand and reduce behaviours that may constitute symptom reinforcement. Family work will intervene as appropriate for any associated family dysfunction, parental psychopathology or other sources of family stress which may impede recovery. Family stresses which are not apparent at initial stages of treatment may become manifest and amenable to intervention in the course of it.

Treatment effectiveness

There have been few satisfactory controlled studies of treatments for childhood somatoform disorders, but a number of clinical reports by hospital paediatricians and child psychiatrists have outlined the beneficial effects of approaches described earlier. Helping parents to understand the links between psychological and physical pain is in itself appreciated by many parents and felt to be influential in making the pain less intense and more manageable.

The best – if still sparse – available evidence of efficacy for unexplained abdominal pains comes from cognitive-behavioural family interventions. Whereas significant improvements on measures of pain intensity and pain behaviour can be achieved by standard paediatric interventions, there are indications that behavioural cognitive family intervention may lead to a higher rate of complete elimination of pain, lower levels of relapse at follow-up and lower levels of interference with activities from pain, as well as more parental satisfaction with treatment. Use by children of active self-coping and changes in maternal care giving strategies are likely to mediate these improvements. A cognitive-family intervention may include:

- discussion of investigations and rationale for pain management
- self-monitoring of pain
- reinforcing well behaviour (and reducing attention to symptoms)
  - promote distracting activities
  - ignore non-verbal pain behaviours
  - avoid modelling sick-role
  - discriminate seriousness of symptoms
- coping skills
  - relaxation
  - positive self-talk
  - distraction
  - positive imagery skills
- problem solving for future pain
- encouragement to participate in routine activities.

A central aspect of treatment is the reduction by parents of attention to the child over physical symptoms, whilst increasing attention and perhaps pleasant joint activities during symptom-free periods. Promising results for the management of chronic fatigue syndrome have been reported using family focused cognitive behaviour therapy, with substantial improvements in fatigue levels, social adjustment and mood and in return to full school attendance.

Work carried out in school settings and in paediatric outpatient clinics for children and adolescentss with migraine and functional headaches has shown that tension headaches can be substantially improved by relaxation training. In some, but not all, studies of adolescents, this is superior to attention placebo control and as effective whether administered at the clinic or as a home base self-administered treatment.

Pharmacotherapy

Anti-depressants can be helpful if there are associated depressive features or because of their sedative effects. The majority of severely affected children are likely to be depressed or in a severe state of anxiety and benefit from medication. Increasingly, serotonin re-uptake inhibitors are used. Through their anti-depressant and sedative effects, anti-depressants can make the rehabilitation process easier to implement.

In-patient admission

Paediatric/psychiatric or psychiatric admission is indicated if the child is very inca-pacitated, for detailed observation of frequent pseudoseizures, if there is associated psychopathology and little progress with outpatient treatment. It may help break the excessive anxious dependency of the child on his parents and focus the child's mind on the rehabilitation process. Specific interventions by physiotherapists, dieti-cian and occupational therapy interventions are often helpful. Therapists need to be specially skilled at motivating ambivalent or scared children to co-operate with treatment. Paediatric wards seldom have the necessary infrastructure and working practices to manage these children, and special procedures need to be put into place for individual cases in close liaison collaboration with psychiatric staff and hospi-tal teachers and through regular multi-disciplinary case discussions. Active family work will be essential. Specialist paediatric/psychiatric units are ideal but rare. Psy-chiatric admission is often appropriate but may not be accepted by families until psychiatrists have done some facilitating preliminary work at the paediatric unit.

In exceptional cases a somatoform disorder will be an expression of severe family disruption and child abuse (including factitious illness). The necessary statutory mechanisms need to be explored to safeguard the child's safety and to allow treat-ment to proceed. As with other disorders, close co-operation between the different doctors involved will be important to avoid different points of view about the condition contributing to protracted investigations and to its continuation.

In cases when there is parental inability or unwillingness to engage in any type of treatment for the child, consideration should be given to whether the child's development and safety are being put at risk and care would be better provided away from the family. This is hardly ever a clear-cut issue and will usually require second opinion from clinicians with special expertise in the area.

Monitoring and evaluation of treatment

The use of scales and specific instruments as described above is helpful in monitor-ing change and in highlighting minor changes which, though not always conducive to subjective improvement, may help motivate further rehabilitation work.

Information to patients and parents

Most parents are involved centrally with the child's problem and a collaborative partnership with the family is called for. Some conditions have strong patient sup-port groups, especially those linked to chronic fatigue syndrome (or ME). Parents and children may derive benefit from the realization that theirs is not an isolated or unique problem and from the information provided. It is also the case, however, that some patient groups hold strong beliefs about the medical nature of symptoms that may reinforce parents in an unhelpful search for a primary medical diagnosis and impede psychiatric involvement and active rehabilitation. Clinicians should be aware of the mixed effects that may derive from patient associations and help parents weigh options in order to engage in the best therapeutic approach for their child.

Problematic issues

The contrasting views by some families and doctors about the nature of somatoform disorders complicates treatment. The same applies to the embarrassment doctors and families may feel about these disorders and about a psychiatric referral, the doubts about malingering, the ambiguities in children's understanding of the nature of their symptoms, and some times also patient support associations as discussed earlier. Nevertheless these complications have to be regarded as intrinsic to somatoform disorders and call for special expertise in assessment and management.

Outcome

Clinical reports indicate that the majority of markedly affected children with somatoform disorders seen in specialist clinics recover or improve in the short term. However, symptoms persist to lesser degrees in a considerable proportion (about one-third in some studies) and some develop psychiatric disorders such as anxiety or eating disorders following recovery. There is also evidence for symptom continuity and increased psychopathology in adulthood. For example, half the subjects in a long-term follow-up study of children with abdominal pains were still symptomatic in early adulthood and associations have been found between recurrent physical symptoms in childhood and adult psychopathology.

Early diagnosis of dissociative/conversion disorder may be linked to better outcome, but some disorders, for example severely impairing chronic fatigue syndrome, can last for years before recovery is achieved. Specific medical precipitants, good pre-morbid personality, lack of parental health problems, good parental psychiatric adjustment and favourable social circumstances may be linked to better outcome.

Prevention

Because of the family aggregation of somatic symptoms and the links between child somatoform disorders and school non-attendance, efforts at prevention might profitably address children of parents with somatoform disorders and those with a history of persistent school non-attendance. Primary care services may be in a good position to guide parents to help children cope with physical symptoms without undue impairment. This may involve supporting children in the use of positive coping strategies, identifying areas of stress and helping them feel in control of situations they find difficult. Once in treatment, addressing the management of personality features (i.e. sensitivity to criticism, conscientiousness, anxiety proneness) as well as of excessive academic and behavioural expectations may help prevent relapse. Somatization can be recognized in young pre-school children, thus offering the possibility of early preventive work.

Conclusion

Recurrent unexplained medical symptoms are common in children and adolescents in the general population. When severe, impairing, related to psychological difficulty and leading to frequent medical help-seeking they form the basis of somatoform disorders.

These disorders tend to be precipitated by physical stressors. Although emotional co-morbidity is common, somatoform disorders are often ascribed by parents to physical pathology in spite of the absence of medical evidence. Child personality features, family health problems and unwitting reinforcement of symptoms by parents are thought to contribute to their maintenance.

Full (but not protracted or extended over time or duplicated) medical examination and investigations, recognition of parental and child views, and strategies to help children and parents reduce the impairment caused by the symptoms (for example, by reducing the attention given to physical symptoms and by establishing mutually rewarding shared activities during well times) are central to management. Psychiatric treatment is required for the often associated emotional co-morbidity and is helpful in setting up a family rehabilitation programme using behavioural cognitive techniques. Engaging families in treatment and psychiatric/paediatric liaison work are both important.

SUGGESTED READING

General reading

J. V. Campo & S. L. Fritz, Somatization in children and adolescents. *Journal of the American Academy of Child and Adolescent Psychiatry*, **33** (1994), 1223–35.

J. V. Campo & G. A. Fritz, A management model for paediatric somatization. *Psychosomatics*, **42** (1994), 46–76.

D. M. Eminson, Somatising in children and adolescents. *Advances in Psychiatric Treatment*, **7** (2001), 267–74, 388–98.

M. E. Garralda A selective review of child psychiatric syndromes with somatic presentation. *British Journal of Psychiatry*, **161** (1992), 759–73.

M. E. Garralda, Somatization in children. *Journal of Child Psychology and Psychiatry*, **37** (1996), 13–33.

M. E. Garralda & L. A. Rangel, Annotation: chronic fatigue syndrome in children and adolescents. *Journal of Child Psychology and Psychiatry*, **43** (2002), 169–76.

S. Taylor & M. E. Garralda, The management of somatoform disorders in childhood. *Current Opinion in Psychiatry*, **16** (2003), 227–31.

Individual studies

J. Apley, The Child with Abdominal Pains, 2nd edn. (Oxford: Blackwell Scientific Publications, 1975).

J. V. Campo, L. Jansen-McWilliams, D. M. Comer & K. Kelleher, Somatization in paediatric primary care: association with psychopathology, functional impairment and use of services. *Journal of the American Academy of Child and Adolescent Psychiatry*, **38** (1999), 1093–101.

H. L. Egger, E. J. Costello, A. Erkanli & A. Angold, Somatic complaints and psychopathology in children and adolescents: stomach aches, musculoskeletal pains, and headaches. *Journal of the American Academy of Child and Adolescent Psychiatry*, **38** (1999), 852–60.

R. Lieb, H. Pfister, M. Mastaler & H. U. Wittchen, Somatoform syndromes and disorders in a representative population sample of adolescents and young adults: prevalence, comorbidy and impairments. *Acta Psychiatrica Scandinavica*, **101** (2000), 194–208.

M. R. Sanders, R. W. Shepherd, G. Cleghorn & H. Woodford, Treatment of recurrent abdominal pain in children: a controlled comparison of cognitive behavioural family intervention and standard paediatric care. *Journal of Consulting and Clinical Psychology*, **62** (1994), 306–14.

Specific assessment instruments

T. Chalder, G. Berelowitz, T. Pawlikowska *et al.*, Development of a fatigue scale. *Journal of Psychosomatic Research*, **37** (1993), 147–53.

J. Garber, L. S. Walker & J. Zeman, Somatization symptoms in a community sample of children and adolescents: further validation of the children's somatization inventory. *Journal of Consulting and Clinical Psychology*, **4** (1991), 588–95.

L. S. Walker & J. W. Greene, The functional disability inventory: measuring a neglected dimension of child health status. *Journal of Paediatric Psychology*, **1** (1991), 39–58.

Appendix 9.1. Diagnostic criteria

ICD-10 criteria

Under ICD-10, somatoform disorders (F 45) are characterized by:
- repeated presentations of physical symptoms
- together with persistent requests for medical investigations
- in spite of repeated negative findings and reassurances by doctors that the symptoms have no physical basis
- if any disorders are present, they do not explain the nature and extent of the symptoms or the distress and preoccupation of the patient.

In the subcategory of somatization disorder the main features are as follows:
- multiple, recurrent and frequently changing physical symptoms of at least 2 years' duration

- most patients have a long and complicated history of contact with both primary and specialist medical care services, during which time many negative investigations or fruitless exploratory operations may have been carried out
- symptoms may be referred to any part or system of the body
- the course is chronic and fluctuating, often associated with disruption of social, interpersonal and family behaviour
- shorter lived and less striking symptom patterns are classified under undifferentiated somatoform disorders and are more likely to be seen in children and adolescents than the full somatization disorder.

In persistent somatoform pain disorder the predominant complaint is:

- persistent, severe and distressing pain, which cannot be explained fully by a physiological process or a physical disorder
- and which occurs in association with emotional conflict or psychosocial problems that are sufficient to allow the conclusion that they are the main causative influences
- the result is usually a marked increase in support and attention, either personal or medical
- pain presumed to be of psychogenic origin occurring during the course of depressive disorder or schizophrenia is not included here.

Dissociative (conversion) disorders (F44) have been classified previously as various types of 'conversion disorder' and are characterized by:

- partial or complete loss of the normal integration between memories of the past, awareness of identify and immediate sensations, and control of bodily movements
- all types of dissociative disorders tend to remit after a few weeks or months, particularly if their onset is associated with a traumatic life event
- more chronic disorders, particularly paralyses and anesthesias, may develop if the onset is associated with insoluble problems or interpersonal difficulties
- they are presumed to be psychogenic in origin, being associated closely in time with traumatic events, insoluble and intolerable problems or disturbed relationships
- the symptoms often represent the patient's concept of how a physical illness would be manifest
- medical examination and investigations do not reveal the presence of any known physical or neurological disorder
- in addition, there is evidence that the loss of function is an expression of emotional conflicts or needs
- the symptoms may develop in close relationship to psychological stress, and often appear suddenly
- only disorders of physical functions normally under voluntary control and loss of sensations are included here

- disorders involving pain and other complex physical sensations mediated by the autonomous nervous system are classified under somatization
- the possibility of later appearance of serious physical or psychiatric disorders should always be kept in mind.

In children most common are dissociative convulsions and loss of ability to move the whole or part of a limb or limbs, but loss of vision or the ability to articulate speech are also seen.

Under Neurasthenia (F-48) it is recognized that considerable cultural variation occurs in the presentation of the disorder and that there are two main types.

- In one type the main feature is a complaint of increased fatigue after mental effort, often associated with some decrease in occupational performance or coping efficiency in everyday tasks. The mental fatigability typically is described as an unpleasant intrusion of distracting associations or recollection, difficulty in concentrating and generally inefficient thinking.
- In the other type, the emphasis is on feelings of bodily or physical weakness and exhaustion after only minimal effort, accompanied by a feeling of muscular aches and pains and inability to relax.
- In both types a variety of other unpleasant physical feelings are common, such as dizziness, tension headaches and feelings of general instability.
- Worry about decreasing mental and bodily well-being, irritability, anhedonia and varying minor degrees of both depression and anxiety are all common.
- Sleep is often disturbed in the initial and middle phrases but hypersomnia may also be prominent.

DSM-IV diagnostic criteria

Diagnostic criteria for 300.81 somatization disorder

A. A history of many physical complaints beginning before age 30 years that occur over a period of several years and result in treatment being sought or significant impairment in social, occupational, or other important areas of functioning.

B. Each of the following criteria must have been met, with individual symptoms occurring at any time during the course of the disturbance:

(1) *four pain symptoms*: a history of pain related to at least four different sites or functions (e.g. head, abdomen, back, joints, extremities, chest, rectum, during menstruation, during sexual intercourse, or during urination)

(2) *two gastrointestinal symptoms*: a history of at least two gastrointestinal symptoms other than pain (e.g. nausea, bloating, vomiting other than during pregnancy, diarrhoea, or intolerance of several different foods)

(3) *one sexual symptom:* a history of at least one sexual or reproductive symptom other than pain (e.g. sexual indifference, erectile or ejaculatory dysfunction, irregular menses, excessive menstrual bleeding, vomiting throughout pregnancy)

(4) *one pseudoneurological symptom:* a history of at least one symptom or deficit suggesting a neurological condition not limited to pain (conversion symptom such as impaired coordination or balance, paralysis or localized weakness, difficulty swallowing or lump in throat, aphonia, urinary retention, hallucinations, loss of touch or pain sensation, double vision, blindness, deafness, seizures; dissociative symptoms such as amnesia; or loss of consciousness other than fainting)

C. Either (1) or (2):

(1) after appropriate investigation, each of the symptoms in Criterion B cannot be fully explained by a known general medical condition or the direct effects of a substance (e.g. a drug of abuse, a medication)

(2) when there is a related general medical condition, the physical complaints or resulting social or occupational impairment are in excess of what would be expected from the history, physical examination or laboratory findings.

D. The symptoms are not produced intentionally or feigned (as in factitious disorder or malingering).

Diagnostic criteria for 300.11 conversion disorder

A. One or more symptoms of deficits affecting voluntary motor or sensory function that suggest a neurological or other general medical condition.

B. Psychological factors are judged to be associated with the symptom or deficit because the initiation or exacerbation of the symptom or deficit is preceded by conflicts or other stressors.

C. The symptom or deficit is not produced intentionally or feigned (as in factitious disorder or malingering).

D. The symptom or deficit cannot, after appropriate investigation, be explained fully by a general medical condition, or by the direct effects of a substance, or as a culturally sanctioned behaviour or experience.

E. The symptom or deficit causes clinically significant distress or impairment in social, occupational or other important areas of functioning or warrants medical evaluation.

F. The symptom or deficit is not limited to pain or sexual dysfunction, does not occur exclusively during the course of somatization disorder, and is not better accounted for by another mental disorder.

Specify type of symptom or deficit:
With motor symptom or deficit
With sensory symptom or deficit
With seizures or convulsions
With mixed presentation

Diagnostic criteria for pain disorder

A. Pain in one or more anatomical sites is the predominant focus of the clinical presentation and is of sufficient severity to warrant clinical attention.

B. The pain causes clinically significant distress or impairment in social, occupational or other important areas of functioning.

C. Psychological factors are judged to have an important role in the onset, severity, exacerbation or maintenance of the pain.

D. The symptom or deficit is not intentionally produced or feigned (as in factitious disorder of malingering).

E. The pain is not better accounted for by a mood, anxiety, or psychotic disorder and does not meet criteria for dyspareunia.

Code as follows:

307.80 Pain disorder associated with psychological factors

Psychological factors are judged to have the major role in the onset, severity, exacerbation, or maintenance of the pain. (If a general medical condition is present, it does not have a major role in the onset, severity, exacerbation, or maintenance of the pain.) This type of pain disorder is not diagnosed if criteria are also met for somatization disorder.

Specify if:
Acute: duration of less than 6 months
Chronic: duration of 6 months or longer

307.89 Pain disorder associated with both psychological factors and a general medical condition

Both psychological factors and a general medical condition are judged to have important roles in the onset, severity, exacerbation or maintenance of the pain. The associated general medical condition or anatomical site of the pain (see below) is coded on Axis III.

Specify if:
Acute: duration of less than 6 months
Chronic: duration of 6 months or longer

Note: The following is not considered to be a mental disorder and is included here to facilitate differential diagnosis.

Pain disorder associated with a general medical condition

A general medical condition has a major role in the onset, severity, exacerbation or maintenance of the pain. (If psychological factors are present, they are not judged to have a major role in the onset, severity, exacerbation or maintenance of the pain.) The diagnostic code for the pain is selected based on the associated general medical condition, if one has been established (see Appendix G), or on the anatomical location of the pain if the underlying general medical condition is not yet clearly established – for example, low back (724.2), sciatic (724.3), pelvic (625.9), headache (784.0), facial (784.0), chest (786.50), joint (719.4), bone (733.90), abdominal (789.0), breast (611.71), renal (788.0), ear (388.70), eye (379.91), throat (784.1), tooth (525.9), and urinary (788.0).

Appendix 9.2. Assessment

Symptom severity scale

Did you have (the symptom) and how bad or severe was it on each of the following days

0	1	2	3	4	5	6	7	8	9	10

not at all   extreme

DATE_____ DAY OF THE WEEK   _____   /_____/

DATE_____ DAY OF THE WEEK   _____   /_____/

DATE_____ DAY OF THE WEEK   _____   /_____/

DATE_____ DAY OF THE WEEK   _____   /_____/

DATE_____ DAY OF THE WEEK   _____   /_____/

DATE_____ DAY OF THE WEEK   _____   /_____/

DATE_____ DAY OF THE WEEK   _____   /_____/

WEEKLY SYMPTOM SEVERITY/ACTIVITY DIARY

NAME _____ WEEK

BEGINNING _____

TIME	MONDAY	TUESDAY	WEDNESDAY	THURSDAY	FRIDAY	SATURDAY	SUNDAY
8–10							
10–11							
11–12							
12–1							
1–2							
2–3							
3–4							
4–5							
5–6							
7–8							
8–12							
Time I went to sleep							

Eating disorders: anorexia nervosa and bulimia nervosa

Hans-Christoph Steinhausen

Department of Child and Adolescent Psychiatry, University of Zurich, Switzerland

Introduction

Most typically, the two eating disorders anorexia nervosa (AN) and bulimia nervosa (BN) have their onset in adolescence and young adulthood. The two disorders in their typical manifestation are thus related to a period of major developmental change. The onset of anorexia nervosa, however, can be seen even before puberty and in rare cases, also at the age of 60 or older. For bulimia nervosa (BN) the typical age at onset is the period of transition from adolescence to young adulthood. It is present in a large proportion of patients in their 20s but also in their 30s and 40s. In a substantial number of cases, anorexia nervosa precedes bulimia nervosa and, in adolescence, the combination of AN with bulimic features is clinically more common than pure BN.

Thus child and adolescent psychiatrists have to deal with a large proportion of anorectic and a smaller proportion of bulimic patients, including a subgroup in which the features of the two disorders combine. Furthermore, the child and adolescent psychiatrist is confronted with a large group of subclinical cases of eating disorders. These cases are marked by a more or less pronounced pattern of dietary attempts with some of them qualifying for the diagnosis of an atypical eating disorder or eating disorder not otherwise specified (EDNOS).

A third category of eating disorders, namely binge eating disorder, is appearing more and more on the map of clinical nosology. However, it has not yet been included in the ICD-10 or DSM-IV systems of classification and most studies so far have dealt with the phenomenon among adult patients.

A Clinician's Handbook of Child and Adolescent Psychiatry, ed. Christopher Gillberg, Richard Harrington and Hans-Christoph Steinhausen. Published by Cambridge University Press.

Table 10.1. Diagnostic criteria of AN according to ICD-10

A. Body weight is maintained at least 15% below that expected (either lost or never achieved), or Quetelet's body-mass index (kg/m^2) is 17.5 or less. Pre-pubertal patients may show failure to make the expected weight gain during the period of growth.

B. The weight loss is self-induced by avoidance of 'fattening foods'. One or more of the following may also be present: self-induced vomiting; self-induced purging; excessive exercise; use of appetite suppressants and/or diuretics.

C. There is a body-image distortion in the form of a specific psychopathology whereby a dread of fatness persists as an intrusive, overvalued idea and the patient imposes a low weight threshold on himself or herself.

D. A widespread endocrine disorder involving the hypothalamic–pituitary–gonadal axis is manifest in women as amenorrhoea and in men as a loss of sexual interest and potency. (An apparent exception is the persistence of vaginal bleeds in anorexic women who are receiving replacement hormonal therapy, most commonly taken as a contraceptive pill.) There may also be elevated levels of growth hormone, raised levels of cortisol, changes in the peripheral metabolism of the thyroid hormone and abnormalities of insulin secretion.

E. If onset is pre-pubertal, the sequence of pubertal events is delayed or even arrested (growth ceases; in girls the breasts do not develop and there is a primary amenorrhoea; in boys the genitals remain juvenile). With recovery, puberty is often completed normally, but the menarche is late.

Atypical anorexia nervosa: This term should be used for those individuals in which one or more of the key features of anorexia nervosa, such as amenorrhoea or significant weight loss, is absent, but who otherwise present a fairly typical clinical picture. Such people are usually encountered in psychiatric liaison services in general hospitals or in primary care. Patients who have all the key symptoms but to only a mild degree may also be best described by this term. This term should not be used for eating disorders that resemble anorexia nervosa but that are due to known physical illness.

Anorexia nervosa

Definition and classification

The main features of AN are:
- a self-induced significant weight loss which is due to
- a weight-phobic psychopathology and accompanied by
- a widespread endocrine disorder with amenorrhoea as the leading symptom and
- a marked body-image distortion. These symptoms are reflected by both the ICD-10 and the DSM-IV-criteria (see Tables 10.1 and 10.2).

The two major classification systems, ICD-10 and DSM-IV, share some similarities with regard to defining criteria of anorexia nervosa. These pertain to the criteria of weight loss, body-image distortion, amenorrhoea and the so-called weight phobia. The two systems are different, however, to some extent with regard to the definition of these criteria. Whereas the ICD-10 makes use of Quetelets's Body Mass Index

Table 10.2. Diagnostic criteria of AN according to DSM-IV

A. Refusal to maintain body weight at or above minimally normal weight for age and height (e.g. weight loss leading to maintenance of body weight less than 85% of that expected, or failure to make expected weight gain during period of growth, leading to body weight less than 85% of that expected).

B. Intense fear of gaining weight or becoming fat, even though underweight.

C. Disturbance in the way in which one's body weight or shape is experienced, undue influence of body weight or shape on self-evaluation, or denial of the seriousness of the current low body weight.

D. In postmenarchal females, amenorrhoea, i.e. the absence of at least three consecutive menstrual cycles. (A woman is considered to have amenorrhoea if her periods occur only following hormone, e.g. oestrogen, administration.)

Specify type:

Restricting type: during the current episode of anorexia nervosa, the person has not regularly engaged in binge eating or purging behaviour (i.e. self-induced vomiting or the misuse of laxative, diuretics, or enemas)

Binge eating/purging type: during the current episode of anorexia nervosa, the person has engaged regularly in binge eating or purging behaviour (i.e. self-induced vomiting or the misuse of laxatives, diuretics or enemas)

(BMI) for the definition of weight loss and therefore considers height as well, DSM-IV uses an absolute weight threshold of 85 per cent of expected weight loss. Both classification systems consider the special situation of pre-pubertal patients who fail to make the expected growth.

There are some advantages of the ICD-10 scheme as compared with those of the DSM-IV. It not only covers the criterion 'self-induced loss of weight' but also provides a clinically useful operational definition of this criterion and links the body-image distortion to the main theme of psychopathology, namely, fear of becoming fat, whereas these two aspects are listed separately among the DSM-IV criteria. In addition, the widespread endocrine disorder in anorexia nervosa is indicated clearly in the ICD-10 set of criteria, whereas the DSM-IV refers only to amenorrhoea, which is more difficult to assess in young patients due to the absence of menstruation in early puberty and the sometimes irregular course soon after menarche.

Finally, both ICD-10 and DSM-IV consider two different types, namely a restrictive type, which refers to patients who exclusively starve, and a binge eating/purging type, which refers to patients who binge-eat and practise self-induced vomiting or misuse laxative, diuretics or enemas. This distinction is meaningful clinically, because bulimic features in anorexia nervosa clearly warrant differential treatment efforts.

In addition to these two major subtypes there are atypical cases of anorexia nervosa that do not fulfil the entire sets of criteria listed in the two major systems of classification. These atypical cases may be marked by an absence of amenorrhoea or significant weight loss or key symptoms that are present only to a mild degree.

Epidemiology

Prevalence and incidence rates

Based on an analysis of a large series of community surveys that were conducted between the late 1970s and the early 1990s, the median prevalence rate for AN was calculated as being 0.13 per 100 females in the age range of 15 to 20 years. However, various more recent community studies indicate that the true prevalence rates are higher, i.e. within the range of 0.2 to 1.3 and that they are specifically higher for adolescents. As a gross estimate, one can expect that less than 1 per cent of adolescent girls in the community suffer from AN.

There is conflicting evidence that incidence rates really have increased in the late twentieth century. An integrative review of the various studies found no increased risk of AN among teenagers, while a near threefold increase was observed among women in their 20s and 30s.

Sex ratios and ethnicity

With a rate of 8:1–40:1, females are predominantly affected by anorexia nervosa. AN is rarely observed among Africans and the Chinese population but it is quite common in Japan.

Implications for clinical practice

During the teenage years, fewer or around one in 100 females in the western world are affected by AN, whereas a considerably higher proportion of adolescent girls experiment with dieting without progressing to the full clinical picture of AN. Boys rarely are affected.

Clinical picture

Main features and symptoms

The core psychopathological feature of anorexia nervosa is the fear of becoming fat or weight phobia, implying that the patient is deeply convinced that the body is too large. Usually, this pursuit of thinness may persist even at times when the patient is extremely emaciated. In the beginning, the patient starts dieting because of concern that she/he is overweight, as measured by the standards of the peer culture. Or perhaps the patient is indeed slightly overweight and is teased by somebody from the family or peer group. This feeling of being overweight may be related to the whole body or to particular parts, such as the thighs or buttocks.

Typically, the diet starts with a reduction of sweets and high-calorific, carbohydrate-rich foods. Weeks or even months may pass before this dieting behaviour is noticed by others. Meanwhile, the patient may have lost control over dieting and the resulting weight loss. Usually, the adolescent anorectic does not recognize the abnormal nature of her/his behaviour and denies the illness. Indeed, the patient feels better being thin and does not seek any help, whereas the parents are most concerned and feel helpless when confronted with the patient's powerful behaviour. This distorted drive for thinness is associated with a disturbance in body image. Despite being emaciated, the patient does not perceive and consider herself or himself thin and also does not accurately identify internal sensations such as hunger, satiety or affective states.

Dieting continues and may be accompanied by further efforts to reduce weight including rigorous exercise, abuse of laxatives or diuretics and vomiting. The purging and vomiting behaviour may progress to binge eating, in which the patient consumes enormous amounts of food within a very short period of time. This bulimic behaviour is followed by either a restrictive period of fasting for several days or else vomiting to prevent weight gain. However, bulimic symptoms within the spectrum of anorexia nervosa, are rather infrequent during adolescence and more frequent among adults.

There are further psychopathological symptoms that are shared with other psychiatric disorders. These include poor self-esteem, a highly restricted realm of interests and cognitions that deal with almost nothing besides food and weight, and the loss of social contacts. Many of these psychopathological features, which also include depressive symptoms like irritability, mood swings and insomnia, are effects of starvation. Furthermore, many patients manifest obsessional behaviour, including compulsive behaviour and obsessive thinking about foods. This pertains not only to peculiar eating habits, for example, eating rituals, but also to other areas such as exercising and food and non-food-related hoarding. Co-morbid obsessive-compulsive disorders are quite frequent.

In addition to these psychopathological symptoms, AN is marked by a number of very specific physical characteristics. Anorectic patients apparently are emaciated and show effects of down-regulation of the autonomic nervous system, indicated by bradycardia, hypotension and hypothermia. Thus complications may arise as a consequence of the effects of the eating disorder on virtually every organ system and deserve careful assessment (see assessment).

The manifestation of AN before menarche is rare. However, the clinical features of the prepubertal cases are essentially similar. Other types of closely related food refusal, selective eating and appetite loss have to be distinguished from anorexia nervosa. Weight loss in these very young patients arrests the process of puberty and interferes with growth in stature and breast development; early diagnosis and competent treatment are vitally important for the child's development.

AN is a rare phenomenon in males, although it may also be underdiagnosed. The combination of prepubertal onset and male sex is extremely rare. Clinically, the illness is strikingly similar in the two sexes. Male patients may show atypical gender role behaviour, more grave symptomatology and poor prognosis.

Differential diagnosis and co-morbidity

Both medical illnesses and psychiatric disorders have to be considered for differential diagnosis. Medical illnesses include tuberculosis, acquired immune deficiency disease, primary endocrine disturbances such as anterior pituitary insufficiency, hyperthyroidism, diabetes mellitus, inflammatory bowel disease, hypothalamic tumours and various malignancies. Weight loss occurs in all of these conditions, whereas the psychological characteristics of anorexia nervosa are lacking. Various drugs can also lead to weight loss and poor appetite.

Other psychiatric disorders have to be considered for both differential diagnosis and as a co-morbid disorder. The very common manifestation of depression in AN is, at least partially, the result of the effects of starvation rather than a true coexistence of two disorders. Similarly, obsessive-compulsive behaviour and obsessional thinking about food in general is a common psychopathological feature in anorexia nervosa, rather than a differential diagnosis or a co-morbid disorder. However, in some cases there is a full-blown clinical picture of obsessive-compulsive disorders (OCD) that goes beyond the obsessive-compulsive component of food and weight concern and deserves special consideration, both in assessment and treatment (see Chapter 6).

Likewise, the distorted drive for thinness resulting from the fear of becoming fat usually is easy to distinguish from phobias and anxiety disorder. However, the full clinical syndromes of anxiety disorders also can co-exist with AN in individual patients. Furthermore, personality disorders can also be observed as a co-morbid condition in a substantial number of patients. Empathy disorders in particular (including Asperger syndrome and other autistic-like conditions) have been observed. In contrast, substance abuse disorders only rarely co-exist with anorexia nervosa.

All these distinctions predominantly reflect the first manifestation of AN. However, the situation may change over time with the more chronic patients who frequently show co-morbidity of various kinds.

Diagnostic instruments

In addition to the clinical interview, both structured interview schedules and various self-report questionnaires can be used in practice. Recommended structured interviews and questionnaires are collected in Table 10.3 and in Appendix 10.1.

Table 10.3. Overview of structured interviews and self-report questionnaires for the assessment of eating disorder

Name of the instrument	Authors	Source
Interviews		
• Eating disorder examination (EDE)	Fairburn, C. G., Cooper, Z.	Oxford University Department of Psychiatry Warneford Hospital, Oxford OX3 7JX, UK
• EDE-children's version (EDE-C)	Bryant-Waugh, R. J. *et al.*	*Int. J. Eating Disorder*, **19**, 391–407, 1996
• Structured interview for anorexia and bulimic disorder (SIAB)	Fichter, M. *et al.*	*Int. J. Eating Disorder*, **24**, *Disorder*, **24**, 227–49, 1998
• Clinical eating disorders rating instrument (CEDRI)	Palmer, R. *et al.*	*European Eating Disorder Review*, **4**, 149–56, 1996
Questionnaires		
• Eating attitude test (EAT)	Garner, D. M.	*Psychological Medicine*, **9**, 273–9, 1979 (see Appendix 10.1)
• Eating disorder inventory (EDI-2)	Garner, D. M.	Psychological Assessment Resources, Inc., PO Box 998, Odessa, FL 33556, USA
• Bulimia test (BULIT)	Smith, M. C., Thelen, M. H.	*J. Consult. Clin. Psychol.*, **52**, 863–72, 1984
• BITE	Henderson, M., Freeman, C. P. L.	*Br. J. Psychiatry*, **150**, 18–24, 1987
• Body-image questionnaire	Steinhausen, H.-C.	*Int'l. J. Eating Disorders*, **12**, 83–91, 1992 (see Appendix 10.2)
Observation scales		
• Anorexia behaviour scale (ABS) Anorectic behaviour observation scale (ABOS)	Slade, P. Vandereycken, W.	*Br. J. Psychiatry*, **122**, 83–5, *Acta Psychiatr. Scand.* **85**, 163–66, 1992 (see Appendix 10.3)

Questionnaires supplement the assessment of psychopathology of a patient with an eating disorder. They should, however, be used with great care as regards the delineation of cut-off scores for clinical cases and the transcultural validity of some of the scales in the adolescent age range. There are rarely any norms so that most of the self-report questionnaires may only help with so-called ipsative measurements, i.e. a comparison of the score of an individual patient across time including the evaluation of treatment effects.

The concept of body image distortions contains two different elements, namely, attitudinal dissatisfactions and perceptual size-estimation inaccuracies. Whereas the assessment of the latter needs relatively expensive techniques and has produced limited effect sizes in controlled studies, the former can be assessed by either questionnaire or self-ideal discrepancy measures. An example is given in Table 10.3 and in the Appendix. These attitudinal measures provide further insight into the specific psychopathology of AN and contribute to the evaluation of change and treatment of the individual patient suffering from AN.

Questionnaires and structured assessment schemes for other co-morbid psychiatric conditions should also be included in the clinical assessment procedures. Examples include the various self-report questionnaires for the assessment of depression (see Chapter 4), anxiety (see Chapter 5) or obsessive-compulsive disorder (see Chapter 6).

Assessment

As with other disorders, anorexia nervosa requires a thorough psychiatric assessment of the history, development of symptoms, psychopathological features and family functioning.

- The behavioural symptoms of both anorectic and bulimic features require a specific focus because of the frequent overlap of the two syndromes. Special emphasis should be placed on issues concerning food intake and eating behaviour, including thoughts and attitudes towards eating and weight.
- Furthermore, the events and emotional states preceding food refusal or binge/purge episodes have to be analysed. Additionally, the assessment should inquire about any attempts the patient might have made to alter eating behaviours.
- National percentile charts appropriate for age and sex should be used for measuring body weight and the Body Mass Index. This is mandatory because the BMI criterion of 17.5 for AN according to ICD-10 is inappropriate for prepubertal and most of the adolescent patients. Large parts of the normal population in the age groups fall under this criteria. The third (or fifth) percentile should be used for the definition of an abnormal BMI. Appendix 10.4 provides percentile charts that are based on a large German population.
- In addition to the defining criteria, significant other clinical symptoms (e.g. features of anxiety depression, obsessive compulsive disorder) should also be addressed.
- Due to the variety of potential medical complications (see Table 10.4), a careful physical assessment and continuous medical supervision, preferably by an experienced specialist of paediatrics or internal medicine, is mandatory.
- The physical examination should also include a list of laboratory investigations, as shown in Table 10.5. There are a number of routine investigations that should be performed with each patient suffering from an eating disorder. Further tests

Table 10.4. Medical complication of the eating disorders

Cardiovascular
- Hypo-tension, bradycardia, prolonged QT interval, arrhythmia
- Decreased heart size
- Attenuated response to exercise
- Myocardial toxicity from emetine
- Pericardial effusion
- Superior mesenteric artery syndrome

Metabolic
- Hypothermia and dehydration
- Electrolyte disturbances, (hypokalaemia, hypomagnesaemia, hypocalcaemia, and hypophosphataemia)
- Hypercholesterolaemia and raised serum carotene
- Hypoglycaemia and raised liver enzymes

Gastroenterological
- Swollen salivary glands, dental caries, and erosion of enamel (with vomiting)
- Delayed gastric emptying, severe constipation and bowel obstruction
- Irritable bowel syndrome, melanosis coli (from laxative misuse)
- Decreased lipase, lactose

Hematological
- Anemia: normochromic, normocytic, or iron deficiency
- Leucopenia, thrombocytopenia
- Hypocellular bone marrow
- Low plasma proteins

Neurological
- Pseudo-atrophy of brain (on MRI or CT scan)
- Abnormal EEG and seizures
- Peripheral neuritis
- Nerve compressions
- Impaired autonomic activity

Endocrine
- Low gonadotropins, oestrogens, testosterone
- Sick euthyroid syndrome
- Raised cortisol and positive dexamethasone suppression test
- Raised growth hormone

Renal
- Pre-renal azotaemia
- Partial diabetes insipidus
- Acute and chronic renal failure

Immunological
- Bacterial infections (staphylococcal lung abscess and tuberculosis)

Musculoskeletal
- Cramps, tetany, muscle weakness
- Osteopenia, stress fractures

are indicated only for particular patients. Finally some laboratory investigations are of academic interest with expected findings only.

- Because of the involvement of the family, both as a victim and perhaps also as an architect, family functioning requires further interviewing and testing.
- As with other child and adolescent psychiatric disorder, all findings of the assessment should be integrated into the multiaxial classification system (MAS) as recommended by the WHO. Thus, diagnoses including co-morbid disorders on axis I should be supplemented by developmental disorders on axis II intelligence

Table 10.5. Laboratory investigations in the eating disorder

Routine
- Full electrolyte profile, including potassium, magnesium, calcium, and phosphates
- Glucose (random)
- Full blood count and ESR (severe sepsis may develop without pyrexia or leukocytosis)
- Total protein, albumin
- Liver function
- Renal function
- Electrocardiogram
- Chest radiograph

Special Indications
- Further hematological studies, iron, folate, and vitamin B12
- Thiamine and other vitamins
- Bone densitometry (for all with a history of emaciation and amenorrhoea of >1 year)
- Abdominal radiographs (for severe bloating)
- Total bowel transit time (for persistent severe constipation)
- Oesophageal sphincter pressure studies (for reflux)
- Lactose deficiency tests (for dairy intolerance)
- Urine and blood osmolality
- Total body nitrogen

Of academic interest

- LH, FSH	*Low (almost invariable)*
- Oestrogens, testosterone	*Low (almost invariable)*
- Cortisol	*Raised (almost invariable)*
- Thyroid function	*Sick euthyroid (likely)*
- Dexamethasone suppression test	*Positive (likely)*
- Amylase	*Raised with vomiting*
- Brain computed tomography /magnetic resonance imaging	*Pseudoatrophy (likely)*

on axis III, physical disorders on axis IV, evaluation of psychosocial circumstances on axis V and global functioning on axis VI.

Aetiology

The causes of AN are complex and not yet well understood. Various theories converge by emphasizing the multifactorial origin coupled with multiple determinants and risk factors and their interaction within a developmental framework. Thus, a complex model has to consider the following predispositions and determinants: individual, familial, sociocultural, biological factors and precipitating events.

Individual factors

There is a strong developmental basis in AN, which is most likely to manifest in adolescence because of the convergence of physical changes and psychosocial challenges with which the adolescent must cope. The increase in body fat, which is more pronounced in adolescent girls than in boys, is frequently associated with increased concern about weight and efforts to control it. Dieting behaviour emerges as the body develops, and as it changes in physical appearance, bodily feelings and reproductive status requires reorganization and transformation of the body image.

While there is a relatively large proportion of female teenagers who engage in dieting, there is also clearly a discontinuity from normal dieting to clinical eating disorders. Certainly, dieting is an important trigger and precondition for eating disorders in susceptible individuals only and there must be further risk factors.

These other risk factors include disturbances of self-perception of body size and of internal affective and visceral states, i.e. poor body image and poor interoceptive awareness. In addition, premorbid obesity may expose the adolescent to humiliation and force her/him to use dieting and other weight-reducing measures.

When taking the clinical history of AN patients, one often finds a premorbid personality pattern of compliance, perfectionism and dependence. Typically, these children present few if any educational problems prior to the onset of the eating disorder. Early eating and digestive problems in childhood may also be present. There is little evidence that psychosexual factors are involved in the causation of eating disorders.

Familial factors

Although the typical AN family does not exist, there is a significant amount of communication and interaction dysfunction in many families with anorectic patients that, however, may not act specifically in the development of eating disorders but rather contributes only indirectly to the vulnerability of developing an eating disorder.

In addition, there are further family risk factors that may play a role in the multi-factorial determination of the eating disorders. These include the higher incidence of weight problems and eating disorders in the family, and the high incidence of physical illness, affective disorders, obsessive-compulsive disorders and alcoholism in the relatives. Furthermore, the adolescent's perceptions of direct pressure from their parents to diet represents a risk factor for the initiation of dieting among adolescent girls.

Sociocultural factors

There is some evidence that sociocultural factors also have to be considered in the aetiology of AN. These factors include the extremely uneven sex distribution, the typical adolescent age of onset and the association of anorexia nervosa to western lifestyle and cultural values. It is assumed that the pressure in western societies to achieve, the importance of physical attractiveness, and the emphasis on slimness and dieting in women all may help contribute to increased risk of the development of eating disorders.

As a result, TV and magazine models and peers' weight-related pressures pertaining to weight concerns have a well-documented effect on adolescent girls. Furthermore, ballet dancers, athletes and modelling students form particular risk groups. It is still unclear whether participation in these activities or sports causes the eating disorder or whether certain individuals with eating problems are drawn to these activities.

Biological factors

Once malnutrition and starvation have started, significant alterations occur in almost all biological domains including the various endocrine systems, the cholinergic, noradrenergic and serotonergic systems, the regulation of immune functions and endogenous opioid activity. Weight loss and starvation lead to a change of the usual mechanisms for the release and inhibition of various regulators of eating behaviour and a new set of regulating mechanisms with many of the pathophysiological alterations serving to sustain the disorder. Furthermore, a small number of genetic studies only allow the conclusion that there may be genetically transmitted dispositional traits in AN.

Precipitating events

As in many other psychiatric disorders, there may be significant life events that precede the manifestation of anorexia nervosa. Frequently, they include separation and loss, disruptions of family homeostasis, new environmental demands, direct threat of loss of self-esteem and, in a small number of patients, physical illness. These events threaten the patients' sense of worth and control over the world, increase the preoccupation with the body, and contribute to the initiation of weight reducing measures.

Development and maintenance of the disorders

Following a general model of the aetiology of almost all psychiatric disorders, it is the interaction between the individual vulnerability to particular risk factors and the operation of protective factors that decide on the development and maintenance of AN. Based on certain hypothetical biological predispositions (e.g. genetic vulnerability), the various individual risk factors develop within the environment of family and culture and may serve as behavioural precursors of the disorder. They probably increase the risk of the development of an eating disorder without making it inevitable.

There is clear evidence that dieting is the most important single factor that precipitates the onset of both anorexia and bulimia nervosa. However, dieting is not yet the early stage of the developing disorder and research still has to show which factors have to be present in order to explain the transition from dieting to frank disorder. Whereas the disorder is transient in certain patients, AN becomes chronic in a considerable number of patients.

The maintenance of the disorder is due to the intensified preoccupation with food, the negative self-concepts and mental state, the reduction of interests and the increased social isolation. In addition, vomiting is another powerful sustaining factor, and delayed gastric emptying and chronic constipation lend the sensation of fullness after meals and serves to prolong dieting.

In addition to these processes there are also certain cognitive factors that continue the chain of detrimental factors. They include positive self-reinforcement resulting from weight loss or phobic avoidance of weight gain and/or personality features such as obsessiveness, the generally restricted ability to cope with stress and the level of impulse control. Furthermore, unresolved predisposing factors from the patient's family or her own biography may also add to chronicity, and secondary gain in terms of receiving considerable attention from the environment is another powerful perpetuating factor.

Finally, unfortunately there are also iatrogenic factors that are responsible for the perpetuation of the illness. These may be characterized by two extremes, namely either rapid weight gain programmes that neglect both provisions for instituting external controls for the patient and attention to other psychosocial issues, or the complete failure to recognize the necessity of weight gain to counteract the effects of starvation.

Treatment

Clinical management and treatment setting

The treatment of AN requires skilled experts and the availability of various treatment modalities. After comprehensive assessment, one has to decide whether a given patient should be an in-patient or outpatient. This decision should be based predominantly on indications as described in Table 10.6. From this table, it is clear that patients with a brief duration of AN and without any major complications are suited for outpatient treatment in the beginning.

However, the patient with delayed referral for assessment and treatment, limited insight into the disorder, insufficient motivation for treatment and a highly

Table 10.6. Treatment setting for AN

Prerequisites for outpatient treatment
- Short duration of the disorder
- No purging or vomiting
- No severe emaciation
- Co-operative family
- No denial of the illness / co-operative patient
- Combination of nutritional counselling and psychotherapy

Indications for inpatient treatment
- Severe emaciation or precipitous loss of weight
- Medical complications
- Depressed mood and/or suicidal thought or intents
- Discouraged family
- Lack of appropriate outpatient facilities

Advantages of inpatient treatment
- Fostering of an otherwise fragile treatment alliance
- Greater awareness of complications
- Direct modification of disturbed eating behaviour
- Multimodal treatment approach

distressed family usually deserves inpatient treatment by a specialized, expert clinical team. Clinical criteria that warrant hospitalization are also outlined in Table 10.6.

Certainly, inpatient treatment has a number of specific advantages in these situations of the more chronic patient due to:
- a higher degree of control and consistency of treatment,
- fostering of the treatment alliance,
- greater awareness of medical complications,
- the availability of various experts in order to provide a multimodal intervention
- and a removal of food and eating-related conflicts from the family.

Inpatient treatment predominantly aims at medical and nutritional stabilization and the initiation of a psychotherapeutic process that should be continued by subsequent outpatient psychotherapy. Inpatient treatment should preferably take place in an adolescent psychiatric ward rather than in a paediatric or medical clinic in order to meet the psychological needs of the patient.

Special units or centres for eating disorders may provide special expertise but do not have to form the basis for service. With skilful training of the staff, adolescent psychiatric wards with different problems and patients can also provide adequate treatment for AN.

Efficient interventions in AN have to follow the principle of multimodal treatment apart from the treatment setting. The various components include psychological interventions, diet, and psycho-educational measures. In a few cases only pharmacotherapy may be considered.

Psychological interventions

Various types of psychotherapy should be provided to the patient suffering from AN. Individual psychotherapy, behavioural interventions, and family therapy have to be considered.

- First, there is good clinical evidence that supportive psychotherapy is an important component in multidimensional treatment strategies for anorectic patients. The provision of empathetic support, insight into conflicts and problems, and the assistance in problem solving is essential for the patient in order to readjust and to prevent relapses. For in-patients, psychotherapy commences during hospitalization and continues after discharge. However, psychotherapy is complicated in many patients due to insufficient motivation, severe emaciation and chronicity, co-morbid disorders, or the patient's very young age.
- In addition, behavioural interventions using operant conditions are an effective short-term method of weight restoration and modification of eating behaviour. Because of their well-documented effects, they should be included in the multimodal inpatient treatment approach.

  Operant conditioning measures use recreational activities, visiting privileges, or freedom of movement within or outside the ward as reinforcers for the target behaviour of normal eating and weight increase. In a stepwise procedure the patient receives more privileges as soon as the targets are met.

  Social skill training programmes may also be used in some patients. Cognitive methods aim at changing dysfunctional beliefs related to food and weight and include the identification and restructuring of these and other dysfunctional thought schemes and thinking patterns. The efficacy of cognitive-behavioural principles in anorectic patients has not been established, in contrast to bulimic patients.
- Similarly, there is also clear empirical evidence that family therapy is beneficial to adolescent anorectic patients with a relatively short history of their illness. Family counselling is as effective as conjoint family therapy. However, an uncritical use of family therapy as the single route to success should be avoided and the treating clinician should be aware of indications and contraindications. Among the latter are chronicity of the disorder, patients with delayed psychosocial development, single-parent families, broken homes, severe psychopathology in one or both parents, physical or sexual abuse of the patient by a parent, highly negative family interactions, or failure of previous family therapeutic attempts.

Diet

- Clearly, weight restoration is the major goal of treatment. The minimum target weight should be specified at the onset of treatment and should be set within 10 per cent or at the 25th percentile of the weight appropriate for age and height. The target weight should be one that the patient can maintain without continued dieting, and it should be approached by a gradual but steady gain averaging about 0.2 kg/day.
- The supervision of the diet should be performed by an experienced dietician with the patient being continuously educated as to the principles of nutrition and healthy diets.
- Tube feeding or parenteral hyperalimentation are very rarely necessary and, because of their psychological and physiological side effects, should be used only as a last resort.

Psycho-educational measures

- During in-patient treatment, one of the cornerstones of clinical management of anorexia nervosa is good nursing. There is sufficient clinical evidence that a supportive and secure relationship with the nurse who is present during mealtimes and can encourage the patient to eat and to ventilate feelings that are related to eating is an essential element of successful interventions.
- Furthermore, counselling of various types is an important part of the multidimensional treatment approach. Nutritional counselling by a skilled dietitian should be combined with outpatient psychotherapy intervention and is also an integral part of any inpatient program in order to establish weight gain and maintenance. Exercise counselling helps the patient to overcome unhealthy exercise practices, to facilitate responsibility for the body, to challenge false beliefs by providing accurate information, and to return to as normal a lifestyle as possible.
- In addition to the individual patient, the family as well requires constant counselling by providing an explanation of the illness and the treatment programme, by encouraging participation in treatment activities, and by helping to bring about a readjustment of family interaction patterns. There is evidence from empirical research that family counselling is as effective as conjoint family therapy sessions.
- In the outpatient phase following hospitalization, individual counselling may also be provided by well-structured manuals relating to dieting and weight regulation.

Pharmacotherapy

In contrast to bulimia nervosa, there is little room for pharmacological intervention in AN. Based on the relatively few controlled trials, one has to conclude that no single drug is of clinically significant use in helping the patient overcome the symptoms of anorexia nervosa. However, pronounced features of depression, anxiety or

Table 10.7. Monitoring and evaluation of treatment in the eating disorders

Specific symptoms

- Weight curve based on percentile charts
- Normalization of eating based on behavioural observation
- Normalization of menstruation based on patient report
- Normalization of eating attitudes and behaviour based on patient questionnaires (e.g. EAT and/or EDI) or interview with patient/parents
- Normalization of body image

Further psychopathology reports

- Mood and feelings questionnaire (MFQ)
- Questionnaires dealing with depression and anxiety
- Children's Yale–Brown Obsessive Compulsive Scale (CY-BOCS)
- Child behaviour checklist (CBCL)
- Youth self-report (YSR)

General evaluation of treatment

- Goal attainment scaling
- Rating scales specific to type of intervention
- Clinical global improvement rating (CGI)
- Children's global assessment of functioning (CGAS)

obsessive-compulsive disorder may warrant antidepressant or anxiolytic treatment. In these instances, treatment with SSRIs is most promising.

Evaluation of treatment

Independent from the treatment setting, all kind of interventions need to be monitored continuously so that treatment of the individual patient can be evaluated. Sources of information include the various staff members or therapists, the patient and the family. Recommendations in addition to laboratory findings as shown in Table 10.5 are further outlined in Table 10.7. In order to conform with quality control expectations, the experienced clinician will use rather more than a few of these recommended measures and add specific documents according to the needs of the individual patient in treatment.

Outcome

Based on an analysis by the author of a total of 117 outcome studies on AN published in the twentieth century and covering the age at onset, a range of prepuberty, adolescence and adulthood, the following statements can be made.

- There is a significantly increased mortality rate in AN averaging around 5–6 per cent with starvation and suicide being the most frequent causes of death.

- Full recovery can only be expected in 45 per cent of the patients, whereas 33 per cent improve and 20 per cent develop a chronic course of the disorder. These figures represent the entire age range and are slightly better for adolescent patients.
- A large proportion of patients show other psychiatric disorders later during their life, i.e. anxiety disorders, affective disorders, obsessive-compulsive disorders, personality disorders and substance abuse disorders. Up to one-quarter of the patients show one of these disorders at follow-up. Thus, many of these patients require long-standing professional help and treatment.
- Approximately one-third does not accomplish employment and normal educational careers and only a minority enter marriage or a stable partnership. The few children of these patients are at an increased risk of malnutrition.
- Among the large list of prognostic factors which have been analysed, only a few are not identified controversially in empirical studies. Favourable prognostic factors include adolescent onset of the disorder, a short duration of symptoms prior to treatment, a good parent–child relationship, histrionic personality features and high socio-economic status. However, one has to keep in mind that these figures represent probabilities and that this list of prognostic factors is not suitable for a prediction of the course of the disorder in any given individual case.

Bulimia nervosa

Definition and classification

The diagnostic criteria of the ICD-10 and the DSM-IV are outlined in Tables 10.8 and 10.9. ICD-10 and DSM-IV are largely comparable with regard to the first two criteria. The DSM-IV criteria are more explicit by specifying a minimum average of 2-weekly episodes of binge eating and compensatory behaviours for at least 3 months. In addition, DSM-IV states that self-evaluation is influenced unduly by body shape and weight and that these disturbances do not exclusively occur in the presence of anorexia nervosa.

DSM-IV also introduces two subtypes, namely a purging type, designating patients who regularly engage in self-induced vomiting or the misuse of laxatives, diuretics or enemas, and a non-purging type. In analogy to AN, this distinction has some clinical relevance also for BN, whereas the validity of these two subtypes still awaits systematic studies.

Both ICD-10 and DSM-IV introduce the category of atypical bulimia nervosa for those cases in which one or more of the key features is absent. Most commonly, this applies to patients with normal or even excessive weight. Among these atypical cases, the DSM-IV also considers the category of binge eating disorder with recurrent

Table 10.8. Diagnostic criteria of BN according to ICD-10

For a definite diagnosis, all of the following are required:

A. There is a persistent preoccupation with eating and an irresistible craving for food; the patient succumbs to episodes of overeating in which large amounts of food are consumed in short periods of time.

B. The patient attempts to counteract the 'fattening' effects of food with one or more of the following: self-induced vomiting; purgative abuse; alternating periods of starvation; use of drugs such as appetite suppressants, thyroid preparations or diuretics. When bulimia occurs in diabetic patients, they may choose to neglect their insulin treatment.

C. The psychopathology consists of a morbid dread of fatness, and the patient sets herself or himself at a sharply defined weight threshold, well below the pre-morbid weight that constitutes the optimum or healthy weight in the opinion of the physician. There is often, but not always, a history of an earlier episode of anorexia nervosa, the interval between the two disorders ranging from a few months to several years. This earlier episode may have been expressed fully, or may have assumed a minor cryptic form with a moderate loss of weight and/or transient phase of amenorrhoea.

Atypical bulimia nervosa: This term should be used for those individuals in which one or more of the key features listed for bulimia nervosa is absent but who otherwise present a fairly typical clinical picture. Most commonly, this applies to people with normal or even excessive weight but with typical periods of overeating followed by vomiting or purging. Partial syndromes together with depressive symptoms are also not uncommon, but if the depressive symptoms justify a separate diagnosis of a depressive disorder, two diagnoses should be made.

Table 10.9. Diagnostic criteria of BN according to DSM-IV

A. Recurrent episodes of binge eating. An episode of binge eating is characterized by both of the following:
   (1) eating, in a discrete period of time (e.g. within any 2-hour period), an amount of food that is definitely larger than most people would eat during a similar period of time and under similar circumstances
   (2) a sense of lack of control over eating during the episode (e.g. a feeling that one cannot stop eating or control what or how much one is eating)

B. Recurrent inappropriate compensatory behaviour in order to prevent weight gain, such as self-induced vomiting; misuse of laxatives, diuretics, enemas or other medications; fasting; or excessive exercise.

C. The binge eating and inappropriate compensatory behaviours both occur, on average, at least twice a week for 3 months.

D. Self-evaluation is influenced unduly by body shape and weight.

E. The disturbance does not occur exclusively during episodes of anorexia nervosa.

Specific type:

Purging type: during the current episode of bulimia nervosa, the person has engaged regularly in self-induced vomiting or the misuse of laxative, diuretics or enemas

Non-purging type: during the current episode of bulimia nervosa, the person has used other inappropriate compensatory behaviours, such as fasting or excessive exercise, but has not regularly engaged in self-induced vomiting or the misuse of laxatives, diuretics or enemas episodes of binge eating in the absence of inappropriate compensatory behaviour characteristic of bulimia nervosa. However, the nosological validity of binge eating disorder and its potential relations to the other eating disorders in terms of continuities is yet unknown.

Epidemiology

Prevalence and incidence rates

Various community surveys converge in their findings that the complete clinical picture of BN may be found in about 1 per cent of adolescent and young adult women during their lifetimes. Thus, it is slightly more common than anorexia nervosa. However, individual symptoms such as binge eating have been found by far more frequently in various community studies of young females. The prevalence rate of BN in adolescents is lower than in adult females; it amounts to approximately 0.5 per cent.

The incidence rates for case detection by general practitioners in the UK was 12.2 per 100 000. It was almost three times higher than that of anorexia nervosa, and the recording of bulimia nervosa increased threefold from 1988 to 1993. Similarly, a sharp rise in incidence was observed in the USA from 1980 to 1983, with relatively constant rates thereafter. However, epidemiological studies conducted between 1980 and 1995 were partly unreliable and did not control for confounding co-morbid disorders. Changes in diagnostic and referral practices were likely to account for the increase in patients seen in specialized treatment centres. Thus, there is no clear empirical evidence for secular changes in the incidence of bulimia nervosa.

Sex ratio

As in AN, in BN females also greatly outnumber males. Although males have been less thoroughly examined in the few well-controlled studies, there is sufficient evidence that males are only seldom affected. The estimated rate is one male among ten females. Whereas the clinical symptoms and demographic features are similar in both sexes, disturbances of psychosexual development and gender identity as well as homosexuality may be observed more frequently in bulimic than in normal males.

Implications for clinical practice

BN is more common than AN in non-clinical populations so that one would expect to find both more adolescent and more adult patients with BM than with AN. The majority of bulimic patients are adults with a peak onset of the disorder around the age of 19 years. Analogous to anorexia nervosa, females by far outnumber males.

In contrast to epidemiological data of the adult population, bulimic patients are under-represented in clinical samples of eating disordered adolescent patients.

Clinical picture

Main features and symptoms

The eating pattern of the bulimic patient is highly typical and is characterized by the rapid consumption of a large amount of food. Estimates of the caloric intake of these eating binges range from 3000 to 20 000 calories. Patients often experience these binges as an altered state of consciousness in which they are out of control of their behaviour. The frequency of binges varies considerably among patients – from several times a day to less than once a week or fortnight – and binges can last from minutes to several hours. Very frequently, they are precipitated by feelings of anxiety, tension, boredom and loneliness. At least in the beginning, the binge itself brings temporary relief from negative mood states. However, the longer the binges continue, the more the patient experiences feelings of guilt, shame and anger.

In addition to binge eating, there are various accompanying or counteracting behaviours. Amongst these symptoms, self-induced vomiting is a very frequent but not a necessary symptom for diagnosis. Whereas not all bulimics are vomiters, most vomiters are probably bulimics. Binge eating usually precedes the vomiting. With increasing duration and severity of the disorder, patients do not require any mechanical device to induce vomiting but, rather, learn to vomit by reflex by contracting their abdominal and thoracic muscles. Other accompanying symptoms like purgative abuse of laxatives or other drugs are used less often than vomiting. However, most purgers also display vomiting.

There are further very specific psychopathological symptoms in BN. These patients are not only preoccupied with constant thoughts about weight, body size and food. The most frequently associated mental state is depression. Other personality characteristics include anxiety, emotional lability, strong needs for approval and external control, impulsiveness and compulsiveness.

With regard to physical characteristics, BN differs from AN. The most obvious sign of differentiation pertains to the fact that the majority of bulimic patients are of normal weight for their height. Menstrual irregularities occur frequently, although amenorrhoea is not as common among bulimics as it is among anorectics. There is a long list of medical complications associated with BN that is largely identical to AN, as shown in Table 10.4. Many of these complications are serious and are often overlooked. However, they may lead to the diagnosis in those patients who do not come into consultation because of bulimia but for other reasons. Thus, a careful physical examination of each patient suffering from bulimia nervosa is mandatory not only for general practitioners, but also for adolescent psychiatrists.

Although BN is rarely observed in males, the symptoms are similar in both sexes. However, disturbances of psychosexual development, gender identity and homosexuality may be observed more frequently than in healthy males, and sexual activity is more frequently inhibited in heterosexually orientated bulimic men than in healthy ones.

Differential diagnosis and co-morbidity

First, BN has to be differentiated from AN due to the absence of emaciation although fluctuation of body weight within normal levels is quite common. Furthermore, amenorrhoea is not as common among bulimics as it is among anorectic patients, whereas menstrual irregularities occur frequently.

The most frequent co-morbid psychiatric disorder is depression. Very frequently, depression results from the vicious cycle of bulimic symptoms and guilt feelings, and there is also a heightened risk of suicidality in these patients. Another quite frequently associated disorder is substance abuse. In a specific subgroup called multi-impulsive bulimia there is a combination of shoplifting, substance abuse and self-harm. Other personality disorders, including histrionic and borderline types, are quite common in BN.

Diagnostic instruments

The diagnostic interviews and questionnaires that were mentioned in the respective section on anorexia nervosa can also be used to assist examination of bulimic patients. There are further questionnaires that were designed specifically for bulimic patients.

Assessment

Due to the fact that many patients themselves do not report their symptoms, a large proportion of cases remain undetected. Some patients may be referred by general practitioners due to medical complications or even by a dentist because of the destruction of the patients' teeth due to constant vomiting.

- Consequently, the physical examination has to be very careful, taking the abnormalities of each organ system into account. The laboratory checks should follow the recommendations of Table 10.5 that were given in the respective section on anorexia nervosa. Thus, in adolescent psychiatric practice, the patient should be advised to consult a specialist in internal medicine.
- The psychiatric assessment should address the typical eating pattern with the frequency of binges, the amount of food consumed during these binges and the accompanying feelings of the patient. Furthermore, the counteracting behaviours of vomiting and purging need to be examined.

- The mental state assessment has to identify to what extent the patient is absorbed by thought about weight, body size and food, and whether or not obsessionality, feelings of depression and abnormal features of personality are present and whether a lack of impulse control or substance abuse may be complicating the disorder.
- Finally, social functioning of the patient should be assessed in order to find out to what extent the patient is socially isolated and withdrawn both within and outside of the family.
- As with other psychiatric disorders, the assessment should end with the delineation of diagnoses and functional states according to the multi-axial system (MAS) of classification on each of the six separate axes.

Aetiology

The model of aetiology of BN is very similar to the one outlined above for AN. It shares the same determinants and risk factors, namely individual, familial, socio-cultural and biological factors.

Empirical studies have addressed various risk factors and shown that early onset cases (at the age of 15 or below), in contrast to typical onset cases, show premorbid overweight and parental lack of care twice as often and that deliberate self-harm is also more common in the younger patients. Furthermore, the exposure to the risk factors of dieting and negative self-evaluation as well as certain parental problems including alcohol use disorder is substantially more common among patients with bulimia nervosa than among control subjects with other psychiatric disorders. Thus one has to conclude that bulimia nervosa is the result of exposure to general risk factors for psychiatric disorders and specific factors for dieting.

Certain life events involving disruption of family or social relationships or a threat to physical safety may play a role in precipitating the onset of the disorder and childhood sexual and physical abuse are also risk factors. The latter, however, are not present in the majority of cases, and are not specific to bulimia nervosa, but are rather risk factors for psychiatric disorders in general.

As shown in Fig. 10.1, the vicious cycle in bulimic patients is perhaps even more pronounced than in patients with anorexia nervosa. Due to suffering from low self-esteem and affective instability, these patients use their bulimic behaviour in order to secure emotional stability and conformity with external standards for weight and shape. However, the resulting feelings of fatigue, irritability and depression and the physical effects in terms of malnutrition, lead again to binge eating behaviour, which in turn induces affective instability.

There is also some limited support for the assumption that genetic factors of vulnerability are important in the aetiology of BN. Higher concordance rates for bulimia nervosa were found in monozygotic twins as compared with dizygotic

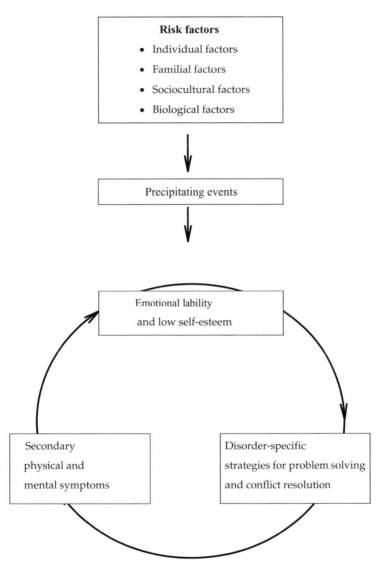

Fig. 10.1.   The aetiology of BN.

twins, and various twin modelling studies indicate that additive genes account for a large proportion of the variance of a lifetime diagnosis of bulimia nervosa and the symptoms of bingeing and vomiting. However, the genetic influences do interact with strong individual-specific environmental factors.

So far, the interpretations of the genetic findings vary among experts. Critical evaluations point to the inconsistencies of findings, with estimates of the heritability of liability to bulimia nervosa from 0 per cent to 83 per cent. These interpretations emphasize that a broad view on the aetiology of the eating disorders should be maintained. In contrast, genetic researchers underline the significant contributions of additive genetic effects and of unique environmental factors in liability to bulimia nervosa whereby the latter are considered to be less prominent than the former.

Treatment

Clinical management and treatment setting

Analogous to the treatment of AN, bulimic patients should also be treated using a multi-modal approach of intervention including psychological methods (i.e. individual and group psychotherapy, cognitive and behavioural treatment) and biological approaches such as medication and nutritional management. Self-help and support groups may offer further opportunities for long-term care and even self-care manuals for guided self-change have been shown to be efficacious.

Hospitalization may be recommended as a method for breaking through the vicious cycle of starvation, binge eating and vomiting. However, the vast majority of patients with BN can be treated on an outpatient basis or in a day clinic and initially inpatient treatment in BN is rarely required. However, hospitalization is indicated in cases in which there are serious medical problems, serious concurrent psychiatric disturbances that would warrant hospitalization in their own right, and unremitting severe symptoms that have not responded to adequate trials of outpatient treatment.

Independent of the treatment setting, individual or group approaches with bulimic patients depend on change motivation of the patient and the absence of complications like laxative or substance abuse, psychosis and suicidal or antisocial behaviour.

Psychological interventions

There are a variety of treatment strategies for BN including individual and group therapies. In contrast to AN, the choice of therapy may be guided to a greater extent by findings from controlled intervention studies.

- Among the individual therapies, cognitive-behavioural interventions have received the widest attention. They centre around the monitoring of eating, weight stimulus control, the provision of information and education and advice regarding eating behaviour. More specifically, cognitive therapeutic strategies aim at modifying dysfunctional thoughts, beliefs and values that perpetuate the eating problem.
- Cognitive behavioural techniques clearly reduce target behaviours and improve the accompanying psychopathology in adult BN patients. However, their application in younger adolescent patients has not been studied systematically.

- The relative efficacy of interpersonal and psychodynamic approaches is less well established, although a few initial studies with adult patients have produced some promising results. The potency of both individual and group therapy may be utilized for adolescent patients with eating disorders in as much as it offers an opportunity to discuss the social isolation in which the disorder takes place to address the irrational beliefs of the patient, to learn alternative ways of coping with conflicts and stress and to ventilate the patients' painful feelings.

Psycho-educational measures

- Although the majority of patients suffering from BN do not show pronounced weight pathologies, nutritional counselling including diary-keeping, self-monitoring of eating behaviour, meals and weight control is an important issue of treatment.
- Furthermore, social activity programmes may be indicated due to the progressing social isolation.
- In addition, job and career counselling is important because many of these older adolescents and young adults are not only confronted with this developmental task, but they fail to master it because of their increasingly handicapped state in which the illness absorbs almost their entire life.

Pharmacotherapy

- Various drugs have been tested in controlled trials. Clearly, the anti-depressants and particularly the SSRIs turned out to be the most promising agents. However, among the effective drugs, no particular anti-depressant is more effective than another. Furthermore, controlled studies have shown that the combination of anti-depressant medication and cognitive-behavioural therapy is not superior to cognitive-behaviour therapy alone.
- In clinical practice, the decision for the application of anti-depressants is restricted due to several facts. First, the effects of treatment are still insufficient because the majority of treated patients remains symptomatic at the termination of treatment. Secondly, the knowledge about matching patients to treatments by well-defined predictor variables is limited and, thirdly, the efficacy of anti-depressants is lower in adolescents than it is in adults.

Monitoring and evaluation of treatment

Unfortunately, both the medical and the psychiatric complications of bulimia nervosa contribute to chronic courses in a substantial number of patients. Continued medical and psychiatric care is therefore mandatory in this disorder. This should consist of regular physical examinations, including laboratory assessment as outlined above in Table 10.5 and many of the evaluation parameters that are documented in Table 10.7. Because of the typical age distribution, mainly adult psychiatrists and psychotherapists rather than adolescent psychiatrists will be involved in the follow-up care.

Outcome

The following statements may be delineated from the author's recent review of 24 follow-up studies of bulimia nervosa patients.

- The mean proportion of full recovery amounts to 47.5 per cent and thus is only slightly higher than for the anorexia nervosa patients. On average, 26 per cent of the patients improve and 26 per cent remain chronic cases at follow-up.
- Crude mortality rates amount to only less than 1 per cent on average. However, follow-up periods in BN patients have been significantly shorter than in AN patients.
- Furthermore, the average rate for other psychiatric disorders is 25 per cent for affective disorders, 15 per cent for substance abuse and 13 per cent for neurotic disorders consisting mainly of anxiety disorders and phobias.
- The study of prognostic factors has not resulted in any non-contradictory finding that could be used in terms of a probability measure.

SUGGESTED READING

P. J. V. Beumont, C. C. Beumont, S. W. Touyz & H. Williams, Nutritional counseling and supervised exercise. In Garner, D. M. & Garfinkel, P. E. (ed.) *Handbook of Treatment for Eating Disorders*, 2nd edn. (New York: Guilford Press, 1997), pp. 178–87.

P. J. V. Beumont, K. Lowinger & J. Russell, Medical assessment and the initial interview in the management of young patients with anorexia nervosa. In Steinhausen, H.-C. (ed.) *Eating Disorders in Adolescence* (Berlin/New York: Walter de Gruyter, 1995), pp. 221–46.

C. G. Fairburn & K. D. Brownell (ed.) *Eating Disorders and Obesity : A Comprehensive Handbook*, 2nd edn. (New York: Guilford Press, 2002).

D. M. Garner & P. E. Garfinkel, *Handbook of Treatment for Eating Disorders*. 2nd edn (New York: Guilford Press, 1997).

D. M. Heebink & K. A. Halmi, Psychopharmacology in adolescents with eating disorders. In Steinhausen, H.-C. (ed.) *Eating Disorders in Adolescence* (Berlin/New York: Walter de Gruyter, 1995), pp. 271–86.

B. Lask & R. Bryant-Waugh, *Childhood Onset Anorexia and Related Eating Disorders* (Hillsdale, New Jersey: Lawrence Erlbaum Associates, 1993).

D. E. Pawluck & K. M. Gorey, Secular trends in the incidence of anorexia nervosa: integrative review of population-based studies. *International Journal of Eating Disorders*, **23** (1998), 347–52.

G. F. M. Russell, Anorexia nervosa of early onset and its impact on puberty. In Cooper, P. J. & Stein, A. (ed.) *Feeding Problems and Eating Disorders in Children and Adolescents* (Chur [Switzerland]; Philadelphia: Harwood Academic Publishers, 1992), pp. 85–112.

U. H. Schmidt & J. L. Treasure, *Getting Better Bit(e) by Bit(e)*. (London: Lawrence Erlbaum Associates, 1993).

H.-C. Steinhausen (ed.), *Eating Disorders in Adolescence* (Berlin/New York: Walter de Gruyter, 1995).

H.-C. Steinhausen, Anorexia and bulimia nervosa. In Rutter, M. & Taylor, E. (eds.) *Child and Adolescent Psychiatry – Modern Approaches*. 4th edn. (Oxford: Blackwell Scientific Publications, 2002).

H.-C. Steinhausen (ed.), Eating disorders. In Steinhausen, H.-C. & Verhulst, F. (ed.) *Risks and Outcomes in Developmental Psychopathology* (Oxford: Oxford University Press, 1999), pp. 210–30.

S. W. Touyz, D. M. Garner & P. J. V. Beumont, The inpatient management of adolescent patients with anorexia nervosa. In Steinhausen, H.-C. (ed.) *Eating Disorders in Adolescence* (Berlin/New York: Walter de Gruyter, 1995), pp. 247–70.

W. Vandereycken, The place of family therapy in the treatment of eating disorders. In Steinhausen, H.-C. (ed.) *Eating Disorders in Adolescence* (Berlin/New York: Walter de Gruyter, 1995), pp. 287–97.

Appendix 10.1. Eating attitudes test (D. M. Garner and P. E. Garfinkel)

Please place an (X) under the column which applies best to each of numbered statements. All of the results will be strictly confidential. Most of the questions directly relate to food or eating, although other types of questions have been included. Please answer each question carefully. Thank you.

	Always	Very often	Often	Sometimes	Rarely	Never
1. Like eating with other people.	( )	( )	( )	( )	( )	(X)
2. Prepare foods for others but do not eat what I cook.	(X)	( )	( )	( )	( )	( )
3. Become anxious prior to eating.	(X)	( )	( )	( )	( )	( )
4. Am terrified about being overweight.	(X)	( )	( )	( )	( )	( )
5. Avoid eating when I am hungry.	(X)	( )	( )	( )	( )	( )
6. Find myself preoccupied with food.	(X)	( )	( )	( )	( )	( )
7. Have gone on eating binges where I feel that I may not be able to stop.	(X)	( )	( )	( )	( )	( )
8. Cut my food into small pieces.	(X)	( )	( )	( )	( )	( )
9. Am aware of the calorie content of foods that I eat.	(X)	( )	( )	( )	( )	( )
10. Particularly avoid food with a high carbohydrate content (e.g. bread, potatoes, rice. etc.).	(X)	( )	( )	( )	( )	( )
11. Feel bloated after meals.	(X)	( )	( )	( )	( )	( )
12. Feel that others would prefer if I ate more.	(X)	( )	( )	( )	( )	( )
13. Vomit after I have eaten.	(X)	( )	( )	( )	( )	( )
14. Feel extremely guilty after eating.	(X)	( )	( )	( )	( )	( )
15. Am preoccupied with a desire to be thinner.	(X)	( )	( )	( )	( )	( )
16. Exercise strenuously to burn off calories.	(X)	( )	( )	( )	( )	( )
17. Weigh myself several times a day.	(X)	( )	( )	( )	( )	( )
18. Like my clothes to fit tightly.	( )	( )	( )	( )	( )	(X)
19. Enjoy eating meat.	( )	( )	( )	( )	( )	(X)
20. Wake up early in the morning.	(X)	( )	( )	( )	( )	( )
21. Eat the same foods day after day.	(X)	( )	( )	( )	( )	( )
22. Think about burning up calories when I exercise.	(X)	( )	( )	( )	( )	( )
23. Have regular menstrual periods.	( )	( )	( )	( )	( )	(X)
24. Other people think that I am too thin.	(X)	( )	( )	( )	( )	( )
25. Am preoccupied with the thought of having fat on my body.	(X)	( )	( )	( )	( )	( )
26. Take longer than others to eat my meals.	(X)	( )	( )	( )	( )	( )
27. Enjoy eating at restaurants.	( )	( )	( )	( )	( )	(X)
28. Take laxatives.	(X)	( )	( )	( )	( )	( )
29. Avoid foods with sugar in them.	(X)	( )	( )	( )	( )	( )
30. Eat diet foods.	(X)	( )	( )	( )	( )	( )
31. Feel that food controls my life.	(X)	( )	( )	( )	( )	( )
32. Display self-control around food.	(X)	( )	( )	( )	( )	( )
33. Feel that others pressure me to eat.	(X)	( )	( )	( )	( )	( )
34. Give too much time and thought to food.	(X)	( )	( )	( )	( )	( )
35. Suffer from constipation.	(X)	( )	( )	( )	( )	( )
36. Feel uncomfortable after eating sweets.	(X)	( )	( )	( )	( )	( )
37. Engage in dieting behaviour.	(X)	( )	( )	( )	( )	( )
38. Like my stomach to be empty.	(X)	( )	( )	( )	( )	( )
39. Enjoy trying new rich foods.	(X)	( )	( )	( )	( )	( )
40. Have the impulse to vomit after meals.	(X)	( )	( )	( )	( )	( )

† The 'X' represents the most 'symptomatic' response and would receive a score of 3 points.

Note: The scoring procedures are described in the following publications: Garner *et al*, *Psychological Medicine*, **9**, 273–9, 1979 and *Psychological Medicine*, **12**, 871–8, 1982.

Appendix 10.2. Body-image questionnaire (NIMH Collaborative Study Group)

Instructions

Your task is to make a number of judgements in relation to your body right now.

Please, place a tick at the appropriate point in terms of whether you liked, disliked, or where in-between you judged your feeling to be about your body right now.

Please remember to place your tick directly <u>on</u> one of the lines, |✓| rather than in the space between two lines.

Thank you very much.

MY BODY RIGHT NOW

(Like)	1 2 3 4 5 6 7	(Dislike)
1. Fat		Thin
2. Beautiful		Ugly
3. Desirable		Undesirable
4. Dirty		Clean
5. Soft		Hard
6. Proportioned		Unproportioned
7. Light		Heavy
8. Powerful		Weak
9. Pleasant		Unpleasant
10. Fragile		Massive
11. Attractive		Repulsive
12. Large		Small
13. Inactive		Active
14. Firm		Flabby
15. Bad		Good
16. Uncomfortable		Comfortable

Note: The scoring procedures are described in the following publication: Steinhausen *et al.*, *International Journal of Eating Disorder*, **12**, 83–91, 1992.

There are two dimensions: attractiveness and massiveness.

These two scales are composed of the following items (* inverted scoring):

Attractiveness: *2, *3, *6, *9, 13, 15, 16

Massiveness: *1, *4, *5, 7, *8, 10, 14

Appendix 10.3. Anorectic Behaviour Observation Scale (ABOS) for parents or spouse (W.Vandereycken)

Name of patient. . . . . Date: . . . .

Completed by: ○ both parents together

     ○ mother

     ○ father

     ○ spouse

     ○ someone else (who? . . . .)

Instructions

Rate the following on the basis of observations of the patient made during the last month at home. Rate an item 'YES' or 'NO' only if you are sure about it (for instance, if you yourself saw it happening). Rate'?' if you are not sure (for instance, if you did not have the opportunity to observe it yourself, if you only heard about it or if you can only suppose that it happened).

		YES	NO	?
1.	Avoids eating with others or delays as much as possible before coming to the dinner table	( )	( )	( )
2.	Shows obvious signs of tension at mealtimes	( )	( )	( )
3.	Shows anger or hostility at mealtimes	( )	( )	( )
4.	Begins by cutting up food into small pieces	( )	( )	( )
5.	Complains that there is too much food or that it's too rich (fattening)	( )	( )	( )
6.	Exhibits unusual 'food faddism'	( )	( )	( )
7.	Attempts to bargain about food (for example, 'I'll eat this if I don't have to eat that')	( )	( )	( )
8.	Picks at food or eats very slowly	( )	( )	( )
9.	Prefers diet products (with low calorie content)	( )	( )	( )
10.	Seldom mentions being hungry	( )	( )	( )
11.	Likes to cook or help in the kitchen, but avoids tasting or eating	( )	( )	( )
12.	Vomits after meals	( )	( )	( )
13.	Conceals food in napkins, handbags or clothing during mealtimes	( )	( )	( )
14.	Disposes of food (out of window, into dustbin or down sink or toilet)	( )	( )	( )
15.	Conceals or hoards food in own room or elsewhere	( )	( )	( )
16.	Eats when alone or secretly (for example, at night)	( )	( )	( )
17.	Dislikes visiting others or going to parties because of the 'obligation' to eat	( )	( )	( )
18.	Has sometimes difficulties in stopping or eats unusually large amounts of food or sweets	( )	( )	( )
19.	Complains a lot about constipation			
20.	Frequently takes laxatives (purgatives) or asks for them	( )	( )	( )
21.	Claims to be too fat regardless of weight loss	( )	( )	( )
22.	Often speaks about slimming, dieting or ideal body forms	( )	( )	( )
23.	Often leaves the table during mealtimes (for example, to get something in the kitchen)	( )	( )	( )
24.	Stands, walks or runs about whenever possible	( )	( )	( )
25.	Is as active as possible (for example, clearing tables or cleaning the room)	( )	( )	( )
26.	Does a lot of physical exercise or sports	( )	( )	( )
27.	Studies or works diligently	( )	( )	( )
28.	Is seldom tired and takes little or no rest	( )	( )	( )
29.	Claims to be normal, healthy or even better than ever	( )	( )	( )
30.	Is reluctant to see a doctor or refuses medical examination	( )	( )	( )

Reprinted from *Acta Psychiatrica Scandinavica*, **85**, 163–6, 1992

Appendix 10.4. Percentile charts for BMI for girls aged 0–18 years (*N* > 17 000) and boys aged 0–18 years (*N* > 17 000) based on a German reference population

(Reprinted from Kromeyer-Hauschild, K. *et al.*, *Montsschr Kinderheilkd*, **149**, 807–18, 2001.)

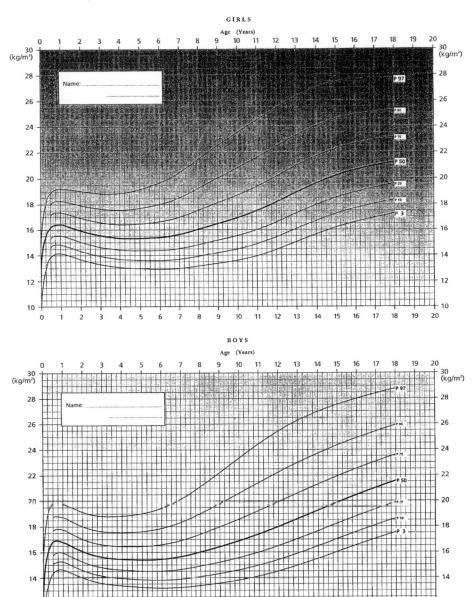

11

Sleep disorders

Gregory Stores

Department of Psychiatry, University of Oxford, UK

Introduction

Sleep disorders in psychiatry

Sleep disorders is not simply a topic comparable to schizophrenia or dissociative disorders. The term covers a very wide range of conditions of diverse aetiology. 'Sleep disorders medicine' is now a multidisciplinary specialty in its own right based on approaches and information from general medicine and paediatrics, child and adult psychiatry, neuropsychiatry, psychology (including developmental aspects) and several other disciplines and specialties. Sleep disorders are by no means only relevant to psychiatry, although there are various important links between them and clinical practice in psychiatry, whatever the age of the patient.

The main connections of this type are as follows.

- Disturbed sleep is a very common feature of many psychiatric disorders in children, adolescents and adults.
- Sleep disturbance is known to be an early sign of serious psychiatric disorder or threat of relapse which, if recognized, might have important preventive value.
- Various psychotropic medications are associated with poor sleep, possibly adding to the patient's coping difficulties.
- Sleep disturbance can affect mood, behaviour, cognitive abilities and performance.
- If severe, such disturbance may cause psychiatric disorder. At least a contributory role has been suggested for some forms of adult depression, and cases of both child and adult attention deficit hyperactivity disorder (ADHD) have been described as a consequence of a primary sleep disorder.
- Some sleep disorders may well be mistaken for primary psychiatric conditions because of similarities in clinical presentation, but also as a consequence

A Clinician's Handbook of Child and Adolescent Psychiatry, ed. Christopher Gillberg, Richard Harrington and Hans-Christoph Steinhausen. Published by Cambridge University Press. © Cambridge University Press 2005.

of clinicians' limited familiarity with the range and manifestations of sleep disorders.

The requirement for reviews such as the following that, as far as possible, statements should be 'evidence based' requires consideration. There are many levels or meaning of 'evidence' ranging from systematic reviews of randomized controlled trials to 'expert opinion'. As in many areas of child and adolescent psychiatry (where the number of methodologically sophisticated studies is generally limited), evidence in support of many of the statements made in the present chapter is at the lower levels. This should not be taken to mean, however, that the value of such evidence is seriously undermined.

Normal sleep in childhood and adolescence

- There are two physiologically distinct forms of sleep: non-rapid eye movement (NREM) sleep and rapid eye movement (REM) sleep.

  NREM sleep is divided into four levels or stages. The first two are light sleep; levels 3 and 4 are called deep sleep because awakening from these levels is most difficult. Stages 3 and 4 NREM combined are also called slow wave sleep (SWS). SWS is largely confined to the first third of the night.

  REM sleep (also called 'dreaming sleep' because most dreaming occurs during it) occurs increasingly as overnight sleep progresses. Brain metabolism is at a high level in this form of sleep, other main features of which are the characteristic eye movements and the virtual absence of skeletal muscle tone.

  As can be seen from Fig. 11.1, NREM and REM sleep alternate with each other several times during overnight sleep.

- Table 11.1 demonstrates that duration of sleep requirements is greatest in infancy (averaging 16–18 hours at full-term birth) and gradually reduces to the usual adult level of 7–8 hours. Post-pubertal adolescents may need at least as much, and possibly more, sleep than they did before puberty.

- The timing of sleep is regulated by the circadian clock in the suprachiasmatic nuclei, which is influenced by melatonin mainly produced in the pineal gland during darkness. This clock also controls other biological rhythms including body temperature and cortisol production with which the sleep–wake rhythm is normally synchronized. From an early age, the sleep–wake rhythm has to be entrained to the day–night cycle. The main cue (or 'zeitgeber') for this process is light perception but social cues (e.g. mealtimes and social activities) are also important.

- Within each 24-hour period the level of alertness and tendency to sleep varies, sleep tendency being greatest in the early hours of the morning and (to a less extent) in the early afternoon (the 'post-lunch dip'). Alertness level is generally highest in the evening before the onset of sleepiness (the 'forbidden zone').

Table 11.1. Average sleep requirements at different ages

Term birth	16–18 hours
1 year	15 hours
2 years	13–14 hours
4 years	12 hours
10 years	8–10 hours
* Adolescence	Possibly 8 hours plus

* Many adolescents are thought to obtain significantly less sleep than this.

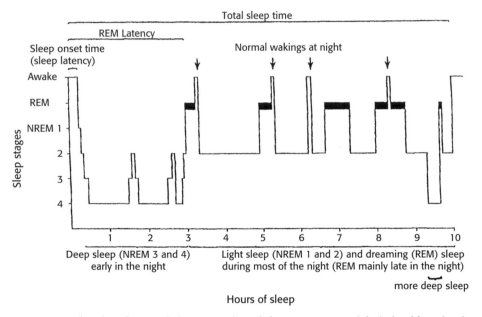

Fig. 11.1.   Hypnogram showing characteristic progression of sleep stages overnight in healthy school-age child. (Reproduced with permission from Stores & Wiggs, 2001.)

However, individual differences are seen even in children. Some people are very alert early in the day ('larks') and others in the evening perhaps until late ('owls').

• Most pre-pubertal children sleep soundly at night and are very alert during the day. This contrasts with post-pubertal teenagers who are sleepy during the day, partly because of lifestyle (including staying up late) but also because of biological changes in sleep at that age.

Types of sleep disturbance

The restorative properties of sleep depend not only on the length of time for which a person sleeps but also the quality of sleep obtained. The timing of the period of sleep is also important.

- There is concern that many young people (especially adolescents) consistently obtain less sleep than they need. Sometimes parents have a mistaken idea of how long their child should sleep, and it can be therapeutic to simply acquaint them with these normal values. There are individual differences in sleep requirements (i.e. in order to function optimally during the day) but, as a rough guide, if a child persistently sleeps at least 1 hour less than the average for the child's age, he may be sleep deprived and likely to benefit from more sleep.
- The most important aspect of sleep quality seems to be the extent to which overnight sleep is consolidated, i.e. free from frequent interruptions. So-called 'fragmented' sleep is caused by repeated awakenings and/or by very brief subclinical 'arousals' in which (as shown by physiological recording) sleep is interrupted without actual awakening. Sleep fragmentation is a particular feature of sleep-related breathing problems.
- The best example of inappropriate timing of the overnight sleep period is shift work. If activities are undertaken at night when the brain is biologically set to be asleep, impaired performance at this time is inevitable and is often accompanied by discomfort and distress. Daytime sleep is often inadequate in both duration and quality. A comparable situation to occupational night-shift work can exist for parents who frequently attend to their child at night.

Combinations of short duration sleep, poor quality sleep and inappropriate timing of sleep are particularly damaging. Ideally, all three possible impairments of sleep should be considered when the restorative value of sleep is assessed.

Sleep problems and disorders

There are three basic and sometimes inter-related sleep problems or complaints: not sleeping enough (sleeplessness or insomnia); sleeping too much (excessive daytime sleepiness or hypersomnia) and episodes of disturbed behaviour during or related to sleep (parasomnias). Although often not attempted, it is essential to try to identify the exact sleep disorder underlying these sleep problems. Treatments based on symptoms alone may well be ineffective and possibly make the sleep problem worse.

Classification of sleep disorders

There is much in favour of using the revised International Classification of Sleep Disorders (or ICSD-R) system, especially to standardize diagnosis in clinical work and research. This system attempts to organize rationally the various ways in which

Table 11.2. Main structure of the International Classification of Sleep Disorders – Revised*

Dyssomnias
Primary sleep disorders causing difficulty getting off to sleep/staying asleep, or excessive daytime sleepiness:
• intrinsic conditions such as sleep apnoea or narcolepsy
• extrinsic factors such as sleep environment or parenting practices
• circadian sleep–wake cycle disorders (mistiming of the sleep period)

Parasomnias
Episodic behaviour intruding into sleep. Grouped according to stage of sleep with which they are usually associated:
• arousal disorders (deep NREM sleep)
  • sleep–wake transition parasomnias
  • REM-related parasomnias
  • other parasomnias

Secondary sleep disorders associated with physical or psychiatric disorders
e.g. as part of dementia
    nocturnal epilepsy
    sleep-related asthma
    associated with depression or anxiety

Proposed sleep disorders
Sleep-related conditions needing further research before being accepted as definitive sleep disorders

* American Sleep Disorders Association (1997).

sleep can be disturbed. The more than 80 different sleep disorders, occurring in adults and children, are grouped as shown in Table 11.2.

ICSD-R contains useful summaries of each of these sleep disorders including main features, associated features and possible complications, course, predisposing factors, prevalence, age at onset, sex ratio, familial pattern, polysomnographic and other laboratory features, and differential diagnosis. Diagnostic, severity and duration criteria are also provided. Each sleep disorder is given a unique code number. By means of a three-axis system, a child's condition and treatment needs can be characterized in terms of the ICSD diagnosis of his sleep disorder, investigations performed and particular abnormalities demonstrated, and accompanying medical and psychiatric disorders. A glossary of basic terms and concepts is also provided.

The advantages of this system over DSM and ICD system are that it provides a more comprehensive, logically structured and regularly revised account of sleep disorders, based on the latest information provided by clinicians and researchers in the field of sleep disorders medicine.

The overall structure of ICSD-R is appropriate for use with children but only some of the disorders described are relevant to them. The pattern of occurrence and/or significance of basically the same disorder can be very different in children compared with adults. For example, many of the parasomnias (e.g. head-banging, sleepwalking and sleep terrors) are more common in childhood where generally they represent a temporary developmental phase without pathological significance. In contrast, it is often said (although not well supported by research) that the same behaviours in adults may well be the result of psychological problems.

General principles of assessment

Basic screening questions should be asked about any child concerning the following.
- Does s/he have any difficulty getting off to sleep or staying asleep?
- Is s/he very sleepy during the day?
- Does s/he have disturbed episodes at night?

Positive answers call for a detailed sleep history.

Sleep history and general review

Parents and also the child (if old enough) should be interviewed and the reasons for any disparities considered. The main aspects to be covered are as follows:
- current sleep problem and its evolution
- past treatments and their effects
- review of the child's current 24-h sleep–wake pattern (see Table 11.3) in order to determine in particular:
  - duration of sleep
  - quality (continuous or disrupted sleep)
  - timing of sleep
  - features suggestive of specific sleep disorders
- sleep environment and arrangements
- development of the child's sleep patterns and problems
- general review of sleep symptoms
- family history of sleep disturbance or other problems.

A sleep questionnaire completed by parents before the interview can provide a useful outline account of these and other aspects. See Appendix 1 for an example of a general, psychometrically sound sleep questionnaire (Owens *et al.*, 2000).

Additional parts of the overall review of children with a sleep problem that are important in order to identify possible contributory factors are as follows.
- developmental history including developmental delays, illnesses, or significant experiences within the family or at school
- review of physical health

Table 11.3. Outline review of child's 24-h sleep–wake pattern (modified according to child's age)

Evening
　Time of evening meal
　Other evening activities
Going to bed
　Preparation for bed, by whom
　Time of going to bed
　Reluctance to go at required time, parents' reactions
　Fears, rituals
　Wanting to sleep with someone, other comforts
　Time taken to fall asleep, experiences during that period
When asleep
　Wakings, frequency, causes, ability to return to sleep
　Episodic events, exact nature, timing, frequency
　Other behaviours during sleep, e.g. snoring, restlessness, bedwetting
　Parents' reaction to night-time events
Waking
　Wakes spontaneously or needs to be woken up
　Time of final waking
　Total duration of sleep period
　Longest period of uninterrupted sleep
　On waking: preoccupations, mood, feeling of being refreshed, other experiences
　Difficulty waking and getting out of bed, time of getting out of bed
Daytime
　Sleepiness, naps
　Lethargy
　Mood
　Overactivity
　Concentration and performance
　Other unusual episodes

- physical examination
- assessment of behaviour and emotional state
- family circumstances.

Sleep diary

Systematic recording each day over a period of 2 weeks or so, using a standardized format, avoids the bias or distortion of retrospective generalizations.

- The occurrence and nature of night-time episodes of disturbed behaviour can be determined.
- Daytime events including sleepiness can be assessed.

- Previously unrecognized patterns of occurrence of sleep phenomena may become apparent including temporal patterns, shift of the sleep phase, or relationships to stressful events or other factors.

Video

Video recordings can be very instructive in the parasomnias, sometimes revealing a very different clinical picture than that provided in the clinic. Home video systems can be used where admission to hospital is not feasible.

Actigraphy

When the details of sleep physiology are not needed, monitoring of body movements by means of wristwatch-like devices ('actigraphs' or 'actometers') can be used at home, or elsewhere, to quantify objectively sleep variables based on the distinction that this procedure broadly provides between wakefulness and sleep. Recordings over several days are easily obtained.

Polysomnography (PSG)

Physiological sleep studies are necessary for diagnosis in only the minority of sleep disorders. Traditionally, this has entailed admission to a sleep laboratory. However, home PSG using portable systems is very appropriate especially for children, although for some disorders it is best seen as only a screening procedure. 'First night effects' are prominent in laboratory recordings. Therefore, to obtain a more representative account of the child's sleep, more than one night of PSG is required to allow adaptation to take place.

Basic polysomnography entails the recording of EEG, an electro-oculogram (EOG) and an electromyogram (EMG). This allows sleep to be staged and a hypnogram (showing sleep architecture) to be compiled. Usually the recording is made overnight but it may be extended during the day if appropriate. Where indicated, basic recording can be extended to include additional physiological measures, such as respiratory variables (and audio-video recordings) for sleep-related breathing problems, additional EEG channels (combined with video) if nocturnal epilepsy is suspected, and anterior tibialis EMG for the detection of periodic limb movements in sleep (PLMS).

The main indications for polysomnography are:
- the investigation of excessive daytime sleepiness including the diagnosis of sleep apnoea, narcolepsy, or PLMS
- the diagnosis of parasomnias where their nature is unclear from the clinical details
- (occasionally) as an objective check on the accuracy of the sleep complaint, or response to treatment.

It is essential that PSG procedure are child friendly and that normative data for children are used in evaluating the results.

Other investigations

As mentioned later, further special investigations may be appropriate depending on the nature of the sleep problem and the purpose of the assessment.

Sleeplessness

Definition and classification

The problem of the 'sleepless' child usually means one or more of the following:
- bedtime difficulties or 'settling problems' (either reluctance to go to bed or difficulty getting to sleep)
- waking up in the night and not being able to return to sleep without his parents' attention or company
- waking early in the morning and not going back to sleep again.

'Sleeplessness' may also be used by parents to mean that their child's sleep is very restless or disturbed by frequent nightmares or other episodic events.

These different problems need to be distinguished from each other because the factors causing or maintaining them can be different and require different types of treatment.

Sometimes, establishing the details of the sleeplessness reveals that the child is, in fact, sleeping normally and that the parents' expectations are mistaken, causing them to worry unnecessarily. If that is the case, explanation and re-assurance may be very therapeutic unless the parents are unable to take a balanced view because they are depressed or emotionally troubled in some other way.

The severity of the sleeplessness can be classified in terms of:
- the frequency with which it occurs
- its duration (different factors are usually involved depending on the duration of the problem)
  - transient (i.e. lasting several days)
  - short term (perhaps several weeks)
  - chronic (months or years)
- the extent of its effects on the child and family (families vary in their tolerance of a child's sleep disturbance).

Within its general category of 'dyssomnias' (by which is meant disorders that produce difficulties initiating or maintaining sleep, or excessive sleepiness) ICSD-R provides a classification of sleep disorders including those underlying sleeplessness. Such sleep disorders are grouped according to whether the cause is intrinsic (e.g. psychophysiological insomnia such as that due to stress), extrinsic (e.g. where the sleep environment is unconducive to sleep) or caused by a circadian rhythm sleep disorder. However, as mentioned previously, the ICSD-R is mainly adult based and needs to be modified to some extent for use with children. Nevertheless, the 34 sleep disorders within the dyssomnia category include a number that are specially relevant to children. These are reflected in the later sections of this chapter where the clinical picture and aetiology of sleeplessness and excessive sleepiness are discussed.

Epidemiology

Prevalence and incidence rates

Sleeplessness (or 'insomnia' as the usual term used for those old enough to complain themselves) is the main sleep problem but prevalence and incidence vary with age. In infants and toddlers it causes concern in about 25 per cent of families. Perhaps 15 per cent of older children have mainly settling problems then the figure rises again to 20 per cent or more of adolescents who have difficulties getting to sleep or staying asleep. Reliable rates for early morning waking are not available.

Particularly high rates of sleeplessness and other sleep problems are consistently described in the following clinical groups (Stores & Wiggs, 2001).

• Children and adolescents with psychiatric disorder in general have very high rates of sleep disturbance.

• Sleeplessness is very common in children with a neurodevelopmental disorder. This can be explained by such factors as parental overpermissiveness or inconsistency, the child's learning disability impairing the acquisition of good sleep habits, or accompanying physical or psychiatric disorder.

• Children with other chronic illness or disorder (e.g. those causing pain or discomfort) are also at special risk of sleep disturbance. This is obviously of importance to psychiatrists involved in liaison work with paediatrics. Some forms of paediatric medication (such as bronchodilators) may affect sleep. Also admission to hospital, especially for intensive care, often causes sleep disturbance that can be persistent.

Sex ratios and ethnicity

No reliable figures are available for sex ratios or different ethnic groups across the age range. In the USA co-sleeping of small children with their parents is said to be more common in black and other ethnic minority families and in lower socio-economic subgroups. Co-sleeping is acceptable to a proportion of families in general.

Implications for clinical practice

The effects of persistent sleep disturbance can have serious consequences for a child's development and for other members of the family.

- Adverse effects on mood and behaviour are reported increasingly comparable to those described in adults, e.g. irritability, impulsiveness, aggression, depression or complaints of exhaustion and other physical ailments.
- Impaired cognitive function and educational performance have also been demonstrated.
- The mood, well-being, general functioning and parenting ability (especially of mothers) are also affected if parents are chronically sleep deprived because of their child's sleeplessness. Marital discord and separation, and even physical abuse of children have been linked to parental sleep loss.
- Other children in the family can be affected by the family upset caused by a child's sleep problem.
- Physical consequences of serious sleep disturbance include impaired growth and failure to thrive in young children and, possibly, other endocrine and immune system abnormalities.

There is evidence that successful treatment of a child's sleep disorder can be followed by reversal of these various adverse effects. Fortunately, it seems that recovery from sleep loss occurs after much less sleep than originally lost although the secondary effects of sleep disturbance my persist longer.

Clinical picture

Main features and symptoms

Clinical presentation varies considerably depending on the cause of the child's sleeplessness and, to some extent, the age of the child. The account given here and in subsequent sections incorporates sleep disorders as listed in ICSD-R. The descriptions of the different sleep disorders emphasize key features that are particularly significant for diagnosis. The breakdown according to age should not be interpreted too strictly as there is some overlap between the different age groups.

Infants and toddlers

- Infantile colic is diagnosed in otherwise healthy infants who, from about 2–3 weeks of age, repeatedly cry inconsolably and cannot fall asleep in the evening supposedly because of intra-abdominal pain (although this has recently been disputed). Typically, this problem resolves by 3–4 months, but sleep problems may continue because of the parents' habitual responses to the child.
- Frequent night wakings in babies who return to sleep only with feeding (leading to the overnight consumption of large amounts of fluid and very wet nappies) suggests the need to promote the circadian pattern of sleeping during the night and feeding during the day. This should be possible by 6 months of age for children

born at term. Gradual reduction of night-time feeding works best and should be effective after about 2 weeks.

- Crying and sleeplessness caused by medical disorders such as cows' milk allergy or otitis media are not confined to particular parts of the day and are likely to be accompanied by failure to thrive, or other evidence of physical illness such as fever. Typically, the child is difficult to console and settle back to sleep.

- In contrast, the more usual settling and night waking problems are characterized by rapid settling and return to sleep when the comforting conditions which the child has come to associate with going to sleep are provided. These 'sleep onset associations' may be objects such as the cot, favourite toys or other transitional objects but, frequently, they involve the parent's presence, i.e. being held, rocked or nursed. At least in most families in western society, a problem arises if the child cannot go to sleep at bedtime, and/or if he cannot get back to sleep after waking during the night without associations that involve the parents' presence and comforting attention.

- Difficulties at bedtime may be related to inappropriate patterns of daytime napping, i.e. too little or too much daytime napping for the child's age or alternatively, a nap too near bedtime.

- Early morning waking (e.g. at 5 am or earlier) may be associated with a nap unusually early in the same day, e.g. at 8.00 am. This nap may, in fact, represent the last sleep cycle detached from the rest of overnight sleep. Alternatively, the sleep phase may be shifted forwards within the 24-hour cycle. If the habit has been established of the child being put to bed very early with early sleep onset, he is likely to wake too early for the parents when his sleep requirements have been met.

Pre-school and school-age children

Bedtime struggles and other settling difficulties often continue after the age of 3 or thereabouts, especially when the child moves from cot to bed and is no longer easily constrained. Many parents are familiar with bedtime delaying tactics in which their child asks for drinks or more stories, expresses fear at the prospect of bed, or steadfastly refuses to go to bed.

- Commonly, the problem is maintained or made worse by parents' inability or unwillingness to establish and enforce rules consistently for going to bed and settling to sleep, i.e. to set limits. A clue to the nature of the problem can be the child's willingness to settle with one parent rather than the other, or with the baby-sitter or with someone else who can set limits. The effects of the parents' inability to set limits are compounded if parents lose their temper, threaten or punish the child who then comes to associate bedtime with upset and fear. The risk of inappropriate parental behaviour at bedtime is increased in parents with marital or psychiatric difficulties.

- Setting limits is only appropriate if the child is physiologically capable of going to sleep at the required time. This is not the case in the so-called 'delayed sleep phase syndrome' (DSPS), which is a cause of settling difficulty at all ages. Characteristically, bedtime struggles do not occur on the occasions when bedtime is delayed because, by then, the child is able to sleep. Both children and adults have a period later in the day when their tendency towards sleep is at its lowest (the 'forbidden zone'). This is followed by a period of least alertness leading to sleep onset. Understandably, if the child is put to bed while still wide awake, he will resist (perhaps vigorously) before eventually falling asleep at the same time whenever attempts to put him to bed began. These settling problems are accompanied by particular difficulty waking in the morning for nursery or school because the child's sleep requirements have not been met in spite of sound sleep. It is easy to see how the child's physiological inability to go to sleep and to get up at the required time can be misconstrued as naughtiness. DSPS may arise in young children from persistent bedtime struggles or from sleep onset disruption due, for example, to illness or holidays.
- Night-time fears are common throughout childhood and may cause difficulty getting off to sleep or disturbance during the night. Their causes, and the way they are expressed, vary greatly with stage of development.
- Restless legs syndrome, now described also in children consists of disagreeable leg sensations with an irresistible urge to move the legs causing difficulty getting to sleep. It is often accompanied by periodic limb movements (see later).
- 'Growing pains', said to be a cause of sleep difficulties in otherwise healthy children, is an ill-defined condition. Where they occur around bedtime, the restless legs syndrome is a possibility.

Adolescents

Older pre-pubertal children are highly efficient sleepers and very alert during the day. Adolescence is characterized by a change in sleep and wakefulness caused by a variety of physiological and psychological factors including late night social activities.

Consistently high rates of insomnia have been described in adolescence, often associated with psychological problems. Various factors may be relevant in the individual case.

- Difficulty getting off to sleep can be the result of worries about daytime demands or other causes of stress.
- The sleep onset problem is very often part of the DSPS, to which reference has already been made concerning young children. This is a form of circadian

sleep–wake cycle disorder (Garcia *et al.*, 2001). Although DSPS occurs at all ages, it is especially common in adolescence. It will be discussed further in relation to daytime sleepiness. The difficulty falling asleep can be severe and often lasts until the early hours, irrespective of the time of going to bed. Concern about not getting sufficient sleep can add to the problem. Again, the insomnia, and the difficulty getting up in the morning, are essentially physiological in nature but are easily interpreted as 'difficult' adolescent behaviour. An irregular sleep–wake pattern (i.e. disorganized and variable episodes of sleep and wakefulness) causes insomnia as well as daytime sleepiness.

- The other psychiatric and medical conditions mentioned earlier may need to be considered as well as medication effects including injudiciously prescribed hypnotics. Possible drug use is particularly relevant at this age. It is capable of producing a range of sleep problems including insomnia.
- The same is true of alcohol, nicotine and caffeine the consumption of which should always be assessed thoroughly. Coffee intake can sometimes be surprising.
- At any age, the possibility should also be investigated that sleeplessness is at least partly the result of factors such as an uncomfortable, noisy, or excessively hot, cold or otherwise unsuitable sleeping environment.

Differential diagnosis and co-morbidity

The issue of differential diagnosis regarding sleeplessness concerns the distinction between the many causes of sleeplessness as just outlined. There is still an unfortunate tendency to not enquire in detail about the underlying cause in the individual case but to try to treat symptomatically with hypnotic or sedative medication (which is rarely effective).

Co-morbity arises in various ways:

- as already illustrated, physical or psychiatric conditions (and their treatment) may be the cause of the sleeplessness
- it was emphasized earlier that various psychological problems and sometimes psychiatric disorder might be caused or worsened by persistent sleep disturbance whatever its origin.

Assessment

The following scheme represents a clinical approach to identifying the cause of sleeplessness in the individual child. Further assessments are not usually required except that actometry can provide a more objective account of sleep-wake patterns, especially if there is uncertainty about the clinic description or where the circadian rhythm sleep disorders need to be documented more precisely. Polysomnography is rarely required.

General

What is the exact nature of the problem when parents say their child does not sleep?

- What form of sleeplessness (e.g. bedtime difficulties, night waking, early morning waking) and how often the problem arises?
- A sleep diary will provide a more accurate account.

Are their expectations reasonable?

- Do they need explanation of what is normal?
- Do they have other problems which are distorting their view?

If the child's sleep pattern is abnormal, consider the underlying sleep disorder and treat it accordingly, rather than:

- simply reassuring parents that it is a passing phase or
- treating it purely symptomatically with medication.

For this and other types of sleep problem, assess the child's sleep adequately including:

- a sleep history
- review of the child's 24-hour sleep–wake pattern
- developmental and family histories
- review of physical and mental health.

Consider general factors which may apply at any age.

- Do the parents handle the child's bedtime and general behaviour inappropriately?
- Are there other family problems that affect the child's sleep?
- Are there other factors preventing satisfactory sleep (i.e. poor sleep hygiene)?
- Does the child have a medical condition (including its treatment) that affects sleep?

Infancy

The child may be of a type who generally cries more than most (including in the evening) without any organic cause.

Frequent waking and only returning to sleep by being fed suggests that the waking has been conditioned by unnecessary frequent feeding at night.

Close relationship of sleeping and other problems with certain types of food suggests allergy.

Early childhood

The number and timing of daytime naps may be inappropriate.

Parental practices and the circumstances surrounding bedtime and waking during the night may be at fault.

- Is there no consistent relaxing bedtime routine?
- Is bedtime unreasonably early?

- Is bedtime and going to sleep associated with pleasant or unpleasant experiences in the child's mind?
- Does the child need his parents' presence to be able to go to sleep?
- Are the circumstances different when the child goes to sleep and when he wakes in the night?
- Do parents give in to their child's delaying tactics at bedtime or demands to be with them if he wakes during the night?
- Does the child readily settle to sleep or go back to sleep in the night with one person but not another (suggesting failure to set appropriate limits)?

Middle childhood

In addition to enquiring about the possible explanations why toddlers may not sleep well, consider the following:

- overarousal from exciting or boisterous activity near bedtime
- night-time fears
- worries about family or school matters which may no longer exist but have set up a habit of not sleeping well
- being put to bed too early causing difficulty getting to sleep or waking early when sufficient sleep has been obtained for the child's age
- the child may be constitutionally unable to get to sleep until late (although other explanations should be considered first).

Adolescence

Some of the above reasons for not sleeping well may still apply but the following possibilities should also be explored:

- changes in lifestyle causing erratic sleep–wake patterns or delay in the timing of the sleep period (easily misinterpreted as 'difficult adolescent behaviour')
- excessive caffeine intake, alcohol, tobacco
- use of illegal substances
- psychiatric disorder.

Aetiology

It is important to consider a whole range of possible explanations in the sleepless child. As illustrated by the following examples, these vary somewhat with the age of the child.

- Physical features have to be excluded, e.g. cows' milk intolerance or middle ear disease in younger children and chronic physical disorders at any age.
- Especially in their early years, most children need their parents' help in coping with night-time separation from them and the potentially frightening experience of the dark or their own thoughts and fantasies. Infants need the comfort of physical

contact. Toddlers are helped by bedtime routines and transitional objects and encouragement to become 'self-soothing' so that they can fall asleep (including getting back to sleep when they awake during the night) without their parents' presence and attention. Children depend on their parents to provide positive attitudes to sleeping and the avoidance of negative association such as disputes, punishment and rejection. Parents also need to set limits if the child 'plays up' at bedtime.

Parents' ability to provide such help depends on their personality and sensitivity, their circumstances and mental state, and possibly also their attitudes to their child's sleep based on their own experiences in childhood.

Sometimes parents are not motivated to improve their child's sleep. For example, a child's presence in the parental bed might be welcomed by one partner as a means of distancing him/herself from the other at night.

- Older children may have bedrooms which are a source of play and entertainment rather than providing an atmosphere conducive to sleep.
- Night-time fears or other stresses, the nature of which can vary with level of cognitive development, may cause difficulty getting to sleep.
- Adolescents may also have difficulty sleeping because of worries associated with their stage of development, poor sleep hygiene, psychiatric illness such as depression, or unsatisfactory lifestyle with irregular sleep habits or substance misuse.

Treatment

This depends on the underlying cause of the sleeplessness problem.

- Drug treatment is rarely justified. Conventional sedative–hypnotic drugs are generally ineffective. The place of melatonin remains uncertain in view of the many unresolved issues surrounding its use (Stores, in press).
- Appropriate attention to underlying physical or psychiatric factors can be expected to improve sleep.
- Advice for parents is required where parenting practices are mainly responsible for the child's sleeplessness. This includes guidance of night-time feeding schedules in infants and satisfactory napping patterns in toddlers.
- The main feature of treatment for sleeplessness caused by inappropriate sleep onset associations is enabling the child to fall asleep without the involvement of a parent. In general, the most appropriate procedure is for the parents to be encouraged to put the child to bed awake and left alone for progressively longer intervals with repeated brief reassurances. The same procedure is followed for night-time wakings. As night-time and sleep onset may have particularly negative associations for psychologically disturbed children, special efforts might need to be made to help them make a smooth transition to restful sleep.
- The basic aim of treatment for bedtime limit setting problems is to introduce a consistent limit setting procedure. Reinforcement of the problem behaviour

Table 11.4. Basic principles of sleep hygiene (relevance varies with age)

Sleeping environment should be conducive to sleep
  Familiar setting
  Comfortable bed
  Correct temperature
  Darkened, quiet room
  Non-stimulating
  No negative associations (e.g. struggles with parents or punishment)
Encourage
  Bedtime routines
  Consistent bedtime and waking up times (weekdays, weekends, holidays)
  Going to bed only when tired
  Thinking about problems and plans before going to bed
  Falling asleep without parents (young children)
  Regular daily exercise, exposure to sunlight, and general fitness
Avoid
  Too much time awake in bed (especially if distressed)
  Overexcitement near bedtime and bedroom as place of entertainment
  Excessive or late napping during the day
  Late evening exercise
  Caffeine-containing drinks late in the day
  Smoking and excessive alcohol
  Large meals late at night

by complying with demands must be avoided; positive reinforcement of good behaviour may also be effective. Help for parents with their other problems may well be necessary before they are able to do what is required.

- Young children's fears of the dark, shadows and monsters require comfort and reassurance. Anxiety about such things may also cause nightmares. If fears and nightmares are frequent, particularly disturbing or not easily amenable to reassurance, the possibility of some underlying serious cause should be considered (e.g. family disruption or trauma) and more intensive help provided.

- The most appropriate management of the delayed sleep phase syndrome is usually to advance the sleep phase gradually, first by bringing the time of waking forward, then the bedtime, including weekends. The prospect of improvement is generally good but totally irregular sleep wake patterns may be one aspect of a lack of routine in family life.

- Good 'sleep hygiene' principles should be observed throughout. This term refers to ways of promoting satisfactory sleep in anyone whose sleep is persistently disturbed. Basic principles for children and adolescents are suggested in Table 11.4. Their appropriateness varies with age. Several of them are particularly relevant to older children or adolescents who complain about lying in bed awake for long periods unable to sleep. It is important that bed does not come to be associated with difficulty sleeping. If someone does not fall asleep after about 20 minutes, it is better to move to another room for a while until they become tired enough to sleep.

Outcome

This depends on the cause of sleeplessness, how amenable it is to intervention, the availability of treatment resources (i.e. professional advice and support facilities for parents) and the appropriateness of the treatment undertaken, as well as the persistence with which interventions are pursued. In general, however, sleeplessness can be seen as a potentially treatable problem (mainly by behavioural means rather than medication), often with a relatively quick response even in severe and long standing cases.

Excessive daytime sleepiness (EDS)

Definition and classification

Clinically, EDS implies a tendency to sleep which is greater than that seen in most other children with the additional connotation that this increased tendency interferes with everyday function to the child's disadvantage.

The severity of EDS is judged as:

- mild: general slowing up of activities and complaint of tiredness without actually falling asleep. The child may yawn, stretch or rub his eyes, have drooping eyelids and complain of tiredness
- moderate: inability to stay awake in circumstances conducive to sleep
- severe: falling asleep when active, e.g. eating or talking.

As in the case of sleeplessness, within the dyssomnias category ICSD-R provides a classification of sleep disorders underlying EDS in terms of whether the cause is intrinsic (e.g. obstructive sleep apnoea), extrinsic (e.g. insufficient sleep) or a circadian-rhythm sleep disorder.

Epidemiology

Prevalence and incidence ratios

Because of different uses of the term 'sleepiness' and the few studies performed, overall rates are unclear but the problem must be common considering the many conditions of which it is a feature. In one study about 20 per cent of school-age children reported frequent daytime sleepiness. There are no reliable figures on sex ratio and ethnicity.

Implications for clinical practice

Experimental findings and clinical reports illustrate a range of adverse effects of EDS:

- impaired cognitive function, especially sustained attention and creativity
- poor school progress
- increased number of accidents and increased risk from hazards
- associated behaviour disturbance including irritability, aggression, depression and ADHD symptoms
- impaired social relationships, activities and opportunities
- family and school problems arising from misinterpretation of pathological sleepiness as laziness or difficult behaviour.

Clinical picture

Main features and symptoms

The clinical picture varies considerably with the cause of the EDS of which there are many possibilities. These can be grouped as insufficient sleep, disturbed overnight sleep and conditions in which sleep tendency is increased.

Insufficient sleep, including circadian sleep–wake cycle disorders

Inadequate sleep (for the many reasons discussed earlier) is a common cause of daytime sleepiness at all ages. However, as mentioned in the last section, adolescents are especially prone to this problem because, although they seem to have a physiological need for more sleep, they often obtain less.

Commonly, the cause of inadequate sleep at this age is late-night and weekend social activities while having to get up for school the following morning. Whereas the delayed sleep phase syndrome (DSPS) mainly presents as a settling problem in young children, inability to get up in the morning is a main difficulty in older children and adolescents. There may also be other causes of difficulty falling asleep, early morning waking and short duration sleep as adolescence is a time of life when sleep disrupting problems or activities are prominent. Inconsistent changes of sleep pattern at weekend and holiday may also contribute to erratic or otherwise unsatisfactory sleep–wake cycles including the so-called 'irregular sleep–wake schedule'. Sometimes the situation is complicated by the use by people of stimulants to stay awake and alcohol or sedative drugs to help them to sleep.

The characteristic features of DSPS, about which specific enquiries should be made, are listed in the later part of this section on the clinical approach to excessive sleepiness.

Disturbed overnight sleep

If duration of sleep appears to be satisfactory, ways in which sleep may be interrupted and its restorative quality reduced have to be considered. Disruptive influences include caffeine-containing drinks (notably cola drinks and coffee); frequent parasomnias (unusual); medical conditions such as nocturnal asthma or epilepsy; medications including hypnotic and sedative drugs (which may produce rebound effects) and possibly stimulants for ADHD; and illicit drug and alcohol abuse including withdrawal effects. Frequent periodic limb movements in sleep are considered to be a cause of excessive daytime sleepiness in adults and have recently been implicated as a cause of behavioural disturbance (including ADHD symptoms) in children because they disrupt sleep.

Increasing attention is being paid to sleep-related breathing difficulties (especially obstructive sleep apnoea) in infants and children in the general population but particularly in children with various neurodevelopmental disorders.

Snoring is common in children, but in perhaps 2 per cent it is part of the obstructive sleep apnoea syndrome (OSAS). As this condition carries a serious risk of psychological and physical complications, its possibility needs to be carefully considered.

In addition to snoring, other night-time features of childhood OSAS should be sought. Observed repeated apnoeic episodes are particularly suggestive of OSAS. However, in spite of the name of the syndrome, in children apnoeas are not an essential feature of significant upper airway obstruction because severe hypoventilation caused by partial obstruction can have the same harmful effects. There may be other evidence of difficult breathing during sleep either from observation of the chest or abdomen (e.g. paradoxical chest–abdomen movements) or grunting, choking, snorting or gasping sounds. Other main features that have been described are cyanosis during sleep, very restless sleep, unusual sleeping positions especially with neck extension, profuse sweating during sleep, sudden awakening following the obstructive event sometimes with distress, and possibly nocturnal enuresis.

Daytime symptoms suggestive of OSAS include those resulting from enlarged tonsils and adenoids (if present) such as mouth breathing with mouth dryness in the morning, and adenoidal facies. The reported psychological features of the syndrome are very wide ranging and are the result of severe disruption of overnight sleep caused by the occurrence of the obstructive apnoeas or hypopnoeas hundreds of times a night. Possible daytime symptoms include bad mood on waking, excessive daytime sleepiness (although this is not a prominent feature in children and may be subtle or absent altogether), difficult behaviour and emotional upset as well as various other neuropsychological problems and poor progress at school. OSAS starting early in life is associated with developmental delay and failure to thrive (obesity is seen in the minority of children with OSAS). In severe cases there is also a risk of cardiopulmonary disease or death.

Conditions in which sleep tendency is increased

There are some conditions of which prolonged or otherwise excessive sleep is an intrinsic part, rather than a consequence. It is important to establish the pattern of occurrence because in some, (such as narcolepsy) the EDS is persistent; in others it is intermittent.

Narcolepsy is an important cause of persistent EDS. Its prevalence has been estimated as 2–5/10 000 with onset in at least a third of cases occurring during childhood or adolescence. The clinical features of the narcolepsy syndrome are largely the result of intrusion of REM sleep phenomena into the waking state ie daytime sleep attacks; hypnagogic hallucinations (produced by the dreaming element of REM sleep) and cataplexy and sleep paralysis, which represent the skeletal muscular paralysis of REM sleep. In addition, overnight sleep is disrupted by frequent awakenings producing a background of daytime sleepiness (sometimes with automatic behaviour) against which the narcoleptic sleep attacks occur.

This full syndrome is not usually seen at the start of the disorder and, especially in children, early recognition can be difficult. Young patients may be distressed by and react to the sleepiness and its social and educational consequences. If and when the other features develop, they may well alarm the child. They can also be a further source of diagnostic uncertainty if they are overlooked or concealed, or if their true nature is not appreciated. For example, cataplexy has been misinterpreted as conversion disorder. Denial, aggression and depression may well result.

Additional causes of persistent EDS in children include certain other neurological disorders of childhood and adolescence, (namely hydrocephalus, post-viral and head injury states each with distinctive clinical features), and idiopathic CNS hypersomnia (unusual in children) in which there is chronic, excessive daytime sleepiness unexplained by medical or psychiatric factors and without the characteristic abnormal REM sleep features of narcolepsy.

The classic example of intermittent EDS is the Kleine–Levin syndrome. This apparently rare condition typically begins in adolescent males, often following an infection or some other type of stressful experience or injury. Periods lasting hours to weeks occur at intervals of weeks to months with return to normality in between. In each episode the patient sleeps for excessively long periods. Overeating (sometimes leading to obesity) and various forms of hypersexual behaviour characterize the awake state in classical cases, together with various other disturbances (including disorientation and hallucinations) suggestive of a mild organic confusional state. At the end of each episode, a short period of depression or elation with sleeplessness may occur. Incomplete forms with only excessive sleepiness are described. There is a tendency towards spontaneous resolution of the condition but this may take many years. The condition is easily misconstrued as something other than an illness.

Other possible causes of intermittent EDS are major depressive disorder (25 per cent of sufferers complain of EDS), intermittent substance abuse, some neurological disorders including status epilepticus, seasonal affective disorder (SAD) and menstruation-related sleep disorders. EDS and other sleep complaints about children in the Munchausen Syndrome by Proxy may occur episodically.

In idiopathic recurring stupor, sometimes described in children, patients have high plasma and CFS levels of an endogenous benzodiazepine-like substance (endozepine-4) and regular episodes of stupor (possibly confused with hypersomnia) with widespread fast activity in their EEG. Episodes are promptly resolved by treatment with flumazenil, a benzodiazepine antagonist.

Differential diagnosis

EDS should be distinguished from:

- other causes of reduced activity such as laziness, boredom, disinterest and depression all of which are common misdiagnoses
- tiredness in the sense of fatigue, exhaustion or lack of energy (without an increased propensity to sleep) for which different explanations are likely including physical illness or depression
- other causes of disturbed mood or behaviour including ADHD symptoms
- simulated EDS as a way of avoiding difficult situations.

Within EDS the differential diagnosis regarding its cause is wide, as already demonstrated.

Co-morbidity

EDS may lead to psychological disorders as a result of the disadvantages that it imposes on the child and the family. This varies with the cause of EDS.

Diagnostic instruments or procedures

- Simple visual-analogue scales from extremely awake to extremely sleepy have been used.
- General sleep questionnaires contain items about sleepiness. Others are more concerned with this particular aspect.
- The main objective measure of sleepiness is the multiple sleep latency test (MSLT), which entails polysomnographic assessment of the onset of sleep in optimal nap conditions. Norms for this and other objective measures are not well established and the measures are inappropriate for young children.

Assessment

The following scheme of clinical enquiry can be helpful in identifying the cause and circumstances of EDS in the individual case. More specific investigations may be appropriate when particular causes of EDS are being considered.

- Polysomnography (PSG) including respiration measures are indicated to assess the nature and severity of upper airway obstruction in cases of OSAS.
- Overnight PSG and multiple sleep latency testing can help confirm a diagnosis of narcolepsy. Conversely a negative human leukocyte antigen test result makes this diagnosis unlikely.
- Toxicology screening is important where substance abuse is suspected.

General

Is the problem really excessive sleepiness, or fatigue or lethargy for which different explanations are likely? Check for physical illness or chronic fatigue syndrome.

Is the complaint of sleepiness genuine or is it simulated?

If sleepiness, how severe is it and what are its effects? Consider behavioural effects including overactivity as a feature of sleep loss or disturbance in young children.

What form of sleepiness (prolonged overnight sleep, daytime sleepiness including sleep attacks)?

Is the sleepiness continuous or intermittent (including being worse in winter)?

Is the child on sedating medication? Has he any neurological disorder associated with sleepiness?

At any age

Is the child's sleep sufficient for his age? (see sleep duration norms at different ages)
- How many hours does he usually sleep?
- Does he get to sleep very late but have to get up at a certain time?
- Does he wake up by himself or have to be woken?
- Is it particularly difficult to wake him up and does he resist strongly?

Does he sleep soundly?
- Is sleep very restless?
- Is it interrupted by frequent wakings or other disturbance?

Is the timing of the sleep period satisfactory?
- Are daytime naps taken inappropriately for child's age?
- Is sleep divided into several periods which are irregular in their distribution or timing (irregular sleep wake schedule)?
- Does the overnight sleep period seem to be shifted with difficulty getting to sleep and sleeping in late when possible, e.g. weekends or holidays (delayed sleep phase syndrome)?

Specific features
- Jerky legs during sleep (periodic limb movements)?
- Snoring or other noisy breathing during sleep (upper airway obstruction)? If so,
- Apnoeic episodes?
- Other evidence of airway obstruction during sleep? (see text)
- Anatomical features predisposing to upper airway obstruction? (see text)
- Discrete episodes of irresistible sleep during the day? Weakness when excited or alarmed? If so, other features of narcolepsy especially hypnagogic hallucinations, sleep paralysis? (narcolepsy syndrome)
- Sleepiness despite apparently satisfactory sleep (idiopathic hypersomnia)?
- Recurrent periods of excessive sleepiness with normality in between? (See various causes for distinctive features.)

Adolescence

Enquire about characteristic features of:
- erratic sleep–wake schedules
- delayed sleep phase syndrome
  - persistently severe difficulty getting to sleep
  - uninterrupted sleep
  - considerable difficulty getting up
  - sleepiness and underfunctioning during the day
  - sleeping in very late at weekends or during holidays.
- Other important considerations:
  - tobacco use, caffeine intake?
  - drugs, alcohol abuse?
  - physical illness disrupting sleep?
  - anxiety or depression?
  - other sleep disorder interfering with sleep?
  - motivated to preserve abnormal sleep pattern (school or family problems)?

Aetiology

This varies considerably with the underlying cause of EDS.
- Where insufficient sleep is responsible, the various aetiological factors discussed earlier in relation to sleeplessness apply.
- Regarding disturbed overnight sleep as a cause, various disruptive influences have already been mentioned such as excessive caffeine intake, medical conditions, medication effects and obstructive sleep apnoea the underlying cause of which in children is usually enlarged tonsils and adenoids although other anatomical features such as craniofacial abnormalities may be responsible.

- Narcolepsy is mainly a disturbance of REM sleep with both genetic and environmental factors playing a part in its development. Recent findings suggest underfunctioning of the hypocretin (orexin) neuropeptide system as a basic fault. Reference has already been made to other neurological causes of persistent EDS.
- The aetiology of Kleine–Levin syndrome remains obscure but the nature of the other possible causes of intermittent EDS listed earlier is clear in most instances.

Treatment

Clearly, treatment needs to be specific to the particular cause of EDS.

- The various psychological interventions appropriate for childhood sleeplessness discussed previously apply if insufficient sleep is the cause.
- Treatment of DSPS has mainly consisted of 'chronotherapy' by which the sleep phase is brought into line with that of others by gradually advancing it, or delaying it stepwise 'round the clock' depending on the size of the initial sleep phase delay. Other treatments have included exposure to bright light when woken and melatonin.
- Chronotherapy requires considerable motivation and cooperation on the part of both patient and family members. In some cases, the young person is not motivated to change preferring the late night activities, or there may be some other psychological reason (including avoidance of school) for not making the effort required. This situation has been called 'motivated sleep phase delay'.
- Treatment of the typical case of sleep apnoea from the general population is removal of enlarged tonsils and adenoids. More complicated causes (e.g. the various congenital upper airway abnormalities in Down syndrome) will be more difficult to treat.
- Treatment of narcolepsy mainly consists of stimulant drugs for the sleepiness and antidepressants for the other manifestations of the syndrome. Regular sleep, adequate sleep routines, planned naps during the day and timing of activities in relation to likely symptoms are important. Explanation of the disorder to all concerned is required, as well as support for what can be a very distressing and limiting condition, often associated with psychological problems.

Outcome

This also depends on cause of the child's EDS. For example, symptomatic control of narcolepsy is usually only partly achieved and treatment generally needs to be lifelong; DSPS, on the other hand, should respond completely to treatment providing there is sufficient motivation on the part of the young person and the family. Significant improvement in the child's psychological condition (also the

Table 11.5. Parasomnias related to stage of sleep

Sleep onset	Sleep starts
	Hypnagogic imagery
	Rhythmic movements
Light NREM sleep	Bruxism
	Periodic limb movements
	Panic attacks
Deep NREM sleep	Arousal disorders
	Confusional arousals
	Sleep walking
	Sleep terrors
REM sleep	Nightmares
	REM sleep behaviour disorder
	(sometimes a secondary parasomnia)
Waking	Hypnopompic imagery
	Sleep paralysis
Various stages of sleep	Nocturnal enuresis
	Sleeptalking
	Nocturnal seizures

family well-being) can be expected following successful treatment of EDS and the other forms of sleep disturbance.

Parasomnias

Definition and classification

Parasomnias is the term used for recurrent episodes of disturbed behaviour, experiences or physiological change which occur exclusively or predominantly in relation to sleep. Two basic types are distinguished:

- primary parasomnias which are sleep disorders in their own right
- secondary parasomnias which are manifestations of physical or psychological disorder.

In ICSD-R the primary parasomnias are classified according to the phase of sleep with which they are usually associated which gives the timing of their occurrence some diagnostic value (see Table 11.5 for some of the more common parasomnias and others of psychological interest).

Epidemiology

Prevalence and incidence

Again, overall rates are not known partly because the less dramatic forms of parasomnia do not come to medical attention. However, parasomnias are collectively very common especialy in middle childhood. No reliable information is available on overall sex ratio and ethnicity.

Implications for clinical practice

- Precise diagnosis is important as different parasomnias may need very different types of treatment.
- The more dramatic forms of parasomnia seem to be a particular cause of diagnostic confusion and imprecision and also quite possibly unnecessary concern about their psychological significance as most are benign.
- Most childhood primary parasomnias remit spontaneously within a few years and therefore children and parents can be reassured although protective measures (e.g. in severe headbanging or sleepwalking) may be required.
- Specific treatment, including medication is needed in only a minority of cases of primary parasomnia but is required for the underlying disorder in many of the secondary parasomnias.
- Although research information on this point is limited, a primary parasomnia might be symptomatic of a psychological problem if it is very frequent, unusually late in onset or persistent or associated with a traumatic experience.
- Parasomnias may lead to psychological disturbance if the child is frightened, embarrassed or otherwise upset by the experience or because of the reactions of other people to the episodes.

Clinical picture

Main features and symptoms

Sleep onset

- Sleep starts usually consist of an isolated sudden jerk but can take a dramatic sensory form (the 'exploding head syndrome').
- Hypnagogic hallucinations (or imagery) may accompany sleep starts but are also common experiences in their own right. The more usual form (unassociated with narcolepsy) can also be frightening, consisting of a combination of a dream-like state and awareness of the environment in which things may be seen, heard, felt, smelled, tasted or distorted. Their counterparts on waking are called hypnopompic hallucinations.
- Rhythmic movement disorder (RMD) refers to recurrent stereotyped movements, mainly of the upper part of the body, usually occurring at sleep onset but also in relation to nocturnal wakings and sometimes at the end of the sleep period. Headbanging in the best known form; head rolling, and rolling or rocking movements of the body are in the same category. These movements may be accompanied by vocalizations. Treatment is not usually needed except perhaps for protective measures such as padding on the cot sides. Unlike sleep-related rhythmic

movements, those which occur during the day are seen in children with severe developmental delay or other serious psychiatric conditions.
• Restless legs syndrome was discussed earlier.

Light NREM sleep (stages 1 and 2)
• Bruxism is forceful grinding and clenching of the teeth in a paroxysmal fashion.
• Periodic limb movements were mentioned earlier.

Deep (stages 3 and 4) NREM sleep (mainly in the first part of the overnight sleep)
The so-called disorders of arousal (i.e. confusional arousals, sleep walking and sleep terrors) are very common parasomnias in childhood. The arousal is, in fact, a partial arousal from deep NREM sleep (SWS) to another lighter stage of NREM sleep or REM sleep. A range of behaviours can occur (from simple to complicated) while the child remains asleep. Some children predisposed to arousal disorders also have such arousals arising from light NREM and REM sleep. Typically, there is only one episode on the night in question but there can be multiple episodes throughout the night, usually less dramatic each time. Arousals can occur during daytime naps. Three basic forms of arousal disorder are described. All have in common a strange combination of behaviour suggesting the child is simultaneously awake and asleep, with confusion, disorientation, unresponsiveness to the environment, automatic behaviour and little or (usually) no recall of events. In later childhood and subsequent ages (unlike earlier) there is a tendency to wake up at the end of an episode. In the individual child there may be a sequence of confusional arousals in early childhood, sleepwalking later and sleep terrors in late childhood and adolescence. Elements of all three can occur at any one stage of development.
• Confusional arousals occur mainly in infants and toddlers with agitated and confused behaviour and crying (which may be intense), calling out, or thrashing about. The child does not respond when spoken to but more forceful attempts to intervene may meet with resistance and increased agitation. Episodes usually last 5–15 minutes before the child and returns to restful sleep.
• Sleepwalking episodes usually last up to 10 minutes or so. The young child may crawl or walk about in his cot; at a later age he may walk around his room or to other parts of the house such as the toilet or his parents' bedroom. Urinating in inappropriate places is common. In later childhood or adolescence, wandering may extend further within or outside the house with an increased risk of accidental injury. Sleepwalking may take an agitated form with an even greater risk of injury from crashing through windows or glass doors, for example.
• Sleep (night) terrors tend to occur in older children and adolescents. Classically, parents are awoken by their child's piercing scream which marks the very sudden onset of the partial arousal. The child appears to be terrified with staring eyes,

intense sweating and rapid pulse and may jump out of bed and rush about frantically, as if pursued, in which case injury from running into furniture or windows is again a serious risk. The event usually lasts no more than a few minutes at most and ends abruptly. At that point the child might wake up and describe a feeling of primitive threat or danger (not the extended narrative of a nightmare).

REM sleep (mainly later in the night)
- True nightmares are characterized by awakening with vivid recall of a sequence of frightening events, (ie. narrative) often with personal involvement. The child may remain frightened after waking and be unable to return to sleep for some time, but reassurance and comforting is usually possible. The dreams may be spontaneous or, precipitated by illness and stress. Nightmares may well co-exist with bedtime fears.
- REM sleep behaviour disorder is characterized by a pathological preservation of skeletal muscle tone during REM sleep and, as a result, the enactment of dreams. If the dream content is violent, self-injury may well result or harm to others nearby. The condition, can be associated with neurological disorders in which case the condition is more appropriately classified as a secondary parasomnia (see below).

Waking
- Hypnopompic imagery was described earlier.
- Sleep paralysis can be very frightening, especially if associated with a feeling of difficulty breathing or inability to speak. Although sometimes part of the narcolepsy syndrome, it is possibly quite common as an occasional, isolated experience.

Parasomnias inconsistently associated with stage of sleep
- Nocturnal enuresis tends to occur in the first half of the night but is possible in any stage of sleep. Voiding of urine at night can also be linked with partial arousals, obstructive sleep apnoea or nocturnal epilepsy.
- Sleeptalking occurs in all sleep stages (mainly REM) and, although often spontaneous, it may occur in association with a number of other parasomnias.
- In parasomnia overlap disorder there are clinical and PSG features of sleepwalking, sleep terrors and REM sleep behaviour disorder.

Secondary parasomnias
The secondary parasomnias illustrate very well that it is important for clinicians in all specialties to be aware of the sleep-related manifestations of psychiatric and other medical disorders.

Nocturnal epilepsies

Sleep disorders can be confused with epilepsy and vice versa.

There are various types of epilepsy, both generalized and localized, in which the seizures are closely related to the sleep–wake cycle. In some the seizures are relatively subtle and may go undetected at night; in others the seizure manifestations are more dramatic creating a greater risk of diagnostic confusion.

- Nocturnal frontal lobe seizures are often misdiagnosed as being non-epileptic because of the complicated motor manifestations (e.g. kicking, hitting, rocking, thrashing and cycling or scissor movements of the legs) and vocalizations (from grunting, coughing, muttering or moaning to shouting, screaming or roaring) which often characterize these seizures.
- Other forms of sleep-related epilepsy at risk of misdiagnosis include seizures of temporal lobe origin with prominent affective symptoms, benign partial epilepsy of childhood with centrotemporal (Rolandic) spikes and benign occipital epilepsy.

Other parasomnias of physical origin

- Headaches of a migrainous type (sometimes related to REM sleep)
- Those associated with respiratory disorders such as asthma or sleep apnoea
- Gastro-intestinal conditions, e.g. gastro-oesophageal reflux
- Nocturnal muscle cramps
- Cardiac arrhythmias
- Both restless legs syndrome and periodic limb movements in sleep can be symptomatic of underlying physical illness.

Parasomnias secondary to psychiatric disorders

- Sleep disturbance (especially nightmares) is prominent feature of post-traumatic stress disorder (PTSD).
- Nocturnal panic attacks in children and adolescents may or may not be accompanied by daytime panic attacks.
- Other psychiatric disorders of which sleep disturbance, including parasomnias, is a common feature include anxiety states (nightmares), and Tourette syndrome (parasomnias). Sleep-related eating disorders, can be associated with daytime psychiatric disorders but more usually they have been linked with a number of other sleep disorders including sleepwalking.
- In pseudoparasomnias, dramatic behaviour, sometimes bizarre or violent, is enacted at night but actually while awake as shown by PSG.

A child may have more than one type of parasomnia. This may be either more than one primary parasomnia or a combination of a primary and secondary parasomnia.

Differential diagnosis and co-morbidity

The various parasomnias need to be distinguished from each other because of their different origins, significance and treatment requirements. Unfortunately, they are often confused because their characteristic features are not known sufficiently. There is a tendency to use the terms 'nightmare' or 'night terror' for any dramatic nocturnal events. In fact, fear or apparently fearful behaviour can occur with very different parasomnias such as true nightmares, agitated sleepwalking, sleep terrors, obstructive sleep apnoea awakenings, some seizures and panic attacks.

Obviously secondary parasomnias are accompanied by physical or psychiatric conditions of which they are part manifestation. In contrast, even dramatic primary parasomnias (e.g. headbanging or sleep terrors) are not intrinsically accompanied by comorbid psychiatric disorder but the child may become disturbed emotionally as reaction to experiencing alarming phenomena (e.g. hallucinatory experiences) because of embarrassment (e.g. sleepwalking when staying with friends or bedwetting) or as a result of parental concern.

Assessment

Detailed clinical assessment is essential for correct diagnosis. There are no diagnostic instruments of particular value. It is necessary to obtain as far as possible the subjective and observed details of the onset of the episode and precise sequence of events until the episode is concluded. The timing and circumstances surrounding the episodes are also very important.

Especially when parents have been alarmed by witnessing the child's night-time episodes, they may be unable to provide sufficient detail, or their account may be distorted with an understandable emphasis on the more dramatic features. In these circumstances, a diary record completed at the time, or the use of home video, may provide helpful diagnostic information. Even so, the diagnosis may remain unclear in which case some form of home-based or inpatient monitoring, combining audio-video and either EEG or sleep recording, will be required.

The following enquiries are likely to identify the nature of the parasomnia in most cases.

General

Enquiries should be made about:
• any daytime attacks (generally favours epilepsy or panic attacks)
• neurological or other physical abnormality
• family history (often positive in arousal disorders).

Consider possible combination of different attacks, each needing separate detailed assessment.

Are there features which raise the possibility that the parasomnias are associated with an underlying psychological problem? In particular:

- high frequency
- unusually late age of onset, recurrence or persistence over many years
- preceding trauma
- accompanying features of a psychological disorder.

Is there evidence of another sleep disorder with which the parasomnia might be linked?

Specific features
Occurrence in first 2 hours of overnight sleep suggests arousal disorder characterized by:

- being inaccessible during episodes
- no recall
- often family history.

Occurrence late in night suggests REM sleep related disorder especially:

- true nightmares

Daytime episodes when awake indicate a secondary parasomnia such as:

- epilepsy
- asthma
- panic attacks.

Aetiology

In contrast to the secondary parasomnias (the aetiology of which should be self evident if the condition is correctly diagnosed), it is difficult to generalize about the cause of the wide range of primary parasomnias. The following further illustrates the aetiological diversity of the parasomnias.

- The aetiology of many primary parasomnias is ill defined and seems to be some form of common temporary predisposition without clear genetic or other familial factors (e.g. rhythmic movement disorders).
- In contrast, factors predisposing to arousal disorders clearly include genetic influences (often there is a family history), sleep loss or sleep disrupting factors such as stress or trauma. Precipitating factors include systemic illness and CNS depressant medication.
- Nightmares can be precipitated by REM suppressing substances including some psychotropic drugs and alcohol. Frequent nightmares may indicated stress or trauma the nature of which might be apparent from their content.

Treatment

Similarly, different parasomnias require different forms of treatment.

- The underlying cause of a secondary parasomnia calls for specific treatment such as antiepileptic medication or psychiatric management of PTSD.

- In most cases of primary parasomnia of the temporary, 'developmental' type, explanation and reassurance are appropriate although protective or safety measures may well be required, e.g. in headbanging against hard surfaces or in view of the risk of accidental injury in sleepwalking.
- Parental education is important in arousal disorders including dissuading them from trying to waken their child in order to comfort him. This is both difficult and likely to be counter-productive.
- 'Anticipatory awakening' before an arousal disorder is due can be helpful.
- Medication has a limited role but can be helpful, e.g. in the treatment of nocturnal enuresis, as a short-term measure for arousal disorders in particularly difficult circumstances, and also for REM sleep behaviour disorder.
- Regular and adequate sleep routines and other sleep hygiene principles are of general value.

Outcome

This also varies widely. As mentioned, many childhood primary parasomnias are self limiting unless maintaining factors continue to operate long-term. The determining factors in secondary parasomnias is the responsiveness to treatment of the underlying disorder.

SUGGESTED READING

Books

G. Stores (2001). *A Clinical Guide to Sleep Disorders in Children and Adolescents.* Cambridge: Cambridge University Press.

G. Stores & L. Wiggs (2001). *Sleep Disturbance in Children and Adolescents with Disorders of Development: its Significance and Management.* London: Mac Keith Press.

Articles

American Sleep Disorders Association (1997). ICSD – *International Classification of Sleep Disorders, Revised: Diagnostic and Coding Manual.* Rochester, MN: American Sleep Disorders Association.

G. Fallone, J. A. Owens & J. Deane (2002). Sleepiness in children and adolescents: clinical implications. *Sleep Medicine Reviews,* **6**, 287–306.

J. Garcia, G. Rosen & M. Mahowald (2001). Circadian rhythms and circadian rhythm disorders in children and adolescents. *Seminars in Paediatric Neurology,* **8**, 229–40.

T. F. Hoban & R. D. Chervin (2001). Assessment of sleepiness in children. *Seminars in Paediatric Neurology,* **8**, 216–28.

N. King, T. H. Ollendick & B. J. Tongue (1997). Children's nighttime fears. *Clinical Psychology Review,* **17**, 431–43.

J. A. Owens, A. Spirito & M. McGuinn (2000). The Children's Sleep Habits Questionnaire (CSHQ): psychometric properties of a survey instrument for school-aged children. *Sleep*, **23**, 1043–51.

J. L. Owens, K. G. France & L. Wiggs (1999). Behavioural and cognitive-behavioural interventions for sleep disorders in infants and children: a review. *Sleep Medicine Reviews*, **3**, 281–302.

G. Stores (2003). Misdiagnosis of sleep disorders as primary psychiatric conditions. *Advances in Psychiatric Treatment*, **9**, 69–77.

G. Stores, Medication for sleep–wake disorders. *Archives of Disease in Childhood*. (In press).

A. R. Wolfson & M. A. Carskadon (1998). Sleep schedules and daytime functioning in adolescents. *Child Development*, **69**, 875–87.

12

Personality disorders

Jonathan Hill, Michaela Swales and Marie Byatt

Child and Development Psychiatry, Royal Liverpool Children's Hospital, UK

Introduction and concepts

'Personality disorder' (PD) is a term that is used in a variety of ways, some helpful and some less so. It can be synonymous with 'not treatable', 'not within the remit of mental health services', or even 'nasty'. This chapter does not refer to any of these. We are referring to relatively persistent maladaptive behaviours and patterns of interpersonal and social role functioning, that are not readily accounted for by discrete episodes of psychiatric disorder.

The available definitions of personality disorder specify that it cannot be diagnosed before age 18. In many respects this simply reflects that many of the identifying features of the personality disorders refer to functioning within adult social roles. It might also be sensible to reserve the term for adults if it were clear that childhood and adolescence is essentially a period of transition and change, contrasted with adult life as a time during which change is unlikely, and if it were to be used to denote that the problems were not open to change. However there is ample evidence for strong continuities in some relevant characteristics, such as aggression and anxious inhibition over childhood and adolescence, and for the possibilities for change during adult life. Furthermore, it is not helpful to include inability to change in the definition of personality disorder. That is an issue that is available for empirical study in relation to different patterns of disorder.

With these considerations in mind, it could be argued that the concept of personality disorder, appropriately modified to take account of adolescent social roles, will be useful in adolescence and even childhood. This may turn out to be the case; however, given the current state of knowledge, that would be premature, because there are major issues to be resolved in relation to personality disorder in adults. If the term is simply imported into practice with younger individuals, those difficulties

A Clinician's Handbook of Child and Adolescent Psychiatry, ed. Christopher Gillberg, Richard Harrington and Hans-Christoph Steinhausen. Published by Cambridge University Press.

will come with it. Equally, the phenomena that the adult concept points to, such as persistent antisocial behaviours, repeated self-injury, or major interpersonal problems, also need a framework of description and explanation before the age of 18. That makes the case for making use, with younger age groups, of what we know about personality disorder mainly from adults.

Standard definitions

Personality disorders in adults are considered to have the following features.

- An enduring condition involving patterns of behaviour and inner experience manifested in the areas of affectivity, cognition, interpersonal functioning or impulse control. These patterns deviate distinctly from the expectations of the person's culture.
- The patterns are pervasive, affecting a considerable range of social and personal situations.
- The onset is in childhood, adolescence or early adulthood.
- The patterns of inner experience and behaviour often cause significant distress and frequently lead to difficulties in social and occupational functioning.
- It is a stable condition that is not limited to episodes of mental illness.
- It is not caused by a general medical condition and is not due to the physiological effects of a substance.

The two main mental health classifications, DSM-IV and ICD-10 share these general criteria for diagnosing personality disorders and then both identify a number of specific personality disorders that generally overlap although they are classified in a slightly different way (see Tables 12.1 and 12.2). For example, DSM-IV lists borderline personality disorder as a distinct personality disorder whereas ICD-10 identifies borderline as a sub-group of emotionally unstable personality disorder. DSM-IV also groups the personality disorders into three 'Clusters', Cluster A – Eccentric, Cluster B – dramatic, and Cluster C – anxious, avoidant.

Both ICD-10 and DSM-IV take the view that a diagnosis of personality disorder usually is not appropriate in adolescence because the behaviour patterns of personality disorder need to be of a long-standing and enduring nature. ICD-10 considers it unlikely that a personality disorder diagnosis will be appropriate before the age of 16 or 17. For a diagnosis in an individual under the age of 18, DSM-IV requires the relevant traits to be present for at least a year, but states that it is unusual for a person in this age group to display pervasive and persistent traits that are not limited to a particular developmental stage or to another mental health problem. DSM-IV does not allow for the diagnosis of antisocial personality disorder under the age of 18. Both ICD-10 and DSM-IV emphasize the importance of considering variations in social norms within different cultures when making judgements regarding personality functioning.

Table 12.1. ICD-10 Disorders of adult personality and behaviour

Paranoid personality disorder
Schizoid personality disorder
Dissocial personality disorder
Emotionally unstable personality disorder
  Impulsive type
  Borderline type
Histrionic personality disorder
Anxious (avoidant) personality disorder
Dependent personality disorder
Anankastic personality disorder
Other specific personality disorders (including narcissistic)
Personality disorder, unspecified

Table 12.2. DSM-IV personality disorders

Paranoid personality disorder Schizoid personality disorder Schizotypal personality disorder	cluster A 'odd or eccentric'
Antisocial personality disorder Borderline personality disorder Histrionic personality disorder Narcissistic personality disorder	cluster B 'dramatic, emotional or erratic'
Avoidant personality disorder Dependent personality disorder Obsessive–compulsive personality disorder	cluster C 'anxious or fearful'
Personality disorder not otherwise specified	

General issues and clinical implications

Controversial issues in the definition of personality disorders

The current controversies in personality disorder are so far reaching in their implications that they need to be reviewed briefly as a background to issues in clinical assessment. References to more detailed discussion are included in the reading list. Currently, there is little consensus regarding the way personality disorders should be conceptualized, nor whether there is an overarching personality disorder entity with subtypes, or fundamentally different kinds of disorder. The term 'personality' in the name of the diagnosis might suggest that the identity of the disorder is firmly rooted in a science of personality and its deviations. However, this is far from the case. There are promising formulations proposing that personality disorders result from combinations of extremes of temperament, such as novelty seeking and lack of behavioural inhibition. However, these do not account well for factors affecting the variability of human behaviours depending on situations and contexts. Other personality theories pay great attention to the nature of interactions between individuals and their environments, however they have not yet contributed substantially to our understanding of personality disorders. In practice it seems that clinicians use criteria that are not closely linked to ideas about normal personality. Studies find that they take account of patients' descriptions of their interpersonal functioning, and their own observations of patients' behaviours in interview. Other clinically based formulations have referred to failures of the self-system, and difficulties in intimate relationships and wider social and occupational interactions. These provide pointers to aspects of functioning to be assessed in adolescents.

There are also doubts regarding the separate identities of hypothesized personality disorders. It is extremely common for an individual to meet criteria for more than one personality disorder and the meaning of this co-occurrence is not clear. This may represent true co-morbidity, the co-occurrence of more than one discrete disorder, but equally may reflect deficits in the current classification. Furthermore co-occurrence of personality disorders and episodic disorders (DSM Axis I) is also very common. It is likely that personality disorders confer risk for Axis I disorders, and that Axis I disorders contribute to impaired personality functioning, and that common factors may underpin both.

We come next to the question of whether it is useful to group diverse symptoms together into a personality disorders. This will be fruitful if it is the case that drawing diverse 'symptoms' together proves effective in understanding causes, course, or response to treatment. In medicine syphilis is an effective example, and developmentally this is also true of autism. However, this approach introduces some definite limitations that are particularly relevant when considering adolescence. For example, unstable relationships and self-harming behaviours are two items in the borderline personality disorder diagnosis. They could therefore be viewed as 'symptoms' of one underlying process. Equally, there may be processes linking the two that can be identified only if they are considered in their own right instead of jointly. For example, there may be particular features of intimate relationships associated with self harm. Investigating possible causal links requires that relationship features and self-harm are identified separately and that temporal associations between the two are established. Clinically, it is important to consider ways in which one symptom of personality disorder may contribute to risk for others, and may therefore be an important target for treatment.

Current concepts of personality disorder suffer from a further crucial limitation, from the perspective of understanding adolescent disturbance, that they do not attend to the nature of the interactions between the individual and his/her environment. Yet there is ample evidence that person–environment interactions are a key to understanding outcomes. Proactive interactions whereby the individual selects particular environments, and evocative interactions in which a person's behaviours affect their environment, can have positive and negative effects. Problem behaviours within personality disorders, such as unstable educational or work performance, often lead to unfavourable occupational and economic environments, which then become part of the overall problem, and major factors in the course or response to treatment. Taking the example of the possible link between features of intimate relationships that might contribute to self harm, these may include characteristics of other people with whom the patient forms relationships, and the behaviours evoked in others to whom he/she is close.

Finally current concepts of PD appear to make developmental assumptions without making them explicit, and this is of considerable importance to assessment of adolescents. For example, the definition of borderline personality disorder refers to instability of intimate relationships, which in practice generally mean romantic relationships. Intimate stable romantic relationships are not common in early adolescence, and so instability may not be a relevant concept. Equally, clinical experience suggests that adolescents with personality difficulties, including those with borderline features, commonly do form intense romantic relationships that break down. However, the pattern of intensity and instability in adolescence may be seen in other relationships, with peers, teachers, or mental health professionals.

Issues in the diagnosis of personality disorders in adolescence

These considerations point to the need for clinical assessments and formulations to consider, not only maladaptive moods, beliefs or behaviours specified by the diagnostic criteria, but also a person's functioning in a range of social domains, and psychiatric symptoms, such as anxiety and depression. Furthermore it is crucial to keep in mind that co-occurring problems may be inter-related, and cannot be assumed simply to be features of one condition. It is therefore important to ensure that a range of problems are evaluated in their own right. Broadly, these fall into three groups of psychological symptoms, abnormal behaviours and social role dysfunction.

Psychological symptoms include markedly depressed or angry mood, affective instability, misattributions of other's behaviours, lack of empathy; abnormalities of behaviour include parasuicide, self-injury, impulsive decision making, or violence; and social role dysfunction educational/occupational failure and persistent avoidance or breakdown of social relationships of varying intensity. The diversity of problems in the personality disorders can place particular demands on detection, assessment and treatment, and this is particularly the case in adolescence. They may be evident in primary care, the accident and emergency department, paediatric outpatients, child and adolescent mental health services, social services residential units, foster care, school and the youth justice service. Establishing that a young person has pervasive difficulties requires both that information is gathered across agencies, and that it is integrated to form a profile of the young person's problems as a whole. For many agencies the idea of doing this within the framework of personality disorder would be seen as stigmatizing or pejorative. However, the view taken in this chapter is that the framework can be used to ensure an adequately holistic assessment, that attends to particular processes, and provides a basis for effective management. Usually, the treatment also has to tackle problems over a broad front, and often the key to a successful outcome is a shared plan and good communication.

The framework outlined here, also emphasizes the need to identify specific areas of dysfunction, and their specific causal factors. For example, in assessing violence the identification of antisocial or borderline personality disorder is a blunt instrument. It provides an indication of the duration and diversity of the problems, and some pointers to a broad set of risks. However, the clinical task is to identify the immediate factors that contribute to the likelihood of violence acts, and the background maintaining factors. This may be informed, for example, by research into executive function and antisocial and borderline personality disorders, but not yet by studies that link specific deficits to specific kinds of violence.

Crucially, the way the individual creates and selects environments through interactions with peers, educational settings, family and therapeutic team needs to be described and understood. The adolescent girl who dresses in a sexually provocative manner, is likely to 'select' an environment of antisocial males, who commonly come from families with several antisocial or borderline members. Thus one set of behaviours, in itself relatively circumscribed, can increase demands substantially on a young person with limited coping strategies. Identifying behaviours that contribute to unfavourable person–environment interactions is therefore an element of assessment, with treatment implications.

In spite of the marked overlap between personality disorder types some distinctions are of value clinically, and influence management. Schizotypal personality disorder in adult life is characterized by a pervasive pattern of social and interpersonal deficits marked by acute discomfort with, and reduced capacity for, close relationships, as well as by cognitive or perceptual distortions and eccentricities of behaviour, beginning by early adulthood. It is likely that the concept of a spectrum of schizophrenic disorders, including schizotypal personality disorder, applies in the pre-adult years, as well as later. Some studies have also indicated that there may be links between schizotypal features in adolescence and pervasive developmental disorders. Sula Wolff described a 'schizoid' disorder in childhood characterized by increased sensitivity, paranoid ideas and an odd style of communicating, with continuities with schizotypal disorder in adult life.

The main features of DSM antisocial personality disorder, in adult life, are unstable work and relationship history, law breaking, fighting, impulsivity and failure to plan, disregard for the safety of self or others, deceitfulness and lack of remorse for antisocial behaviours. DSM IV requires that these behaviours are preceded by conduct disorder before the diagnosis can be made. The ICD definition is, in many ways, similar and specifies callous unconcern for the feelings of others, low tolerance to frustration and low threshold for aggression, incapacity to experience guilt and to profit from experience (including punishment), and proneness to blame others or offer rationalizations for antisocial behaviours. ICD states that dissocial personality disorder is usually preceded by conduct disorder, and this is supported by a substantial body of evidence from prospective studies, finding continuities from early onset antisocial problems to adult antisocial disorders. If antisocial problems in adolescence are characterized in terms of conduct disorder, it is important for the clinician to keep in mind commonly associated difficulties, included in the personality disorder diagnosis, such as poor peer relationships. However, currently there are no strong reasons to consider antisocial problems in adolescence in terms of personality disorder rather than conduct disorder, which is described in Chapter 18. The remainder of this chapter will focus on borderline personality disorder.

Borderline personality disorder

Borderline personality disorder is described in adults as a severe and chronic disorder characterized by a pervasive instability of affect and interpersonal relationships, and impulsivity. Behaviours that commonly lead to distress and impairment include suicide attempts, self-harm and substance misuse. Co-occurring anxiety and mood disorders are common. Estimates of its prevalence in the general population range between 0.4 per cent and 2 per cent.

Definition and classification

Overwhelmingly, recent research in this area has made use of the DSM IV criteria for borderline personality disorder (BPD). There are nine criteria of which five or more need to be present:
- frantic efforts to avoid real or imagined abandonment
- a pattern of unstable and intense interpersonal relationships characterized by alternating between extremes of idealization and devaluation

- identity disturbance: markedly and persistently unstable self-image or sense of self
- impulsivity in at least two areas that are potentially self-damaging (e.g. spending, sex, substance abuse, reckless driving, binge eating).
- recurrent suicidal behaviour, gestures or threats or self-mutilating behaviour
- affective instability due to a marked reactivity of mood (intense episodic dysphoria, irritability or anxiety)
- chronic feelings of emptiness
- inappropriate or intense anger or difficulty controlling anger (e.g. frequent displays of temper, constant anger, recurrent physical fights)
- transient stress-related paranoid ideation or severe dissociative symptoms.

In ICD-10, the diagnosis is 'emotionally unstable personality disorder' which includes impulsivity, emotional instability and outbursts of anger. The 'borderline type' refers to disturbance of self-image, chronic feelings of emptiness, liability to become involved in intense and unstable relationships, excessive efforts to avoid abandonment and self harm. Thus the only substantive difference is that ICD-10 does not include transient paranoid or dissociative symptoms.

Clinical picture

In practice, the problems of unstable mood and relationships, and impulsive behaviours, especially of self-harm, are the ones that alert the clinician to the possibility of borderline personality disorder. The prototypic profile of a person with borderline personality disorder refers to a young woman with intense unstable intimate relationships, marked rapid changes of mood, impulsive behaviours including self-harm and a markedly and persistently unstable self-image or sense of self. It might be argued that this is less likely to be discriminating in adolescence, which itself has been characterized as a period of instability of relationships, mood swings and identity crisis. However, in practice it is not difficult to identify, even young, adolescent males and females who show the same or similar problems to a degree that clearly sets them apart from most of their peers.

The DSM profile envisages instability of romantic relationships, whereas it is unusual for young adolescents to have any but relatively superficial boyfriend/girlfriend relationships. However, there are patterns of relating in early adolescence that appear to be forerunners of the adult pattern. Sometimes, the young person is already forming intense romantic attachments, either ones that break down rather like those in adults, or ones that are more stable but in which there is a greater intensity and reliance than is common in early adolescence.

Irrespective of whether there are intense romantic relationships, intensity and instability are generally seen in other intimate relationships. This is evident particularly in relationships with parents, and with peers. One of the few studies to examine, prospectively, family relationships associated with the emergence of borderline disorder during adolescence found that maternal inconsistency and high maternal overinvolvement were key processes. Further work is needed to establish to what extent these maternal behaviours not only played a causal role, but also reflected to some degree intense unstable relating in the young people that was already present prior to the emergence of borderline disorder that met DSM criteria.

Relationships with peers can also form rapidly and intensely, thereby more resembling romantic relationships, and then are either dropped suddenly or breakdown. When borderline young people are in care, they often form rapid and intense attachments with residential staff or foster parents, which are also prone to becoming rapidly negative. Another feature commonly observed in adolescents and adults is the tendency to form intense relationships, or attachments, with inappropriate people, for example with a teacher or a caretaker in a residential unit. This is consistent with the research evidence that borderline adults are likely to have a preoccupied or entangled form of insecure attachment. It suggests that borderline functioning is also associated with a low threshold for perceiving attachment cues in others' behaviours, and seeking the care and attention normally associated with established attachment figures either prematurely or inappropriately.

Repeated self-harm may already be prominent in adolescence, either as overdoses with varying degrees of suicidal intent, or self-injury without any suicidal motives. Most commonly, this involves cutting, which varies between superficial scratching and serious disfiguring injury. However, there are many other methods including swallowing objects, or placing objects up the vagina or anus. Young people with chronic physical conditions such as diabetes or renal failure may mismanage their condition to self-harm. Other behaviours that are not so self-evidently motivated by self-harm sometimes appear to have that function. Examples include running away, having sex with strangers and prostitution. This may be linked to confusion about identity. A young adolescent girl may dress at times in a sexually provocative way that puts her at risk, but at other times like a younger child implying a need for a greater than usual level of care from adults.

It is as important to focus on the aspects of functioning that are not emphasized in the borderline formulation as those that are. Strikingly, problems in the management of day-to-day living and in work are not generally considered in the diagnosis of borderline personality disorder, but they are commonly present. Similarly, although some adolescents manage to maintain academic functioning and self-care, many do not. School performance can be disrupted by peer difficulties and by effects of mood swings on attention and motivation in school and on school attendance.

A key feature of borderline personality disorder, not included in the diagnostic items, but very familiar to clinicians, is a distinctive pattern of responding among those who have attempted to provide support or treatment. This is characterized by exceptional efforts, unusual practices and markedly contrasting opinions. Often the network is large and includes professionals who have dedicated more time, or made more commitments, to the young person than they do for most. Sometimes this seems to happen without any particular motivation, but often those involved are drawn by their perception of the extent of the young person's vulnerability coupled with a sense that they personally can do something that others cannot. Equally, it is common for others in the network to take a very negative view, feeling for example that too much is being offered, that those who take a sympathetic view are being deceived or manipulated, or that apparent change is illusory.

Differential diagnosis

Differential diagnosis with other personality disorders may appear to be a redundant concept given that multiple disorders is so common. However, in practice, characterizing the predominant pattern can be very informative. This is particularly the case in relation to antisocial personality disorder. It is very common for adolescents who meet BPD criteria also to be seriously antisocial. However, clinically there often appear to be core features of the condition that point in one rather than the other direction, for example differences in the quality of the instability of close relationships. In some instances it appears to arise from a lack of personal or emotional investment in particular relationships, and this seems more characteristic of the antisocial pattern. Where this amounts to callousness, the difference from the borderline pattern is clear; however it may be more subtle, where the individual claims a strong attachment but also behaves with indifference or cruelty. In other instances the drive for intensity and attachment predominates, with the formation of idealized relationships, and bitter disappointment when they fail to come up to expectations. This suggests borderline functioning.

It is a moot point as to whether consideration of the number of comorbid personality disorders is of clinical value. Certainly, these often cross the boundaries of the DSM 'Clusters' so that the young person with borderline features (Cluster B) may also be anxious and avoidant in social situations (Cluster C). However the key to treatment is identifying domains with problematic functioning and those where functioning is good, and assessing the factors and processes contributing to dysfunction.

Studies of adults indicate that individuals with personality disorders generally also have symptoms of episodic disorders, referred to in DSM as Axis I Disorders. It is common also for adolescents with personality dysfunction to suffer from depression, one or more anxiety disorders, post-traumatic stress disorder, alcohol or drug abuse or dependence, or an eating disorder. It is essential to identify these disorders, to integrate their treatment with the overall management of the young person's difficulties. In doing this it is important to keep in mind that we know very little of the way in which the symptoms and underlying processes in episodic disorders interact with personality problems. This is the case with respect to the origins of the disorders, and their treatment. Sometimes, the effective treatment of an episodic disorder such as depression also leads to a substantial improvement in wider dysfunction that had been attributed to personality difficulties. This is consistent with the developmental evidence that not only do personality difficulties increase the risk for episodic disorders, but also episodic disorders increase the likelihood of subsequent personality disorders. Equally, the effective treatment of an episodic disorder may have no beneficial effects on the wider functioning of the young person. In other cases there can be substantial improvement of Axis I symptoms as personality difficulties are tackled. Generally, however, any treatments for Axis I disorders need to be embedded in the wider management which is guided by the principles outlined earlier.

Differentiation of borderline difficulties from the social and communication difficulties referred to variously as autistic spectrum disorders or Asperger syndrome can be difficult, but very important. Misdiagnosis is particularly likely to occur where the young person's deficits have been missed prior to puberty, but become much more prominent as he/she makes serious misinterpretations in social and especially sexual interactions. The lack of social awareness can lead to inappropriate attachments, and there can be rapid changes of mood and self-harm especially where the young person experiences repeated rejections or sexual exploitation.

Assessment

Many of the key tasks in carrying out an assessment are implied by the issues reviewed in the previous section. Generally, when a young person with borderline problems is referred to a child and adolescent mental health team several other agencies are already involved. Indeed, the extent of that involvement alerts the clinician to the possibility that he/she has these problems. It is not possible to be prescriptive about the order in which things are done, however, generally, early contact with key people in the network of professionals who are already involved is helpful. This is particularly the case where he/she is in contact with social services or the courts, but even where that is not the case, teachers or school support workers, and various medical professionals may already have a prominent role. At the same time, it is essential to work within a framework that takes account of who has parental responsibility, and who should be informed and can give consent, making sure that at all times the young person is fully engaged.

This means that commonly the processes of assessment, and of engagement go hand in hand. For example, the team may receive a telephone call from a worried support worker in a school about a 14-year-old girl who has told her that she is cutting herself, and does not want her parents to know. Such a call is usually about the young person's problem and the anxiety of the support worker. The clinician needs to ask questions such as does the girl know about the phone call, who has the support worker talked to in the school, and what is the support worker's view regarding telling the parents? It may be helpful to know about the support worker's role in the school, and about the usual lines of communication and decision making. The answers to these questions provide information about processes in the young person's professional network and therefore also about the young person herself. At the same time, by asking such questions, the mental health worker positions his/her self to providing a helpful response. If these topics are not clarified, in the tangled web of unclear communications that often surrounds the young person with borderline difficulties, such phone calls can rapidly lead a helpful child and adolescent mental health team into further compounding the confusion. Clearly, not all young people who cut themselves have borderline difficulties, and phone calls of this kind may be made about young people with a wide range of clinical problems. Equally, an awareness of the confusions that often surround the young borderline helps a clinical team to reflect early on the need to clarify each step of the referral and assessment process.

The ultimate aim of the first steps is to ensure that assessment can be carried out with the agreement of those who have parental responsibilities, and the full knowledge of the young person. In practice, this can involve difficult decisions, for example where the young person threatens serious self-harm if parents or social workers are informed. Even once this has been established, the task of assessment is often one that has to take account of the young person's particular difficulties or vulnerabilities. In line with the assessment of psychiatric disorders in adolescence generally, the process should include interviews with the young person, with those close to him/her, and teachers. Family interviews, tests of academic attainment, of IQ, and of specific neuropsychological functions each should be considered. However, each has to be timed carefully, paying attention to the young person's responses to what is being offered.

Commonly, the adolescent with borderline difficulties is ambivalent about help that is offered, at the same time behaving in ways that communicate a need to be helped, and rejecting that help, at least from some people. This may mean that individual interviews, however sensitively carried out may be counter-productive, and that many of the early steps entail gathering information from various informants, combined with circumscribed contacts with the young person. Where the young person is happy to be seen alone, the interviewer needs to be sensitive to the way he/she experiences his/her self and others. This is particularly important in relation to the process described by Kleinian psychoanalysts as splitting. This refers to the tendency to perceive the self and others either in an entirely positive light, or as completely useless or/and hopeless. As a consequence, the interview may appear inappropriately bland or positive, tempting the interviewer to press for discussion of the problems, in an attempt to assess the young person's view of them. This may under some circumstances be appropriate and informative, and under others lead to a sudden change of mood and behaviour that undermines the engagement.

Standardized assessments for personality disorders in adults are well established. These include the Structured Clinical Interview for DSM-IV Personality Disorders, and the Personality Disorder Examination. Several studies of personality disorders in adolescence have made use of these measures, and report patterns of symptoms similar to those found in adults. They are semi-structured interviews in which the interviewer works systematically through the DSM criteria for each personality disorder, asking whether the subject suffers from the problem. For many of the items the interview requires examples of affected behaviours, and the interviewer should attempt to establish that they occur in several settings. Crucially, the symptoms should be long standing and not simply a function of an episodic disorder such as depression.

Many adolescents with personality difficulties do not find it easy to work through a standardized interview lasting an hour or more, and then informant accounts may be needed. In our experience carers and professionals are often able to answer most of the questions in a standardized interview for the personality disorders. Furthermore, features of borderline personality disorder, such as mood instability and identity disturbance, may affect the sufferer's ability to provide an accurate account of their own difficulties, in which case informant accounts may be more valid.

It will have been evident from previous sections that making the diagnosis of one or more DSM or ICD personality disorders forms only one element of an adequate assessment of the treatment needs of an adolescent with borderline problems. Crucially, one cannot place a strong emphasis on whether or not the patient meets the requirement to fulfil five criteria in making clinical judgements. Fewer than the required criteria may be met at a high level of intensity or frequency leading to marked impairment, and that should not lead the clinician to conclude that a personality disorder is not present. For example, most clinicians would regard evidence of repeated intense idealized attachments across a range of relationships, coupled with a low threshold for perceiving rejection or neglect, as indicative of borderline problems, irrespective of the patient's diagnostic status.

With these caveats in mind, standardized assessments do have the advantage of ensuring that a range of relevant problems is covered, and enable different patients' problems to be compared systematically. Given the paucity of studies in the field, they may also be used to establish much needed prospective studies of clinical samples.

Aetiology

Many theories of the origins of borderline personality disorder have proposed a central role for adverse, and in particular traumatic, experiences in childhood. Among referred adults with borderline personality disorder the rate of recalled sexual abuse and neglect is very high; above 90 per cent in some studies. While it is likely that childhood trauma and neglect have a role in the development of borderline personality disorder, very little is known regarding their importance compared with other risk factors, nor of possible causal mechanisms. A meta-analysis covering 21 studies into possible associations between child sexual abuse and borderline personality disorder found there was only a moderate pooled effect size. Childhood sexual abuse and neglect are experienced by at least 20 per cent of girls before the age of 16 contrasted with general population prevalence estimates of borderline personality disorders (BPD) of 0.4–2 per cent. Therefore, even if abusive or neglectful experiences were necessary for borderline personality disorder, they would not be sufficient, and it is likely that more specific aspects of childhood adversities together with other vulnerability factors need to be identified.

Identification of the role of specific aspects of childhood adversity is likely to require more precise specification of the phenomena to be explained. For example, individuals with borderline personality disorder also report more dissociative experiences and these may have their own antecedents, or may share them with borderline problems more generally. There is currently no consensus on psychological mechanisms in borderline personality disorder that might provide a link with adverse experiences in childhood; however emotional dysregulation and failure of reflective function are both promising candidates. Several studies have suggested that intrusive and inconsistent mother–child interactions may contribute to the risk for borderline personality disorder, and links with hypothesized psychological mechanisms can be envisaged. Intrusive parenting is likely to lead to intense affect from which the child takes evasive action to reduce affect, hence leading to the experience of extremes of emotional intensity. Inconsistent mother–child interactions are likely to inhibit the child's capacity to read the intentions or states of mind of the parent, and hence limit his/her ability to think of others' behaviours in mental state terms. If, as is often the case, the parent also has been abusive, and therefore conceiving of the parent's motives includes understanding motives for abusive behaviour, the child is likely to inhibit reflection regarding the parent, with implications for reflectiveness more generally.

These speculations may be of value clinically; however it is crucial to keep in mind how little we know about the development of borderline personality disorder. In contrast to the substantial body of prospective findings on the nature and causes of the childhood antecedents of antisocial personality disorder, we know very little about the functioning of borderline individuals before puberty. It is possible, given the co-morbidity discussed earlier, that some antisocial adolescents and young adults with histories of conduct problems and attention deficit/hyperactivity disorders as young children, might also be considered to have borderline pathology. However clinical experience suggests that, although some adolescents with clear borderline features have had overt behavioural and social problems as young children, many have not. We do not yet understand the nature of the early vulnerabilities.

One consequence of this paucity of evidence is that our knowledge of the early biological and psychological risks is very limited. By definition these cannot be assessed retrospectively. However, our working assumption must be that there are individual vulnerabilities that interact with environmental risks. Temperamental characteristics of emotional lability and impulsiveness are likely candidates, as are prefrontal cortex deficits leading to difficulties, for example, in making adaptive responses to changing situations.

Treatment

The assessment, and above all, the treatment of borderline personality difficulties in young people provide a challenge not only to individual clinicians, but to child and adolescent mental health teams, and to the wider organization of services. Currently services for young borderline adolescents are provided across a wide range of settings including residential adolescent units, day facilities, and therapeutic fostering projects. One common feature of all of these, and of similar facilities for young adults, is the close integrated working of professionals, to create an intensive coherent approach. Generally, it is helpful for the professionals to have a shared 'model' that informs their work together, and provides a basis for working with the divisions that are often engendered by borderline processes. Crucially, a treatment team also must relate to a wide range of professionals who are likely to be unfamiliar with the model. Sometimes it is possible, especially if a collaboration can be established over time, to share the model with other agencies. Equally, it is essential that such a process is respectful of differences, otherwise it is vulnerable to the communication difficulties described earlier. Where it is not possible to explicitly share models of working, it is essential for treatment teams to convey a capacity to think about and respect contrasting perspectives, and to display a quiet insistence on the clarity of communication, responsibility and decision making. The aim is to create a platform from which the specific problems of the young person can be addressed.

No one treatment has been established as the standard approach, because adequately powered randomized controlled trials have not been conducted. In this chapter we have focused on dialectical behaviour therapy (DBT) because it embodies the principles discussed that appear to be necessary for all treatments for borderline problems, and it has been used extensively with adults. Clinical experience and small non-randomized trials suggest that it is well suited to the treatment of borderline adolescents.

Dialectical behaviour therapy (DBT)

DBT considers the primary problem to be one of affect regulation (lability of mood and problems with anger). As a consequence of this difficulty, both adolescents and adults who meet the criteria have difficulty regulating interpersonal relationships (chaotic relationships and fear of abandonment); in controlling behaviour (suicidal and impulsive behaviours); in regulating the sense of self (identity disturbance and inner emptiness); and in regulating cognition (paranoid ideation and dissociative symptomatology). Problems arising in these other domains, of course, exacerbate affect dysregulation and lead to a perpetuation of the problematic behaviours. The treatment directs its therapeutic endeavour to all five systems of dysregulation to impact directly on those behaviours leading to a diagnosis.

Inherent in the treatment and an essential component of it, is a biosocial theoretical perspective that emphasizes the impact of both biological and social processes in the aetiology and maintenance of the problematic behaviours that constitute the diagnosis. The biosocial theory suggests that individuals who meet criteria for BPD are vulnerable to the development of these problems as a consequence of a degree of emotional vulnerability, i.e. they are highly sensitive and reactive to emotional stimuli and in addition have a slow return to baseline levels of arousal. These characteristics may be fundamentally innate, but they may also be developed early in life following on from, or as part of, poor or abusive attachment experiences. The theory then emphasizes that this vulnerability transacts with a certain type of environment, namely an invalidating environment. Such environments are thought to reject communication that the individual makes regarding private experience as being an invalid (inaccurate) perception of the way the world is. This environmental response often leads to an escalation of emotional distress.

One of the major consequences of this response is that children raised in these environments do not learn to identify emotional states and occasionally physical states accurately nor do they learn to regulate affect as it is more often than not denied. In addition, invalidating environments also intermittently reinforce escalations of emotional displays. This results in two opposing responses to affect being shaped. The first is the inhibition or denial of emotional states, whereas the second is an extreme response, which often appears to be inappropriate to the level of the stimulus that elicited it. This pattern of oscillation between two contrasting styles is one that perpetuates into adulthood. The invalidating environment also has a tendency to oversimplify the ease of solving problems and to have inappropriate developmental expectations of the child. Consequently, the child does not learn to set realistic goals for solving everyday problems nor learn to tolerate the distress that is a necessary part of learning new skills.

All three responses of an invalidating environment only serve to exacerbate the sensitivity that the child already possesses. The enhanced emotional sensitivity tends to 'pull' further invalidation from the environment. This transaction iterates throughout development leading to the development of entrenched behaviour patterns. Many of the impulsive behaviours leading to the diagnosis of borderline personality disorder are conceptualized within the model as either a direct consequence of emotional sensitivity in conjunction with an invalidating environment or as an indirect consequence of finding alternative means to regulate both affect and the environment as all other means have been ineffective.

Principles of dialectical behaviour therapy

Dialectics as a world view permeates the treatment. Some of these dialectics have already been discussed; for example, the transaction between biological vulnerability and the invalidating environment. Nowhere is the dialectical approach of the treatment more evident, however, than in the treatment strategies. The central dialectic is between change on the one hand and acceptance on the other. For adolescents with the extent and complexity of problems presented, change is essential; however, to focus exclusively on change is to fundamentally invalidate the value of what is. It is the task of the therapist to help the adolescent find a synthesis to this dialectic – to change what needs to be changed yet to accept that which is valid in the way the adolescent currently is.

At its centre, DBT expresses this main dialectic in the form of two opposing treatment strategies; problem solving focused at changing target behaviours and validation that focuses on accepting things as they are. Problem solving in DBT is the main change strategy and fundamentally is no different to problem solving in any other cognitive-behavioural treatment. Once the target behaviour is identified the therapist assists the adolescent in identifying vulnerability factors, prompting events and the complex series of emotions, cognitions and actions that both led up to and followed the target behaviour. The adolescent and the therapist then focus on the generation, evaluation and implementation of strategies to solve the problematic links in the chain of events surrounding the identified behaviour. Solutions are drawn from a range of sources. If the problem is due to a capability deficit, then the new skills that adolescents are learning in the skills group (these are themselves dialectically arranged into skills focussing on change – interpersonal effectiveness skills, emotion regulation skills – and those focusing on acceptance – mindfulness and distress tolerance) are drawn upon. If the skills are present but not utilized, owing to the interference of problematic emotions, then exposure to the cues eliciting the problematic emotion is the relevant intervention. If the difficulty is a result of dysfunctional cognitions, then cognitive restructuring is employed. If the problem is one of the required behaviour being too low in the response hierarchy, however, then contingency management strategies are introduced.

Validation, in contrast, centres on accepting the adolescent as he or she is and assisting the adolescent in identifying those aspects of behaviour, emotion and cognition that are a valid response to the current situation. The dialectical synthesis of these two contradictory therapeutic strategies lies in helping the adolescent validate those aspects of the problematic behaviour that are valid whilst at the same time working to change those aspects of behaviour that are not. For example, self-mutilation can be considered a 'valid behaviour' in a number of respects. First, for many adolescents it is valid in terms of its antecedents. This is often the only way adolescents have learned to handle problematic affects and therefore, relying on this behaviour makes sense from their own learning history. Secondly, the behaviour is valid in that it is often highly effective in regulating unpleasant affect and, therefore, the behaviour is valid in terms of its goal. The behaviour is invalid, however, in that it is not effective in reaching the adolescents ultimate goal of feeling better about themselves as in the longer term the behaviour often leads to further shame and distress.

The central dialectic of problem solving and acceptance is complemented by others involving therapeutic style (where a responsive, genuine and self-involving style is counterpoised with an irreverent, confrontational style) and case management (where the rare intervention in the environment on the patients behalf by the therapist, is complemented by a style of consultation-to-the-patient, which aims to teach the adolescent how to become more effective in managing both her treatment and her personal network). These different strategies are woven together with a number of dialectical strategies that embody both the acceptance and change dialectic within them. For example, the strategy of making lemonade out of lemons which concentrates on the advantages of difficult and problematic situations for enhancing learning. To truly make lemonade, however, you first must accept that what has occurred is truly a lemon (acceptance) before being able to move on to add water and sugar in the form of new skills and strategies (change) to produce the lemonade.

Treatment of adolescents with these behaviours is often an exercise fraught with conflict and often leads to staff splitting, with different professionals taking opposed views regarding the understanding of the adolescents' problems and the proposed solutions. It is in working in such situations that a further aspect of the dialectical philosophy proves beneficial. The dialectical nature of the treatment rests on an assumption that reality as a whole is complex and oppositional and that no one position has a monopoly on the truth. So, when tensions arise within the adolescent, between the adolescent and the therapist or between different members of the treatment team or the treatment team and the family, the dialectical stance encourages the identification of that which is valid in the two opposing positions so as to facilitate a synthesis that moves both the understanding of the adolescent and their treatment on.

For example, it is not uncommon in working with adolescents presenting with behaviour patterns of the borderline type for some staff involved with them, or some family members, to see the adolescent as a vulnerable victim of tragic circumstances. Often, staff and family members on this end of the dialectic believe that support, care and understanding are required to resolve the difficulties and that the adolescent must not be pushed too hard to overcome their problems. On the other end of the dialectic, however, there may be staff or family members who see the adolescent's behaviour as manipulative, intentionally aimed at changing others' behaviour in an attempt to avoid the consequences of their own behaviour. Staff and family members in this position often want to push hard for change and to be more confrontative with the adolescent. Rather than either one pole being an accurate description of the adolescent and their behaviour, there is some truth in both ends. Thus, the adolescent who has been sexually abused is likely to be highly emotionally vulnerable and will require support, care and understanding from his or her family and the treatment team. Nevertheless, aspects of their behaviour, for example, aggressive behaviour, whilst originally solely a product of emotional dysregulation, may have come to also have an interpersonal function in that by being aggressive the adolescent has learnt that distressing tasks may be avoided. It does not follow, however, that the aggressive behaviour is intentionally engaged in to compel the other person to withdraw. In this circumstance the adolescent needs both understanding and assistance in changing their behaviour pattern in order to reduce the impact of the behaviour on others.

Structuring the treatment programme

In accordance with the complexity and severity of the problems presented by these adolescents, the treatment is multi-functional and multimodal. There are five functions of comprehensive DBT, each of which is emphasized in one mode. These are as follows.

- Capability enhancement: the aim here is simply to enhance the adolescents' basic capabilities of affect regulation, distress tolerance and interpersonal skills. This function is most often delivered by a skills training group.

- Motivational enhancement: adolescents with this degree of disturbance experience numerous difficulties in the application of new skills to the complex problems that beset them. This function is aimed at assisting adolescents to apply their newfound skills to their own life problems, in particular attending to cognitions, emotions or reinforcement contingencies that interfere with the implementation of skilful behaviour. This function is most commonly delivered via individual DBT psychotherapy.
- Generalization: it cannot be assumed that even with the addition of individual psychotherapy that adolescents will generalize new found skills to their non-therapy environment. There are often many additional challenges required in the integration of skilful repertoires of behaviour. This function offers explicit coaching in the application of problem-solutions to the adolescent's real world situations. This may be delivered by between session skills coaching, by telephone, by case management or by training family members in the same skills that the adolescents are learning.
- Enhancing therapist capabilities and motivation to treat effectively: adolescents, like their adult counterparts with these problematic behaviours, present a challenge to even the most experienced therapist. Therefore, aspects of the therapeutic programme are devoted to monitoring the application of the treatment and supporting therapists in the therapeutic task. A consultation team most often delivers this function where all therapists involved in the treatment programme receive supervision and support.
- Structuring the environment: delivering a treatment of this degree of complexity requires some management within both the treatment environment and the non-therapy environment of the adolescent. This can be delivered in a number of ways. For example, a programme director may liaise with the rest of the health system about referral criteria or programme limits or by having structured family therapy sessions to ensure that the family are reinforcing more adaptive behaviours.

Structuring progress through therapy

Treatment in DBT follows a series of stages and the first two are described here to illustrate the process. Stage 1 of treatment has as its primary goal the establishment of safety and stability; this is achieved by a concrete focus on targeted behaviours that present threats to life and to effective therapy. Once the adolescent is stable and is no longer engaging in suicidal or other impulsive behaviours, stage 2, which focuses on the processing of past events, is commenced.

There are two key issues for effective treatment to highlight here. The first is that although many of these adolescents will have a history of abuse this does not form part of the initial focus of treatment. Addressing these issues early in treatment is likely to enhance affect dysregulation and impulsive behaviours that may precipitate early termination of therapy. The second point to note is that it is vital that the treatment system does not punish effective resolution of stage 1 issues by terminating or reducing support when the adolescent is presenting fewer challenges to the system. Whilst it is not essential that the same therapist and treatment team provide both stage 1 and stage 2 input, the contingencies around the cessation of problematic behaviours need to ensure that adolescents can move through stage 2 rather than being left with a range of past issues unresolved. The outcome of this contingency will be a return to the behaviours seen in stage 1. In treatment systems that are often overstretched there may be a tendency to withdraw support when the adolescent is presenting with fewer extreme behaviours – this may be the moment to increase involvement and support.

Within stage 1 the treatment takes a structured approach to the amelioration of current difficulties by utilizing a target hierarchy to order treatment interventions. Problematic behaviours are grouped according to priority. Top priority is given to 'life-threatening behaviours', which comprise suicidal, parasuicidal, other high lethality behaviours, such as very low weight in anorexia nervosa, which are acutely life-threatening and, in forensic populations, homicidal behaviours. Following from these, so-called 'therapy-interfering behaviours' are prioritized, as following suicide, the gravest risk to this client group is treatment dropout. Therapy-interfering behaviours are any behaviour engaged in by either the adolescent or the therapist that impact on the effectiveness of the therapy in resolving the adolescents' difficulties. The focus on behaviours of the adolescent that reduce treatment effectiveness is particularly useful for adolescents who often engage in a range of behaviours in session that make therapy a challenge. The therapist's behaviour is highlighted here in recognition of the important transaction between the adolescent and the therapist in making an effective working alliance.

With adolescents with complex and distressing behaviours, there is a risk that the therapist may engage in strategies that are ineffective in the long term at resolving problems but which in the short term may ease the therapeutic tension. For example, not pressing the adolescent to address self-mutilation as whenever this is attempted the adolescent becomes verbally aggressive. Whilst avoiding the topic solves the immediate therapeutic problem, the adolescent does not learn how to stop self-mutilation or how to tolerate the shame elicited when problematic behaviours are discussed. One of the main functions of the consultation team, as highlighted above, is to assist therapists in selecting and adhering to the most effective therapeutic strategies in such circumstances. By discussing the likelihood that they will engage in therapy-interfering behaviours, the therapist can facilitate the adolescent in discussing areas that may be problematic on their side. Following on from these behaviours, quality-of-life-interfering behaviours are targeted. Here behaviours that have a serious impact on the adolescents' quality of life are addressed such as other Axis 1 diagnoses, forensic behaviours, other impulsive behaviours, and serious interpersonal difficulties.

The provision of treatment in non-specialist settings

Dialectical behaviour therapy has been described in some detail, not only because of its promise in the treatment of borderline problems in adolescents, but also because the principles are relevant no matter which approach is used. In particular, it is probably essential that treatment has several modalities. Experience from adult approaches in therapeutic communities or day hospital provisions, as well as DBT, suggest that individual psychotherapy alone is not capable of addressing the diversity of problems. The young person with borderline problems commonly says different things to different professionals, so that the therapist may not hear about self-destructive or disruptive behaviours, and so cannot work with them. Furthermore sessions at fixed times in the week are not well suited to the need to respond to crises, or impulsive behaviours. If there is not a therapeutic team available to inform the response, it is likely to occur in an uninformed way.

However, there are ways of establishing a therapeutic team even where there is not a specialist service. For example, it is common for adolescents with borderline difficulties to be in the care of social services, either in residential units or foster families. Close working with social workers, support workers, residential staff and foster carers, using the principles reviewed earlier in the chapter can lead to very effective treatment approaches. Generally, this is achieved where there is support at a senior level, and the contributions of staff of different levels of skill and experience are valued. For example, it is common for the borderline adolescent in a residential unit to form a close relationship with a young inexperienced member of staff, perhaps along the lines that they are more like friends than staff and resident. At the same time, senior members of staff form a more sceptical view of the young person, that is also critical of the young staff. Differences of view such as this may be resolved within a hierarchy in favour of the senior staff, and the link with the younger staff member ended. Where there is an opportunity to work with a residential staff group, these patterns of relationships can be anticipated and understood, in which case the views and relationships of staff either side of the 'split' can be brought into the treatment plan.

DBT also embodies a spirit of respect that is often difficult to engender in the face of extreme behaviours and emotions, and yet is essential. Whatever the treatment approach, it is crucial that this is evident in clinicians' attitudes to the young person. This will be reflected in the way clinicians talk to the young person about their difficulties. The emphasis is on identifying specific areas of difficulty and competence and working with them. In our view the status of 'personality disorder' as a diagnosis is so unsatisfactory, even in adults, that reference to it with patients is difficult to justify. Nevertheless, it is important to convey that the problems are well recognized, and to provide a description of the clinician's understanding of them and of how that will be linked with treatment. It is also often helpful to make clear that the aim is to help the young person make long term changes, and that this may take some time.

An area of therapeutic work that has been relatively neglected in translating therapeutic approaches to borderline personality disorder from adults to adolescents concerns the family of the patient. The role of the family changes markedly over adolescence and this has to be respected during assessment and treatment. Responsibility for the young adolescent who is not in the care of the local authority rests substantially with parents, and they need to be involved actively at each stage. Clinical judgement has to be used regarding the role of parents with older adolescents. Tense, intense and turbulent relationships between the adolescent and family members are common and the clinician's response cannot be prescribed simply. It is essential at the outset to avoid assumptions regarding the origins of such difficult relationships, and in particular the assumption that the parents' behaviours have caused the young person's problems. For reasons reviewed earlier it is generally the case that they arise from many years of mutual influence, and often angry and hurt feelings on both sides.

There are two key questions: what should the parents be told about the young person's difficulties, and how should they be involved in the treatment? The decision regarding communication with parents depends on the age of the child, the clinician's formulation regarding the family as well as the young person, and who is present. The same principles used in talking to the young person should guide conversations with parents. It will be rare for parents or even the family not to be actively involved with the treatment of a young adolescent, but quite common in later adolescence. However, parental or family involvement does not necessarily mean family therapy. The key issue is whether work with the family aims primarily to promote their support of the therapeutic work and to prevent it being undermined by family relationships, or whether change of family relationships is a key element of the therapeutic approach.

Although there are reports of the integration of individual and family approaches, there is currently no evidence base that can assist in making this judgement. If involvement of the family focuses primarily on support for the treatment with the individual young person, the emphasis will be on making sure parents understand the treatment approach, discussing ways in which that may be challenging to their child and hence how they can be supportive, and how their responses to his/her behaviours can be consistent with those of providing the treatment. This will be reviewed in regular, but not necessarily frequent, meetings. Where family therapy is seen as integral to the treatment, the goals generally include altering interaction and communication patterns in such a way as to foster more adaptive functioning. A wide range of family therapy techniques may be employed to achieve this. For example, drawing on functional family therapy, the therapist may identify and discuss with the family interdependencies and contingencies between family members in their day-to-day functioning and in relation to the young person's problem behaviours. Once this has been done, the therapist and family consider alternatives that may be less likely to reinforce those behaviours, and may promote more harmonious interactions. Where it appears that problematic behaviours have been a form of communication, alternative less problematic and generally clearer communications can be established.

Recent reviews of drug treatments for borderline personality disorder in adults have concluded that serotonin re-uptake inhibitors and monoamine oxidase inhibitors may contribute to improvement independent of their antidepressive effects. However, the evidence is not sufficiently strong to point to clear treatment recommendations. Pharmacotherapy may occasionally be considered in the treatment of borderline problems in adolescents; however, it is not established practice. The risks of suicidal thoughts and self harm associated with the use of a range of serotonin re-uptake inhibitors in adolescents under the age of 18 are particularly relevant to young people with borderline problems.

SUGGESTED READING

A. W. Bateman & P. Fonagy, Effectiveness of psychotherapeutic treatment of personality disorder. *British Journal of Psychiatry*, **177** (2000), 138–43.

D. F. Becker, C. M. Grilo, W. S. Edell & T. H. McGlashan, Diagnostic efficiency of borderline personality disorder criteria in hospitalized adolescents: comparison with hospitalized adults. *American Journal of Psychiatry*, **159** (12) (2002), 2042–7.

S. Bezirganian, P. Cohen & J. S. Brook, The impact of mother-child interaction on the development of Borderline Personality Disorder. *American Journal of Psychiatry*, **150** (12) (1993), 1836–42.

M. J. Block, D. Westen, P. Ludolph, J. Wixom & A. Jackson, Distinguishing female borderline adolescents from normal and other disturbed female adolescents. *Psychiatry*, **54** (1) (1991), 89–103.

J. Hill, Disorders of Personality. In M. Rutter and E. Taylor (eds.), *Child and Adolescent Psychiatry*, *4th edn.* (Oxford: Blackwell, 2002).

A. James, M. Berelowitz & M. Vereker, Borderline personality disorder: study in adolescence. *European Journal of Child and Adolescent Psychiatry,* **5** (1) (1996), 11–17.

L. Y. Katz, B. J. Cox, S. Gunasekara & A. L. Miller, Feasibility of dialectical behavior therapy for suicidal adolescent inpatients. *Journal of the American Academy of Child and Adolescent Psychiatry,* **43** (3) (2004), 276–82.

A. L. Miller, J. Glinski, K. A. Woodberry, A. G. Mitchell & J. Indik, Family therapy and dialectical behavior therapy with adolescents. Part I: Proposing a clinical synthesis. *American Journal of Psychotherapy,* **56** (4) (2002), 568–84.

13

Mental retardation/learning disability

Christopher Gillberg

Department of Child and Adolescent Psychiatry, University of Göteborg, Sweden

Introduction

Many children, adolescents (and adults) have 'learning problems'. Some need a lot of extra attention and support to be able to learn new things in fairly well-circumscribed areas, such as reading, writing and mathematics, but do not have similar needs in other areas. Such individuals should be considered for a diagnosis of a specific developmental disorder. Yet others appear to have problems in learning across the board. If they have not been identified as having a learning disability already in the first few years of life – in which case their learning disability is usually severe – it is high time to consider the possibility during the first school years.

Mental retardation (MR) – recently referred to as learning disability in the UK – is neither a medical condition, nor – strictly speaking – a medical diagnosis. It is not a psychiatric disorder, but is usually listed in psychiatric disorder diagnostic manuals. It is still often referred to as a 'developmental disorder', but even such terminology is inappropriate. While not basically a medical problem, MR has very strong links to medical conditions, and psychiatric and developmental disorder. MR as an important 'knowledge niche' of medicine was not acknowledged until about 150 years ago. In 1850, the first medical periodical devoted to MR was published ('Observations on Cretinism'). Sixteen years later John Langdon Down wrote his landmark paper on the heterogeneous nature of mental retardation. Psychometric tests were developed in France by Binet and Simon in 1905, and intelligence quotients (IQs) came to be accepted as an adequate measure of intelligence.

Definition and classification

MR is an administrative label, which is applied in individuals who consistently test below a certain IQ level (usually 70) and who show functional impairment

A Clinician's Handbook of Child and Adolescent Psychiatry, ed. Christopher Gillberg, Richard Harrington and Hans-Christoph Steinhausen. Published by Cambridge University Press. © Cambridge University Press 2005.

and deficits in social adaptation as a consequence of low IQ. While there is no generally accepted definition of intelligence, there is good evidence that the concept of 'general intelligence' or a 'g-factor' has good validity. In addition, there is mounting support for the notion of individual IQ differences being linked to differences in information-processing speed. Executive functions – especially inhibitory processes – are a likely basis for the development of intelligence. Visuo-spatial skills are often an important part of intelligence testing. Some such skills, including memory for spatial locations, may reflect automatic processes rather than 'general intelligence'. This could be one reason why some 'savants' with severe MR may have islets of visuo-spatial abilities.

ICD-10 criteria

The ICD-10 diagnostic category for conditions associated with IQ under about 70 and deficits in social adaptation is mental retardation (Box 13.1). However, in recent years the term learning disability (LD) has come to be used in the UK, where it has become the official term. MR is subdivided into 'mild' (IQ 50–69), 'moderate' (IQ 35–49), 'severe' (IQ 20–34), and 'profound' (IQ<20).

Box 13.1. Diagnostic criteria for mental retardation (ICD-10)

A condition of arrested or incomplete development of the mind, which is especially characterized by impairment of skills manifested during the developmental period, skills which contribute to the overall level of intelligence, i.e. cognitive, language, motor, and social abilities. Retardation can occur with or without any other mental or physical condition.

Degrees of mental retardation are conventionally estimated by standardized intelligence tests. These can be supplemented by scales assessing social adaptation in a given environment. These measures provide an approximate indication of the degree of mental retardation. The diagnosis will also depend on the overall assessment of intellectual functioning by a skilled diagnostician.

Intellectual abilities and social adaptation may change over time, and, however poor, may improve as a result of training and rehabilitation. Diagnosis should be based on the current levels of functioning.

The following forth-character subdivisions are for use with categories F70–F79 to identify the extent of impairment of behaviour:

.0   **With the statement of no, or minimal, impairment of behaviour**
.1   **Significant impairment of behaviour requiring attention or treatment**
.8   **Other impairments of behaviour**
.9   **Without mention of impairment of behaviour**

Use additional code, if desired, to identify associated conditions such as autism, other developmental disorders, epilepsy, conduct disorders, or severe physical handicap.

F70   Mild mental retardation

Approximate IQ range of 50 to 69 (in adults, mental age from 9 to under 12 years). Likely to result in some learning difficulties in school. Many adults will be able to work and maintain good social relationships and contribute to society.

Includes: feeble-mindedness
mild mental subnormality

F71   Moderate mental retardation

Approximate IQ range of 35 to 49 (in adults, mental age from 6 to under 9 years). Likely to result in marked developmental delays in childhood but most can learn to develop some degree of independence in self-care and acquire adequate communication and academic skills. Adults will need varying degrees of support to live and work in the community.

Includes: moderate mental subnormality

F72   Severe mental retardation

Approximate IQ range of 20 to 34 (in adults, mental age from 3 to under 6 years). Likely to result in continuous need to support.

Includes: severe mental subnormality

F73   Profound mental retardation

IQ under 20 (in adults, mental age below 3 years). Results in severe limitation in self-care, continence, communication and mobility.

Includes: profound mental subnormality

F78   Other mental retardation

F79   Unspecified mental retardation

Includes: mental:
- deficiency NOS
- subnormality NOS

DSM-IV criteria

The DSM-IV category is also called mental retardation. This is the term adopted in most countries. In a sense, it is inappropriate, in that it does suggest that mental development is retarded rather than restricted; in the majority of individuals given a diagnosis of mental retardation 'catch-up' will not occur, and so it is not really an issue of slowed development as suggested by the word retardation. Parents and other people for whom the psycho-educational process of coming to terms with the child's diagnosis is of paramount importance, misleading concepts can cause a lot of problems. False hope that, with appropriate intervention and education, the child will eventually become free of learning problems can lead to devastating consequences, including charlatan treatments and parental self-blame after envisaged progress does not come about.

Subdivision of cases into mild, moderate, severe and profound is accomplished in a fashion similar to that of the ICD-10, although the borderlines are defined less strictly. Sometimes mental retardation is subdivided only on the rather crude measure of IQ 50 (higher IQ labelled 'mild', lower IQ labelled 'severe'). Many studies suggest that, in clinical practice, this may have advantages from the point of view of aetiological classification. However, clinical studies and experience indicate that further subdivision has important implications for teaching, training and outcome.

Epidemiology

Prevalence rates

The reported prevalence of MR varies substantially across studies, which is often due to the heterogeneity of definitions, instruments used and study designs. According to the assumed normal distribution of IQs, prevalence would be expected to be about 2–3 per cent, plus cases due to medical conditions. There is general agreement that severe mental retardation occurs in 0.3–0.5 per cent of the general population of school-age children. This figure is relatively stable across time and region. Mild mental retardation is reported at much more variable prevalence rates, ranging from 0.5–2.0 per cent. Borderline intelligence (IQ about 70–84) associated with major adjustment and behavioural problems is even more common, but exact prevalence rates are difficult to establish, given the variable cut-off level for 'major adjustment problems' used.

Incidence rates

The incidence of mental retardation, particularly milder variants, is difficult to study, given the problems or early ascertainment, which are more pronounced the closer one gets to the IQ 70 level.

Sex ratios

Clinical studies show a fairly high boy:girl ratio for mental retardation. This drops to considerably lower levels in the general population (about 1.3:1). The male preponderance is generally attributed to X-linked genetic mechanisms.

Implications for clinical practice

In many western cultures service development – particularly when it comes to diagnostic and early intervention programmes – has been better than in other fields of child psychiatry. Nevertheless, for those with mild MR – and particularly for those with borderline MR – the situation is often problematic. These cases are often missed or misdiagnosed in spite of there being major behaviour, emotional, adjustment and academic problems. There is a widespread reluctance to 'test' children in many countries, and 'IQ-testing' is especially contentious. Children, whose main 'underlying' problem is really MR, are often brought to clinics only at the age of 10 to 15 years with referral diagnoses of depression or ADHD/conduct disorder. Others may have been in individual psychotherapy for years without a proper assessment or test of intellectual functioning. It is of paramount importance that clinicians working with children are aware of the relatively high frequency of MR in the general population and the even higher rate among children presenting with any kind of behavioural or emotional problem. All child psychiatric patients need to be assessed clinically as regards their overall level of intellectual functioning.

Clinical picture

Main features and symptoms

No symptoms can be said to be typical of mental retardation *per se*. Some children have such obvious physical signs (e.g. Down syndrome or various other chromosomal syndromes) that the possibility of MR is entertained from birth.

For those with severe and profound levels of MR, a diagnosis is usually made in the first 4 years of life. However, in cases with autism spectrum disorders and severe ADHD, the additional diagnosis of MR may be missed for another few years (all the problems shown by the child being attributed to these disorders), unless expert clinicians are involved in the very early diagnostic process. The failure to pass the expected developmental milestones is usually what alerts parents and doctors to the possibility of the diagnosis. Children with epilepsy, cerebral palsy and other neurological disorders are known to have a very high rate of concurrent MR, and so a diagnosis is often considered early on in the evaluation process of these conditions. Those with IQs under 20 usually speak little if at all, and almost never learn to read or write (except when there is associated hyperlexia).

Those with moderate mental retardation usually are now recognized long before starting school, even though the occasional case with relatively better verbal than performance skills may be missed for another several years. Some of the individuals affected will learn to read and write, but others will not. Unless there is autism or a specific language disorder, they also, usually, have some speech and language skills.

Mild mental retardation is often missed well into the school years and even into adolescence and adulthood (see above). The developmental delays and symptoms are usually much less striking than in more severe cases and are often ascribed to familial developmental lag, or various individual ('attention deficits', 'dyslexia', 'language delay', 'personality') and/or environmental factors ('understimulation', 'lack of peer group') rather than being suspected immediately of being associated with MR. Clinically, unless there is associated autism, dyslexia or speech and language disorder, children with mild MR usually will acquire relatively good expressive language skills and some reading and writing skills.

Differential diagnosis and co-morbidity

There are many problems of differential diagnosis in the field of MR including those that pertain to recognizing that there may be an important intellectual problem at all. It is also important to keep in mind that MR is associated almost always with other behavioural, social cognitive or medical problems. Many of the diagnoses considered under the heading of differential diagnosis can equally be regarded as common 'co-morbidity' conditions (Box 13.2).

Box 13.2. Differential diagnosis in Mental Retardation

Suspicion of MR because of general developmental delay, speech-language delay, extreme ADHD or autism spectrum problems : IQ-testing

IQ 50–69:
- Consider the full range of possible psychiatric co-morbidity (in particular ADHD, autism spectrum disorder, depression, bipolar disorder, schizophrenia, and catatonia)
- Exclude (either through expert clinical evaluation or genetic testing) fetal alcohol syndrome, 22q11deletion, Williams, the fragile-X, Prader–Willi, and Down syndrome
- Consider neurocutaneous, and neurometabolic disorders (particularly hypomelanosis of Ito and neurofibromatosis)
- Expect to find a likely cause in about 40% of cases

IQ<50
- Consider autism spectrum disorders, self-injury, violent behaviours, pica, rumination, confusional and other psychotic states, including bipolar swings
- Consider fetal alcohol syndrome, Angelman, Rett, Smith–Magenis, Williams, Prader–Willi, fragile-X, Down, and other chromosomal syndromes
- Consider neurocutaneous (particularly tuberous sclerosis), and neurometabolic disorders (particularly if signs or symptoms of deterioration)
- Expect to find a likely cause in about 80% of cases

All IQ levels
- Rule out/diagnose visual and hearing impairments, epilepsy and motor control disorders (including cerebral palsy) in all MR cases

---

Language delay and language disorder

In young children, language delay is an almost universal phenomenon associated with MR. Language disorder, like virtually any other condition, can occur in MR, but it is important to recognize that language delay *per se*, if on a par with the child's overall developmental level, should not prompt a separate diagnosis of language delay. Unfortunately, it is not uncommon for children to be diagnosed with language delay/language disorder without the underlying MR being recognized for months or years.

Behavioural and emotional problems and psychiatric disorder

LD is associated strongly with a whole host of behavioural and emotional problems and psychiatric disorders in children and adolescents. There is a clear link with the degree of MR, in that as IQ goes down so the rate of psychiatric disorder goes up. Several studies show a rate of about 50 per cent of all children and adolescents with MR having psychiatric disorders. There are particularly strong links with autism and ADHD, and, in those with severe MR, with self-injurious behaviours, pica, and rumination. Virtually any psychiatric problem seen in people of normal intelligence can be encountered in MR, even though it is often difficult to apply the DSM-IV/ICD-10 diagnostic criteria in those with the most severe and profound levels of intellectual disability. Depression, anxiety and 'psychosis' commonly are diagnosed, but possibly also often missed. Bipolar disorder should be considered in all cases of MR showing severe mood or behavioural 'swings', particularly if associated with 'new' sleep problems and a family history of bipolar disorder or mania.

Medical disorders

As in autism, the diagnosis of MR is only the beginning phase of assessment. Medical disorders of various kinds are so frequent in MR that they must receive priority in the search for underlying causes. This is especially true of those with an IQ of about 50 or under, where a clear or likely cause can be found in about 80 per cent of cases, but even in those with IQ in the 50–70 range, a reasonable cause can be found in about 40 per cent of all affected individuals. The cause is related very often to a specific medical disorder. Almost all the behavioural phenotype syndromes have a large subgroup with MR, including many cases with severe and profound MR.

Epilepsy occurs at a rate of about 30 per cent in those with severe and profound MR, and in about 10 per cent of those with moderate and mild variants. It is often complex, consisting of a variety of seizure types, some of which can be very difficult to treat.

Many other neurological disorders are also much overrepresented in MR (including all the variants of cerebral palsy and the range of neuromuscular disorders).

A whole host of genetic syndromes (see below) need to be considered as soon as a diagnosis of MR has been made. In those with IQs under 50, some of the most important of these are Down syndrome (which – albeit rarely – can be missed – especially in mosaicism cases – during the newborn period), other major chromosomal disorders, the Fragile-X syndrome, Angelman syndrome, Rett syndrome, Smith–Magenis syndrome, tuberous sclerosis and Prader–Willi syndrome. In those with mild MR, there is, in addition, a need to screen out the 22q11-deletion syndrome (CATCH-22), hypomelanosis of Ito, neurofibromatosis, and the sex chromosome aneuploidies (which, in the case of those with supernumerary chromosomes, are often associated with learning, behavioural, emotional problems and unexpectedly tall stature).

Fetal alcohol syndrome (FAS) and fetal alcohol effects (FAE) need to be considered across the board of cases with a low level of intellectual functioning.

Genetic syndromes ('behavioural phenotype syndromes')

The so-called behavioural phenotype syndromes have recently come to the forefront as an important area of research and development of clinical services. 'Behavioural phenotypes' are conditions with a known, usually genetic, aetiology, and a relatively characteristic behavioural presentation. Down syndrome, 22q11-deletion syndrome, the Fragile-X syndrome, Prader–Willi syndrome, Angelman syndrome, Rett syndrome, tuberous sclerosis and Smith–Magenis syndrome are some of the best-known examples of behavioural phenotype syndromes. Each of these syndromes is rare (usually occurring in 1 in 1000 or much fewer individuals), but together they comprise about 0.5 per cent of the general population of children and, hence, a very considerable fraction of all those with MR.

- Down syndrome occurs in about 1 in 600 live-born children. It accounts for up to one-third of all cases with severe and profound MR, and for a much smaller, albeit considerable, fraction of those with moderate and mild MR. A large proportion of all Down syndrome cases develop the clinical features of Alzheimer's disease as they grow older, usually in their mid-40s. Both children and adults with Down syndrome have a rate of psychiatric disorder of about one in three. Down syndrome is associated with a relatively low risk of atherosclerosis. This might be linked to a decreased risk for the insulin resistance syndrome (at least in women with Down syndrome). Conversely, there is a very high risk (about one in four) for epilepsy in adult age (but not in childhood), and seizure onset is often linked to onset of Alzheimer's disease.

  Prenatal screening for Down syndrome is now often done in two steps in the second trimester. Using a so-called triple or quadruple serum test, those women at increased risk for an affected pregnancy are identified. In addition to Down syndrome, such tests tend to preferentially identify fetal trisomy 18, Turner syndrome, Smith–Lemli–Opitz syndrome, triploidy, trisomy 16 mosaicism and fetal death. Screen positive women may go on to have more precise antenatal diagnostic procedures performed.

- 'CATCH-22' or 22q11-deletion syndrome has received widespread attention in the recent past. The combination of cardiac problems, anomalous face, thymus hypoplasia (causing proneness to infections in early life), cleft (soft) palate (leading to a nasal tone of voice) and hypocalcemia (in the early years) is typical, and associated with a large mutation on chromosome 22q11.3 (='CATCH-22' syndrome).

  Early studies suggested a strong link with schizophrenia, but this has now been disputed by new findings from studies of larger and possibly more representative samples. Next to Down syndrome, the 22q11-deletion syndrome is one of the most common genetic syndromes associated with MR, and it is believed to affect 1 in 3000 (or even 1 in 2000) children. IQ can be in the normal range and severe MR is uncommon. About half of all cases with this syndrome are believed to suffer from mild MR. Attention deficits, lack of energy, 'non-verbal learning disability' and autistic-type features are very common. Some specific (and some unspecific) brain changes have been demonstrated at MRI examination, particularly in the (left) cerebellum, insula, and frontal and (right) temporal lobes.

- The fragile-X syndrome which is caused by a trinucleotide expansion of the distal part of the long arm of the X chromosome, is probably the third most common behavioural phenotype syndrome with a prevalence of about 1 in 3000. Given its rather specific phenotype, life-time trajectory, and inheritance pattern, it is important to establish the diagnosis in all affected individuals. A phenotype checklist consisting of 28 items (7 physical and 21 behavioural characteristics) has been shown to have excellent ability to pick out those individuals with developmental disabilities who need to undergo genetic testing for the syndrome.

  Young boys with the syndrome are differentiated from other boys with MR by showing more motor skills deficits, increased initial avoidance, attention deficits and hyperactivity, but also by having a more positive mood after warming up. Autism is common in the fragile-X syndrome (both boys and girls). Interestingly, this may be linked to the much delayed expressive language development typical of the group with the fragile-X syndrome. Tangential language during conversation – possibly linked to social anxiety, hypersensitivity to social and sensory stimuli, and inhibitory control deficits – is a highly characteristic phenomenon in the fragile-X syndrome. This phenomenon is not encountered in autism or non-fragile-X MR.

- Prader–Willi syndrome, which is caused by loss of the paternal contribution of the proximal portion of the long arm of chromosome 15 (i.e. deletion or maternal disomy/imprinting of 15q11–13), is associated with distinct physical (muscular hypotonia, a characteristic face, overweight, small stature and hypogonadism) and behavioural characteristics (including overeating and 'skin-picking') as well as a very high rate of MR (often moderate). Obsessive and repetitive activities are common as are stubbornness, mood instability and self-mutilation.

Autism is relatively rare in this condition, which is in stark contrast to Angelman syndrome (see below) in which autistic features are almost universal. The chromosome 15 location is currently one of the 'hot spots' in autism research. Obsessive desire for sameness is a common autism feature shared across the Prader–Willi and Angelman syndromes. It is possible that the genetic dysfunction at 15q11–13 is linked specifically to obsessive compulsive behaviours rather than to autism '*per se*'. Among the likely neurochemical mediators are GABA, serotonin and neuropeptides, which are all influenced by genes in the affected chromosomal area.

- Angelman syndrome is caused by loss of maternal contribution to the same proximal portion of chromosome 15 that is affected in Prader–Willi syndrome. It is associated with severe or profound MR, much delayed onset of independent walking, ataxia, obsessions and compulsions (see above), lack of speech, overactivity, restlessness, eating and sleep problems and a multitude of autistic symptoms (e.g. fascination with water). Epilepsy or epileptogenic discharge on the EEG (usually of a characteristic type) are almost universal. Episodes of inappropriate laughter, once believed to be the hallmark of the syndrome, occur only in about half of all affected individuals.

- Smith–Magenis syndrome is a rare syndrome caused by a lesion on chromosome 17. It is associated with severe to mild MR, extreme behaviour problems, including violent behaviours, self-injury, hyperactivity, autistic features and major sleep problems. Levels of attainment and of adaptive behaviour are often strikingly low. Dependence on others in adult life is much greater than might have been expected from the general level of intellectual functioning.

- Rett syndrome is a curious condition of stunted head growth, loss of acquired hand use, development of stereotypic hand movements, and overall developmental arrest (after a period of normal or almost normal infancy development). Rett syndrome received widespread recognition only in the 1980s. All affected individuals have profound or severe (occasionally moderate) MR, and have no or little speech. However, there is a rare preserved speech variant which can be difficult to separate from autistic disorder. It occurs almost exclusively in females, but it has been described in a male with Klinefelter syndrome.

The so-called MECP2 gene was found to be associated with the disorder in the late 1990s and was at first believed to be the cause of Rett syndrome. After it was discovered that only about 80 per cent of all classical cases have the gene defect, and it was shown that some males with non-Rett type MR also have the MECP2 gene, theories were revised. It is now hypothesized that disruption of the

MECP2 gene alters the normal developmental expression of various other genes, some of which must account for the peculiar phenotypic manifestations of Rett syndrome.

• Fetal alcohol syndrome (FAS) and fetal alcohol effects (FAE) are perhaps the most common of all (albeit environmentally caused) behavioural phenotype syndromes affecting about 1 in 600 (FAS) to 1 in 200 (FAE) of all children. Ethyl alcohol may have devastating effects on the developing brain. During the intrauterine synaptogenic period (roughly the last trimester of pregnancy), alcohol has the capacity to trigger widespread neuronal apoptosis. It appears to do so by blocking NMDA-glutamate receptors and stimulating some GABA receptors. Many anticonvulsants and sedatives have similar pharmacological properties and could be partly responsible for some of the behavioural and cognitive symptoms associated clinically with 'the fetal alcohol syndrome'. Animal studies further suggest that ethanol may have a specifically toxic effect on astroglial cells.

Prospective longitudinal studies of children whose mothers had been documented to abuse alcohol in pregnancy show a trend towards a dose–response relationship between level and length of pregnancy alcohol exposure and MR/behaviour problems in the offspring many years later. Smoking and alcohol in pregnancy have been associated recently with ADHD. Whether smoking, like alcohol, is also associated with increased risk of MR in the offspring remains to be tested in empirical studies.

Visual and hearing impairments

Reduced visual and auditory capacities are both over-represented in MR, separately or in combination. It is easy to miss out on diagnoses associated with such problems (including refraction errors, retinopathies, middle ear abnormalities and sensorineural hearing deficits), particularly in those with severe and profound levels of MR.

Decision tree

The diagnosis of MR should always prompt the search for co-morbid problems and underlying causes/risk factors (Box 13.2). The first step is to determine what level of MR applies.

Cases with mild MR are often associated with genetic, social and/or cultural factors, and a specific cause (such as a genetic behavioural phenotype syndrome) can only be identified in about 40 per cent of the cases. Mild MR is also associated with much the same range of behavioural and psychiatric co-morbidities encountered in children with low normal or normal IQ. However, autism spectrum disorders, catatonia and ADHD are over-represented meaning that a screen for these disorders is always called for. If diagnostic criteria for any of these apply (and please note that symptoms have to be out of keeping with child's overall level of IQ) and the child is handicapped by the problems, a dual (or triple) diagnosis should be made. Of the behavioural phenotype syndromes, 22q11-deletion syndrome, the fragile-X syndrome, Williams syndrome, Prader–Willi syndrome and Down syndrome (including mosaic cases), should always be considered (see below).

In those with IQs under 50, a specific cause/likely aetiology can be identified in up to 80 per cent of cases. Autism spectrum disorders, self-injurious behaviours, violent behaviours, pica, rumination and various psychotic states are very common in this group, and screens for all of these are essential. Individuals with severe and profound MR (with IQs under 35) should always be considered for DNA/chromosomal tests for Angelman, Rett, Williams, Prader–Willi, the fragile-X, and Smith–Magenis syndromes to mention but a few (see below), and for a possible underlying neurocutaneous or metabolic (including neurometabolic) disorder.

Given that epilepsy and motor control disorders (including cerebral palsy) are so common, a thorough history and a neuromotor examination are essential in all cases.

Diagnostic instruments

Rating scales specifically for individuals with MR can be subdivided roughly into those that cover general symptomatology often encountered in people with low IQ, and those that are geared more specifically at identifying problems typical of behavioural phenotype syndromes. One of the best researched instruments in the former class is the Developmental Behaviour Checklist (DBC). Examples of the latter variant are the Behavioural Phenotype Postal Questionnaire and the Down Syndrome checklist.

Detailed clinical interview with a close carer (usually one of the parents) combined with a psychometrically reliable and valid psychological IQ test and a medical–psychiatric examination of the child provide the cornerstones for the diagnosis of MR. There are no instruments (other than the IQ-tests per se) geared specifically to the diagnosis (including differential diagnosis) of MR. However, use of the Vineland Adaptive Behaviour Scale (an interview schedule probing in some depth into the 'Activities of Daily Life' of the individual), is widespread, and does provide an important tool for assessing overall functioning in children with disabilities including those with a main diagnosis of MR.

Assessment

The diagnosis of MR should only be seen to be the first, albeit important, portion of the full assessment to which all children with much below average IQ should be entitled. MR is never a sufficient diagnosis in and of itself. It is exceptionally rare for a child (or an adult for that matter) with MR to have none of: a co-morbid psychiatric disorder, major behavioural or emotional problem, a neurological or other physical disorder, or a known underlying cause or major risk factor associated with the MR. Thus, just as in other neurodevelopmental disorders, a full assessment by a MR medical 'expert' (be he/she a child neuropsychiatrist, child neurologist or developmental paediatrician) is always required. The examination/assessment performed by this expert, along with the detailed clinical interview with the affected individual and a close carer (usually one or both of the parents and including a detailed family and developmental history), plus a psychometric evaluation with an appropriate IQ (or developmental/social functioning) test, will be essential in all cases (Box 13.3).

Box 13.3. Assessment of individuals with mental retardation/learning disability

Examinations	Relevant clinical questions at issue and possible conditions targeted by the method
Neuropsychological test assessments	
Wechsler scales (WPPSI, WISC-III, WAIS-R), Leiter, Raven, Griffiths scales, or Vineland-interview (see References)	General level, verbal/visuospatial differences, specific peaks or troughs
History taking	
Family history of developmental, neurological, and/or psychiatric disorder	Familiarity, hereditary conditions
Developmental history	Early motor, language and cognitive development
Clinical examination	
Height, weight, hypo/hypergenitalism	Sex chromosome aneuploidies, Prader–Willi syndrome, fragile-X syndrome
Head circumference	Autism, Sotos syndrome, Microcephalus, Rett syndrome
Minor physical anomalies	Chromosomal/genetic syndromes
Skin (including Wood's light)	Tuberous sclerosis, Ito's hypomelanosis, neurofibromatosis, Sturge-Weber syndrome
Scoliosis/kyphosis	Rett syndrome
Heart murmur	Williams syndrome, 22q11-deletion, Down syndrome
Eyesight (including fundus) Hearing	FAS, intrauterine infections such as toxoplasmosis, Spielmeyer-Vogt syndrome, homocysteinuria, CMV, Rubella embryopathy
Hand and overall motor function, tonus and neurological aberrations	Rett syndrome, Prader–Willi syndrome, neuromuscular disorders, frontal lobe dysfunctions, central nervous system immaturity

Autism screening

Dysfunctions in social interaction, communication and flexibility, assessed according to the DSM-IV, ICD-10, or by use of specific rating scale	Autism spectrum disorders

Behavioural characterization (examples only)

Gaze-avoidance, turning away on greeting	Fragile X syndrome
Over-eating, skin-picking, temper tantrums	Prader–Willi syndrome
Social chatting, garrolousness, anxiety	Williams syndrome
Aggression, violent behaviours	Y chromosome aneuploidies

Basic laboratory assessments (all newly diagnosed cases)

Thyroid hormones	Hypothyroidism
Hematologic and electrolytic markers	Vitamin or other nutrition deficiencies, endocrine disorders
Karyotype	All sorts of ancuploidies, translocations, deletions, rearrangements

Special laboratory assessments (as indicated by basic work-up)

Sexual steroids	Inborn errors in sexual hormone metabolism
Parathyroid hormone	Hypoparathyroidism
HIV	AIDS or AIDS-related complex including cognitive dysfuntion and dementia
DNA-tests	Fragile-X, Angelman, Prader–Willi, 22q11-deletion, Williams syndrome, MECP2
MRI	Malformations, scarring, enlargement of ventricle system, cortical atrophy, white mater changes, migration disturbances, tuberous sclerosis
EEG	Slow waves or epileptiform activity
Auditory Brainstem Responses (ABR)	Deafness
Metabolic screen, blood/urine	Inborn errors of metabolism, e.g. PKU, Sanfilippo syndrome, other mucopolysaccharidoses
Lumbar puncture; protein electrophoresis, gangliosides, amino acids, monoamine metabolites, tau protein, growth associated protein-43, GFA-protein	Non-ketotic hyperglycinemia, infections, nerve cell degeneration, synaptic de- and regeneration

The psychometric evaluation must be done in all cases. One of the Wechsler scales will usually be appropriate for borderline and mild MR cases. In those with more marked MR, other tests are often required. The Leiter scale is appropriate for non-verbal children (even though, because of its strong loading on visuo-spatial skills, it tends to overestimate IQ in children with MR and autism), and one of the Griffiths scales will often be useful in those with severe and profound levels of MR. The Vineland Adaptive Behavior Scales test does not provide IQ estimates, but the social quotients derived provide rough estimates of the overall level of intellectual functioning and a good measure of social adjustment.

As in cases of autism, the medical–neurological examination (which must always include head circumference, height, weight and evaluation of minor physical anomalies, skin abnormalities and hearing and visual problems) in MR is important for deciding on what further laboratory investigations to make (see below). The clinical examination must include a systematic neurological and psychiatric screen for epilepsy, motor control problems including cerebral palsy, autism spectrum disorders, self-injurious behaviours, ADHD, tics, sleep disorders and feeding/eating problems including pica and rumination (which may cause severe undetected gastrointestinal problems/bleedings and anaemia and lead to self-injury/violent behaviours). The results of the medical–psychiatric examination and the tests performed should be conveyed to all concerned both orally and in writing.

Laboratory investigations

- All individuals with IQ under about 50 should be screened for neurometabolic disorders, including PKU and hypothyroidism. All girls with an IQ under 35 should be screened for the gene associated with Rett syndrome (the so-called MECP2 gene located on the long arm of the X-chromosome).
- All those with IQs under 35, in addition, need to be screened for the Angelman gene on chromosome 15.
- All with IQs under 50, and those who have a multitude of minor physical anomalies, and those who are unexpectedly tall should receive a chromosomal screen (karyotype), and a test for the FMR-1-gene diagnostic of the fragile-X syndrome.
- An EEG should often be performed in cases with IQ under 50, and, of course, in all who raise suspicion of having epilepsy.
- All with the combination of MR, autism spectrum disorder and epilepsy should be given a brain imaging examination (MRI usually to be preferred), as should those with any skin indication of a neurocutaneous disorder (tuberous sclerosis, neurofibromatosis, hypomelanosis of Ito).
- The MR expert clinician should determine if, and when, other laboratory investigations, including urine, blood and cerebrospinal fluid screens need to be done.

A full assessment of the type of day-care or schooling the child/adolescent is getting should be made, so as to ensure proper 'developmental-level-appropriate' training. It is also important to assess the degree to which parents and other family members understand the child's needs.

Aetiology

There are many different causes of MR, including genetic and a variety of environmental factors (which, in turn, vary from purely biological to biopsychosocial).

Genetic factors

The genetics of MR is becoming better understood. Nevertheless, with advances in genetic research it is also becoming obvious that there are very few straightforward solutions in the field of MR. IQ regardless of level is a strongly heritable trait. Average heritability rates are reported at about 0.5. Genetic factors may play an even larger role in MR, even though the mechanisms involved vary considerably.

- Mutations in X-linked genes are likely to account for much of the discrepancy across the genders which is encountered in virtually all studies of MR.
- Imprinting may be an important cause of differential expression of symptoms in conditions affecting the same portion of the genome but with widely discrepant phenotypes (see under Prader–Willi and Angelman syndrome).
- Trinucleotide repeat expansion is a mechanism underlying a number of specific behavioural phenotype syndromes including the Fragile-X syndrome.
- Rearrangements involving subtelomeric regions have been implicated recently as a major cause of MR. While such rearrangements are relatively frequent in MR, current estimates suggest that they account for no more than about 5–10 per cent of all idiopathic MR cases. They do not appear to be the cause of multiple miscarriages, as has been suggested by several authors on theoretical (not empirical) grounds.
- Specific chromosomal and defective gene syndromes are a very common cause of MR, particularly among those with severe and profound MR. However, recent research has demonstrated that, even among those with mild MR and borderline intelligence such syndromes are quite common. They include the Fragile-X syndrome, 22q11-deletion syndrome, and the various gonosomal aneuploidies, such as Klinefelter syndrome. Even though Klinefelter syndrome may only account for about 1 per cent of all cases of mild MR (as compared with fewer than 0.1 per cent of those with IQs above 70), it has been suggested that cytogenetic testing of all prepubertal males with 'idiopathic' cognitive impairment should be performed, even in the absence of dysmorphic features. Nevertheless, the presence of multiple minor physical anomalies in any child with any degree of MR, is a much stronger indication that karyotyping or other genetic testing should be carried

out. Mosaicisms and chimaerisms may also be more common than appreciated previously.

Biological environmental factors

Many environmental biological factors can cause, lead to or be associated with increased risk of MR.

- Various environmental neurotoxicants contribute to MR. Lead and methylmercury poisoning can cause MR, and attention problems even at low-dose chronic exposure. Other proven or suspected environmental developmental neurotoxicants include PCB, dioxins, pesticides, tobacco smoke, maternal use of tobacco, marijuana, and cocaine and thalidomide. The fetal alcohol syndrome is a fairly specific variant of an environmental neurotoxicant behavioural phenotype syndrome. Other teratogenic syndromes include thalidomide embryopathy and fetal valproic syndrome.

- Prematurity (in particular, birthweight around or under 1000 g) is a well-known risk factor. Survival rates for infants born in neonatal care centres increase with each week of gestational age from 22 (0–21%) to 26 weeks (75–93%). The majority of the survivors will be free of major disability, even though about 20 per cent will later be diagnosed as having MR and another 40–50 per cent may have subtle neurodevelopmental or neuropsychiatric disabilities in the school and teenage years. Even birthweights under about 3000 g confer an increased risk for school-identified disability including MR.

- Hydrocephalus, even if properly surgically treated during the neonatal period, is associated with a markedly increased risk of MR.

- Meningitis and encephalitis in infancy and early childhood are still important causes of MR and other major disabilities, even though the vast majority of those affected have excellent outcomes.

- Traumatic brain injury increases the risk for MR as well as for a number of adverse behavioural outcomes. Children exposed both to violence (often leading to traumatic brain injury) and trauma-related psychological distress may suffer significant reductions of IQ.

- Radiation, chemotherapy, and intrathecal corticosteroid treatments have all been implicated in MR and borderline intelligence. More recent studies report that children surviving acute lymphoblastic leukemia have very few indications of cognitive impairments several years after finishing treatment. This may be due to the use of 'chemotherapy only' in the very latest studies.

Psychosocial environmental factors

Psychosocial factors interact with biological environmental factors in a variety of ways to produce a range of clinical presentations in the field of MR. Some such adverse factors have transient effects that will be counteracted by positive changes in the psychosocial environment. Others will have had such devastating effects in early development that permanent changes in brain activity and functioning have resulted.

- Psychosocial deprivation can lead to reduction in IQ. The effects can be transient in some cases where the psychosocial environment is changed for the better at an early stage. However, they can also be long-term, possibly permanent, in cases of long-standing deprivation (including in children raised in extremely understimulating orphanages). In such cases, the effects on IQ are likely to be mediated through permanently altered brain function. Psychosocial deprivation is much more likely to account for an important proportion of MR variance in underdeveloped countries, and in slums and ghettos of various kinds.

Treatment

Clinical management and treatment setting

There is no pharmacological, psychological or educational treatment available for MR. However, claims have been made that a class of drugs categorized as 'nootropics' may enhance cognitive performance and there has been at least one study suggesting a significant increase in IQ after 15 months of amphetamine treatment of ADHD. These results, of course, do not translate to treatment recommendations for MR, but they do suggest that pharmacological therapies for increasing IQ are not the far-fetched alternative they would seem at first glance.

Also, it needs to be acknowledged from the very beginning that there is usually no 'growing out of' MR. Therefore, individuals affected, need constantly revised intervention plans throughout childhood and adolescence into adult life.

Virtually everybody with an intellectual disability will need special education or considerable adjustment of the school situation so as to provide opportunity for optimal learning. They will also usually need the service of an interdisciplinary team consisting of doctors, psychologists, occupational therapists, physiotherapists and speech and language experts. Those with IQ under 50 usually benefit most from attending a special class (which is not equivalent to a special school) for individuals with intellectual disability.

Treatment algorithms and decision trees

Interventions in mental retardation need to be adopted in accordance with a number of associated factors including the level of retardation, expressive and receptive language competence, severity and type of behaviour problems, specific interest patterns, other co-existing conditions (including medical disorders, ADHD, tic disorders, depression, anxiety and eating disorders) and symptoms (including severe sensory/perceptual abnormalities, self-injurious and violent–explosive behaviours).

Psychological interventions

Psychoeducation is perhaps the most important part of any intervention scheme for MR. Children and adults with MR will need education tailored to their individual level of intellectual functioning usually throughout the lifespan. They need the support of teachers knowledgeable about matters to do with MR, who understand the need to adjust expectations and demands (including regarding reducing stress, time pressure, overstimulating environments as well as understimulation and the need always to inidividualize all interventions in accordance with the unique person's unique potential). They also need a life-long perspective on the part of those planning ahead.

Under optimal circumstances the person with MR and his/her close family/relatives should be scheduled for regular doctors' visits (ranging from monthly to yearly depending on degree of associated – including behavioural and emotional – problems). The MR-specialist doctor (be he a specially interested GP, a neurologist, psychiatrist, or a 'learning disability specialist') and/or a specially trained psychologist could be the 'spider-in-the-web' person regularly overseeing the needs of the person with MR in collaboration with the family and making certain that those needs are met in the best possible way.

Psychological, psychosocial, and educational interventions for deprived children with low IQ have been demonstrated to have positive effects on behaviour, overall adjustment, and possibly also on IQ. Behavioural treatment methods for self-injurious behaviours in MR – and possibly for autism with MR – are effective if used in a systematic fashion in a well-educated environment. Nevertheless, even with good behavioural interventions, the MR persists, suggesting that a greater emphasis should be placed – if at all possible – on prevention.

Pharmacotherapy

No currently known drugs are likely to affect the ultimate outcome of MR. However, many pharmacological interventions are available for symptoms and disorders often encountered in MR.

Neuropsychopharmacological medication very often is given to people with MR. This may be because of marked behaviour problems in autism, depression or various kinds of challenging behaviour. For the latter kind of problems, antipsychotics are most often used, but hypnotics and anxiolytics are often given also, perhaps particularly in cases with anxiety, sleep problems and various kinds of challenging behaviours including self-injury. These medications appear to be somewhat helpful, but they only rarely produce dramatic symptom reductions. In fact, physically exhausting training might sometimes work better.

Children with autism often have MR but are given only rarely medications when in their pre-adolescent years. However, after adolescence, about 40 per cent are given psychotropic medications, mostly of the antipsychotic type. There is a great risk that people with MR will be kept on psychotropic medications for long periods of time if there is not a regularly recurring medical–psychiatric review of the need to use them. Some medications have been proposed to be effective for particular psychiatric symptoms and behavioural problems associated with MR. Overall, so-called challenging behaviours in people with MR are often reviewed clinically with a view to some kind of medication treatment.

Only a few randomized controlled trials have been performed, and these provided no evidence of whether antipsychotic medication helps or harms adults with the combination of MR and challenging behaviours. However, risperidone appears to be effective (and have relatively few side effects apart from weight increase) for disruptive behaviours in school-age children with MR. Olanzapine has been tried in stereotyped self-injury in MR and found to be helpful in some cases but side effects can occassionally be severe. Other treatment suggestions include lithium or other mood stabilizers, naltrexone and serotonergics, but the empirical support for most of these is weak.

Monitoring and evaluation of treatment

Monitoring of interventions in the field of mental retardation usually is best carried out at regular visits to an outpatient clinic specializing in the field of neuropsychiatric disorders with childhood onset. Rating scales can be useful in some cases but many such scales have not been developed for the purpose of measuring treatment effects and are more appropriate for diagnostic purposes.

Information to parents and patients

As has already been outlined, information to all those concerned is extremely important. Nevertheless, the extent and type of information that can or should be shared with people concerned will have to vary according to a wide variety of factors that cannot always be predicted beforehand.

Patient information leaflets were tested on measures relating to medication knowledge and satisfaction in a randomized-examiner blind study of people with mild to moderate MR and a mental illness. Participants with mild MR in the leaflet group showed significant deterioration over a 5-week period indicating that written information may actually be confusing to this patient group, at least in the short term.

Coaching

Direct 'hands-on' support and coaching of young people with MR and other disabilities are efficient tools for improving employment integration and increasing wages. This probably applies in other developmental disabilities also, but is a sadly neglected intervention approach that has not been put to the test sufficiently in scientific study.

Attitudes to people with MR

Negative attitudes to people with MR can be changed through 'attitude training'. Adolescent females and those who have frequent contacts with individuals with MR have more positive attitudes than males and those who rarely meet people with MR. A most important aspect of negative or ignorant attitudes towards people with MR is reflected in the tendency – clinically and in research – to produce acquiescence (yea-saying) in interviews with people who have MR. Submissiveness/desire to please on the part of the person with MR, and question complexity on the part of the interviewer may be the most important reasons for yea-saying. In police interrogations this may prove disastrous for the individual with MR. Both of these can be reduced substantially (and interview result reliability correspondingly increased) by using interviewers who show respect and have sufficient knowledge about the implications of MR.

Problematic issues

There are many problems pertaining to intervention in mental retardation. First of all, MR is usually life-long and, while this is generally accepted, it does not always pervade the provision of services. Many families get reasonably good diagnostic and early intervention service provision, but are then left without regular follow-up or continued help after the child reaches adolescence or early adult age. Creating a service that is consistent with the needs of individuals with MR over time is difficult. In the last several years, the issue of follow-up into adult age has come under debate. Many argue that multidisciplinary teams working with children and adolescents should be working in close liaison with, maybe even in the same clinic as, those providing continued care for adults with developmental disabilities. Such teams, while having expertise in MR, should probably not focus exclusively on individuals with low IQ, but on all those with neurodevelopmental problems, including speech–language disorders, autism, ADHD and tic disorders.

Outcome

Short- and long-term outcome

Of all available measurements in child psychiatry/developmental pediatrics, IQ is the one that is most stable over time. The study of the long-term prognosis for individuals with low IQ has been relatively neglected. The severity of childhood MR is probably the most powerful predictor of adult adaptive functioning, quite regardless of underlying etiology. However, a differential prognosis can be made usually with much better prediction if the underlying cause is known. A majority of adults with MR have very limited economic resources, even when earnings from employment and benefits from governmental income support programmes are included. In the recent past there have been several more papers published on the outcome of autism than on MR/mental retardation *per se*. The autism studies usually include quite a large subgroup with MR, but no control group with MR without autism. Classic autism has a very poor outcome from the psychosocial point of view. Even though cases with severe MR have a particularly poor outcome, those with mild MR and low normal levels of intelligence also do poorly from the adaptive functioning point of view.

Quality of life

One recent study looked at costs and quality of life for adults (most of whom had MR) living in supported living residences, small group homes and large group homes. Taking individual participant characteristics into account, there were no differences as regards costs. However, those in small group homes had larger social networks, and more contacts with people who were not staff or family. These residents were considered at less risk of abuse.

Effects on the family

LD increases the risk that parents (mothers especially) may score in the depressed range on depression inventories such as the Beck scale. Mothers of children with autism score higher (50% score in the depressed range) than other parents of children with MR.

Mortality

There is excess mortality in individuals with MR. However, disease mortality may be very high up to 40 years of age, but does not seem to increase thereafter. Cause-specific mortality also differed from that of the general population in that deaths from neoplasms and external causes were encountered less frequently in those with MR. Non-mobile children and those incapable of self-feeding may be at particular risk of short life expectancy. Both the scope and pattern of disease mortality and cause specific mortality tend to become increasingly similar to those of the general population after age 40 years.

Prognostic factors

It goes almost without saying that the lower the IQ the poorer the prognosis. This has been shown in many studies, but there are several caveats that should be observed before arriving at generalised conclusions. It should also be recognized that quality of life is not necessarily completely dependent on higher IQ.

Appendix

Diagnostic instruments in the public domain

Questionnaires

The DBCL (Developmental Behavior Checklist) (Einfeld & Tonge, 2002) is an adaptation of the CBCL for use with children and adolescents with MR. It has been validated fairly well psychometrically, and is useful for screening behavioural and emotional problems in young people with IQ under about 70.

Diagnostic interviews

There are no diagnostic interviews specifically geared at eliciting information for diagnosing MR. The Vineland Adaptive Behavior Scale (Sparrow et al., 1984) is a very useful interview (with a carer) instrument for assessment of the child's overall level of social and adaptive functioning which allows the calculation of a 'social quotient', which has been shown to roughly correspond to IQ-level derived by other tests, particularly in children with severe and profound MR (who are usually difficult to test on specific IQ tests).

There are excellent investigator-based diagnostic interviews for autism (with or without MR).

Observation schedules/rating scales and clinical checklists

There are many checklists for individuals with behavioural phenotype syndromes, (e.g. the Maes et al., 2000 fragile-X checklist). The interested reader is referred to several publications by O'Brien (1992, 1995, 2002).

Medical work-up

The medical work-up required in MR obviously will differ from case to case. An individual decision has to be made by the expert child neuropsychiatrist, child neurologist or developmental paediatrician well acquainted with the many medical disorders known to often underlie MR.

Psychological tests

A wide variety of psychological tests are useful in the work-up of individuals with MR. One of the Wechsler scales is often appropriate, but with non-verbal individuals or when IQ is in the 50-and-below-range, then other tests may have to be used (Leiter, 1997; Raven et al., 1986; Griffiths, 1970).

SUGGESTED READING

J. A. Burack, R. M. Hodapp & E. Zigler (eds.), *Handbook of Mental Retardation and Development.* (Cambridge: Cambridge University Press, 1998).

C. Gillberg, *Clinical Child Neuropsychiatry.* (Cambridge and New York: Cambridge University Press, 1995).

J. C. Harris, *Developmental Neuropsychiatry. Assessment, Diagnosis and Treatment of Developmental Disorders.* (New York and Oxford: Oxford University Press, 1995).

J. W. Jacobson & J. A. Mulick (eds.), *Handboook of Mental Retardation and Developmental Disabilities.* (London: Kluwer Academic/Plenum Publishers, 2003).

G. O'Brien & W. Yule (eds.), *Behavioural Phenotypes.* (London: MacKeith Press, 1995).

G. O'Brien, Measuring behaviour in developmental disability: a review of existing schedules. In *Developmental Medicine and Child Neurology.* (London: MacKeith Press, 2001).

G. O'Brien ed., *Behavioural Phenotypes in Clinical Practice.* (London: MacKeith Press, 2002).

K. Slaggert, E. Arthur & J. Jongsma (eds.), *The Mental Retardation and Developmental Disability Treatment Planner.* (Chichester: Wiley, 2000).

REFERENCES

Einfeld, S. L. & Tonge, B. T. (In press). *Manual for the Developmental Behaviour Checklist* (2nd edn) – *Primary Carer Version (DBC-P) and Teacher Version (DBC-T).* University of New South Wales: *Melbourne and Sydney: Monash University Centre for Developmental Psychiatry and Psychology and School of Psychiatry.*

Griffiths, R. (1970). *The Abilities of Young Children. A Study in Mental Measurement.* London: University of London Press.

Maes, B., Fryns, J. P., Ghesquiere, P. & Broghgraef, M. (2000). Phenotypic checklist to screen for fragile X syndrome in people with mental retardation. *Mental Retardation*, **38**, 207–15.

O'Brien, G. (1992). Behavioural phenotypes and their measurement. *Developmental Medicine and Child Neurology*, **34**: 365–7.

(ed.) (2002). *Behavioural Phenotypes in Clinical Practice.* London: MacKeith Press.

O'Brien, G. & Yule, W. (eds.) (1995). *Behavioural Phenotypes.* London: MacKeith Press.

Raven, J. C., Court, J. H. & Raven, J. (1986). *Coloured Progressive Matrices.*

Roid, G. H. & Miller, L. J. (1997). *Leiter International Performance Scale-Revised.* Wood Dale, IL: Stoeling Co.

Sparrow, S. S., Balla, D. A. & Cicchetti, D. V. (1984). *The Vineland Adaptive Behavior Scale.* Circle Pines, MN: American Guidance Service.

14

Specific developmental disorders of speech and language

Carla J. Johnson[1] and Joseph H. Beitchman[2]

[1] Department of Speech and Language Pathology, University of Toronto, Canada
[2] Child and Family Studies Centre, Ontario, Canada

Introduction

The communication skills of listening and speaking are basic to virtually every aspect of human life because they permit the sharing of feelings, thoughts, ideas and information with others. Most children acquire listening and speaking skills effortlessly in the course of development. A few children, however, experience significant problems in acquiring these key communication abilities, despite seemingly normal development in other areas. These children are considered to have specific developmental disorders of speech and language and are at risk for other associated learning, emotional and behavioural disorders.

The ICD-10 designates several types of specific developmental disorders of speech and language (see Table 14.1). A key distinction central to the typology is that between speech, the complex and rapid motor movements that translate ideas into spoken words, and language, the conventional code used to understand and express ideas. The ICD-10 explicitly recognizes one type of speech disorder, specific speech articulation disorder, and three types of language disorders, expressive language disorder, receptive language disorder and acquired aphasia with epilepsy (Landau–Kleffner). Other speech and language difficulties are classified as one of two remaining types: other or unspecified. In all types, the normal acquisition of speech and/or language skills is delayed or disrupted early in infancy or childhood, while other aspects of development proceed in a relatively normal fashion. Moreover, the speech or language difficulties are not attributable to obvious sensory, structural, cognitive or neurological problems. This chapter will focus primarily on the three types of speech or language disorder most likely to be encountered by child and adolescent psychiatrists: specific speech articulation disorder, expressive language disorder and receptive language disorder.

A Clinician's Handbook of Child and Adolescent Psychiatry, ed. Christopher Gillberg,
Richard Harrington and Hans-Christoph Steinhausen. Published by Cambridge University Press.
© Cambridge University Press 2005.

Table 14.1. ICD-10 diagnostic criteria for specific developmental disorders of speech and language

Specific speech articulation disorder

A. Articulation (phonological) skills, as assessed on standardized tests, are below the 2 standard deviations limit for the child's age.

B. Articulation (phonological) skills, as assessed on standardized tests, are at least 1 standard deviation below non-verbal IQ as assessed on standardized tests.

C. Language expression and comprehension, as assessed on standardized tests, arewithin the 2 standard deviations limit for the child's age.

D. There are no neurological, sensory, or physical impairments that directly affect speech sound production, nor is there a pervasive developmental disorder.

E. *Most commonly used exclusion clause.* Non-verbal IQ is below 70 on a standardized test.

Expressive language disorder

A. Expressive language skills, as assessed on standardized tests, are below the 2 standard deviations limit for the child's age.

B. Expressive language skills, as assessed on standardized tests, are at least 1 standard deviation below non-verbal IQ as assessed on standardized tests.

C. Receptive language skills, as assessed on standardized tests, are within the 2 standard deviations limit for the child's age.

D. Use and understanding of non-verbal communication and imaginative language functions are within normal limits.

E. There are no neurological, sensory, or physical impairments that directly affect use of spoken language, nor is there a pervasive developmental disorder.

F. *Most commonly used exclusion clause.* Non-verbal IQ is below 70 on a standardized test.

Receptive language disorder

A. Language comprehension, as assessed on standardized tests, is below the 2 standard deviations limit for the child's age.

B. Receptive language skills, as assessed on standardized tests, are at least 1 standard deviation below non-verbal IQ as assessed on standardized tests.

C. There are no neurological, sensory, or physical impairments that directly affect use of spoken language, nor is there a pervasive developmental disorder.

D. *Most commonly used exclusion clause.* Nonverbal IQ is below 70 on a standardized test.

Acquired aphasia with epilepsy [Landau–Kleffner syndrome]

A. Severe loss of expressive and receptive language skills occurs over a period of time not exceeding 6 months.

B. Language development was normal before loss.

C. Paroxysmal EEG abnormalities affecting one or both temporal lobes become apparent within a time span extending from 2 years before to 2 years after the initial loss of language.

D. Hearing is within the normal range.

(cont.)

Table 14.1. (*cont.*)

E. A level of non-verbal intelligence within the normal range is retained.

F. There is no diagnosable neurological condition other than that implicit in the abnormal EEG and presence of epileptic seizures (when they occur).

G. The disorder does not meet the criteria for a pervasive developmental disorder.

Other developmental disorders of speech and language Developmental disorder of speech and language, unspecified.

This category should be avoided as far as possible and should be used only for unspecified disorders in which there is significant impairment in the development of speech or language that cannot be accounted for by mental retardation or by neurological, sensory, or physical impairments that directly affect speech or language.

Reprinted with permission from World Health Organization: *The ICD-10 Classification of Mental and Behavioural Disorders: Diagnostic Criteria for Research.* © World Health Organization, Geneva, 1993.

Child and adolescent psychiatrists need to be alert to the possible presence of developmental speech and language disorders because these disorders:

- are relatively common in children
- often go undetected in clinical populations
- frequently co-occur with other psychiatric and learning problems
- may interfere with a child's ability to participate in or benefit from psychiatric assessments or interventions that rely heavily on verbal communication (e.g. clinical interview, psychotherapy), and
- may impact significantly on a child's long-term prognosis for adequate social, emotional, academic and vocational outcomes.

The astute and well-informed clinician plays a key role in ensuring that a child's individual needs are adequately recognized and addressed.

Specific speech articulation disorder

Definition and classification

Specific speech articulation disorder is characterized by a significant delay or difficulty in learning to correctly produce the sounds of speech in the absence of significant expressive or receptive language problems. The problems in production of speech sounds must be greater than expected for the child's mental age. The category excludes speech articulation impairments that are due to aphasia, apraxia, hearing loss or mental retardation. There is a range of severity. In the most severe cases, speech may be unintelligible even to family members. Other terms for specific speech articulation disorder include phonological disorder, dyslalia, lalling or functional articulation disorder.

The ICD-10 category of specific speech articulation disorder is similar, but not identical, to the DSM-IV-TR classification of phonological disorder, which appears under the heading of communication disorders. The ICD-10 and DSM-IV-TR categories differ in two main ways. First, the ICD-10 category is more restrictive, in that it encompasses only developmental speech sound production difficulties, whereas DSM-IV-TR also includes speech problems attributable to certain structural and neurological problems. Secondly, in the ICD-10 scheme, the various speech and language disorders are mutually exclusive. Specific speech articulation disorder can be diagnosed only when expressive and receptive language skills are not impaired significantly. The DSM-IV-TR scheme (see Table 14.2), however, allows for a diagnosis of phonological disorder to co-occur with a diagnosis of language disorder.

Discussion of clinical applicability

Child and adolescent psychiatrists should be aware that the ICD-10 scientific criteria for specific speech articulation disorder are more restrictive than the criteria employed in much of the clinical and scientific literature on speech disorders. Thus, the DSM-IV-TR criteria may be more compatible with general clinical practice. However, in this chapter, the ICD-10 criteria will provide the main organizational framework to maintain consistency with other chapters in this book.

Epidemiology

Prevalence rates

By definition, using the ICD-10 criteria, the prevalence rate for specific speech articulation disorder should be slightly less than 3 per cent of children because this is the percentage that should score below 2 standard deviations on a test of speech sound production. However, estimates employing other criteria vary from 2 per cent to 6 per cent of children at preschool and early school ages, in part reflecting differences in criteria and test procedures across studies. Speech eventually normalizes for most affected children, resulting in a prevalence decline to less than 1 per cent in the late teen years.

Sex ratios

Specific speech articulation disorders occur more often in boys than girls, with ratios in the range from 4:1 to 2:1, depending on the study sample and diagnostic criteria. Familial aggregation has also been reported, but interpretation is not straightforward because researchers have not always carefully ruled out possible confounded language problems.

Table 14.2. DSM-IV-TR diagnostic criteria for phonological disorder, expressive language disorder, and mixed receptive–expressive language disorder

Phonological disorder

A. Failure to use developmentally expected speech sounds that are appropriate for age and dialect (e.g. errors in sound production, use, representation or organization such as, but not limited to, substitutions of one sound for another [use of /t/ for target /k/ sound] or omissions of sounds such as final consonants).

B. The difficulties in speech sound production interfere with academic or occupational achievement or with social communication.

C. If mental retardation, a speech–motor or sensory deficit, or environmental deprivation is present, the speech difficulties are in excess of those usually noted with these problems.

Coding note: If a speech–motor or sensory deficit or a neurological condition is present, code the condition on Axis III.

Expressive language disorder

A. The scores obtained from standardized individually administered measures of expressive language development are substantially below those obtained from standardized measures of both non-verbal intellectual capacity and receptive language development. The disturbance may be manifest clinically by symptoms that include having a markedly limited vocabulary, making errors in tense, or having difficulty recalling words or producing sentences with developmentally appropriate length or complexity.

B. The difficulties with expressive language interfere with academic or occupational achievement or with social communication.

C. Criteria are not met for mixed receptive–expressive language disorder or a pervasive developmental disorder.

D. If mental retardation, a speech–motor or sensory deficit, or environmental deprivation is present, the language difficulties are in excess of those usually noted with these problems.

Coding note: If a speech–motor or sensory deficit or a neurological condition is present, code the condition on Axis III.

Mixed receptive–expressive language disorder

A. The scores obtained from a battery of standardized individually administered measures of both receptive and expressive language development are substantially below those obtained from standardized measures of non-verbal intellectual capacity. Symptoms include those for expressive language disorder as well as difficulty understanding words, sentences, or specific types of words, such as spatial terms.

B. The difficulties with receptive and expressive language significantly interfere with academic or occupational achievement or with social communication.

C. Criteria are not met for a pervasive developmental disorder.

D. If mental retardation, a speech–motor or sensory deficit, or environmental deprivation is present, the language difficulties are in excess of those usually noted with these problems.

Coding note: If a speech–motor or sensory deficit or a neurological condition is present, code the condition on Axis III.

Implications for clinical practice

Child and adolescent psychiatrists may encounter children for whom specific speech articulation disorder is suspected. Although it may not be the primary referral concern, the disorder must be considered in the overall process of assessment and treatment planning.

Clinical picture

Main features and symptoms

A slowed rate of speech sound development is the characteristic feature of children with specific speech articulation disorders. Usually, the sequence of speech sound development parallels that shown by children who are developing typically, but occasionally, a child will show idiosyncratic or unusual developmental patterns. In order to diagnose this disorder, it is essential to appreciate the typical course of speech development, as shown in the first column of Table 14.3.

Speech sound development involves both linguistic and motor learning. Children must learn the specific vowels and consonants that make up a particular language and their permissible combinations in syllables and words. They must also learn to make the rapid and coordinated muscle movements that are required to produce these sounds and combinations in a consistent and recognizable fashion. Because each language has its own sound system, the specific patterns of normal development vary somewhat from language to language. Accordingly, judgements about articulation disorders must be made with respect to language-specific developmental expectations. The situation is complicated further in the case of children who are exposed regularly to more than one language. Speech sound differences that are the result of the normal interferences that occur in the process of learning two or more languages must be distinguished carefully from the delays in speech development that characterize articulation disorders.

The normal course of speech sound development is gradual, with noticeable individual differences among children. Although each language has certain characteristic features, a general sequence of development can also be discerned across languages. An early milestone is the onset of canonical babbling, which occurs at about 6 months of age. At this point, children begin to produce simple syllable-like vocalizations, consisting of both vowel-like and consonant-like sounds. These babbled vocalizations gradually increase in frequency, length and variety, and begin to take on the rhythmic and melodic characteristics of the specific language that is being learned. Some time between 12 and 18 months, children begin to use vocalizations that are recognizable as first words. These early words typically are formed from a restricted set of consonants and vowels that are fairly consistent, both within and across languages.

Table 14.3. Typical development of speech articulation, expressive language and receptive language abilities

Typical age	Speech articulation	Expressive language	Receptive language
1 year	• Babbles continuously. • Mixes words and jargon sounds. • Imitates pitch.	• Uses two to three words meaningfully (may not be clearly pronounced). • Responds to simple questions • Uses gestures for communication (e.g. pointing, showing). • Repeats some words upon request or spontaneously.	• Understands 3–50 words. • Follows simple directions accompanied by gestures. • Recognizes own name. • Inhibits action in response to 'no'. • Responds to 'bye-bye'.
2 years	• Produces speech that is 50 per cent intelligible. • Produces 70 per cent of consonants correctly. • Uses some consonant–vowel–consonant syllables and two-syllable words.	• Uses 200–300 words. • Puts two words together (e.g. 'papa go'). • Names most common objects. • Uses a few prepositions (e.g. in, on), pronouns (e.g. you, me), verb endings (e.g. -ing, -s, -ed) and plurals (-s), but not always correctly. • Asks 'what's that?' questions.	• Follows simple commands not accompanied by gestures. • Points to objects in response to 'show me' (e.g. body parts). • Understands familiar action verbs. • Understands simple questions.
3 years	• Produces speech that is 75 per cent intelligible and usually understood by family members. • Begins production of simple rhymes. • Simplifies complex speech sounds (e.g. 'kiss' pronounced as 'tiss'; 'spider' as 'pider').	• Uses 900–1000 words. • Produces 3–4 word simple sentences. • Answers where, who and what questions. • Uses 'no' or 'not' in speech. • Produces possessive form of nouns (e.g. mummy's).	• Understands what, why, who questions. • Understands common spatial terms (e.g. in, on, under, above). • Follows two-step commands.
4 years	• Decreases use of speech simplification processes. • Uses speech that is usually understood by strangers.	• Uses 1500–1600 words. • Uses when and how questions. • Uses conjunctions (e.g. if, but, because) to conjoin sentences. • Recounts stories and events from recent past. • Expresses future occurrences.	• Understands words for basic colours, shapes, and sizes. • Understands when and how questions. • Understands most questions about immediate environment. • Carries out series of two unrelated commands.

Table 14.3. (*cont.*)

Typical age	Speech Articulation	Expressive language	Receptive language
5 years	• Uses speech that is 100 per cent intelligible, although minor errors may occur. • Segments words into syllables.	• Uses 2100–2300 words. • Uses compound and complex sentences with at least two clauses. • Uses contractions (e.g. can't, won't). • Discusses feelings. • Prints own name.	• Know some letter names, numbers. • Follows three-step commands. • Understands passive sentences (e.g. 'The dog was hit by the boy'). • Understands most prepositions referring to space (e.g. above, beside, toward) and time (e.g. before, after, until).
6 years	• Segments words into phonemes. • Makes very few speech sound errors.	• Uses 5000 words. • Uses well-formed complex sentences with all parts of speech (e.g. nouns, conjunctions, adverbs). • Tells address and telephone number. • Tells daily experiences and simple jokes. • Answers why questions with an explanation.	• Understands letter–sound associations in reading. • Understands exceptions to basic grammatical rules.
8 years	• Produces most speech sounds in adult-like manner. • Makes occasional errors on complex words (e.g. aluminium). • Segments and manipulates sounds in a word.	• Verbalizes ideas and problems readily. • Produces figurative language (e.g. metaphors, idioms, proverbs).	• Understands indirect requests (e.g. 'It's cold in here' understood as request to close window). • Understands that some words have multiple meanings. • Reads simple books for pleasure.
10 years	• Produces complex words correctly.	• Explains relationships between meanings of multiple-meaning words. • Uses language to explain, converse, persuade and tease.	• Acquires abstract vocabulary and new information from written texts. • Understands common idioms (e.g. 'Did the cat get your tongue?').

Early words do not match adult forms in a precise fashion, at least in part because children do not yet have well-developed control and coordination of the many muscles and structures (e.g. lungs, jaw, lips) that are involved in speech production. Accordingly, children often simplify the production of words in predictable ways. For example, they may repeat syllables (e.g. 'baba' for bottle), delete final consonants (e.g. 'daw' for dog), or substitute certain sounds for others (e.g. 'tee' for key). These error patterns, called phonological processes, are a normal part of early development and are overcome gradually as children learn more words and acquire more proficiency in rapidly articulating the sounds of the language they are learning. Children also gradually expand their repertoire of different consonant and vowel sounds, mastering increasingly difficult sounds and sound combinations. In general, girls progress somewhat faster than boys in acquiring speech articulation and language skills.

By age 3, family members usually understand the speech of a child who is developing typically; by age 4, strangers usually understand a child's speech. Still, the typical 4-year old does not produce all sounds in a completely correct, adult-like, manner. The mastery of certain difficult sounds and sound combinations in a language may not be achieved fully until the age of 8 years.

A few children are identified with specific speech articulation disorders as early as the age of 2, but identification at about 4 years is more common. The child with an articulation disorder may be late in starting to talk. The repertoire of speech sounds, especially consonants, may be limited and more characteristic of a younger child. Error patterns involving sound omissions and substitutions may persist long after the age at which they are typically overcome. Speech may be difficult to understand, even for familiar listeners. On occasion, a child may become self-conscious about speech and begin to withdraw from speaking situations.

Differential diagnosis and co-morbidity

The primary issue in differential diagnosis is to distinguish whether speech alone is affected or whether language development is also compromised, thereby justifying a diagnosis of expressive or receptive language disorder instead of specific speech articulation disorder. This is a crucial distinction because, as discussed later in this chapter, the long-term prognosis for children with language disorders is less favourable than for those with articulation disorders only.

It is also necessary to rule out possible organic factors that might be responsible for the speech production difficulties. Normal findings in the case history and in a neurological examination will rule out speech difficulties that reflect aphasia, apraxia or dysarthria attributable to congenital or acquired neurological conditions.

Similarly, normal results in a hearing test and in an intellectual assessment will rule out sensory causes and mental retardation, respectively.

Diagnostic instruments

An articulation test is a common diagnostic instrument. Children are asked to name pictures or objects that have been chosen carefully to require the production of the various speech sounds found in a particular language. Ideally, the test will contain normative information from a large sample of children to which an individual child's performance can be compared. Some common articulation tests are listed in Table 14.4.

Assessment

A comprehensive assessment for any of the developmental speech and language disorders will include:

- a careful developmental and medical history
- an intellectual assessment
- a hearing test
- an examination of the structures involved in speech (e.g. tongue, lips, palate), and
- a detailed assessment of both speech and language functioning.

Table 14.5 outlines the purposes and procedures for each part of the assessment. Referrals to appropriate specialists should be made as required. Usually, the detailed assessment of speech and language will require the expertise of a professional who specializes in speech and language disorders, variously known as a speech–language pathologist, speech–language therapist, logopedist, orthophoniste, or other similar titles.

The speech–language specialist will compare the child's speech patterns carefully in both single words and connected speech. Results from other procedures will suggest the relative contribution of motor and linguistic issues to the observed patterns of speech sound production, thereby helping to develop an appropriate treatment plan.

For children exposed to multiple languages, the assessment is complicated by the need to collect information concerning the child's proficiency in each language. Information is required about the timing, circumstances, and amount of the child's exposure to each language. The speech sound systems of the languages also need to be compared carefully to identify sound confusions and interferences that are a normal result of acquiring two or more languages. A diagnosis of articulation disorder is appropriate only if there is clear evidence that speech sound acquisition is delayed in all languages relative to those of other children in similar

Table 14.4. Some diagnostic instruments commonly used to assess speech articulation, expressive language and receptive language abilities

Instrument	Author/year	Publisher	Age range	Areas assessed
Bankson-Bernthal Test of Phonology (BBTOP)	Bankson N. W., Bernthal J. E.1990	Pro-ed, Austin, TX	3 to 9 years	Speech articulation
British Picture Vocabulary Scales	Dunn L. M., Dunn L. M., Whetton C. W., Burley J. 1997	NFER Nelson, Windsor, UK	3 to 15;8 years	Receptive language
Clinical Evaluation of Language Fundamentals – 4th edn. (CELF-4)	Semel E., Wiig E., Secord W. 2003	Psychological Corporation, San Antonio, TX	6 to 21 years	Expressive and receptive language
Communication and symbolic behaviour scales-developmental profile (CSBS-DP)	Wetherby A., Prizant B. 2001	P. H. Brookes Publishing, Baltimore, MD	6 months to 2 years	Expressive and receptive language
Expressive vocabulary test (EVT)	Williams K. T. 1997	American Guidance Service, Circle Pines, MN	2;6 to 90 years	Expressive language
Goldman–Fristoe test of articulation 2nd edn. (GFTA-2)	Goldman R., Fristoe M. 2000.	Pro-ed, Austin, TX	2 to 21 years	Speech articulation
Hodson assessment of phonological processes – 3 (HAPP-3)	Hodson B. 2004	Pro-ed, Austin, TX	3 to 8 years	Speech articulation
MacArthur-Bates communicative development inventories (CDI)*	Fenson L., Dale P., Resnick J., Thal D., Bates E., Hartung J., Pethick S., Reilly J. 1994	P. H. Brookes Publishing, Baltimore, MD	12 to 27 months	Expressive and receptive language
Peabody picture vocabulary test 3rd edn. (PPVT-III)	Dunn L. M., Dunn L. M., Williams K. T. 1997	American Guidance Service, Circle Pines, MN	2;6 to 90 years	Receptive language
Photo Articulation Test 3rd edn. (PAT-3)	Lippke B. A., Dickey S. E., Selmar J. W., Soder A. L. 1997	Pro-ed, Austin, TX	3 to 8 years	Speech articulation
Preschool language scale-4 (PLS-4)**	Zimmerman, I. L., Steiner V. G., Pond R. E. 2002	The Psychological Corporation, San Antonio, TX	Birth to 6; 11 years	Expressive and receptive language

Table 14.4. (*cont.*)

Instrument	Author/year	Publisher	Age range	Areas assessed
Test of language development-intermediate, 3rd edn. (TOLD-I.3)	Hammill D. D., Newcomer P. L. 1997	Pro-ed, Austin, TX	8 to 12 years	Expressive and receptive language
Test of language development-primary (TOLD-P.3)	Newcomer P. L., Hammill D. D. 1997	Pro-ed, Austin, TX	4 to 8 years	Expressive and receptive language, speech articulation
Test for reception of grammar – 2nd edn. (TROG-2)	Bishop D. V. M. 2003	Psychological Corporation, London, UK	4 years to adult	Receptive language

Note: Standardization samples for each test include at least 50 children for each year in the normative range. Most tests are available in English only, with exceptions noted as follows: *the CDI is available in more than 30 different languages [see www.sci.sdsu.edu/cdi/cdiwelcome.htm for details; **the PLS-4 is available in a Spanish version (US norms).

language learning environments. Obviously, such a decision is not always straight forward.

Aetiology

The aetiology of specific speech articulation disorder is not known. Multiple biological and environmental factors most likely play a role. Some of those that have been suggested include:

• genetic factors
• impoverished language input
• brain abnormalities
• neurodevelopmental immaturity
• subtle auditory problems
• linguistic factors, and
• speech mechanism or motor control problems.

Each factor enjoys some support in the literature but none appears to be common to all cases.

Treatment

Clinical management and treatment setting

Professionals who specialize in speech and language disorders typically are responsible for the treatment of specific speech articulation disorders. Treatment may be provided on an outpatient basis in hospitals or clinics or as part of the educational programme in schools or preschool settings. The speech–language specialist

Table 14.5. Recommended procedures in assessment of specific disorders of speech and language

Procedure	Purpose
Case history	Identify referral concerns; obtain specific information on child's development of speech, language and other abilities
Hearing test	Rule out hearing loss as contributing factor to speech–language problem or identify and manage hearing problem
Oral mechanism examination	Assess structural and functional integrity of systems required for speech production or identify and manage problems
Intellectual testing	Determine whether cognitive abilities are or are not within expectations for child's age
Speech and language testing	Determine whether speech articulation, expressive language, and receptive language skills are or are not within expectations for child's mental age; if speech or language disorder identified, determine goals for intervention
Neurological history and examination	Obtain neurological history to rule out neurological conditions such as birth injury, head trauma, hydrocephalus, cerebral palsy, epilepsy and other conditions as contributing factors to speech–language problem. Identify and manage neurological condition. Check for muscle tone, reflexes, and asymmetrical tone, strength or reflexes, including an examination of the symmetry and movement of the tongue. Check head circumference to rule out microcephaly.
Behavioural observation and history from parents or caregiver.	Use as necessary to • rule out pervasive developmental disorder, elective mutism, or other related diagnoses, or • identify common co-morbid conditions such as reading or other learning disabilities, anxiety disorders, attention deficit/ hyperactivity disorder or other behavioural and psychiatric disorders

may deliver the treatment directly to the child or may teach parents, teachers or others to deliver the intervention with consultative support. For children learning multiple languages, a decision must be made concerning the language in which treatment should be delivered. Fortunately, there is some evidence to suggest that, with careful planning, gains made in one language may transfer to the other.

Treatments

The primary goal of all treatments is to facilitate the child's learning of age-appropriate speech sound production. Factors considered in choosing a type of treatment include the age of the child and the nature and severity of the problem. Although a variety of treatment techniques and programmes are available, they generally represent two main approaches. Both approaches have been shown to facilitate speech sound learning.

The first general approach, termed phonological intervention, is appropriate for children whose multiple speech error patterns appear to reflect difficulties in learning the linguistic regularities that underlie the sound system of their language (e.g. when and how sounds contrast or combine with each other). The intervention activities are designed to help children expand and elaborate their knowledge and use of the linguistic features of the speech sound system that they have not yet acquired. With improved knowledge, children then reduce the error patterns in their speech, with corresponding improvements in intelligibility and overall communication success.

The second general approach, termed traditional intervention, is appropriate for children whose speech difficulties appear to reflect problems in executing the motor gestures required for the correct production of a few specific sounds. The intervention activities focus on helping the child analyse and reproduce the auditory characteristics and motor gestures (e.g. tongue positioning, lip movements) required for a particular sound. Systematic practice helps to ensure that correct production becomes well established in everyday speech.

Pharmacotherapy

Pharmacotherapy is not indicated except as needed for co-morbid disorders.

Monitoring and evaluation of treatment

The speech–language specialist will typically monitor the effects of an ongoing treatment through periodic assessments of speech sound production skills. Thus, reports from the speech–language specialist and the parents should assist the psychiatrist in monitoring a child's treatment progress.

Information for patients and parents

Parents of children with specific speech articulation disorders should receive general information about the nature of the disorder and the long-term prognosis, which is generally quite favourable if no other co-morbid conditions are present. Parents should be encouraged to participate in the child's treatment, as instructed by the speech–language specialist.

For children with a history of frequent ear infections, it is also important to educate parents about the possible detrimental effects of such intermittent infections on hearing ability and, therefore, on the child's speech sound development and treatment progress. Parents should be taught to watch for signs of infection and associated hearing loss and to seek prompt medical attention for those infections.

Problematic issues

There is no evidence to suggest that exposure to multiple languages makes the learning of speech or language skills more difficult than exposure to just one language. Thus, it is not necessary or desirable for parents to limit a child's exposure to multiple languages. It is, however, critical that parents use a language in which they are fluent when speaking to their child in order to maximize the success of parent–child communications and to provide the best possible speech and language models for the child.

Outcome

Short- and long-term outcome

For most children with specific speech articulation disorders, speech sound production eventually normalizes by ages 8 to 9. Normalization generally occurs even without treatment, although treatment usually accelerates the process. Mild, residual problems in the precision and consistency of sound production may remain into adulthood, but usually do not have significant effects on intelligibility. When present in isolation, specific speech articulation disorder is associated with few adverse long-term academic, social, psychiatric, or behavioural outcomes. Articulation difficulties, however, are often noted in conjunction with language disorders, which have less favourable long-term prognoses. Hence, early articulation problems may serve as a marker for these more serious disorders, which generally have more adverse long-term consequences.

Prognostic factors

Children with severe articulation disorders that persist to the school-age years are at risk for poorer outcomes than those with milder forms of the disorder. Those with severe speech problems may not develop adequate phonological awareness (the ability to perceive, identify and mentally manipulate speech sounds), an ability crucial to learning to read and spell. If necessary, explicit instruction in phonological awareness may be required.

Expressive language disorder

Definition and classification

Expressive language disorder (see Table 14.1 for the ICD-10 criteria) is characterized by a significant delay or difficulty in using spoken language relative to mental age expectations. Language comprehension, however, is not affected, at least not to the same degree. Speech articulation may or may not be affected. The category excludes expressive language problems that are due to acquired aphasia with epilepsy, receptive language disorder, dyphasia and aphasia (NOS), elective mutism, mental retardation or pervasive developmental disorders. There is a range of severity. In the most severe cases, children show markedly reduced speaking vocabularies and use much shorter, less elaborate sentences than other children of the same age.

Other terms for expressive language disorder include developmental dysphasia or aphasia, expressive type. The most comparable DSM-IV-TR classification is also termed expressive language disorder (see Table 14.2 for criteria). The DSM-IV-TR category, however, is more inclusive, encompassing expressive language difficulties that are attributable to acquired neurological problems. DSM-IV-TR also allows for co-occurrence of phonological and language disorders; ICD-10 does not allow for co-occurrence. In both schemes, expressive language disorder does not overlap with receptive language disorder (mixed receptive–expressive language disorder in DSM-IV-TR), in which both expressive and receptive language skills are impaired.

Discussion of clinical applicability

Readers are reminded that the information found in the literature and presented here may better reflect the DSM-IV-TR criteria than the more restrictive ICD-10 criteria.

Epidemiology

Prevalence rates

Again, strict application of the ICD-10 criteria should yield prevalence estimates of less than 3 per cent. Most studies, however, use more liberal criteria, resulting in prevalence estimates for expressive language disorder ranging from 3–7 per cent of preschool and school-aged children. Moreover, approximately 10–15 per cent of young children are late in starting to talk, but 50–80 per cent of these will eventually overcome their slow start to acquire language skills in a typical fashion.

Sex ratios

Expressive language disorder is more common in boys than in girls, with ratios ranging from 5:1 to less than 2:1, depending on the sample and criteria employed. Familial aggregation is commonly reported and probably reflects both environmental and genetic influences.

Implications for clinical practice

The possibility of expressive language disorder should be considered for any child with a history and current presentation of slow language development.

Clinical picture

Main features and symptoms

Children with expressive language disorders are usually late in starting to talk and slow in expanding their repertoire of spoken language skills. However, the sequence of expressive language development usually parallels that shown by children who are developing typically (see Table 14.3). Children with expressive language problems eventually acquire language skills but they do so at a slower rate than their peers. Thus, the specific manifestations of expressive language disorder change with maturation.

Expressive language disorders may be evident in the areas of content, form, or use of language. Problems with content may result in a small speaking vocabulary and a restricted ability to express complex or abstract ideas. Difficulties with the form of language may be reflected in short, incomplete, or ungrammatical sentences and in severe delays in learning to correctly use certain grammatical forms. In English, these difficulties may result in errors in use of verb tense endings (e.g. -ing, -s, -ed), auxiliary or modal verbs (e.g. are, was, should), plurals (e.g. feet, dresses), or pronouns (e.g. she, his, they). In other languages, errors may occur on various other grammatical features that are difficult to learn. Limitations in the use of language may be evident in a restricted range of communicative functions (e.g. question, explain, comment) or in difficulties in maintaining and extending conversations. Connected discourse, such as that used for telling stories, relating events, or giving explanations, may be particularly uninformative, disorganized and difficult to follow. Approximately 40 to 60 per cent of those identified with expressive language disorder also have speech articulation problems.

Differential diagnosis and co-morbidity

The key distinction in differential diagnosis is to determine whether only expressive language is affected or whether receptive language is also involved, thereby indicating a diagnosis of receptive rather than expressive language disorder. This distinction is important because the long-term prognosis for children with expressive language disorders is more favourable than for those with receptive language disorders. In clinical practice, cases of pure expressive language disorder may be relatively rare. The clinician therefore, should always be alert to the possibility of co-morbid conditions that may accompany expressive language disorder, such as reading or other learning disorders, developmental coordination disorder, attention deficit/hyperactivity disorder, or other behavioural or psychiatric conditions.

The clinician must also rule out other conditions that might be responsible for the expressive language problems. As with speech articulation disorders, the possible influences of neurological conditions, sensory problems, and mental retardation will be ruled out by normal findings in the case history and neurological examination, the hearing test and the intellectual assessment, respectively. Acquired aphasia with epilepsy will be ruled out by a history of slow development from the beginnings of language acquisition. Elective mutism will be ruled out by the observation that language difficulties are consistent across all communication situations. Pervasive developmental disorder will be ruled out by the absence of abnormal social interactions and stereotypical behaviours.

Diagnostic instruments

One or more well-standardized language tests are required for accurate diagnosis. The test(s) chosen must assess both expressive and receptive aspects of language functioning. For a comprehensive assessment of expressive language, evaluation will ideally encompass production of spoken language in single words (e.g. naming pictures, actions, or categories), sentences (e.g. repeating or formulating sentences with various grammatical structures) and connected discourse (e.g. telling a story or explaining a familiar procedure). Standardized tests of expressive language may also be supplemented by collection and analysis of samples of spontaneous language use in specific situations, as compared to age-level expectations. Some commonly used language tests are listed in Table 14.4.

Assessment

As discussed earlier, a comprehensive assessment for all speech and language disorders includes the procedures outlined in Table 14.5. A speech and language specialist will usually perform the assessment of communication abilities, taking account, if necessary, of the child's exposure to multiple languages. Because standardized language tests are not available in all languages, it may be necessary to rely on systematic observation of communication skills to identify children who may have expressive language disorders.

Aetiology

The aetiology of expressive language disorder is unknown, but it is probable that multiple biological and environmental factors are implicated. Some proposed causal factors include:
- genetic factors
- impoverished language input
- brain abnormalities
- neurodevelopmental immaturity
- subtle auditory problems
- specific linguistic factors, and
- general cognitive factors.

Each proposal has some empirical support but none accounts for all cases.

Treatment

Clinical management and treatment setting

Speech–language specialists in a variety of settings treat children with expressive language disorder, either directly or indirectly via trained parents, teachers, or others. For multi-lingual children, careful consideration is given to choosing the language of treatment.

Treatments

Treatments are behavioural in nature, with a focus on expanding expressive language skills by promoting verbal exchanges, increasing vocabulary usage, encouraging varied and correct sentence formulation and fostering coherent expression of ideas in a variety of communication situations. When necessary, speech articulation skills may also receive attention.

A variety of treatment techniques and programmes, both direct and indirect, have been shown to be effective in promoting short-term gains in the use of specific expressive language features. However, it remains to be determined whether language intervention can close or narrow the gap in overall expressive language growth on a long-term basis.

Pharmacotherapy

Pharmacotherapy is needed only for co-morbid disorders.

Monitoring and evaluation of treatment

Regular reports from the speech–language specialist and the parents will enable the clinician to monitor treatment progress.

Information for patients and parents

The parents of children with expressive language disorders will benefit from general information about the nature of the disorder and the long-term prognosis, which may be relatively favourable when there are no other co-morbid conditions. Parents should also be encouraged to speak regularly and often to their children during the course of daily activities and to follow any other specific recommendations provided by the speech–language specialist. Further, they should be taught to identify symptoms of ear infections and associated hearing loss and to seek prompt medical attention for them. Parents should use the language in which they are most fluent to foster effective interactions with their child.

Outcome

Short- and long-term outcome

As mentioned earlier, 50–80 per cent of children who are slow in starting to talk eventually acquire normal language skills. Those who are, instead, diagnosed with expressive language disorder typically continue to develop expressive language skills, but at a slower rate than their unaffected peers. By school age, most children with expressive disorders have acquired sufficient expressive language to participate in simple, social conversations but they may continue to experience significant difficulty in more demanding expressive tasks, such as those that require precise vocabulary and complex explanations. Such expressive language difficulties may persist into adulthood.

Some children with severe expressive problems may also experience other difficulties, such as reading or other learning disorders, attention deficit/hyperactivity disorder, or other psychiatric or behavioural problems (anxiety disorder, depression). Generally, however, adverse outcomes and co-morbid difficulties are less common for children with expressive language disorders than for those with receptive disorders.

Prognostic factors

Prognosis is best for children with strong receptive language skills, high levels of nonverbal intelligence, and no accompanying co-morbid conditions.

Receptive language disorder

Definition and classification

Receptive language disorder (see Table 14.1 for ICD-10 criteria) is characterized by a significant delay or difficulty in understanding spoken language relative to mental age expectations. These problems in comprehension of language must be greater than expected for the child's mental age and are usually accompanied by difficulties in expressive language. Speech articulation may or may not be affected. The category excludes language comprehension problems that are due to acquired aphasia with epilepsy, autism, dyphasia and aphasia (NOS or expressive type), elective mutism, language delay due to deafness or mental retardation. There is a range of severity. In the most severe cases, children may have marked difficulties in understanding even simple spoken language at the single word, sentence and discourse levels.

Other terms for receptive language disorder include congenital auditory imperception, developmental dysphasia or aphasia (receptive type), developmental Wernicke's aphasia, or word deafness. The most comparable DSM-IV-TR classification is mixed receptive-expressive language disorder (see Table 14.2 for criteria).

Discussion of clinical applicability

As with the speech and language disorders discussed earlier, the DSM-IV-TR scheme is better represented in the clinical and scientific literature on receptive language disorder than the ICD-10 scheme.

Epidemiology

Prevalence rates

Prevalence estimates of less than 3 per cent should result from the ICD-10 criteria. In available studies, however, more liberal criteria resulted in prevalence estimates for receptive language disorder of about 5 per cent in preschool children and 3 per cent in school-aged children.

Sex ratios

Boys are more likely than girls to have receptive language disorder, with sex ratios ranging from as high as 4:1 to less than 2:1. As in the case of expressive language disorder, the reported familial aggregation presumably reflects both genetic and environmental influences.

Implications for clinical practice

Any child with a history and current presentation of slow language development, reading problems, or other academic difficulties should also be assessed for possible receptive language disorders.

Clinical picture

Main features and symptoms

Like their peers with expressive language disorders, children with receptive language disorders are usually late to start talking and slow to expand their repertoire of spoken language skills. More importantly, however, they are also slow to develop understanding (comprehension, reception) of spoken language. Children with receptive disorders may have difficulty in learning new words and in understanding verbal messages of all types (e.g. questions, descriptions, instructions, explanations). Their misinterpretations of verbal messages may lead them to draw inappropriate conclusions or give nonsensical responses. These comprehension failures may not be recognized and may, instead, be attributed erroneously to laziness, inattention or stubbornness. Children with receptive language problems generally follow a sequence of receptive language development similar to that shown by children who are developing typically (see Table 14.3), albeit at a slower rate. Thus, the specific characteristics of receptive language disorder vary with age.

Like expressive disorders, receptive disorders may be evident in the content, form, or use of language. Difficulties with content may result in a small comprehension vocabulary and a limited understanding of complex or abstract ideas. Problems with the form of language may hinder understanding of lengthy or grammatically complex sentences in daily conversations and academic situations. Limitations in understanding the use of language may be evident in misinterpretations of the main ideas or communicative intentions expressed by others (e.g. not recognizing humour or irony). These comprehension difficulties are usually accompanied by expressive language difficulties similar to those shown by children with expressive language disorder. Moreover, speech articulation problems may occur in as many as 40 to 60 per cent of those identified with receptive language disorder.

Differential diagnosis and co-morbidity

After receptive language deficits are confirmed, the clinician must then rule out the presence of several other conditions, as outlined in the section on expressive language disorder. Occasionally, a child with receptive language disorder, particularly if anxious, will show language interactions so disorganized and incoherent that they might be considered thought disordered and symptomatic of schizophrenia. In such a case, the clinician may need to take extra care in diagnosis, paying careful attention to the presence and absence of co-morbid symptoms. Children with language disorders are also at risk for co-morbid learning and behavioural problems, particularly reading disabilities, anxiety disorders and attention deficit/hyperactivity disorder. Children with a history of a childhood language disorder are at significantly increased risk for young adult anxiety disorders and, for boys only, an increased risk of antisocial personality disorders.

On occasion, a child diagnosed with high-functioning autism may also have speech articulation problems, which are not usually considered part of the syndrome of high functioning autism. In such a case, a co-morbid diagnosis of speech articulation disorder may be appropriate.

Diagnostic instruments

Diagnostic instruments (see Table 14.4) are similar to those outlined earlier for expressive language disorders.

Assessment

Similarly, assessment procedures parallel those described previously for expressive language disorders (see Table 14.5).

Aetiology

The aetiology of receptive language disorder is unknown, but the proposed causal factors are similar to those suggested for expressive language disorder. A plausible hypothesis, given current evidence, is that language disorders are multiply determined.

Treatment

Clinical management and treatment setting

As for other speech and language disorders, speech–language specialists provide direct or indirect behavioural treatments for receptive language disorders, carefully selecting the language of treatment if a child is multilingual. For children with accompanying reading or other academic problems, other educational treatments may also be warranted. Common co-morbid conditions, such as attention deficit/hyperactivity disorder, may also require treatment.

Treatments

Treatments for receptive language disorder focus on improving language comprehension skills by teaching new vocabulary, improving understanding of various sentence types, and fostering understanding of other's communicative intentions. Special efforts may also be required to foster language comprehension skills in other relevant contexts, such as the home and school. Speech articulation and expressive language skills may also be addressed in treatment, if required.

Both direct and indirect treatments are known to enhance comprehension of specific receptive language features. However, language intervention has not yet been shown to foster long-term growth in receptive language or ameliorate the adverse long-term effects of language comprehension deficits on academic progress and social interactions. Explicit instruction in phonological awareness skills (e.g. mental identification and manipulation of the sounds of the language), however, may help to prevent early difficulties in learning to read.

Pharmacotherapy

Pharmacotherapy is not indicated except as required for co-morbid disorders.

Monitoring and evaluation of treatment

The clinician can monitor treatment progress via reports from the parents and the speech–language specialist. For school aged children, academic progress should also be monitored via teacher report, with special education support sought for children who are not progressing satisfactorily.

Information for patients and parents

In addition to information about the nature of receptive language disorder, parents should be advised regarding possible warning signs of the associated academic, social and behavioural difficulties that often accompany this disorder. Parents should be encouraged to participate in their child's language treatment, during which they will be taught how to facilitate comprehension, promote language development and foster communication. Parents should also be supported in seeking other services that may be required to alleviate accompanying academic, social, and behavioural difficulties. Finally, as for expressive language disorders, parents should be advised to seek prompt treatment for ear infections and to communicate in a language in which they are fluent to enhance their child's language growth.

Outcome

Short- and long-term outcome

Children with early receptive language disorders are less likely to eventually acquire normal language skills than those with early expressive disorders. As they mature, children with receptive disorders continue to acquire language comprehension and expression skills, but at a slower rate than children who are developing in a typical fashion (see Table 14.3 for language development milestones). By school age, many children with receptive disorders will be able to understand and respond to simple, social conversations but will fail to comprehend and participate in the more complex language activities required for academic success.

Because adequate language comprehension is so crucial to all aspects of academic learning, children with receptive disorders typically become increasingly disadvantaged relative to their peers with adequate language skills. In at least 40–50 per cent of cases, oral language problems hinder the development of the written language skills of reading, writing and spelling. Concomitant academic difficulties may lead to frustration, withdrawal, inattention or reduced motivation. Both oral and written language difficulties may persist into adulthood, limiting career options, earning potential, social adjustment and quality of life.

Prognostic factors

Prognosis is affected primarily by the severity of the receptive language difficulties, with more severe comprehension difficulties resulting in less favourable long-term outcomes. Co-morbid conditions also are a negative prognostic factor, whereas high non-verbal intelligence is a positive prognostic indicator.

Acquired aphasia with epilepsy (Landau–Kleffner syndrome)

Definition and classification

Acquired aphasia with epilepsy (Landau–Kleffner syndrome) is characterized by a period of normal language development, followed by an abrupt loss of previously acquired skills in both expressive and receptive language (see Table 14.1 for ICD-10 criteria). The sudden language loss is associated with paroxysmal abnormalities in the electroencephalogram (EEG) and, often, with epileptic seizures. The loss of language and onset of seizures may occur in close temporal proximity or in an asynchronous fashion, with either one preceding the other by as much as 2 years. Hearing and non-verbal intelligence remain within normal limits and the condition is not attributable to a known neurological condition, other than that implied by the abnormal EEGs and seizures. Further, the disorder does not meet criteria for a pervasive developmental disorder, but autistic-type symptoms are common.

The ICD-10 classification scheme lists acquired aphasia with epilepsy as a separate disorder, whereas DSM-IV-TR categorizes it as a mixed receptive–expressive disorder of the acquired type. Other terms for the disorder include acquired epileptiform aphasia, word deafness, and auditory agnosia. Some confusion in terminology exists, because some of these same alternate terms may also be used for receptive language disorder, emphasizing that comprehension deficits are a key feature common to both disorders.

Epidemiology

Prevalence rates and sex ratios

Acquired aphasia with epilepsy is a rare disorder. Since described by Landau and Kleffner in 1957, approximately 200 cases have been reported. Familial aggregation has not often been observed. Affected males outnumber females 2:1.

Clinical picture

Main features and symptoms

The hallmark of acquired aphasia with epilepsy is a marked loss of expressive and receptive language skills after a period of normal language acquisition. Onset is typically between 3 and 7 years of age, but may range from 1 to 13 years. The loss of language may be so dramatic that the child appears to have suddenly become deaf. Hearing acuity, however, remains normal. Abnormal EEG activity is always present. Clinical seizures occur in about 80 per cent of cases, often during sleep. They can be rare and can disappear in adolescence. The onset of seizures may precede or follow the onset of language loss by as much as 2 years.

Both expressive and receptive language skills are typically affected. Language loss may occur gradually or precipitously. Comprehension deficits are usually evident first, with expressive problems developing later. There is a range of severity, with the most severe cases becoming completely non-verbal. Oral language skills may fluctuate somewhat over a period of months or years. If the child has already developed reading and writing skills, these are sometimes preserved and can be used to augment or replace oral language for communication purposes.

Differential diagnosis and co-morbidity

A report of language loss after a period of normal acquisition will alert the diagnostician to the possible presence of this disorder. The EEG abnormalities are diagnostic. They include bilateral temporal or temporoparietal spikes or spike and wave and wave discharges. A sleep EEG will document abnormal brainwave activity. Because language loss and seizures may also occur in autistic regression, some cases will require the clinician to devote extra attention to evaluation of the social and behavioural characteristics of the child in order to make the correct diagnosis.

Assessment

Recommendations for the assessment of communication skills and related abilities, as outlined in Table 14.5, should also be followed for children suspected of this disorder. In addition, EEG and other imaging approaches, such as magnetoencephalography, in conjunction with magnetic resonance imaging or single photon emission computed tomography (SPECT) can be used to help localize the source of the lesion.

Aetiology

The cause of acquired aphasia with epilepsy is not known, but it does not appear to be inherited, as there is limited evidence of familial history. Some have proposed that an inflammatory encephalitic process may be responsible, while others suggest that the syndrome may have multiple possible causes. Some classify the disorder as part of the syndrome called electrical status epilepticus of sleep (ESES).

Treatment

Clinical management and treatment setting

Speech–language treatment and, often, special education will be needed for children with acquired aphasia with epilepsy. Medical treatment is indicated for control of seizures.

Treatments

For cases with mild degrees of language loss, speech–language treatment may be implemented, as outlined for receptive language disorders. For more severe cases, the speech–language specialist may introduce sign language or another alternative system to enable these children to maintain communication and interaction with others. The introduction of another communication system will not hinder recovery of oral language and may, in fact, facilitate it.

Pharmacotherapy

Corticosteroids have been associated with the greatest successes, although incomplete. High initial doses (prednisone 1 mg/kg/day) given early in the course of LKS and for extended periods (> 6 months) appear to be most effective. Although empirical evidence is lacking on the most effective approach, some clinicians prefer to give 5–7 mg/kg/week in a once weekly dose. Typically, anti-convulsants are prescribed to control seizures and abnormal EEG activity although they have not been known to alleviate the language deficit, or lead to sustained improvements in the EEG abnormality. When seizures are intractable and pharmacological interventions are ineffective in control of seizures or abnormal EEG activity, surgery sometimes is recommended.

Monitoring and evaluation of treatment

Speech–language and other behavioural treatments can be monitored via reports from parents or from professionals providing the treatments. These children should be followed closely until their clinical condition stabilizes.

Information for patients and parents

Parents of children with acquired aphasia with epilepsy may require counseling to assist them in dealing with the sudden and devastating nature of this disorder. They will also require information and support concerning the variability in the course of the disorder and its long-term prognosis. Parents should receive careful instructions about the administration and monitoring of any drug treatments that are prescribed. Parents should also be encouraged to communicate with their child using alternative strategies such as pictures, written messages, or sign language, which may be recommended by a speech–language specialist. Because this disorder is so rare, parents should also be helped to take a role in educating others about the disorder and advocating for their child's needs. In this regard, parents may use the Internet to contact self-help organizations for children with this disorder.

Outcome

Short- and long-term outcome

Outcomes are variable in this disorder. Most children recover some language functioning relative to their most acute stage of language loss. This recovery may occur quickly over a period of days or slowly over many years. The majority of cases, however, do not recover normal language functioning. Persistent language problems continue into adulthood and range in severity from mild problems in comprehension and expression to total inability to communicate with oral language. In contrast, the abnormal EEG findings and seizures usually disappear by adolescence.

Prognostic factors

Age of onset is a prognostic indicator, with earlier onset of language loss associated with poorer prognosis for recovery of language functioning. Recovery does not appear to be associated with the extent of language loss or the presence or absence of seizures.

SUGGESTED READING

J. Bauman-Waengler, *Articulatory and Phonological Impairments: A Clinical Focus, 2nd edn.* (Needham Heights, MA: Allyn & Bacon, 2004).

J. Beitchman, D. Cantwell, S. Forness, K. Kavale & J. Kauffman, Practice parameters for the assessment and treatment of children and adolescents with language and learning disorders. *Journal of the American Academy of Child and Adolescent Psychiatry*, **37** (10 Suppl.) (1998), 46S.

J. H. Beitchman, B. Wilson, C. J. Johnson *et al.*, Fourteen-year follow-up of speech/language-impaired and control children: psychiatric outcome. *Journal of the American Academy of Child Adolescent Psychiatry*, **40** (2001), 75.

N. J. Cohen, M. Davine, N. Horodezky, L. Lipsett & L. Isaacson, Unsuspected language impairment in psychiatrically disturbed children: Prevalence and language and behavioral characteristics. *Journal of the American Academy of Child and Adolescent Psychiatry*, **32** (1993), 595.

H. Kolski & H. Otsubo, The Landau–Kleffner Syndrome. *Advances in Experimental Medicine and Biology*, **497** (2002), 195–208.

J. Law, J. Boyle, F. Harris, A. Harkness & C. Nye, Prevalence and natural history of primary speech and language delay: findings from a systematic review of the literature. International *Journal of Language and Communication Disorders*, **35** (2000), 165.

L. B. Leonard, *Children with Specific Language Impairment.* (Cambridge, MA: Bradford, 1998).

J. H. Menkes & H. B. Sarnat (eds.) *Child Neurology*, 6th edn. (Lippincott Williams & Wilkins, 2000).

L. Olswang, B. Rodriguez & G. Timler, Recommending intervention for toddlers with specific language impairment: we may not have all the answers, but we know a lot. *American Journal of Speech and Language Pathology*, **7** (1998), 23.

R. Paul, *Language Disorders from Infancy through Adolescence: Assessment and Intervention.* 2nd edn. (St. Louis, MO: Mosby, 2001).

R. O. Robinson, G. Baird, G. Robinson & E. Simonoff, Landau–Kleffner syndrome: course and correlates with outcome. *Developmental Medicine and Child Neurology*, **43** (2001), 243.

L. Shriberg & J. Kwiatkowski, Developmental phonological disorders. I: A clinical profile. *Journal of Speech, Language and Hearing Research*, **37** (1994), 1100.

L. Shriberg, D. Austin, B. Lewis, J. McSweeny & D. Wilson, The speech disorders classification system (SDCS): extensions and lifespan reference data. *Journal of Speech, Language and Hearing Research*, **40** (1997), 723.

C. Toppelberg & T. Shapiro, Language disorders: a 10-year research update review. *Journal of the American Academy of Child and Adolescent Psychiatry*, **39** (2000), 143.

D. Weindrich, Ch. Jennen-Steinmetz, M. Laucht, G. Esser & M. H. Schmidt, Epidemiology and prognosis of specific disorders of language and scholastic skills. *European Child and Adolescent Psychiatry*, **9** (2000), 186.

15

Reading and other learning disorders

Margaret J. Snowling[1] and Barbara Maughan[2]

[1]Department of Psychology, University of York, UK
[2]Institute of Psychiatry, De Crespigny Park, London, UK

Introduction

The majority of children who have adequate educational opportunity learn to read without difficulty, and this provides access to the wider curriculum. For a significant minority, however, specific learning difficulties represent a major obstacle to progress, initially with reading, spelling and writing processes and subsequently (as a consequence) with many other aspects of schooling. Reading and spelling difficulties are often accompanied by problems with numeracy, but some children have difficulties with arithmetic or mathematics in the absence of reading problems. Specific learning difficulties are commonly described as 'dyslexia' if they affect reading and spelling processes, and 'dyscalculia' if arithmetic is specifically affected. In addition the term 'non-verbal learning difficulty' or 'syndrome' (NVLS) is sometimes used to describe children whose main scholastic difficulty is with mathematical thinking but who may have accompanying problems with motor skills, attention and social relationships. There is a substantial body of evidence to guide clinical practice with respect to dyslexia, and to a lesser extent dyscalculia. In contrast, there is a paucity of research on NVLS, and it is not currently recognized in the diagnostic systems although similarities with Asperger syndrome have been noted. In view of the lack of consensus about this syndrome, we do not discuss it further here.

Definition and classification

ICD-10 classifies specific learning difficulties as 'specific disorders of scholastic skill'. The following disorders are included: specific reading disorder, specific spelling disorder, specific disorder of arithmetic skill and mixed disorder of scholastic skills. The use of two further entries is discouraged: other developmental disorders of

A Clinician's Handbook of Child and Adolescent Psychiatry, ed. Christopher Gillberg,
Richard Harrington and Hans-Christoph Steinhausen. Published by Cambridge University Press.
© Cambridge University Press 2005.

scholastic skills and developmental disorder of scholastic skills, unspecified. In general, specific learning difficulties are diagnosed if a child's achievement, as measured by individually administered standardized tests of reading, maths or written expression, is substantially below that expected for his or her age and intelligence, and provided that school experiences have been in the expectable range. ICD-10 advocates a conservative criterion of attainment falling 2 standard errors of prediction below the level expected on the basis of the child's chronological age and general intelligence, with all tests administered on an individual basis. Furthermore, there must be no external factors that could account for underachievement. ICD-10 notes that in these disorders the normal process of skills acquisition is disturbed from the outset, due to abnormalities in cognitive function, largely the result of some form of biological dysfunction. It also emphasizes that there is a need to take the developmental course of the disorder into account. Retardation of one year (e.g. in reading) at age 7, for example, is much more severe than a similar level of retardation at age 14; in addition, the nature of associated impairments may change with age (see below).

DSM-IV classifies specific learning difficulties as 'Learning Disorders' and includes the following: reading disorder, mathematical disorder, disorder of written expression and learning disorder not otherwise specified. The diagnosis should be used if the disorder interferes with academic achievement or with activities of daily living that require reading, writing or mathematical skills. DSM-IV is less specific than ICD-10 in terms of the attainment levels to be included, only requiring that measured attainments (in reading, maths, or writing) should be 'substantially below' those expected for the individual's age, IQ and schooling. If a sensory deficit is present, the learning difficulties must be in excess of those usually associated with the disorder. DSM-IV also notes that low self-esteem, demoralization and social problems are frequently associated with learning disorders and that there is a high degree of co-morbidity with disruptive disorders and depression. In adulthood, many individuals with learning disorders have difficulties in employment or social adjustment.

The key features of the different disorders, according to the classification manuals, are summarized in Tables 15.1 and 15.2. However, the diagnosis of specific learning difficulties is more often the domain of psychologists and educators than of psychiatrists. Arguably, therefore, the formal diagnostic criteria have been tempered by educational policy and practice. There has, for example, been considerable concern in recent years about adherence to the 'discrepancy definition' of reading disorders that prescribes that reading attainment should be low relative to age and intelligence. The main reasons for these concerns are that (a) the correlation between IQ and reading skill is relatively low; (b) there are few cognitive differences relevant to reading between poor readers of high and low IQ; and

Table 15.1. Diagnostic criteria for specific developmental disorders of scholastic skills according to ICD-10

Specific reading disorder (F81.0)
A. Either of the following must be present:
  (1) a score on reading accuracy and/or comprehension that is at least 2 standard errors of prediction below the level expected on the basis of the child's chronological age and general intelligence, with both reading skills and IQ assessed on an individually administered test standardized for the child's culture and educational system;
  (2) a history of serious reading difficulties, or test scores that met criterion A(1) at an earlier stage, plus a score on a spelling test that is at least 2 standard errors of prediction below the level expected on the basis of the child's chronological age and IQ.
B. The disturbance described in criterion A significantly interferes with academic achievement or with activities of daily living that require reading skills.
C. The disorder is not the direct result of a defect in visual or hearing acuity, or of a neurological disorder.
D. School experiences are within the average expectable range (i.e. there have been no extreme inadequacies in educational experiences).
E. *Most commonly used exclusion clause.* IQ is below 70 on an individually administered standardized test.

Specific spelling disorder (F81.1)
A. The score on a standardized spelling test is at least 2 standard errors of prediction below the level expected on the basis of the child's chronological age and general intelligence.
B. Scores on reading accuracy and comprehension and on arithmetic are within the normal range (± 2 standard deviations from the mean).
C. There is no history of significant reading difficulties.
D. School experience is in the average expectable range (i.e. there have been no extreme inadequacies in educational experiences).
E. Spelling difficulties have been present from the early stages of learning to spell.
F. The disturbance described in criterion A significantly interferes with academic achievement or with activities of daily living that require spelling skills.
G. *Most commonly used exclusion clause.* IQ is below 70 on an individually administered standardized test.

Specific disorder of arithmetical skills (F81.2)
A. The score on a standardized arithmetic test is at least 2 standard errors of prediction below the level expected on the basis of the child's chronological age and general intelligence.
B. Scores on reading accuracy and comprehension and on arithmetic are within the normal range (± 2 standard deviations from the mean).
C. There is no history of significant reading or spelling difficulties.
D. School experience is in the average expectable range (i.e. there have been no extreme inadequacies in educational experiences).
E. Arithmetical difficulties have been present from the early stages of learning arithmetic.

(cont.)

Table 15.1. (*cont.*)

F.   The disturbance described in criterion A significantly interferes with academic achievement or with activities of daily living that require arithmetical skills.

G.   *Most commonly used exclusion clause.* IQ is below 70 on an individually administered standardized test.

Mixed disorder of scholastic skills (F81.3)

This is an ill-defined, inadequately conceptualized (but necessary) residual category of disorders in which both arithmetical and reading or spelling skills are significantly impaired, but in which the disorder is not solely explicable in terms of general mental retardation or inadequate schooling. It should not be used for disorders meeting the criteria for F81.2 and either F81.0 or F81.1.

Developmental disorder of scholastic skills, unspecified (F81.9)

This category should be avoided as far as possible and should be used only for unspecified disorders in which there is a significant disability of learning that cannot be solely accounted for by mental retardation, visual acuity problems, or inadequate schooling.

(c) given appropriate provision, the prognosis for children with specific reading disorders and more general reading difficulties is similar. In addition, it is not clear what aspects of IQ should be measured (verbal or performance), and the degree of under-achievement to be regarded as significant is arbitrary. It has therefore been argued by some that the measurement of IQ is not central to the diagnosis of reading disorders (although practice still varies with regard to this issue, as acknowledged by ICD-10). The criteria used to diagnose the other learning disorders have been less contentious (primarily because these diagnoses are seldom used); in fact, there is not a one-to-one mapping between the categories of disorder specified in the diagnostic manuals and those typically used by school systems or by researchers in the field.

Table 15.3 summarizes the similarities and differences between the DSM-IV and the ICD-10 classifications of learning disorders and shows the relationship between these and some of the more commonly used terms in educational practice and in the extensive research literature. Variation both among professionals involved in the diagnosis and management of these disorders, and among the school systems in which they work precludes a definitive classification, but the Table is nonetheless informative. It highlights a number of key points. First, the disorders primarily affect two domains of learning: literacy and numeracy. While finer cuts in the classification of learning disorders are possible, these two sorts of learning problem (which in some cases are co-morbid) capture the majority of difficulties that interfere with academic achievement or daily life skills. Second, ICD-10 and DSM-IV deal differently with children who face learning difficulties in more than one domain: in

Table 15.2. Diagnostic criteria for learning disorders according to DSM-IV

Reading disorder

A. Reading achievement, as measured by individually administered standardized tests of reading accuracy or comprehension, is substantially below that expected given the person's chronological age, measured intelligence and age-appropriate education.

B. The disturbance in Criterion A significantly interferes with academic achievement or with activities of daily living that require reading skills.

C. If a sensory deficit is present, the reading difficulties are in excess of those usually associated with it.

Coding note: If a general medical (e.g. neurological) condition or sensory deficit is present, code the condition on Axis III.

Mathematics disorder

A. Mathematical ability, as measured by individually administered standardized tests, is substantially below that expected given the person's chronological age, measured intelligence and age-appropriate education.

B. The disturbance in Criterion A significantly interferes with academic achievement or with activities of daily living that require mathematical skills.

C. If a sensory deficit is present, the difficulties in mathematical ability are in excess of those usually associated with it.

Coding note: If a general medical (e.g. neurological) condition or sensory deficit is present, code the condition on Axis III.

Disorder of written expression

A. Writing skills, as measured by individually administered standardized tests (or functional assessments of writing skills), are substantially below those expected given the person's chronological age, measured intelligence and age-appropriate education.

B. The disturbance in Criterion A significantly interferes with academic achievement or with activities of daily living that require the composition of written texts (e.g. writing grammatically correct sentences and organized paragraphs).

C. If a sensory deficit is present, the difficulties in writing skills are in excess of those usually associated with it.

Coding note: If a general medical (e.g. neurological) condition or sensory deficit is present, code the condition on Axis III.

Learning disorder not otherwise specified

This category is for disorders in learning that do not meet criteria for any specific Learning Disorder. This category might include problems in all three areas (reading, mathematics and written expression) that together significantly interfere with academic achievement although performance on tests measuring each individual skill is not substantially below that expected given the person's chronological age, measured intelligence and age-appropriate education.

Table 15.3. DSM-IV and the ICD-10 classifications of learning disorders in relation to common terms used to describe children's special educational needs

Core Deficit	ICD-10	DSM-IV	Educational Practice	Psychological Research
Reading skill (accuracy)	Specific reading disorder	Reading disorder	Specific learning difficulties (SpLD) or Dyslexia	Specific reading difficulties; Developmental dyslexia
Reading comprehension		–	–	Poor comprehender
History of reading difficulties with current spelling disorder		–	Dyslexia	Dyslexia (compensated)
Spelling skill (no history of reading difficulties)	Specific spelling disorder	–	Specific spelling difficulties	Developmental dysgraphia
Arithmetical skills (without reading/spelling difficulties)	Specific disorder of arithmetic skills	–	Specific difficulties in mathematical learning (numeracy)	Dyscalculia
Mathematical skills		Mathematics disorder		Non-verbal learning difficulty or syndrome (NLVS)
Writing skills (difficulties in composition)	Other developmental disorder of scholastic skills	Disorder of written expression	Would typically be noted as an accompanying feature of SpLD	–
Reading, spelling and arithmetic	Mixed disorder of scholastic skills		SpLD or dyslexia	Sp LD

Notes: The term 'specific' refers to the fact that the deficit is observed in an individual whose IQ is in the normal range; for educational and research purposes, an IQ of 85 or above is usually assumed. ICD-10 recommends that an IQ < 70 should be taken as an exclusion factor.

DSM-IV diagnoses can be made in each area where disorders are observed, while ICD-10 imposes a hierarchy whereby specific spelling disorder is only diagnosed in the absence of significant reading problems, and specific disorder of arithmetic skills is only diagnosed in children without marked reading or spelling difficulties.

Literacy problems

Under the umbrella of problems of literacy come reading, reading comprehension, spelling and writing difficulties. Neither ICD-10 nor DSM-IV separates out problems of reading accuracy from problems of reading comprehension, although this difference is very important in educational practice (where comprehension difficulties are frequently overlooked). Moreover, although it is possible to find spelling difficulties in the absence of reading problems, this is rare and most times reading and spelling difficulties stem from the same core cognitive deficits (and of course failure to read exacerbates spelling difficulties). It is also noteworthy that the term 'disorder of written expression' is rarely used, although most practitioners are aware that in almost all cases where literacy is affected, the production of written work is the most seriously affected skill. Finally, implicit in the classification of learning disorders is the assumption that the diagnosis of reading disorder should be made only when there is no mathematical or arithmetic learning problem. Yet research has shown that reading and arithmetic processes share, to some extent, the same cognitive base, making the dissociation of the two disorders less likely than their association.

Numeracy problems

Similar to literacy problems, children experience different kinds of difficulty with mathematics, and these are not well differentiated either in the classification manuals or in practice. In principle, arithmetic difficulties (affecting computation) can occur without problems in understanding mathematical concepts, such as numerosity, magnitude, commutativity or geometry, and may reflect verbal short-term memory problems. However, arithmetic tests differ in the extent to which they assess different aspects of numeracy, and this leads to an unhelpful tendency to categorize all mathematical difficulties together. In a similar vein, whether or not the mathematical learning difficulty co-occurs with a reading problem is not usually uppermost in a practitioner's mind, yet this can give important clues as to the nature of the problem; when they co-occur it is important to assess the extent to which simply being unable to read and write well (including organizing one's work on the page) is preventing progress in written maths. When there is no reading disorder, it is more likely that the numeracy problem is due to a difficulty with mathematical thinking *per se*.

In the light of the above discussion, and the nature of the evidence base, we divide the remainder of this chapter between developmental disorders of reading and spelling (literacy), and disorders of number skills (numeracy).

Epidemiology

As will be apparent from the previous discussion, findings from epidemiological studies of learning disorders are likely to be sensitive not only to the diagnostic criteria selected for the survey, but also to the precise tests chosen to assess attainments. A further complicating factor is the educational context in which learning takes place. Taken together, these factors make it very difficult indeed to compare prevalence and incidence figures across age groups, and more significantly across countries. With this in mind, the focus here is on population studies of English-speaking cohorts; such data need to be interpreted cautiously with respect to other linguistic and cultural contexts, where differences might include the age of school entry and the type of reading instruction.

Reading difficulties and dyslexia

Prevalence and incidence

In English-speaking countries reading disorders affect between 4 per cent and 8 per cent of school-aged children. Using an IQ-discrepancy criterion of 2 standard errors of prediction below expected performance, early epidemiological studies in England reported prevalence rates of just over 3 per cent (3.1% on tests of reading accuracy, and 3.6% on tests of reading comprehension) among 9- and 10-year olds in a non-metropolitan area. Using exactly comparable screening and assessment procedures, rates were more than doubled (at 6.3% for reading accuracy and 9.3% for reading comprehension) in an inner city area, suggesting that social factors play a key role in risk for reading disability. At this level of severity the great majority of these 'IQ-discrepant' poor readers also read very poorly for their chronological age, and were if anything more impaired in spelling than in reading.

Not unexpectedly, rates of reading disability vary with age. Incidence rates rise sharply over the early school years; estimates based on IQ-discrepancy criteria peak at around ages 9 to 11 years, while low achievement formulas continue to identify additional poor readers in the early teens. Children first identified at different ages may have differing patterns of cognitive deficits (see Clinical Picture for a more detailed discussion). Problems with word decoding are likely to predominate in the earliest years of schooling. A second, later-emerging group of poor readers appear to have adequate decoding skills (and so cope with the initial stages of learning to read) but face problems at older ages when the curriculum requires a heavier emphasis on comprehension. Later still, in the teens and into adulthood, individuals who have overcome (or compensated for) early reading difficulties may still face problems with spelling or written expression. In addition, it is important to remember that (like all other types of psychological assessment) classifications of reading disorders inevitably involve measurement error. As a result, repeated assessments of the same child at different ages may not be entirely stable: some children will fall just below a chosen threshold at one age, but just above at another. Enquiring about the history of a child's literacy difficulties, as well as about current performance levels, is central to a comprehensive assessment.

The language in which children learn to read appears to affect the likelihood of reading disorders (though evidence remains somewhat anecdotal on this issue). European languages vary markedly in the consistency or transparency of their writing systems. Many (including Dutch, Italian, German, Spanish, Czech, Greek and the Nordic languages) show very regular correspondences between speech sounds and their written expressions, while others – most notably English, but to a lesser extent Danish and French – are much less regular (or more opaque). Opaque orthographies present all children with more challenges in learning to read, and normally developing young readers learn to read and spell more quickly in languages with more transparent writing systems. However, such comparisons are confounded by differences in teaching regime. For example, languages that have transparent orthographies tend to favour phonic approaches to the teaching of reading. Such regimes facilitate the development decoding skills but not reading fluency, which appears to be a source of reading difficulty in such languages.

Sex ratios

Boys are considerably more likely to be referred for reading difficulties than girls, but epidemiological studies suggest that this is not simply a matter of referral bias. Sex ratios of between 1.5:1 and 3:1 males: females have been reported in large-scale community studies, confirming that boys are indeed at increased risk.

Mathematical difficulties and dyscalculia

Prevalence

The prevalence of arithmetic and mathematical disorders is less well documented than for reading, and little is known about incidence rates. Overall prevalence rates of around 6–7 per cent have been reported from the USA and Europe, but few studies have separated pure arithmetic difficulties from disorders involving both numeracy and reading. In one UK study that did so, the prevalence of specific arithmetic difficulties was recorded as only 1.3 per cent in an epidemiological sample of 9 to 10 year olds. Although this estimate seems low, it is rare in clinical experience to find a child referred because of arithmetic difficulties (possible dyscalculia) who does not also have dyslexia.

Sex ratios

Unlike reading disorders, specific numeracy problems are as common (if not slightly more common) in girls as in boys.

Implications for clinical practice

Although boys are much more likely to present with reading disorders than girls, it is important not to overlook the possibility of a reading disability in girls who are struggling in literacy-related aspects of schoolwork. In addition, because reading and arithmetic difficulties often overlap, it is wise to consider the possibility of associated mathematical or reading difficulties even when a child is primarily referred because of concerns in just one aspect of academic skills.

Clinical picture

Reading difficulties and dyslexia

Before discussing the clinical presentation of dyslexia and related disorders, it is necessary to briefly describe what is known about the process of learning to read (and spell), to provide a context for understanding the relationship between the core symptoms and their impact. The most widely accepted current view is that reading requires the child to understand that the letters of printed words map to the sounds of spoken words – the so-called alphabetic principle. (In Chinese languages, the reading process is different and will not be discussed here.) A pre-requisite is that the child should know the letters of the alphabet and their sounds, and that they should be able to reflect on the sound structure of words, an ability referred to as phonological awareness. Phonological awareness is measured by tasks such as deciding whether or not two words rhyme (*boat-coat* vs *boat-trip*), deciding which is the odd one out in a set of spoken words (such as sack, set, moat, sort) or deleting a sound from a nonword to give a word (*bice*, take away the /b/ is '*ice*'). Phonological awareness tasks are very difficult for young children, especially when they require the manipulation of phonemes (the smallest units of speech); dealing with rhyming units (e.g. –*oat*) is easier, but arguably less directly related to learning to read.

Once children have acquired the alphabetic principle, they begin to read (and write) words using a phonic approach. However, they still have a long way to go before their reading skills are automatic. English, an inconsistent writing system in which many words have irregular spellings, takes many years for children to master (this is also true of Danish and to a lesser extent of French). The challenge is less marked for readers of more transparent writing systems in which letter–sound correspondences are predictable with few exceptions.

Regardless of the language that has to be learned, fluent reading is required if reading comprehension is to be adequate. Poor readers of transparent orthographies, such as German or Italian have been reported to be accurate but slow in reading, placing them at risk of problems of reading comprehension because of a 'bottleneck' in processing capacity. It is important to note, however, that reading comprehension draws on additional skills to those involved in decoding. Specifically, in order to understand what has been read, an individual has to have adequate vocabulary knowledge, good working memory resources, the ability to make inferences and various other processes specific to text integration (such as monitoring what has been read). It is for this reason that problems of reading comprehension can occur even when basic decoding skills are well developed. Such specific reading comprehension deficits are usually associated with wider language difficulties than are observed in dyslexia.

Developmental course of dyslexia

Table 15.4 outlines the primary presenting characteristics of dyslexia at different ages and summarizes what is known about the different manifestations in transparent and opaque languages.

Pre-school manifestation

Because learning disorders are defined in relation to scholastic attainments, clinicians will seldom be required to diagnose them in the pre-school years. Nonetheless, since dyslexia runs in families, it is worth the clinician who is involved with an older child asking about younger siblings, with a view to providing relevant advice. Recent research shows that the precursors of dyslexia in the pre-school period which serve as useful indicators that the child is 'at risk' include:

- slow speech development
- speech difficult to understand (an older child may translate)
- understanding in advance of the ability to express him or herself in words
- difficulty learning nursery rhymes
- slow to learn letters (e.g. from alphabetic friezes)
- often a lack of interest in activities such as drawing and colouring.

This list makes clear that (regrettably) 'dyslexia' will be easier to detect in a middle-class household and may be overlooked more easily in a first-born child (where there is no one with whom parents can compare his or her development).

Early school years

School systems differ in the age at which children begin to receive formal reading instruction (at the present time, this is at the age of 5 years in the UK and about a year later elsewhere in the European community). Cardinal symptoms of dyslexia in the early school years are slow mastery of letters and difficulty acquiring phonological

Table 15.4. Presenting characteristics of dyslexia at different ages, with differences between dyslexia in English and in more transparent languages in italics

Developmental phase	Symptom in English	Symptom present in transparent languages
Preschool	Delayed speech	Delayed speech
	Poor expressive language	Poor expressive language
	Poor rhyming skills	Poor rhyming skills
	Little interest in letters	Little interest in letters
	Poor letter knowledge	*Not usually taught before school*
Early school years	Poor letter knowledge	Poor letter knowledge
	Poor phonological awareness	Poor phonological awareness
	Poor memory for verbal instructions	Poor memory for verbal instructions
	Poor word attack skills	*Phonic skills develop relatively well; reading is slow*
	Idiosyncratic spelling	*Phonetic spelling*
	Problems copying	Problems copying
Middle school years	Difficulty learning tables and number facts	Difficulty learning tables and number facts
	Word finding difficulties and subtle speech problems	Word finding difficulties and subtle speech problems
	Subtle speech problems (e.g. on polysyllabic words)	Subtle speech problems (e.g. on polysyllabic words)
	Slow reading	Slow reading
	Poor decoding skills when faced with new words	*Decoding is accurate but slow*
	Phonetic spelling	Phonetic spelling
Adolescence and adulthood	Poor verbal memory affects performance	Poor verbal memory affects performance
	Lack of reading fluency	Lack of reading fluency
	Slow speed of writing	Slow speed of writing
	Organization and expression in written work	Organization and expression in written work
	Naming difficulties	Naming difficulties

awareness (particularly phoneme skills). Although the child may be able to build a reasonable sight vocabulary of words if their memory for what they see is good, their phonic skills typically lag behind. They also have difficulty spelling because this skill is more demanding on phonological skills than reading; it requires the ability to segment words into phonemes, to hold these in mind whilst also trying to remember how to write the letters. Many parents report a rapid decline in the confidence of a child with dyslexia during the first two years in school. Sometimes, the problem may come to light because behaviour deteriorates at school or because the child becomes easily upset, particularly at home.

Middle school years

It is in the middle school years that the problems of dyslexia come to the fore. Even the intelligent and well-supported dyslexic child, who may have managed to keep up during the infant school years, can be expected to run into difficulty as the reading and writing demands of the classroom increase in grades 2 to 6. The presenting picture depends, however, on the language of instruction (see Table 15.4). For children learning to read English, word decoding difficulties associated with poor phonics knowledge persist and slow down the development of the sight vocabulary. Since it is almost never the case that words that cannot be read can be spelled, spelling becomes an increasing problem, with errors being both phonetically accurate (e.g. *skool* for *school*) or dysphonetic (e.g. *aventer* for *adventure*). Particularly where there is a preponderance of dysphonetic errors, written work is difficult to decipher. In addition, there is an increasing discrepancy between the child's ability to express him or herself orally and in writing. This may be for a number of reasons: the effort of spelling might be such that the creative use of language is stifled, words and word-endings (e.g. grammatical inflections) may be omitted because attentional resources are devoted to spelling, the child may be excessively slow, or the child may have additional language difficulties, such as vocabulary limitations, that are reflected in their writing.

Research on children learning to read in transparent languages suggests that the behavioural manifestation of dyslexia is rather different or, at least, that the decoding difficulties so typical of dyslexia in English are more easily overcome. By the middle school years, most children with dyslexia have reasonable mastery of the alphabetic principle (arguably because the orthographic system supports it). Their reading is therefore relatively accurate, at least compared with that seen in their English-speaking counterparts, though it is not perfect. The main presenting symptom is a lack of reading fluency, although some may complain about reading comprehension, presumably because of a bottleneck in text processing caused by their slow reading. In most of the European languages, spelling is less predictable than reading. Thus, dyslexic children tend to have spelling difficulties in these languages, as they do in English.

Outside of literacy processes, children with dyslexia present with a range of other deficits that can affect both their behaviour in the classroom and their morale. Dyslexia is a controversial field and several different hypotheses concerning its causes have been proposed. These include deficits in rapid auditory processing, magnocellular deficits and cerebellar impairments. Common to all these theories is the prediction that children with dyslexia will experience phonological (speech) processing impairments. Indeed, the most widely accepted contemporary view is that many of the difficulties observed in dyslexia stem from an underlying cognitive deficit that, theoretically, has been described as a deficit at the level of phonological representations (literally, how the brain encodes the speech sounds of words). This deficit provides a parsimonious explanation for the following problems:

- poor verbal short-term memory (a component of the working memory system that is used in mental arithmetic)
- word finding difficulties (may affect written language expression)
- subtle speech problems, particularly with the pronunciation of long words (e.g. statistical, preliminary)
- poor new word learning (affects second language learning and learning of subject-specific vocabulary, such as terms used in biology).

Ironically, the problems that are a consequence of the phonological deficit are often less easy to compensate than reading and spelling deficits (where teaching and intensive practice can help). Hence problems of short-term memory, word-finding difficulties, and difficulties with novel words in spoken and written language are hallmarks of dyslexia across the lifespan.

Secondary school years and young adulthood

By the time children with dyslexia reach adolescence, a range of different outcomes can be expected depending upon the severity of the disorder, the integrity of other cognitive and linguistic skills, and the reading intervention, teaching and family supports that the child has received. In the most favourable circumstances, the adolescent with dyslexia will be able to read adequately for academic purposes and their spelling will be phonetically acceptable. Most will use a word processor (and spell-checker) to prepare their work. The main presenting symptom will be slowness in reading and in written expression; both of these difficulties can have a deleterious effect on performance in many curriculum areas, particularly literary ones. In addition, many young people with dyslexia complain about having to learn a foreign language, though some take well to second language learning. Examination preparation is problematic for many with dyslexia not only because of poor verbal learning skills, but also because of the anxiety these situations provoke.

In less auspicious circumstances (where less progress has been made in reading and spelling, or where school and family supports have been more limited), reading disorders can adversely affect young people's progress across the school curriculum. Not surprisingly, self-esteem and attitudes to schooling often suffer as a result, and many poor readers become disengaged from education at this stage. Risks of unexplained absence and truancy increase, and some young people will opt to leave school at the earliest opportunity, with minimal or no qualifications.

For those who go on to further or higher education (where it should be borne in mind, they are studying their chosen academic discipline), the main complaints are:

- difficulties with note taking
- the time taken by reading assignments
- difficulties with the organization of written work
- difficulty in meeting deadlines (often because of slowness in working)
- forgetting appointments, such as tutorials
- examination anxiety
- lack of confidence.

Adulthood

Dyslexia can be very stressful in the workplace, not least because of literacy demands, but also because associated difficulties such as problems with working memory, organization and time management may have a significant impact on performance. Many adults with dyslexia prefer not to disclose their difficulties to employers, making it difficult for adequate support to be put in place. In such cases, disciplinary action or dismissal is the worst scenario. A diagnostic assessment can be invaluable in helping employees recognize their own strengths and difficulties and hence, not only to choose an appropriate work setting suited to their abilities, but also to seek further training.

Mathematical difficulties and dyscalculia

In comparison with the wealth of research on the development of literacy, much less is known about the development of numeracy through the school years. It is generally believed that children have an in-built number sense such that, shortly after birth, they can detect the difference between one object in the visual world and two or more objects. Starting from this innate understanding of numerosity, pre-school children learn to count and thereby lay down an important foundation for the subsequent development of their mathematical thinking. At school, they are introduced to conventional number systems including mathematical symbols and formal mathematical procedures, such as addition and subtraction.

Most research attention has been focused on the process of addition which, for young children, builds directly on the child's understanding of the count sequence and cardinality (that the last number counted describes the quantity that is there). In adding two quantities, children first use a strategy called 'count all'; they count one set of items and then carry on to count the next. The next stage is to use the 'count on' strategy; here they start with the number describing the first set and then

Table 15.5. Mathematical disorders: the clinical picture

Verbal mathematical difficulties	Non-verbal mathematical difficulties
Counting	Number sequence
Learning names of number symbols	Magnitude judgements (basis of number concepts)
Learning number bonds	Understanding place value
Learning and using multiplication tables	Selecting the correct algorithm
Subtraction (counting backwards)	Estimation
Mental arithmetic	Spatial concepts (e.g. in geometry)

count on each of the items in the second set. A more sophisticated use of this strategy involves starting first with the larger number, so that a smaller number of items have to be counted (added) on. As children perfect these strategies, they gradually begin to build up their memory for the number bonds, for example, that 2 + 3 equals 5. At a later stage of proficiency, they will begin to directly retrieve these number facts so that they no longer have to add, at least not to solve addition problems involving additions of single digit numbers. Children initially start out using their fingers to aid their addition. As they begin to use direct retrieval strategies, finger-counting normally drops out of their repertoire, though it may be retained for counting backwards (to solve subtraction problems) or for the use of repeated addition as a strategy for multiplication.

In principle, there are two main forms of mathematical learning difficulty. Children can have low-level computational difficulties (with arithmetic) or they can have higher-level conceptual difficulties with maths. Arithmetic difficulties are usually associated with limitations of verbal short-term memory and verbal learning problems, whereas mathematical difficulties can be non-verbal and affect reasoning and spatial imagery processes. However, there is one feature of teaching and learning in the domain of number that means the two 'subtypes' of difficulty are difficult to distinguish; this is that mathematical development is cumulative. In short, basic addition, subtraction, and multiplication processes are involved in higher-level mathematics, such as geometry, algebra and calculus. Hence, a basic deficit in computation seldom remains circumscribed; rather, it is likely to have a pervasive effect on mathematical performance, and even on the acquisition of mathematical concepts within the grasp of the individual. Moreover, high levels of anxiety are often associated with mathematics and these can exacerbate difficulties.

Table 15.5 summarizes the types of problem that are reported by school-age children with mathematical difficulties. The Table separates the problems that are primarily verbal in origin from those that may be considered to have a basis in non-verbal learning difficulties. The verbal type are arithmetic in nature and often associated with dyslexia. The non-verbal type may be seen in children who do not

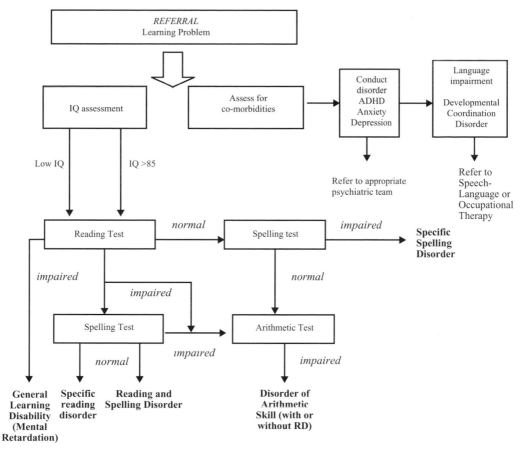

Fig. 15.1.   Assessment of learning problems: decision tree.
(Essential components of an assessment for learning disorders are shown in bold)

have reading problems and who may have quite good rote knowledge of arithmetic facts, such as number bonds.

Differential diagnosis and comorbidity

The main issues for differential diagnosis in numeracy disorders parallel those for literacy disorders and therefore they will be discussed together (see Fig. 15.1 for a decision tree). In practice, it is more likely that a psychiatrist will be consulted about a learning disorder when there are associated emotional or behavioural difficulties than when the disorder occurs in pure form. In the rare case of a 'pure' referral, this is most likely to be when a desperate parent feels unable to convince the education authorities of her child's difficulties and then, the presenting condition is more likely to be dyslexia than dyscalculia (because the latter less often attracts parental concern).

Co-morbidity

Many reading disorders are the sequelae of speech and language disorders. Although signs of persistent speech or language difficulty may be subtle, comprehensive language assessment often reveals significant concurrent co-morbidity. Co-morbidity with disruptive behaviour disorders is also common, and some children with learning disorders are at increased risk of emotional difficulties. Among children of primary school age, co-morbidity with attention deficit hyperactivity disorder (ADHD), especially the inattentive subtype, will frequently be encountered: community surveys show that approaching 20 per cent of children with reading/spelling disorders meet criteria for ADHD, and that rates may be even higher among children with numeracy problems. Conduct disorder also shows strong overlaps with literacy difficulties, sometimes contributing to elevated risks of delinquency in the teens. Finally, although evidence in relation to emotional difficulties is less extensive, co-morbidity with anxiety disorders occurs at higher than expected rates among children with reading disorders, and they also seem prone to low mood.

Associated behaviour problems are often prominent in the concerns of referrers, can adversely affect children's school adjustment, and may exacerbate their learning problems. As a result it is useful for clinicians to ask the parents and teachers of a referred individual to complete a standard rating scale, such as the Strengths and Difficulties Questionnaire (SDQ) before they are seen in order to make a preliminary judgement about possible comorbidities. It is also helpful to ask for sight of school reports to gauge the developmental course of the learning disorder and its accompanying features. Case history taking, particularly focusing on family factors, pre-school language development and early reading acquisition can be very informative. In particular, note should be taken of any persisting difficulties with speech, language or motor skills, and where these are significant, referral to speech–language therapy or occupational therapy may be appropriate.

Assessment

While there are a number of screening instruments for dyslexia available, these should be used with circumspection. Many suffer from the problem of false positives, and in particular, they do not differentiate well between children with specific learning difficulties and children with more general developmental delay (learning disabilities). This is a key question that must be addressed if appropriate management advice is to be given. Formally, the best way of determining this is with the use of an IQ test. When assessing adults, an IQ test can provide a particularly helpful way for a psychologist to assess an individual's strengths and difficulties and also to provide a preliminary assessment of the fit between the person and their current (or hoped for) job.

Once a decision has been made as to whether a referred person has a specific or a more general learning difficulty, the assessment should proceed to diagnose reading, spelling and/or arithmetic problems. A clear issue is the extent to which the psychiatric team, specifically their psychologist, should be involved in this further assessment. For some teams, the more appropriate course of action might be to refer a child on to the relevant educational professionals. For an adult, an occupational psychologist may be able to provide a more relevant job-centred assessment. However, for a diagnosis to be made, the assessment need not take long and will not only provide invaluable advice to the patient, but will also act as a stepping stone to further assessment and appropriate management of the learning disorder.

A brief diagnostic assessment can be undertaken within about one hour, if a shortened IQ test is used. The basic components of an assessment that would give an accurate indication of whether or not a child or adult had a learning disorder would comprise:

- IQ test (short form)
- single word reading and spelling test
- test of written arithmetic (optional in the case of referral for dyslexia)
- test of verbal short-term memory
- test of phonological awareness.

Suggested tests in English are listed in Appendix 15.1. A more comprehensive assessment would be required before setting up a teaching programme, however. This would usually include, in addition to the above, tests of decoding skills, reading fluency, reading comprehension, written expression, arithmetic skills and quantitative reasoning.

Aetiology

Reading difficulties and dyslexia

Although we are far from having a complete understanding of the causes of reading disorders, aetiological influences have been explored at a variety of levels: in terms of underlying cognitive deficits, neurobiological influences and possible environmental concomitants.

Cognitive deficits

The task demands of reading are so complex that reading difficulties may arise for a wide variety of reasons. Dyslexia was initially referred to as 'word blindness', and many parents still assume that it stems primarily from problems in visual processing. Some children with dyslexia do show mild to moderate impairments in visual and auditory perception, and sometimes with motor coordination, and these may well exacerbate their difficulties. The overwhelming balance of evidence now suggests that the core deficits facing most children with reading and spelling difficulties lie in the language system, and more specifically in the realm of phonological processing. Preschool phonological skills predict later reading progress, and deficits in phonological processing are still detectable in adult dyslexics who have largely overcome overt problems with reading and spelling. Phonological difficulties affect children with reading problems irrespective of IQ, and are now viewed as a main cause of impaired word recognition and decoding. In addition, dyslexia is associated with problems in verbal learning, working memory (a system for storing and manipulating information) and listening comprehension.

Where problems centre on poor comprehension, children typically show poor vocabulary knowledge and syntactic skills, and limitations in working memory. In the early school years, poor comprehenders may have adequate decoding skills; over time, however, they may also face declines in reading accuracy. This underscores a key issue for any consideration of the links between specific cognitive skills and reading disorders. Fluent reading is a complex process, relying not only on decoding but also on vocabulary and on comprehension and semantic skills. In normally developing readers progress in each of these skills supports and facilitates growth in others. In children with reading disorders these reciprocal processes are compromised; as a result, initially relatively circumscribed deficits can contribute to wider-ranging patterns of difficulty over time.

Genetic influences

It has long been known that reading difficulties run in families. For a boy, the risk of having a reading problem if his father is dyslexic is as high as 50 per cent (around 40% if his mother is dyslexic); for a girl, risks are somewhat lower. Twin studies have shown that this familiality reflects a significant genetic component: both reading disorders and general reading performance show clear genetic influences. Different reading component sub-skills show different patterns of heritability; heritability estimates also vary with age, so that, for example, genetic influences on word recognition decline as children get older, while genetic effects on spelling increase. In addition, there is evidence that heritability estimates vary with IQ, such that genetic factors are more important contributors to reading disorders among more able children than for those with below average IQs. Currently, reading disorders are attracting extensive attention in molecular genetic research. Replicated gene markers for dyslexia have been identified on chromosomes 1, 2, 3, 6, 15 and 18, though the precise genetic mechanisms that are involved are not yet understood. Finally, there is evidence that the co-morbidity between ADHD and reading disorders is partly attributable to shared genetic effects.

Reading and the brain

Studies of dyslexic readers using functional brain imaging techniques have also burgeoned in recent years. Taken together, these studies suggest that regions of left-hemisphere temporal cortex function differently in dyslexic and normal readers, with dyslexic readers showing under-activation of these areas during reading and phonological processing tasks. Interestingly, minor structural abnormalities have been documented in these regions and a recent report suggests there is a reduction in the volume of gray matter here among dyslexic readers. In addition, dyslexia may be the result of biological factors that are environmental in origin but much less is known about these.

Psycho-social influences

In addition to these cognitive and biological influences, it is clear that school and home environmental factors – either alone, or in combination with individual vulnerabilities – also contribute to a child's risk of developing reading problems. At the most broad-brush level, reading disorders show a strong social gradient that is not entirely attributable to differences in phonological skills or general intellectual abilities, and poor readers often come from large families, where later-born children may face delays in language development.

Direct literacy-related activities in the home will also be important. Perhaps surprisingly, reading with young children has relatively modest effects on later literacy development, though contributions to vocabulary and phonological skills appear larger. From very early in development, however, children differ in their interest in books, and children at risk for dyslexia may well be among those who are more difficult to interest and engage. Where parents themselves have literacy problems, this might also set the stage for less than optimal reading-related experiences in the home. In practice, however, many reading disabled parents are acutely conscious of the need to support their children's literacy development, and anxious for advice on the best approaches to do so.

Reading disorders primarily become apparent at school, and school experiences can undoubtedly be influential. Classroom studies have shown that low and high ability reading groups often provide very different contexts for learning: skilled readers tend to be attentive, and to benefit from each others' successes in oral reading, while their less skilled counterparts often face disruptions in lessons (so reducing the time spent on reading), and are more likely to be exposed to reading errors by their peers. This is just one example of what have been described as 'Matthew effects' in the classroom – rich-get-richer and poor-get-poorer mechanisms whereby the difficulties of struggling readers, and the successes of their more skilled peers, are amplified by their classroom experiences. If, as sometimes happens, reading materials are too difficult, reading can quickly become an unrewarding or anxiety-provoking experience for at-risk children. Over time, the cumulative impact of such processes leads to massive variations in children's 'exposure to print' – a factor known to have an independent effect on reading progress.

Mathematical difficulties and dyscalculia

Much less is known about the causes of mathematical difficulties, and no consensus on aetiology has yet been reached. Some of the main cognitive models focus on the role of working memory: children with mathematical difficulties have problems on simple working memory tasks, on more complex tasks involving the central executive (control processes), and on working memory tasks that require the spatial transformation of non-verbal stimuli. The involvement of executive processes means that children with attentional difficulties are especially likely to face problems in mathematics. Family studies have shown that approximately half of all siblings of children with developmental dyslexia also have mathematical difficulties, and evidence from twin studies also points to a role for genetic effects. As yet, neuroimaging studies have focused mainly on normal individuals engaged in arithmetic tasks. These have shown left frontal lobe activation on relatively simple, over-learned arithmetic tasks (which presumably are language dependent), but that for more complex calculations that involve both visual and numerical magnitude representations, both parietal lobes are activated. At this stage it thus appears that mathematical skills are predicated on a neural network that involves frontal and parietal areas of both hemispheres of the brain. As with reading disorders, environmental factors – and in particular the problems faced by children with arithmetic difficulties in all-ability classrooms – have also been implicated in the development of dyscalculia. Finally, there is emerging evidence that dyscalculia is associated with emotional disorders. More generally, children who are anxious about maths tend to perform poorly on basic arithmetic tasks because they sacrifice accuracy for speed; psychological interventions for such anxiety can improve competence in mathematics significantly.

Treatment

There is now a considerable body of research evaluating interventions for reading disability. In recognition of this, in the USA, the National Reading Panel has recently produced a detailed report of best practice in the teaching of reading. There is no comparable body of knowledge relating to the teaching of mathematics to children with impairments, although there are certainly very good maths teachers and their instruction manuals provide advice on how best to manage children with arithmetic disorders.

Educational management and treatment setting

Decisions about the management of children's learning disorders are, by necessity, shaped by the current educational climate. At the present time, the climate is one of inclusion; it follows that the main aim is to educate children with learning disorders along with their peers in mainstream classrooms. Although this is a laudable aim, many professionals who work with such children are concerned that, as evidence shows, their needs are best met by intensive individualized programmes $z = s$ of intervention, and these cannot easily be delivered in a mainstream setting. Thus, whilst every effort should be made to keep a learning disabled child with his or her peers for social reasons, in the most severe cases, special placement may need to be considered.

In the most ideal scenario, a child's learning difficulty will be identified early and appropriate support given in the classroom. If the difficulty persists or the current management arrangements are insufficient to keep the difficulties at bay, then a staged process of management usually begins. An example is outlined below:

- classroom support and monitoring, ideally with input from home
- withdrawal for small group teaching
- withdrawal for individual support (it would be rare for a child with dyscalculia in the absence of literacy problems to proceed further than this stage)
- placement in a special unit (or rarely, in specialist schools).

In further and higher education settings, there is sometimes a resource for students who require learning support. In the UK, students with dyslexia are eligible for a Disabled Student's Allowance from their local education authority, which they can use to pay for extra teaching support or for equipment such as a dictaphone. They may also, in severe cases, use the fund to pay for a note-taker in lectures or a proof-reader to assist them to correct their work.

As an adult with a learning disorder, support can be more difficult to find. When seeking a job, it is best to disclose any dyslexic (or arithmetic) difficulties that might affect performance and take steps to ensure that the appropriate support is in place. It is worth finding out about government-funded schemes to improve literacy levels in the workforce where these exist, and also possibly alerting potential employers.

Interventions

During the past 20 years, there have been two important influences on the teaching of reading and spelling to children with difficulties. The first, associated with Marie Clay in New Zealand, was Reading Recovery; the second, associated with Lynette Bradley and Peter Bryant in the UK was phonological awareness training. Both approaches were successful in helping failing readers whose problems were identified early. Following on from this, it has been demonstrated that a combination of these two approaches provides a powerful intervention for poor readers.

The combined approach, devised by Peter Hatcher, UK, has been used successfully by trained teachers with poor readers from the age of 6 years, with older dyslexic children and with children with moderate learning disabilities.

The main elements of this approach include:

- training in letter knowledge
- teaching concepts of print
- training to manipulate the sounds of words, particularly phoneme awareness
- applying letter and sound knowledge to word reading and writing (phonics)
- reading text at an easy level (for reinforcement, practice and confidence)
- reading text at an instructional level (to practice decoding words in context, with teacher support)
- writing a simple story (could be just one word or one sentence, with support).

Lessons are individual and last for 30 minutes, at least twice a week. More recently, the approach has been adapted for delivery by mainstream teachers to whole classes, and by teaching assistants to small groups. The effects of the mainstream approach were not found to be significant for children who were learning to read normally (they did not need the phonological training). However, it was particularly helpful for children at risk of reading difficulties on school entry. For these children, supplementing their reading curriculum with phoneme awareness training during the first five terms of school prevented a decline in reading attainment (relative to their peers) that was seen in controls who did not receive such training. The second adaptation was used by trained teaching assistants, working with groups of six 6-year-old children whose reading was progressing slowly. The programme, which was delivered on a daily basis (for 12 weeks), was effective in moving their reading skills from the low average to the average range for their age.

It is important to emphasize that dyslexic children with severe phonological deficits can respond very slowly even to the most effective of teaching approaches. Indeed, initial phonological skill is one of the best predictors of responsiveness to intervention. It is perhaps because of their slowness of response, and in some cases, the intractable nature of the disorder, that some families turn to alternative or complementary therapies to help their dyslexic children. These may be useful in individual cases but the evidence base for their efficacy is almost totally lacking. For children who do not respond to conventional treatments, the best advice at the present time is to consider more intensive therapies, including special school placement. In addition, information technologies have a lot to offer. Ideally, students with dyslexia should be taught to become fluent keyboard users, with special instruction in the use of a spell-checker. In addition, some children with dyslexia can use voice-to-text synthesis as an aid to written work successfully.

In formal assessments and examinations, people with dyslexia should normally be eligible for allowances and accommodations. Usually these would be granted following an assessment by a psychologist or specialist teacher. The most common allowance is extra time in written examinations, and dispensation for spelling errors. If the student has particularly poor reading skills, then they may be allowed someone to read the questions to them. Similarly, an emanuensis can be granted in the case of severe difficulties with the production of written work. In addition, if the student has been using a computer routinely in the classroom, then they may apply to use one in examinations. A more usual course of action is for the student's examination papers to be typed up at the end of the assessment, before they are marked. It needs to be emphasized, however, that allowances are granted on the assumption that (a) the student wishes for them (b) the student is used to having them. They may be counter-productive for the student who does not want to stand out as 'different', who may get excessively tired in examinations or who does not know how to use extra time or an emanuensis wisely.

Monitoring and evaluation of treatments

Best practice dictates that procedures should be in place within school systems for the assessment and management of learning disorders in children of school age. Multi-professional assessment is often needed in the case of complex difficulties, particularly where there are co-morbid emotional or behavioural disorders. As outlined earlier, learning disorders are frequently co-morbid with ADHD and other disruptive behaviour disorders, and to a lesser extent with anxiety and depression. Detailed guidelines for the treatment and management of these conditions are set out in other chapters in this volume. Although academic outcomes may show some modest improvements from the successful management of co-morbid emotional/behavioural disorders, evidence is too sparse at this stage to recommend specific treatments for co-morbid disorders on grounds of their likely benefits for learning; as a result, the management of co-morbid conditions should proceed as appropriate given the nature of the presenting emotional/behavioural problems and associated impairments. It is good practice for there to be within-school reviews of progress towards educational objectives at least once per term. Formally, there needs to be a multi-professional review of the learning disorder on an annual basis.

Practice is more variable with respect to learning disorders in adolescence and adulthood. The main aim of diagnosis should be to provide an explanation of what may be a history of underachievement, and an understanding by the patient of their strengths and difficulties. This should place the patient in the best position to seek relevant advice, support and training and in the longer term, to seek improved career and employment options.

Outcome

There have now been a considerable number of follow-ups of reading disabled children into the teens, and a smaller number into adulthood. By contrast, very little is known about the prognosis for dyscalculia; as a result, this section focuses primarily on outcomes of reading problems.

Reading disorders and dyslexia

Three main issues have been explored in follow-up studies of developmental reading problems: (i) the persistence of reading and spelling difficulties; (ii) the impact of those difficulties on other aspects of adolescent and adult functioning; and (iii) the long-term implications of the co-morbidity between reading problems and disruptive behaviours in childhood.

Persistence of reading problems

Longitudinal studies have consistently shown that developmental reading problems persist. As a group, poor readers continue to lag behind their peers in reading and spelling skills throughout the school years, unless they are the recipients of very effective teaching. IQ-discrepant and generally backward readers make similar progress, and initial severity, along with general intellectual skills, seem the most important predictors of reading levels in the teens. Comprehension and word recognition skills do improve, but the underlying phonological deficits found in dyslexic children are often highly resistant to change; as a result, later reading is less automatic, more effortful, and slow. As in childhood, there will be a spread in later reading and spelling skills. In representative samples, around 20 per cent of severely disabled readers can be expected to achieve normal reading levels by adulthood, and that proportion is often higher in clinic samples. Spelling may be more severely affected: in one adult follow-up 75 per cent of poor readers fell in the bottom 10 per cent of scores in a comparison group, and none scored above the median. For a sizeable minority of disabled readers, continuing problems with reading and spelling will be severe enough to affect progress in many aspects of the school curriculum. For the most severely affected, even the most basic everyday reading materials may prove difficult to access well into adult life.

For clinicians, these findings provide a valuable basis for advising children and families on the likely outlook for young people with dyslexia: realistically, most will need to recognize that their difficulties will persist at some level, and may require ongoing accommodations. What the bald follow-up findings fail to capture is the subjective experience of facing continuing difficulties in a core skill area that most children master soon after they start school. Many adolescents with dyslexia retain a lingering sense that they are lazy or slow, and find schooling either anxiety-provoking or aversive. Even in adulthood, a proportion of individuals with reading disorders will continue to face problems with the literacy demands of day-to-day life – filling in forms, writing letters, even signing cheques can be troublesome, and, if they need to be done in public, a source of real worry and embarrassment. As access to computers and spell-checkers expands, these difficulties are becoming less pressing; even so, a minority of adults with dyslexia rely heavily on others to help them in literacy-related tasks, and some effectively avoid them.

Educational attainments and pychosocial functioning

On-going literacy problems inevitably impact on broader patterns of educational attainment. Here, however, social background also seems central to progress. In more favoured samples, most dyslexics appear to complete their schooling satisfactorily, and many go on to college or higher education. Though they may take longer than non-disabled readers to achieve qualifications, and may – advisedly – focus on less reading-intensive areas of study, many able poor readers from socially advantaged homes can expect to attain good qualification levels in time. In less favoured circumstances, outcomes are often much less positive. Negative attitudes to schooling can result in disaffection, non-attendance and early drop-out at the secondary stage, with inevitable consequences for qualifications. Training schemes after school-leaving age, especially in vocational courses, can prove an important later route to qualifications in groups of this kind.

Educational attainments are among the strongest predictors of occupational outcomes. Books on dyslexia frequently list eminent artists or business people who had reading or spelling problems in childhood. As they suggest, a history of dyslexia is no necessary bar to occupational success; equally importantly, parents and young people need to be aware that not everyone with reading difficulties is destined to follow in their footsteps. In middle class samples many dyslexic young people enter management positions, the arts, or the less 'reading-intensive' professions, and rely on word-processors and other supports to help with literacy-related tasks; on average, SES levels tend to be rather lower than for their parents. In less favoured samples, occupational outcomes are predictably less positive. Disabled readers are likely to enter manual occupations, some with low pay and limited job security; indeed, studies have consistently shown that adults with a history of reading problems face higher risks of unemployment than their peers, and may be especially vulnerable to job losses when labour market conditions are poor. Those from working class backgrounds are less likely to achieve upward social mobility than their contemporaries, and those from non-manual backgrounds are more likely to be downwardly mobile. By mid-life, the cumulative impact of these various factors can leave some disabled readers in poor material circumstances.

Evidence on other psychosocial outcomes is more limited, but important in light of the high rates of co-morbidity between reading difficulties and psychiatric problems in childhood. Most studies have concluded that reading difficulties have little impact on the persistence of childhood disorders into adolescence, but that poor readers may be at some increased risk of depressed mood and trait anxiety in the teens. The still scattered findings in adulthood suggest some (relatively non-specific) increased risk for psychiatric morbidity, though at much lower levels than in childhood. Low mood seems more associated with IQ than with reading disorders *per se*, but one area of concern for some dyslexics may be social phobia, possibly reflecting a more generalized form of the severe anxieties experienced by a minority of adults when faced with reading and writing tasks in any 'public' setting.

Problems in adult social functioning may be more common, though these seem to owe as much to the sequelae of poor qualifications and adolescent conduct problems as to reading difficulties as such. Perhaps predictably, employment and day-to-day coping are the areas most likely to present difficulties for poor readers later in life, while patterns of interpersonal relationships are relatively unaffected. Where employment options are (or are perceived to be) limited, some studies have reported that young women with histories of reading problems move into relationships and parenthood at young ages; once again, however, the key precursors here seem to lie in associated behaviour problems rather than in reading disorders alone. For young people without co-morbid behaviour problems, current evidence suggests that psychosocial functioning in adulthood is likely to be good.

Anti-social behaviour

Later indicators of anti-social behaviour are of particular interest given the strong overlap between reading problems and disruptive disorders in childhood. Although findings remain limited, follow-ups of both referred and community samples have found no excess of aggression, criminality or other aspects of antisocial behaviour among disabled readers in adult life. Any increased rates of adolescent delinquency seem to be of an 'adolescence-limited' kind, largely associated with truancy and disaffection from schooling in the teenage years. Later criminality, reported in retrospective studies of young 'anti-social' people, appears to be predicted not by early reading disorder but by ADHD and conduct disorder.

More generally, the follow-up evidence suggests that many of the adjustment problems faced by dyslexic children and adolescents may be exacerbated by the impact of their learning difficulties on functioning at school. Perhaps inevitably, learning disorders present young people with major challenges in the school setting, that can fuel both anxiety and frustration. Later in life, when environments can be selected, literacy demands are lower, and opportunities to exploit other strengths are maximized, it is encouraging to note that many of these early difficulties seem likely to remit.

Mathematical difficulties and dyscalculia

Outcome findings for dyscalculia are restricted to relatively short-term follow-ups (of 2–3 years at most), and have focused almost exclusively on the persistence of mathematical difficulties *per se*. At the very start of schooling, classifications of mathematical problems may not be stable: some children show difficulties in first grade that no longer are apparent by second grade, and isolated arithmetic weaknesses also seem less stable than more pervasive problems. If mathematical difficulties are still apparent in middle childhood, they seem likely to persist into the teens: in one sample 47 per cent of children with dyscalculia at ages 10/11 continued to show similar difficulties three years later, and the group as a whole scored in the lowest quartile of the range for their non-disabled peers. Initial severity, IQ and the presence of arithmetic problems in siblings have all been found to predict later progress. Where reading disorders have been assessed alongside mathematical problems, children with combined maths and reading problems progress more poorly in mathematics than those with mathematical problems alone.

SUGGESTED READING

Review articles and books

B. Butterworth, *The Mathematical Brain.* (London: Macmillan, 1999).

S. E. Fisher & J. C. DeFries, Developmental dyslexia: genetic dissection of a complex trait. *Nature Reviews: Neuroscience*, **3** (2002), 767–80.

E. L. Grigorenko, Developmental dyslexia: an update on genes, brains and environments. *Journal of Child Psychology and Psychiatry*, **42** (2001), 91–126.

F. Ramus, S. Rosen, S. C. Dakin, *et al.* Theories of developmental dyslexia: insights from a multiple case study of dyslexic adults. *Brain*, **126** (2003), 841–65.

R. S. Shalev & V. Gross-Tur, Developmental dyscalculia. *Pediatric Neurology*, **24** (2001), 337–42.

M. J. Snowling, *Dyslexia.* (Oxford: Blackwell, 2000).

F. R. Vellutino, J. M. Fletcher, M. J. Snowling & D. M. Scanlon. Specific reading disability (dyslexia): what have we learned in the past four decades? *Journal of Child Psychology and Psychiatry*, **45** (2004), 2–40.

Books with practical advice

D. Bartlett & S. Moody, *Dyslexia in the Workplace.* (London: Whurr, 2000).

N. Goulandris, *Dyslexia in Different Languages: Cross-linguistic Comparisons.* (London: Whurr, 2003).

E. Grauberg, *Elementary Mathematics and Language Difficulties.* (London: Whurr, 1997).

V. Muter, *Early Reading Development and Dyslexia.* (London: Whurr, 2003).

M. J. Snowling & J. Stackhouse, *Dyslexia, Speech and Language: A Practitioner's Handbook.* (London: Wiley, 2005).

Appendix 15.1. **Diagnostic instruments in the public domain**

Suggested protocol suitable for client with suspected learning disorder (English-speaking):

General cognitive ability

D. Wechsler, *Wechsler Abbreviated Scale of Intelligence.* (San Antonio: The Psychological Corporation Ltd, 1999) [suitable for children and adults].

Reading and numeracy

J. K. Torgeson, R. K. Wagner & C. A. Rashotte, *Test of Word Reading Efficiency.* (Austin, Texas: Pro-Ed, 1999) [suitable for school age child and young adult].

D. Wechsler, *Wechsler Objective Reading Dimensions.* (London: The Psychological Corporation, 1993) [suitable for school-age child].

D. Wechsler, *Wechsler Objective Numerical Dimensions.* (London: The Psychological Corporation, 1996). [suitable for school age child].

G. Wilkinson, *Wide Range Achievement Test 3.* (Delaware, USA: Wide Range Inc., 1993) [suitable for adult and school age child].

Phonological skills

N. Frederickson, U. Frith & R. Reason, *Phonological Assessment Battery.* (Slough: NFER-Nelson, 1997) [suitable for school age child].

V. Muter, C. Hulme & M. Snowling, *The Phonological Abilities Test.* (London: The Psychological Corporation, 1997) [suitable for 5–7 year-old].

Information for parents and children

Adult Dyslexia Organisation www.futurenet.co.uk/charity/ado/adomenu/adomenu.htm

British Dyslexia Association www.bda-dyslexia.org.uk

British Dyslexics www.dyslexia.uk.com

Department for Education and Skills

Dyslexia Institute www.dyslexia-inst.org.uk

European Dyslexia Association www.bedford.ac.uk/eda/

Information for Parents www.parentcentre.gov.uk

The Council for the Registration of Schools Teaching Dyslexic Pupils (CreSTeD). www.crested.org.uk

The Website for Parents of Dyslexics and SpLD www.dyslexichelp.org

16

Autism spectrum disorders

Christopher Gillberg

Department of Child and Adolescent Psychiatry, University of Göteborg, Sweden

Introduction

Some children are less socially interactive and communicative than others. When the combination of social and communication problems takes on the quality of a clinically severely impairing condition one needs to consider the possibility of a disorder of social interaction, particularly one that may fall under the diagnostic umbrella of 'autism spectrum disorders'.

Autism was first delineated as a syndrome of childhood onset by Leo Kanner in the US in the 1940s. Long before that – at the turn of the eighteenth century – classic autism cases had been described by John Haslam in the UK and Jean Itard in France. The word autism (from the Greek *autos* for self) was introduced by Eugen Bleuler to depict the self-centred thinking believed to be typical of schizophrenia. Considered by Kanner to be a discrete disease entity, early infantile autism was conceptualized as an extremely rare disorder, and one which would be easy to identify and diagnose. It was only in the early 1980s that the concept of autism spectrum disorder was introduced by Wing and Gillberg. Wing put forward the notion of a fairly specific triad of impairments of social, communicative and imaginative functioning as being at the basis of all autism spectrum disorders. She also coined the term Asperger's syndrome for the kind of 'high-functioning' autism spectrum disorder described originally by Hans Asperger (who used the term autistic psychopathy) at about the same time that Kanner described his more 'low-functioning' variant of autism.

It is now clear that autism spectrum disorders existed in the Middle Ages and probably long before that. It is not a new group of disorders, even though awareness about its existence and clinical manifestations has a fairly brief history.

A Clinician's Handbook of Child and Adolescent Psychiatry, ed. Christopher Gillberg,
Richard Harrington and Hans-Christoph Steinhausen. Published by Cambridge University Press.
© Cambridge University Press 2005.

Definition and classification

The terminology in the field of autism spectrum disorders is fraught with problems. The diagnostic manuals do not use the term autism spectrum, but instead refer to pervasive developmental disorders (PDD). PDD is a misnomer in that not all autism spectrum disorders are pervasive. Furthermore, profound mental retardation, the most pervasive of all developmental disorders, is not considered a PDD. In clinical practice, autism spectrum disorders remains the preferred term. However, some authorities in the field speak of autism and autism (or 'austistic') spectrum disorders, whereas others include the core syndrome of autism (childhood autism/autistic disorder) as a subgroup within the autism spectrum disorders. The latter definition will be used here. Under this model, autism spectrum disorders and PDD can be seen as synonymous concepts. Both the ICD-10 and DSM-IV list five different subtypes of PDD: the core syndrome of autism, Asperger syndrome, childhood disintegrative disorder, atypical autism or PDD not otherwise specified (PDD NOS) and Rett syndrome. The inclusion of Rett syndrome as one specific variant of autism spectrum disorder makes little sense as Rett syndrome is one of the many medical disorders that are often associated with autistic symptomatology. It belongs on the medical disorder axis of the multiaxial classification system.

ICD-10 criteria

The ICD-10 category for the core syndrome of autism is childhood autism (Box 16.1). The definition is based upon the simultaneous presence of all three of the triad of severe impairment of reciprocal social interaction, severe impairment of reciprocal communication (including but not exclusive to problems with language use), and severe restriction of imagination and behavioural repertoire. The problems need to be at a level that is out of keeping with the child's overall chronological and developmental age. Problems must have been present before age 3 years. There is also an exclusion criterion which leads to diagnostic confusion if strictly adhered to and prevents clinicians from making appropriate diagnoses and interventions for comorbid problems. This criterion should be disregarded in clinical practice.

The ICD-10 category of Asperger syndrome has been shown to be a theoretical construct not consistent with clinical realities. For instance, Asperger's own cases do not meet criteria for this category. The criteria for social and behavioural impairments are the same as for childhood autism. Nothing is said about the communication impairment (so striking in the typical case of Asperger syndrome). The major problem with this set of criteria resides in the requirement for normal development in the first three years of life, something almost unheard of in autism spectrum disorders. In clinical practice, the criteria by Gillberg & Gillberg

Box 16.1. Childhood autism (ICD-10)

F84.0 Childhood autism

A. Abnormal or impaired development is evident before the age of 3 years in least one of the following areas:

    (1) receptive or expressive language as used in social communication;

    (2) the development of selective social attachments or of reciprocal social interaction;

    (3) functional or symbolic play.

B. A total of at least six symptoms from (1), (2), and (3) must be present, with at least two from (1) and at least one from each (2) and (3):

    (1) Qualitative abnormalities in reciprocal social interaction are manifest in at least two of the following areas:

        (a) failure adequately to use eye-to-eye gaze, facial expression, body posture and gesture to regulate social interaction;

        (b) failure to develop (in a manner appropriate to mental age, and despite ample opportunities) peer relationships that involve a mutual sharing of interests, activities and emotions;

        (c) lack of socio-emotional reciprocity as shown by an impaired or deviant response to other people's emotions; or lack of modulation of behaviour according to social context; or a weak integration of social, emotional, and communicative behaviours;

        (d) lack of spontaneous seeking to share enjoyment, interests, or achievements with other people (e.g. a lack of showing, bringing, or pointing out to other people objects of interest to the individual).

    (2) Qualitative abnormalities in communication are manifest in at least one of the following areas:

        (a) a delay in, or total lack of, development of spoken language that is not accompanied by an attempt to compensate through the use of gesture or mime as an alternative mode of communication (often preceded by a lack of communicative babbling);

        (b) relative failure to initiate or sustain conversational interchange (at whatever level of language skills is present), in which there is reciprocal responsiveness of the communications of the other person;

        (c) stereotyped and repetitive use of language or idiosyncratic use of words or phrases;

        (d) lack of varied spontaneous make-believe or (when young) social imitative play.

    (3) Restricted, repetitive and stereotyped patterns of behaviour, interests, and activities are manifest in at least one of the following areas:

(a) an encompassing preoccupation with one or more stereotyped and restricted patterns of interest that are abnormal in content or focus; or one or more interests that are abnormal in their intensity and circumscribed nature though not in their content or focus;

(b) apparently compulsive adherence to specific, non-functional routines or rituals;

(c) stereotyped and repetitive motor mannerisms that involve either hand or finger flapping or twisting, or complex whole body movements;

(d) preoccupations with part-objects or non-functional elements of play materials (such as their odour, the feel of their surface, or the noise or vibration that they generate).

C. The clinical picture is not attributable to the other varieties of pervasive developmental disorder: specific developmental disorder of receptive language (F80.2) with secondary socioemotional problems; reactive attachment disorder (F94.1) or disinhibited attachment disorder (F94.2); mental retardation (F70–F72) with some associated emotional or behavioural disorder; schizophrenia (F20–) of unusually early onset; and Rett's syndrome (F84.2).

(Box 16.2) are the ones most commonly used. Many individuals meet criteria both for autism and Asperger syndrome. It is often best in such cases to make the diagnosis of autism but equally to provide the information that it is the variant referred to as Asperger syndrome.

Childhood disintegrative disorder (Box 16.3) is an autism spectrum disorder with the typical clinical presentation emerging only after a period of a few/several years of normal/near normal development. It is referred to as 'Other childhood disintegrative disorder' in the ICD-10 ('other' because the ICD-10 considers Rett syndrome to be a disintegrative PDD variant).

Atypical autism (Box 16.4) is an autism spectrum disorder which cannot be classified as childhood autism, Asperger syndrome or childhood disintegrative disorder.

DSM-IV criteria

The DSM-IV category autistic disorder is virtually identical to the ICD-10 childhood autism concept except as regards exclusion criteria. Thus, the DSM-IV does not completely rule out making additional diagnoses such as ADHD.

The DSM-IV category of Asperger's disorder is almost identical to that of the ICD-10, and, hence of little use in clinical practice.

Box 16.2. Asperger syndrome (Gillberg & Gillberg)

1 **Social impairment (extreme egocentricity)**
 (at least two of the following):
 (a) difficulties interacting with peers
 (b) indifference to peer contacts
 (c) difficulties interpreting social cues
 (d) socially and emotionally inappropriate behaviour.

2 **Narrow interest**
 (at least one of the following):
 (a) exclusion of other activities
 (b) repetitive adherence
 (c) more rote than meaning.

3 **Compulsive need for introducing routines and interests**
 (at least one of the following):
 (a) which affect the individual's every aspect of every-day life
 (b) which affect others.

4 **Speech and language peculiarities**
 (at least three of the following):
 (a) delayed speech development
 (b) superficially perfect expressive language
 (c) formal pedantic language
 (d) odd prosody, peculiar voice characteristics
 (e) impairment of comprehension including misinterpretations of literal/ implied meanings.

5 **Non-verbal communication problems**
 (at least one of the following):
 (a) limited use of gestures
 (b) clumsy/gauche body language
 (c) limited facial expression
 (d) inappropriate facial expression
 (e) peculiar, stiff gaze.

6 **Motor clumsiness**
 Poor performance on neuro-developmental examination

Box 16.3. Other childhood disintegrative disorder (ICD-10)

A. Development is apparently normal up to the age of at least 2 years. The presence of normal age-appropriate skills on communication, social relationships, play and adaptive behaviour at age 2 years or later is required for diagnosis.

B. There is a definite loss of previously acquired skills at about the time of onset of the disorder. The diagnosis requires a clinically significant loss of skills (not just a failure to use them in certain situations) in at least two of the following areas:
 (1) expressive or receptive language
 (2) play
 (3) social skills or adaptive behaviour
 (4) bowel or bladder control
 (5) motor skills.

C. Qualitatively abnormal social functioning is manifest in at least two of the following areas:
 (1) qualitative abnormalities in reciprocal social interaction (of the type defined for autism)
 (2) qualitative abnormalities in communication (of the type defined for autism)
 (3) restricted, repetitive and stereotyped patterns of behaviour, interests and activities, including motor stereotypies and mannerisms
 (4) a general loss of interests in objects and in the environment.

D. The disorder is not attributable to the other varieties of pervasive developmental disorder, acquired aphasia with epilepsy (F80.6); elective mutism (F94.0); Rett's syndrome (F84.2); or schizophrenia (F20).

Childhood disintegrative disorder in the DSM-IV is similar but not identical to the syndrome described in the ICD-10.

PDD NOS is the DSM-IV equivalent of the ICD-10 atypical autism category. However, it is even more loosely defined.

Clinical applicability

The ICD-10/DSM-IV definitions for childhood autistic disorder are fairly straightforward and easy to apply in clinical practice. Problems arise when considering whether or not to make additional comorbid diagnoses. When there are clinically impairing conditions, such as ADHD, the exclusionary criteria of the diagnostic manuals should be disregarded.

Major problems pertain to the diagnosis of the other subgroups within the autism spectrum. For instance, the boundaries between atypical autism and childhood

Box 16.4. Atypical autism (ICD-10)

A. Abnormal or impaired development is evident at or after the age of 3 years (criteria as for autism except for age of manifestation).
B. There are qualitative abnormalities in reciprocal social interaction or in communication, or restricted, repetitive and stereotyped patterns of behaviour, interests and activities. (Criteria as for autism except that it is unnecessary to meet the criteria for number of areas of abnormality.)
C. The disorder does not meet the diagnostic criteria for autism (F84.0).

Autism may be atypical in either age of onset (F84.10) or symptomatology (F84.11); the two types are differentiated with a fifth character for research purposes. Syndromes that are atypical in both respects should be coded F84.12.

F84.10 Atypicality in age of onset

A. The disorder does not meet criterion A for autism (F84.0); that is, abnormal or impaired development is evident only at or after the age of 3 years.
B. The disorder meets criteria B and C for autism (F84.0).

F84.11 Atypicality in symptomatology

A. The disorder meets criterion A for autism (F80.0); that is, abnormal or impaired development is evident before the age of 3 years.
B. There are qualitative abnormalities in reciprocal social interactions or in communication, or restricted, repetitive, and stereotyped patterns of behaviour, interests and activities. (Criteria as for autism except that it is unnecessary to meet the criteria for number of areas of abnormality.)
C. The disorder meets criterion C for autism (F84.0).
D. The disorder does not fully meet criterion B for autism (F84.0).

F84.12 Atypicality in both age of onset and symptomatology

A. The disorder does not meet criterion A for autism (F84.0); that is abnormal or impaired development is evident only at or after the age of 3 years.
B. There are qualitative abnormalities in reciprocal social interactions or in communication, or restricted, repetitive and stereotyped patterns of behaviour, interests and activities. (Criteria as for autism except that it is unnecessary to meet the criteria for number of areas of abnormality.)
C. The disorder meets criterion C for autism (F84.0).
D. The disorder does not fully meet criterion B for autism (F84.0).

disintegrative disorder are not clear, and it is difficult to determine the difference between a non-autism spectrum disorder case and PDD NOS.

Further diagnostic complications stem from the use of the term 'high-functioning' autism, often applied to cases meeting ICD-10/DSM-IV criteria for autism and who test at near normal, normal or even superior levels of IQ. Most clinicians would argue that such cases fit better under the diagnosis of Asperger syndrome, particularly if the level of spoken language is superior. The term 'high-functioning' is inappropriate in that it suggests that the affected individual is 'well functioning', which is certainly almost never the case in an individual with a clinically diagnosed autism spectrum disorder.

In clinical practice it would seem reasonable to diagnose children and adolescents as having an autism spectrum disorder if and only if there are severe problems in at least two of the three triad domains, or if there are mild-moderate problems in two domains and severe problems in a third domain. Subgrouping according to ICD-10/DSM-IV could then be achieved for autism, childhood disintegrative disorder and atypical autism/PDD NOS. If the clinical gestalt of Asperger syndrome is invoked, then going through the Gillberg criteria might be helpful before concluding that this category is applicable. The word autism (such as in autism spectrum disorder) should always be mentioned in the diagnostic formulation. Many countries require this diagnostic label for the provision of adequate services.

Epidemiology

Prevalence rates

There is general agreement that autistic disorder and the other conditions referred to in the autism spectrum disorder/PDD category are much more common than held up until the 1990s. The prevalence for all autism spectrum disorders is in the range of 0.5–1.0 per cent of the general school age population. Core autism cases account for about one-third of this proportion and Asperger syndrome/atypical autism for the vast majority of the remainder. Childhood disintegrative disorder is extremely rare. Most of the available evidence suggests that the relatively high rates now reported for autism spectrum disorders are due to increased awareness, new autism concepts/diagnostic criteria, and that, in the past diagnostic overshadowing often occurred (i.e. that if there was already a diagnosis of, e.g. epilepsy, mental retardation or tuberous sclerosis, an additional diagnosis of autism was less likely to be made) rather than to any real increase in the population.

Incidence rates

Autistic disorder incidence has only been studied in a few register-based surveys. These studies show a tendency towards an increase over time in the 1990s, but this appears to be at least partly accounted for by a parallel drop in the incidence of registered mental retardation.

Sex ratios

Clinical studies show a very high boy:girl ratio for autism. This drops to considerably lower levels (around 1.5–3:1) in the general population. Several studies now suggest that girls with autism spectrum disorders are underdiagnosed and receive other diagnoses such as depression, personality disorder, or eating disorder. It further appears that girls may be much less likely than boys to be referred for help at an early age. Girls in the general population show less of hyperactive and violent behaviours (commonly encountered in autism spectrum disorders and often part of the reason for referral) and talk more and at an earlier age. Therefore, it would take a more severe variant of an autism spectrum disorder to produce the 'full-blown' clinical picture manifested by boys at an early age. Girls who receive an early diagnosis of autism are often among those most severely affected and with major signs of brain dysfunction (including epilepsy). The more moderate and milder variants of autism spectrum disorders in girls tend to show up in clinics at a much later age, sometimes not until adulthood. It is only if they encounter clinicians well trained in child neuropsychiatry that they will receive the 'correct' diagnosis of an autism spectrum disorder.

Implications for clinical practice

The fact that autism spectrum disorders (including autistic disorder) are so much more common than previously held means that service development has not been able to keep up with the increasing demands for intervention. This is particularly true for adolescents and adults, but there is a considerable degree of unmet need even for young children. Children with any kind of major behavioural, social or learning problem should always be considered for a possible diagnosis within the autism spectrum. It is perhaps particularly important that this diagnostic possibility not be overlooked in girls.

Clinical picture

Main features and symptoms

The triad of impairments typical of all autism spectrum disorders affect social, communicative (including language) and behavioural/imagination functioning (Box 16.5). There are usually additional symptoms, including a whole range of perceptual abnormalities, but these are not currently considered necessary features for the diagnosis.

Box 16.5. Main features and symptoms in autism spectrum disorders

The autism triad of impairments (typical of all autism spectrum disorders) are:

- *Severe impairment of reciprocal social interaction*

  The *social* 'style' may vary from 'aloofness', through 'friendly and passive' to impulsive, intruding 'active but odd'.

- *Severe impairment in reciprocal communication affecting spoken language and non-verbal communication*

  This can present as complete muteness or the reduction of spoken language down to a few words or sentences, but it may also show as extremely repetitive complex language. Non-verbal aspects of communication (gestures, facial expression) are also affected, as is comprehension of communicative intent.

- *Severe restriction in the behavioural repertoire and lack of flexible imaginative skills*

  In children with mental retardation, stereotypics are the rule. Such behaviours may occur in those with higher IQ also, but usually to a less conspicuous degree. Fixation on routines, rituals, and pedantry, are almost universal. Those with IQs in the normal or superior range very often develop *narrow interests*.

Not part of the triad but extremely common in autism are perceptual distortions/abnormalities of various kinds

One (or more) of oversensitivity to touch, certain sounds, smell, taste or visual stimuli is an almost universal phenomenon.

The early course and clinical presentation of autism spectrum disorders differ quite considerably from one case to another

About two in three of all cases have shown some social, communicative or typical behavioural change already before their first birthday. Others appear to develop normally up until 12–24 months and then suffer real or seeming regression, sometimes, but not always in temporal association with onset of seizures.

All problems have to be out of keeping with overall developmental level

In clinical practice diagnose children and adolescents as having an autism spectrum disorder if there are severe problems in at least two of the three triad domains or if there are mild–moderate problems in two domains and severe problems in a third domain. Subgrouping according to ICD-10/DSM-IV can then be achieved for autism, childhood disintegrative disorder and atypical autism/PDD NOS. If the clinical gestalt of Asperger syndrome is invoked, then going through the Gillberg criteria (Box 16.2) might be helpful before concluding that this category is applicable. The word autism (such as in autism spectrum disorder) should always be mentioned in the diagnostic formulation. Many countries require this diagnostic label for the provision of adequate services.

The severe impairment of reciprocal social interaction

This feature may be observed in the staring, fixed or 'wide-open' gaze which is not used to regulate social interaction, the reduced ability to take the cognitive and emotional perspective of another person, disregard for needs of age-peers and adults alike, a complete lack of turn-taking in social interactions or games, and failure to understand the need for social overtures. Many are perceived as lacking in empathy, even though this does not necessarily imply 'coldness'. Many have strong affects, but with their problems understanding the perspective of the other person, they misinterpret social signals, as, in turn, others misunderstand their affects. Some are 'sweet', 'naive', and 'easy to love' so long as demands are kept to a minimum or within an accepted routine.

The social 'style' may vary from complete 'aloofness'/autistic aloneness, through a 'friendly and passive' interactive style to an impulsive, intruding 'active but odd' pattern of interaction. The group showing the active but odd style (and sometimes those who are aloof) may be severely hyperactive from a very early age. They may receive a diagnosis of ADHD or hyperkinetic disorder, and it is only when the hyperactivity has come under control with treatment or at a later age that the underlying severe social interaction impairment of autism comes to attention. The child with an autism spectrum disorder usually has no 'real' friend, even though, occasionally, he or she may be a passive member of a group where very little interaction is demanded. The lack of concern about the absence of friends is sometimes the most striking feature, even though, in other cases or at a later age, the person with an autism spectrum disorder may have come to realize that it is 'normal' for young people to have friends and therefore may worry about 'not being normal' because there are no friends. Some may insist that their parents call up a 'friend and bring him over' and will go on and on about the time the friend will arrive, only to ignore the 'friend' completely once he or she has arrived in the house.

The severe impairment in reciprocal communication

This can present as complete muteness or the reduction of spoken language down to a few words or sentences, but it may equally show as extremely repetitive complex language. About one-third of those with the core syndrome of autism never speak in communicative phrases. Some acquire single word skills at the expected time but then do not progress beyond this stage for many months or years. This is often perceived as a 'set-back' even in cases where there have been some documented abnormalities in the social domain at an earlier age. Even those with the clinical presentation of Asperger syndrome (who often progress to a stage of elaborate, even 'perfect' language) often go through such a stage of plateauing language development and may be perceived as very late speakers (particularly perhaps as compared with brothers or sisters), only to 'explode' in their acquisition of spoken language skills around age 3–5 years, when, within a period of only some months they go from 'almost mute' to 'adult type' expressive language. The vast majority – even those with the clinical presentation of Asperger syndrome – have great difficulty understanding the meaning of what other people tell them or ask them in conversation, even when they themselves are able to speak in grammatically perfect sentences. Again, their reduced capacity for taking the other person's cognitive and emotional perspective is severely limiting for their ability to grasp the meaning of communication.

In those with good verbal expressive skills, the ability to participate in conversation is usually severely restricted. They fail to use social overtures, and burst in on other people without regard for their point of view. They start talking 'in mid-thought' taking it for granted that the other person knows exactly what they are talking about. They get fixated on something very concrete and go on and on about this rather than following the overall theme. They fail to listen to the other person's point of view, or are just too slow processing the underlying message that the conversational partner is trying to convey. It is this failure to really communicate in the presence of good or superior expressive skills that is referred to as pragmatic disorder (sometimes, often erroneously, termed 'semantic pragmatic disorder' – see below).

Non-verbal aspects of communication are also affected. There is usually little or unvaried use of gestures and facial expressions. Body language may be described as 'awkward' and 'clumsy'. Many 'stand off' and have great difficulty mixing with other people. Others come up too close and may pat other people's heads, smooth down their hair, feel their cheeks or touch their private parts in a naive way.

The severe restriction in the behavioural repertoire

This feature is seen by many to reflect the lack of flexible imaginative skills. In children with marked degrees of mental retardation, repetitive motor behaviours (e.g. stereotypies such as hand-flapping, finger flickering, body rocking, head banging) are the rule. Such behaviours may occur in those with higher IQ also, but usually to a less conspicuous degree. Fixation on routines, rituals, pedantry, and a variety of symptoms that might equally be described as obsessive-compulsive are almost universal, but may be obscured or lacking in those with severe co-morbid inattention and hyperactivity. Some throw extreme tantrums when routines are broken or demands of any kind are made. In older individuals, these are often referred to as 'violent outbursts' (or even 'aggressiveness', a term that should usually not be employed, because it is very difficult to determine whether the violence is intentional or not). Play is almost always rigid, stilted, or lacking altogether. Hard objects are often much preferred over soft and cuddly things. Because, at least when very young children with autism do not seem to appreciate the existence of other people's minds, they do not go to them for comfort or for sharing positive or negative experiences. Many have elaborate routines involving feeding behaviours (e.g. will only eat one particular type of food and only if seated on a particular stool with one elbow resting on the table), bathroom activities (e.g. can only brush teeth in front of mirror at home, cannot manage in front of other mirrors in other bathrooms).

Those with IQs in the normal or superior range very often develop narrow interests (e.g. in meteorology, dinosaurs, opera singers, Chinese pottery, Rommel's desert wars, the Paris Metro system, train time tables, telephone directories, or computers to mention some of the countless possibilities) that come to occupy so much of their time that there is little left over for any other kind of meaningful activity. They tend to talk endlessly about these special interests and appear to be unaware that others may not share them. Many are extremely interested in details and are very astute in memorizing matters concerned with the observable world. They may remember in the most astounding detail what people were wearing ten years ago or the particulars of a building not visited for more than a few minutes many years previously. Those with the highest levels of IQ are often expert at picking up other people's 'weak spots'. They may also have 'emotional radar' and observe minute change in social atmosphere even while not being able to make the slightest sense of what is going on. Such skills may lead the clinician to erroneously exclude even considering a diagnosis in the autism spectrum.

Not part of the triad but extremely common in autism are perceptual distortions/abnormalities of various kinds

One (or more) of oversensitivity to touch, certain sounds, smell, taste or visual stimuli is an almost universal phenomenon. The abnormal reactions to auditory stimuli (e.g. strong reactions to barely audible sounds and little or no reaction to loud noise) are often among the presenting symptoms of autism in the first year of life. Decreased pain cold/heat sensitivity is another common symptom which may or may not be accompanied by a whole range of self-injurious behaviours. These can be the most debilitating problem in the whole set of symptoms shown by a child with autism. As already mentioned, hyperactivity, often amounting to full symptomatic diagnostic criteria for ADHD or hyperkinetic disorder, is a very common handicapping symptom, especially in the pre-school child. The ICD-10 has a special category for children with mental retardation, hyperactivity and stereotypies, but it is unclear whether this should be regarded as a specific subgroup rather than autism with a certain kind of 'co-morbid'/overlapping problem. In other cases hypoactivity can be the major problem with lack of initiative, lack of interest in new things (which may be shown, e.g. in relation to presents which may trigger extreme temper tantrums), and 'resistance to change and learning'. Sleep problems are also very common, and constitute a handicapping problem in about one in three of all pre-school children with one or other of the autism spectrum disorders.

Subjectively, children with autism spectrum disorders may be extremely psychologically frustrated by overstimulating environments, perceptual overreactions, verbal interactions, common demands for social interaction and, in some cases, demands of any kind. In a structured, calm environment with predictable routines they are usually 'happy', even though they tend not to share this experience with others in a spontaneous fashion. Some of those with very high IQ seem to have little memory of their lives up to around – perhaps – age seven, eight or nine years. Others appear to have the opposite problem of not being able to forget anything they ever experienced.

The early course and clinical presentation of autism spectrum disorders differ quite considerably from one case to another

About two in three of all cases have shown some social, communicative or typical behavioural change already before their first birthday. Others appear to develop normally up until 12–24 months and then suffer real or seeming regression, sometimes, but not always in temporal association with onset of seizures. Until recently it was considered very rare for autism not to present with the full-blown clinical picture before age 5 years, but new studies of adults and follow-up studies of children with atypical autistic features and language disorders in early childhood indicate that not infrequently autism emerges more clearly only after the first years. Children with very early onset extreme hyperactivity and motor control problems constitute other risk groups in whom the clinician must be prepared to assess for features of autism at later follow-up.

Differential diagnosis and comorbidity

There are many problems of differential diagnosis in the field of autism including those that pertain to differentiating between the various forms of conditions within the spectrum. The most common comorbid or overlapping syndromes are ADHD, developmental coordination disorder (DCD), tic disorders, depression, bipolar disorder, anxiety disorders and eating disorders. Common associated symptoms are hyperactivity, hypoactivity, inattention, perceptual abnormality, violent outbursts, self-injury, sleep problems and catatonic features (Box 16.6). Medical disorders are very commonly associated with autism spectrum disorders and should be coded on a separate diagnostic axis (Box 16.7).

ADHD

Hyperactivity, inattention and handicapping impulsiveness are almost universally occurring problems in all autism spectrum disorders. When, from the point of

---

Box 16.6. Co-morbid and overlapping psychiatric/developmental problems

The most common co-morbid/overlapping psychiatric and developmental syndromes are
- Mental retardation
- Speech–language problems
- ADHD
- DCD
- Tic disorders
- Depression
- Bipolar disorder
- Anxiety disorders
- Eating disorders
- Selective mutism
- Semantic pragmatic disorder
- Non-verbal learning disability

The most common co-morbid symptoms are
- Perceptual problems
- Sleep problems
- Violent behaviours
- Self-injurious behaviours
- Hyperactivity
- Hypoactivity
- Catatonic features

---

view of symptom threshold, they amount to combined ADHD (and especially when symptom criteria for hyperkinetic disorder are met), a separate diagnosis for this category should be considered. Many children with autism spectrum disorders, perhaps particularly those with IQs above 50, may benefit from the same type of intervention approaches that are advantageous for other children with ADHD (see Taylor, this volume). Children with the combination of ADHD and DCD have a relatively high risk of also meeting criteria for an autism spectrum disorder. It is not always appropriate to give the autism spectrum disorder diagnosis priority over ADHD. The syndrome that, from the point of view of intervention need, is the most handicapping should be named as the primary diagnosis. Thus, one child might, correctly, receive the diagnosis of ADHD at age 3 years, of ADHD with atypical autism at age 4 years, and autistic disorder with ADHD at age 9 years.

Box 16.7. Medical disorders in autism spectrum disorders

Epilepsy

About one in three of all with childhood autism is affected; two peaks, one in the first four years and another around the time of adolescence, small number of new cases in adult age; low but possibly raised rate in Asperger syndrome; early onset cases are usually difficult to treat, adolescent onset cases often relatively benign.

Hearing deficits

Much over-represented and often missed in autism spectrum disorders.

Acoustic hypersensitivity

More than half of all with childhood autism; common in Asperger syndrome also.

Visual deficits and strabismus

Refraction errors common and often missed; severe visual deficits over-represented; some congenitally blind children have autism.

Specific medical disorders

Several specific medical disorders are much overrepresented in childhood autism (and possibly more common in Asperger syndrome than in the general population) and need to be ruled out in each case examined, either at assessment by expert in the field or after specific testing; some of the most important disorders are listed here (do not forget that autism occurs in about 10% of Down syndrome cases):

  Tuberous sclerosis
  Fragile-X syndrome
  Partial tetrasomy/trisomy 15 syndrome
  Rett syndrome
  Hypomelanosis of Ito
  Moebius sequence
  Angelman syndrome
  CHARGE association
  Smith–Magenis syndrome
  22q11 deletion syndrome
  Sex chromosome aneuploidies
  Rubella embryopathy
  PKU
  Sotos syndrome (and other variants of macrocephalus)

DCD

In the past, children with autism were believed to be exceptionally talented in the field of motor performance. This is now known to be a mistaken notion. To the contrary, the vast majority have mild, moderate or severe motor control problems, and many meet criteria for DCD. The motor control problems are usually most strikingly present in those with higher IQ, perhaps as a consequence of the higher demands for more 'normal functioning' usually made on this group. Mild DCD problems are part and parcel of the Asperger syndrome diagnosis, but when the motor control problems are moderately or severely debilitating, they may require specific intervention and a separate diagnosis of DCD should be made.

Tic disorders

Tics are very common in children in the general population, but are definitely much overrepresented among those with autism spectrum disorders. They may be motor tics (in which case they can be very difficult to separate from motor stereotypies), vocal tics, simple or complex (in which case they can be indistinguishable from complex stereotypies or stereotyped utterances), transient or chronic. When motor and vocal tics occur together and are handicapping in their own right (as separate from autism), a separate diagnosis of Tourette syndrome might be warranted. Having said this, it also needs to be added that tics are only rarely severely handicapping, and that, therefore it is uncommon for a tic disorder (including Tourette syndrome) to be the primary diagnosis.

Depression

Depression is common in teenagers with autism spectrum disorders. A change in behaviour (such as hyperactivity turning to hypoactivity), loss of appetite or severely disrupted sleep patterns may all indicate depression in autism. Loss and bullying are common precipitants of depression in autism spectrum disorders. For instance, the death of a parent might not seem to affect the child with autism at all early on. However, as weeks pass and the child gradually realizes that the routine of having someone catering to his/her particular and peculiar needs has disappeared, depressive symptoms set in. As in the case of the child being victimized by bullies, he/she is unlikely to communicate anything about his feelings to other people, and the depressed mood may therefore go relatively unnoticed or at least undiagnosed for longer periods of time.

Bipolar disorder

It seems likely that bipolar disorder is overrepresented in families who have children with autism and clinical experience suggests that bipolar disorder is a not uncommon comorbidity in autism and Asperger syndrome. Mood swings, periods of extreme hyperactivity, 'intermittent explosive behaviours' and abrupt sleep disturbance are all possible indicators of bipolar disorder, especially in the presence of a positive family history for such disorder.

Anxiety disorders

Children with autism spectrum disorders are often anxious, particularly in situations when they do not know what is expected of them. 'Panic attacks' amounting to confusional states are often seen in settings of perceptual overload such as in the middle of a busy street or in crowds of people making all sorts of verbal demands. The individual with autism might then cover his ears and start screaming, hitting himself or running out in front of oncoming vehicles. DSM-IV panic disorder or generalized anxiety do occur occasionally and are most commonly diagnosed in those with higher IQ, but it is unclear whether the rate of such problems is increased over and above that of the general population. Selective mutism – often categorized as an anxiety disorder – is strongly associated with autistic features. Any individual diagnosed with this condition should be assessed with a view to finding possibly comorbid or underlying autism.

Eating disorders

Food fads, food refusal and overeating are all common, perhaps almost universal phenomena in autism spectrum disorders. Anorexia nervosa has been shown to be associated with autism spectrum disorders. Ten to twenty per cent of a general population group of adolescent girls with anorexia nervosa meet full criteria for an autism spectrum disorder and continue to do so five and ten years after onset of the eating disorder. Such cases are usually missed cases of early onset autism/Asperger syndrome who develop extreme routines and rituals around food in teenage (as part of a lifelong proclivity for rituals and routines). They meet diagnostic criteria for anorexia nervosa, but will not be benefited by typical eating disorder interventions unless the underlying autistic problems are acknowledged.

Other developmental, psychiatric and personality disorder diagnoses

In young adult age, many individuals with autism spectrum disorders apply for help within adult psychiatric services. It is then very common for them to receive diagnoses of 'schizophreniform disorder' or of 'personality disorder'. The underlying autism diagnosis may be disregarded or missed altogether. Those with high IQ – with the support of an understanding family and good teachers – may have managed without psychiatric intervention for many years until the demands of living alone and coping with 'normal' activities of daily life become overwhelming. It rarely, if ever, adds anything to say that a person with an autism spectrum disorder also meets criteria for a personality disorder. Even if this is often true, nothing is gained in terms of better understanding or better treatment. Schizophrenia-like symptoms (including 'psychotic breakdown', confusion and concrete 'ideas of reference') are not uncommon in people with autism spectrum disorders who are subjected to stressful experiences. Once the stress is removed they quickly return to their usual style and functioning.

Catatonic features are not uncommon and may develop into frank catatonia in a minority of adolescents and adults.

Selective mutism is a relatively rare condition in which children speak freely in some situations (often at home) but refuse to speak at all in other settings (often at school). It is not rare for the clinical presentation of selective mutism to disguise an underlying autism spectrum disorder.

Semantic pragmatic disorder is a diagnostic label used mostly by speech–language therapists. Many individuals in the autism spectrum suffer from semantic pragmatic disorder or, at least, pragmatic disorder (see above under 'The severe restriction of reciprocal communication'). It is unclear what proportion of those with so-called semantic pragmatic disorder meet some or all criteria for an autism spectrum disorder.

Non-verbal learning disability is a neuropsychological concept used in cases with much poorer results on performance than on verbal portions of IQ-tests, e.g. who score 20 points or more lower on the performance than the verbal part of the WISC. This test profile is common in Asperger syndrome. It is believed often to reflect right hemisphere dysfunction. As with semantic pragmatic disorder, it is unclear what proportion of those who do show this particular kind of test profile do not have an autism spectrum disorder.

Medical disorders

In classic autism in the general population, as many as one in four individuals may have a medical disorder which, in one way or another is strongly associated with the autistic symptomatology. In specialized autism clinics, to which those with an already 'overshadowing' medical disorder diagnosis (such as tuberous sclerosis or the fragile X syndrome) are less likely to be referred, the rate may be lower, but certainly not negligible there either. Indeed, recent studies of autism spectrum disorder cases with normal or high IQ, show that as many as one in six in such groups may have an important associated medical disorder. This means that all individuals with a diagnosis of an autism spectrum disorder will need a medical assessment by a clinician well trained in the field, who knows which disorders to look out for (Box 16.7).

Epilepsy is very common in childhood autism and in atypical autism cases with mental retardation, occurring in 25–40 per cent of all cases depending on the duration of follow-up. Slightly under half of this proportion is contributed by cases with seizure onset in the first five years of life. The epilepsy in such cases is often severe and presenting with a combination of several different types of seizures. The majority of the remainder have adolescent onset of seizures, which are usually of a more benign type. A small number of additional cases of epilepsy emerge in early adult life. Epilepsy is much rarer in Asperger syndrome, but it does occur at rates considerably higher than in the general population.

Macrocephalus occurs in about one in five of all children in the autism spectrum. This can sometimes be associated with a particular syndrome (Such as Solot syndrome), but is often 'idiopathic'.

Moderate hearing deficits occur in about 10 per cent of all individuals with childhood autism and complete deafness is present in a few per cent (which is much higher than in the general population). Extreme acoustic hypersensitivity is very common and occurs in 30–50 per cent of all cases. Visual deficits are also much overrepresented. Certain kinds of congenital blindness with brain damage (e.g. retinopathy of prematurity) are strongly associated with autism spectrum disorders.

Tuberous sclerosis, the fragile-X syndrome and the partial tetrasomy 15 syndrome are probably the most common specific brain disorders encountered in autism cases with an IQ of about 50 and below. Together they account for 10–15 per cent of all such cases. Other relatively common medical conditions in autism spectrum disorders, across the board of intellectual functioning, are Moebius syndrome, 22q11 deletion syndrome, Angelman syndrome and sex chromosome aneuploidies. In the past, rubella embryopathy and PKU yearly contributed quite a considerable number of new autism cases, but with primary and secondary prevention measures, these are now almost never encountered in Europe or other industrialized parts of the world.

Differential diagnosis varies considerably depending on the age at which the child presents for assessment. In children under the age of about four years many present with a suspicion of deafness, language delay, general delay, or extreme hyperactivity.

If a hearing test reveals normal hearing in a child who 'appears deaf', autism should be suspected, even though some children with ADHD, or specific speech–language disorders (including Landau–Kleffner syndrome) can present in a similar way. It is important that autism still be considered a possibility even if hearing is reduced or the child is deaf.

Mental retardation occurs in about 70–80 per cent of children with childhood autism and should usually not be considered an 'either–or' diagnosis in autism. However, it is essential to make note of the fact that it is only when symptoms are out of keeping with the overall developmental level of the child that they should be taken to indicate autistic problems. There is an ongoing controversy regarding the appropriateness of making the diagnosis of autism in individuals with very low developmental levels. Some authorities would not make the diagnosis of autism in people with a mental age under about 18 months.

Language delays are part and parcel of childhood autism. Children presenting with language delay may have mental retardation, autism (or both), or they may have 'isolated' language delay. However, many children with so-called specific language disorders do have mild, moderate or even marked autistic features.

Hyperactivity in very young children, especially when associated with language or general delays, can be the most alarming symptom in autism. Sometimes, the autistic symptoms emerge more clearly only after the hyperactivity has subsided (either after medical–psychological treatment or with age).

In recent years, parents have become much more informed about autism, and it is not uncommon that they themselves bring the child to medical attention suspecting that he/she might suffer from autism.

In older children with the clinical picture of Asperger syndrome or atypical autism, it is much more common for the odd social style and 'personality' to be the presenting feature. However, attention deficits, hyperactivity, and 'inexplicable' academic failure could be the reason for referral in other cases.

Once a diagnosis of an autism spectrum disorder has been established, this usually receives priority over other diagnoses. However, given the extremely high rate of overlap and comorbidity with other conditions, it is important that the autism diagnosis does not lead to the exclusion of other diagnoses. Rather, a diagnosis within the autism spectrum should always prompt a careful search for all of the possible conditions that might be linked to it. It is reasonable always to consider the condition whose symptoms are the most impairing and form the basis for the most severe handicaps in the primary diagnosis. Autism is usually the most impairing of all conditions. If diagnostic criteria for ADHD are met and the child is impaired to the extent that specific treatment for ADHD is needed, a separate diagnosis of this condition should be made. There may well be a need for one or two further diagnoses to be made, e.g. it is not uncommon for one child to meet criteria for Asperger syndrome, ADHD, DCD and Tourette syndrome all at the same time, and all conditions needing to be treated. In clinical practice, as has already been mentioned, one should usually disregard the exclusion criteria of the DSM-IV/ICD-10. Medical disorders, including epilepsy, should be coded on a separate axis for medical diagnoses.

Diagnostic instruments (Box 16.8)

Rating scales

Rating scales – for screening or preliminary diagnosis – of autism can be subdivided into those that have been developed for the purpose of screening typical cases, and those that are geared rather towards finding cases of 'high-functioning' autism, Asperger syndrome and atypical autism. The most widely used scale for people in the autism spectrum with IQ under 70 is the *Autistic Behavior Checklist* (ABC) which provides a good measure of the level of symptoms and severity. It takes about 30 minutes to complete for somebody who knows the child well

---

Box 16.8. Diagnostic instruments

Rating scales (for screening or preliminary diagnosis)
Autistic Behavior Checklist (ABC) (Krug *et al.*, 1980)
Autism Screening Questionnaire (Berument *et al.*, 1999) based on the ADI-R (see below).
Childhood Autism Rating Scale – Revised (CARS-R)(Schopler *et al.*, 1988)
Autism Spectrum Screening Questionnaire (ASSQ) (Ehlers & Gillberg, 1993) – see Appendix
Asperger Syndrome Diagnostic Interview (ASDI) (Gillberg *et al.*, 2001) – see Appendix

Detailed clinical interview with a close carer (usually one of the parents)
Diagnosis of social and communication disorders (DISCO) (Wing *et al.*, 2002) developed for clinical and research purposes; covers the whole autism spectrum
Autism Diagnostic Interview Revised (ADI-R) (Lord *et al.*, 1994) is another excellent investigator-based interview for tapping into classic autism cases, but has been developed specifically for research
Use of the DISCO-10 and ADI-R requires diploma training

Observation of the child's behaviour
Autism Diagnostic Observation Schedule (ADOS) (Lord *et al.*, 1989) and the Pre-Linguistic ADOS (PL-ADOS) (DiLavore *et al.*, 1995)

Psychological tests
Are not required for the diagnosis of autism as such, but they are necessary components of the diagnostic evaluation. One of the Wechsler scales for estimation of IQ (or the Leiter scale in non-verbal children) should be tried in all cases. Occasionally in very learning disabled children one has to settle for an estimate of overall functioning based on Vineland interview.

(or for the clinician interviewing that person). Scores of about 70 or above are indicative of autism. There is also a brief autism screening questionnaire, see Appendix reference list, based on the ADI-R (below). A mixture of observation and interview is usually required for the completion of the Childhood Autism Rating Scale – Revised (CARS-R). This scale, which takes about 45 minutes to complete, is the instrument most widely empirically studied in the autism field. It provides a summary score in the range of 15–60, with cut-off for a preliminary diagnosis of autism at 30 and for severe variants of autism at 36. For individuals in the autism spectrum with an IQ of about 60 and above, the best validated screening instrument in school age children is the Autism Spectrum Screening Questionnaire (ASSQ) for completion by parents or teachers in under 10 minutes. Scores range from 0–54 and children attending clinics are likely to have an autism spectrum disorder if they score above about 20. Finally, there is the Asperger Syndrome Diagnostic Interview (ASDI), which takes about 40 minutes to complete and which provides a very good indication whether or not an individual meets diagnostic criteria for Asperger syndrome (or another autism spectrum disorder with IQ of about 60 or above).

Detailed clinical interview

An interview with a close carer (usually one of the parents) is the most important single measure of any in the diagnostic process. This is often best accomplished by using a structured or semi-structured psychometrically tested investigator-based diagnostic interview. One of the best clinical interviews of this kind is the DIagnosis of Social and COmmunication Disorders (DISCO), which covers not only autism spectrum disorders but also symptoms of many of the overlapping/comorbid conditions as well as providing a detailed picture of the individual's early development. The Autism Diagnostic Interview Revised (ADI-R) is another excellent investigator-based interview for tapping into classic autism cases, but has been developed specifically for research, not clinical, purposes, and does not cover all of the spectrum disorders or comorbidities. Use of the DISCO and ADI-R requires diploma training.

Observation of the child's behaviour

This is a most important component of the diagnostic process, but unfortunately one which is often overlooked. It is still not uncommon for children to be diagnosed as having an autism spectrum disorder without there having been a proper observation of the child itself. The Autism Diagnostic Observation Schedule (ADOS) and the Pre Linguistic ADOS (PL-ADOS) are excellent research instruments for structured rating of social interaction and communication behaviours in the child, but again have been developed for research, rather than clinical purposes. Nevertheless, if used as a complement to other instruments (including semistructured clinical observation of the child in the doctor's office or at psychological testing) and clinical judgement, this scale can provide important insights into the individual child's particular symptom constellation. Observation of the child in a naturalistic setting (such as in preschool or school, at home or in the playground) may sometimes be the best, and only, way of definitely determining whether he/she actually meets criteria for autism or not.

Box 16.9. Assessment

Expert medical evaluation by child neuropsychiatrist, child neurologist or developmental pediatrician should include:
head circumference
height and weight
evaluation of minor physical anomalies
skin abnormalities screen
brief neurological screen
hearing and visual assessment
Those with IQs under 50 need to be screened for the Angelman gene.

Girls with an autism spectrum disorder and IQ under 50 should be screened for the MECP2 gene associated with Rett syndrome.
A chromosomal screen (karyotype) and an FMR-1-test to screen for the fragile-X syndrome should be done in those with IQs under 85, and those who have a multitude of minor physical anomalies, and those who are unexpectedly tall.

EEG should be performed in all cases with IQ under 70 and in all who raise suspicion of suffering from any kind of epilepsy.

Brain imaging examination (MRI usually to be preferred) should be done in all with the combination of autism spectrum disorder, mental retardation and epilepsy as well as in those with any skin indication of a neurocutaneous disorder (tuberous sclerosis, neurofibromatosis, hypomelanosis of Ito)

Psychological tests are not required for the diagnosis of autism as such, but they are necessary components of the diagnostic evaluation. One of the Wechsler scales for estimation of IQ (or the Leiter scale in non-verbal children) should be tried in all cases. Occasionally in very learning disabled children one has to settle for an estimate of overall functioning based on Vineland interview.

Assessment

The diagnosis of an autism spectrum disorder is only the beginning phase of assessment (Box 16.9). The multifactorial nature of autism makes it mandatory to perform an expert medical evaluation by a doctor (child neuropsychiatrist, child neurologist or developmental paediatrician) with state-of-the-art skills in syndromology, mental retardation, autism and the comorbidities so often associated with autism. This is currently not done in all cases, and it is unacceptable. Psychometric evaluation, including a measure of the child's overall intellectual level of functioning, must be done in all cases.

The clinical medical–neurological examination

The clinical examination must always include head circumference, height, weight, and evaluation of minor physical anomalies, skin abnormalities, a brief neurological screen, and hearing and visual problems. This examination is crucial for deciding on what further laboratory investigations need to be performed.

Genetic/chromosomal analyses

All girls with an autism spectrum disorder and IQ under 50 should be screened for the MECP2 gene associated with Rett syndrome. All those – boys and girls – with IQs under 50, in addition, need to be screened for the Angelman gene on chromosome 15. All with IQs under 85 and those who have a multitude of minor physical anomalies and those who are unexpectedly tall should receive a chromosomal screen (karyotype) and an FMR-1-test to screen for the fragile-X syndrome.

EEG

An EEG should be performed in all cases with IQ under 70 and in all who raise any suspicion of suffering from any kind of epilepsy.

Brain imaging examinations

All with the combination of autism spectrum disorder, mental retardation and epilepsy should be given a brain imaging examination (MRI usually to be preferred), as should those with any skin indication of a neurocutaneous disorder (tuberous sclerosis, neurofibromatosis, hypomelanosis of Ito).

Other laboratory examinations

The expert clinician's judgement is needed to determine if and when other laboratory investigations, including urine, blood and cerebrospinal fluid screens need to be done.

Screen for psychiatric comorbidity

The clinical examination must also include a systematic psychiatric screen for ADHD, tics, motor control problems, sleep disorders, self-injurious behaviours, eating disorders and the other common comorbidities listed in the foregoing. The results of the medical–psychiatric examination and the tests performed should be conveyed to all concerned both orally and in writing.

Educational assessment

As always, it is necessary to evaluate whether or not the type of day-care or schooling the child is getting is in keeping with his/her abilities, developmental level, and personality. The extent to which parents and other family members understand the child's needs is, of course, also, important to judge.

Aetiology

There are multiple causes of autism spectrum disorders.

Genetic factors

Genetic factors are very important in autism. The sibling rate for the core syndrome given a proband with core syndrome autism is about 5 per cent, but the rate for an autism spectrum disorder in such cases is probably in the order of 15 per cent to 25 per cent. This, of course, is much above the level expected by chance in the general population. Twin studies have shown concordance rates of 60–89 per cent in monozygotic twins and under 5 per cent in dizygotic twins (similar to non-twin siblings), suggesting a heritability of close to 100 per cent in cases which are not associated with specific medical disorders. It is not clear exactly what it is that is inherited, but it now seems likely that aberrant or variant genes may act in concert, that more than 30 different genes are likely to be involved, and that the individual genes may increase liability for a particular autism feature rather than for the full syndrome of autism. Genome scan and candidate gene studies of autism have suggested a number of chromosomal regions of interest (particularly chromosomes 2, 6, 7, 15, 16, 18, and X), but – with the exception of neuroligin X-linked genes – at the time of going to press with this book, few specific genes or gene products have been identified in autism.

Mental retardation and epilepsy

The links between autism spectrum disorders on the one hand and mental retardation and epilepsy on the other are strong, especially in the childhood autism subgroup. The prevalence of autism spectrum disorders in severe mental retardation is about 35 per cent, in mild retardation about 10–25 per cent, and in individuals with IQ above 70 under 0.5 per cent. These rates, and the rate of about 35 per cent epilepsy in core childhood autism, suggest strong links between autism and brain dysfunction.

Types of brain dysfunction

The frontotemporal portions of the brain are often dysfunctional in autism (bilaterally or, typically in more 'high-functioning' cases in the right hemisphere). The brainstem and cerebellum have also been shown to be abnormal in relatively large subgroups of individuals with autism. Autopsy studies have revealed abnormalities in the amygdala and cerebellum in particular. Megalencephalus is much overrepresented in autism spectrum disorders, apparently more so among those with IQs above 70.

Hyperserotonemia in the blood, dopamine and endorphin dysfunction, and excess of protein in the cerebrospinal fluid have all been shown to be associated with autism in group studies, but it is not clear what relevance, if any, these 'markers' may have for the understanding of autism aetiology.

It has been demonstrated convincingly in many case studies that certain acquired brain lesions, such as in connection with herpes encephalitis, can cause autism without there being any known genetic susceptibility. However, many of the associated medical disorders which are currently believed to be aetiologically related to autism (such as tuberous sclerosis) are themselves genetic. Also, some studies suggest that, even when there is an associated medical disorder that is believed to be important in the pathogenetic chain of events, interaction with autism susceptibility genes may occur. It has been suggested that, in certain cases, there might have been genetic predisposition for a 'mild autistic-like condition' ('broader autism phenotype') but that additional (pre-, or perinatal) brain damage has led to the full-blown syndrome of autism.

Psychosocial factors

It is unlikely that psychosocial factors themselves cause autism, but conditions with some similar symptomology have been reported in children exposed to severe emotional and psychosocial deprivation in the first years of life. If such factors play a role in some autism cases, they would do so by impinging (perhaps irreversibly) on brain systems that are crucial for social and communicative functioning.

It is likely that autism spectrum disorders will be shown to be the 'final common behavioural presentation' of a multitude of different etiologies, and that only after more sophisticated subgrouping than can currently be achieved, will it be possible to find the cause in an individual case.

Neuropsychological dysfunction

Neuropsychologically, children in the autism spectrum usually have executive function deficits showing clinically as poor planning ability, low motivational level, difficulty with time concepts, and problems maintaining a strategy for reaching a goal. Sustaining attention may be very difficult, and there appear to be general problems with shifting of attention from one object of focus to another.

Mentalizing ('theory of mind') deficits are almost universally occurring, particularly in pre-school children. These deficits are connected to the lack of empathy and inability to take the cognitive and emotional (though not necessarily perceptual) perspective of other people.

There is also usually a decreased drive for central coherence, meaning that individuals with autism may have no difficulty remembering details or amassing concrete factual knowledge about the observable world, but may have major problems fitting the details into a coherent 'whole' or to make sense of all the facts.

Problems of procedural learning may be linked to the decreased coherence drive and show as difficulty acquiring a new sequence of skills while having no or little problem acquiring the individual part skills of that sequence. Neurophysiological studies have suggested that decreased connectivity between neurons and between brain regions might account for some of these findings.

Several recent studies indicate that people in the autism spectrum tend to look more at the lower portions of other people's faces when processing their facial expressions. These findings could go some way towards explaining the unusual/avoidant gaze contact encountered in many individuals with autism spectrum disorders.

Overall cognition and/or cognitive profile is almost always affected. On cognitive tests those with a diagnosis of childhood autism (and of atypical autism) usually fall below IQ of about 80, whereas the majority of those with Asperger syndrome test at or above IQ 70. The former group frequently do better on performance than verbal parts of tests, whereas the opposite pattern is more likely to be encountered in those with Asperger syndrome (which may be referred to as 'non-verbal learning disability). On the Wechsler scales, core autism cases often have relatively better results on the subtest of block design, while showing a trough on the comprehension subtest. Those with a diagnosis of Asperger syndrome often show a similar pattern when young (even though, unlike those with classic autism, the better result on block design may well be coupled with a poor result on object assembly), but as they grow older (and are laboriously taught the 'rules of the real world'), they tend to do better and better on the comprehension subtest. Slow processing appears to be typical of Asperger syndrome. Many individuals with this diagnosis would pass on most tasks if they were not timed.

Treatment

Clinical management and treatment setting

The evidence base for interventions in autism spectrum disorders is limited. No one treatment will lead to a cure, and it is unlikely that a single mode of intervention will ever dominate the arena, given the multifactorial contribution to autism pathogenesis. A child with a diagnosis within the autism spectrum and his/her family will need the continued support of an expert team consisting of a medical doctor, psychologist, and a special education expert (at the very least) for many years, usually throughout childhood and into early adult life. It is usually to be preferred that this service is offered within a slightly broader child neuropsychiatric or developmental paediatric clinic rather than in a highly specialized autism centre, in which the experts may not have enough skills in the neighbouring fields of co-morbidity.

Treatment algorithms and decision trees

Interventions in autism need always be individualized and adopted in accordance with a number of associated factors including IQ level, expressive and receptive language competence, severity and type of behaviour problems, specific interest patterns, other co-existing conditions (including medical disorders, ADHD, tic disorders, depression, anxiety and eating disorders) and symptoms (including severe sensory/perceptual abnormalities, self-injurious, and violent-explosive behaviours). There can be no overall decision trees for the treatment of autism. In fact, it may not even be appropriate to be speaking of 'treatment' in autism, but rather to refer to education, habilitation and intervention.

Education

Those with childhood autism and an IQ of 70 or under almost always need to attend specialist autism classrooms, whereas those with Asperger syndrome may well benefit from attending a mainstream classroom. Nevertheless, in this intellectually better functioning group it is important to be able to offer a choice, and some, for instance many of those who are victims of bullying, will do much better and have a better quality of life in a classroom for intellectually normal, able or gifted children with autism spectrum disorders. Others may do better in mixed special education classrooms. Decisions about education are important for all children, but perhaps more so for those with autism than for anybody else. The most important aspects pertain to the knowledge of autism on the part of the teachers. All children in the autism spectrum will need a considerably greater amount of structure, concreteness, and systematic, well-planned skills training (both as regards school day structure and overview and in all individual subjects) than is usually considered required (or even helpful) for other children. Without skills training, no (or almost no) skills will emerge in autism; this is what makes autism so different from all other conditions. Other children will seek out help, ask when they do not understand and will be able spontaneously to find solutions to problems that had not been envisaged. Not so for those with autism: unless an adult well versed in the many facets of autism is there and can plan ahead and make the environmental demands more predictable for the child, little or no learning of new facts or skills will come about.

Specific education programmes, such as that developed under the acronym of TEACCH ('Treatment and Education of Autistic and Communication handicapped Children'), are available and provide a very good basis for training teachers and parents to become proponents for and providers of an 'autism-friendly' environment. This may comprise a calm and predictable setting rich in structure, concreteness, and, usually, though not always, including much more visual material including so-called 'Picture Exchange Communication' system (PECs) than ordinarily provided in education. Change (of routines or introduction of new materials) is often best accepted and accomplished if introduced gradually. Continuity as regards time, place and people is a most important aspect of autism education, and one which is strongly emphasized in the TEACCH philosophy. It is usually best for a child in the autism spectrum to have a small number of teachers who know the child very well rather than being exposed to what others might perceive of as a 'stimulating range of personalities'. Children with autism usually have a hard time if left with a choice in the academic setting. An autism-friendly teacher will know to 'read' the signals and either make the choice for the child or gently coach him/her to make a good decision.

Psychological interventions

Psychoeducation is perhaps the most important part of any intervention scheme for autism spectrum disorder. Parents, siblings, and, depending on the intellectual capacity, the affected individual, all need detailed up-to-date information about autism, its causes, prognosis and possible intervention strategies. They need to be well informed about relevant support groups, books, pamphlets, videos, CDs, DVDs, conferences, Internet addresses and other ways to access information. Considering the family (including the extended family of aunts and uncles, grandmothers and grandfathers) the child's most important helpers will usually provide the best support framework for the future. In the past, it was often felt that parents of children with autism were over-protective. We now know that (over)protectiveness is very much what is needed if the person with an autism spectrum disorder is to achieve a good quality of life in adult age. Psychoeducation also must involve educating 'society' in a broader sense. Teachers, health-care staff and the general public need to be well informed about autism in order that autism friendly environments be thought of as a salient part of the interventions and that attitudes to people with autism be changed in positive ways.

'ABA' (applied behaviour analysis) has been shown to effectively reduce some problem behaviours in autism and to improve social and communication skills. What is still disputed is how many hours a week such programmes need to be applied in order to be optimally effective. Some parents want to have their children in a stringent ABA-protocol for 40 hours a week or more, and seem to find this very helpful. Others would not be happy with such a demanding and time-consuming intervention, and would rather have their child involved for 10–15 hours a week, or in a behaviourally orientated education programme of the TEACCH variant.

Individual talks with teenagers with autism spectrum disorders of the Asperger variant can be beneficial so long as the psychologist/doctor is well acquainted with the basic problems typical of autism. Psychoanalytically orientated psychotherapies have little place in the overall intervention programme for people in the autism spectrum.

Pharmacotherapy

No currently known drugs are likely to affect the ultimate outcome of autism spectrum disorders. However, many pharmacological interventions are available for symptoms associated with autism spectrum disorders.

ADHD

Severe ADHD or hyperactivity will often respond favourably to typical stimulant treatment (see Taylor this volume) in autism spectrum disorder cases with IQs above 50. In those with severe and profound mental retardation, a positive response is not impossible, but the odds are not very favourable. The common inability to shift attention so often seen in autism can sometimes become even more marked during stimulant treatment, and may lead to the clinical impression that withdrawal and aloofness has increased. One has to strike a balance here as to what is the most handicapping symptom: hyperactivity, inattention, or 'withdrawal'. In any case, tapering the stimulant will usually – within a day or two – lead to the child becoming exactly as he/she was like before stimulant treatment started.

Hyperactivity, violent outbursts and self-injury

Severe hyperactivity when combined with violent behaviours and self-injury is more likely to respond to an atypical neuroleptic, such as risperidone (often in doses of 0.5–3.0 mg/day once a day for children under 12 years, increasing to about 1.0–4.5 mg/day for older individuals).

Depression

In depression and social withdrawal, particularly in autism spectrum disorder with normal IQ, and especially when there is also a high degree of obsessionality/ritualism, a trial of a serotonin reuptake inhibitor such as fluoxetine (10–40 mg/day in one dose for those under 12 years, 20–80 mg/day for those of about 13 and above).

Epilepsy

Those with epilepsy should be treated for their seizure disorder in close collaboration with a child neurologist. Lamotrigine and valproic acid sometimes appear to have beneficial effects not only on the seizure disorder, but also on mood swings and violent behaviour. Carbamazepine is probably the antiepileptic drug most widely used in the treatment of epilepsy in autism. It is often effective, but there is a tendency for perseverative symptoms to become more pronounced in some individuals. Other antiepileptic drugs, perhaps particularly the benzodiazepines, are associated with a high rate of behavioural toxicity in autism (including cognitive blunting, violent outbursts, self injury, hyperactivity, and confusional states).

Bipolar disorder

Associated bipolar disorder, not exceedingly rare in autism, is often best treated with risperidone in doses as suggested, followed by the addition of a mood stabilizer such as valproic acid, or, in some cases, lithium.

Tic disorders

Tics only rarely require separate pharmacologic intervention in autism, but if they are extreme, risperidone, again, is quite likely to be effective.

Sleep disorders

Sleep disorders are difficult to treat. Melatonin (3 mg half an hour before projected sleep onset) – according to clinical experience – can be very effective in inducing sleep, but if used on a regular basis, tends to lose its effect. After a 'drug holiday' of a few months, parents report that the drug can be used again with good effect for a similar amount of time, whereafter a new break is needed.

Monitoring and evaluation of treatment

Monitoring of interventions in the field of autism are usually best carried out at regular visits to an outpatient clinic specializing in the field of neuropsychiatric disorders with childhood onset. Rating scales can be useful in some cases but many such scales have not been developed for the purpose of measuring intervention effects and are more appropriate for diagnostic purposes. Initially, a family may have to come for visits several times a month, but, in the longer perspective, doctor's visits can usually be reduced to once a year. However, it has to be appreciated from the outset that management is long term, and that no intervention will lead to complete disappearance of further service needs.

In many countries, children with autism spectrum disorders are under special service provision acts and may need an expert diagnosis of autism in order to access such services. Parents may be entitled to specific financial support because of the handicapping nature of the child's condition. Acts, laws, support conditions and services change over time. The psychiatrist catering to the family's needs will have to keep abreast of developments in these fields so as to be able to provide an optimal coordinating medical–psychiatric–education service.

Information to parents and patients

As has already been outlined, information to all those concerned is extremely important. Very often, the easiest way of accessing good information about autism is through a support group such as the National Autism Society. Having said that, it is also important to be aware that some information about autism is unscientific and, occasionally, outright unhelpful, spreading myths about the causes and cures. Rather than trying to persuade parents to avoid such information, one should inform them of their existence, so that, when they come across it, they may be better prepared to form their own opinion, distance themselves from it or come back asking about it.

Problematic issues

There are many problems pertaining to intervention in autism. The word treatment in itself implies the possibility of a cure. Some parents are desperate for a cure and will go for second and third opinions in order to find a doctor/'specialist' who will come up with a suggestion for one. There are charlatans in the field of autism. Almost every year sees the emergence of a new miracle cure with no empirical evidence to support it (three of the most promulgated therapies for which scientific support is lacking are holding therapy, facilitated communication, and secretin therapy, all of which are not recommended). An in-depth diagnosis with careful consideration of comorbidities and possible causes and open sharing of all information with the family will go a long way towards avoiding a situation in which parents feel at a loss, and may save them a lot of psychological suffering (and economic hardship) at the hand of unscrupulous self-appointed 'experts'. Autism is usually a lifelong condition. Organizing and providing a service that makes sense over time is difficult, but in the long run, rewarding for all concerned. In the last several years, the issue of follow-up into adult age has come under debate. Many argue that multidisciplinary teams working with children and adolescents should be working in close liaison, maybe even in the same clinic, as those providing continued care for adults with autism spectrum disorders.

Outcome

Short- and long-term outcome

Diagnoses of conditions within the autism spectrum are stable over the shorter term. In the very long term perspective they are also relatively stable, even though conditions diagnosed as atypical or as falling just outside the spectrum are more likely to be considered typical at the later evaluation.

Of those with classic autism, it is likely that, in adult life, the majority will continue to be dependent on other adults for work, activities and dwelling. Even the most recent follow-up studies, in which, at least partly adequate interventions have been provided from early childhood, suggest that only a few per cent of all affected individuals will be completely independent at age 20–40 years. However, these studies also suggest that with good early programmes, the number needing medication or long-term stay in psychiatric hospitals may be greatly reduced. Quality of life in an autism-friendly environment can be good even when independence has not been achieved.

Mortality is increased in the classic group. This can usually be attributed to epilepsy, a severe associated medical disorder, or accidents (including drowning). One study showed 5 per cent had died before age 30 years, which is much higher than in the general population. Nevertheless, it seems that the vast majority of all people with autism will live to be old.

Outcome in Asperger syndrome is much less well understood. However, it varies enormously, some people doing very well indeed in adult life and may have made excellent careers for themselves, living with a partner and even having children. Unfortunately, some of these children themselves have autism spectrum disorders. A large subgroup of those with Asperger syndrome have major psychiatric and academic problems in adult life. This includes a subgroup who attempts or actually commits suicide. The outcome studies in the longer term are only beginning to appear, and it is currently unknown what proportion of all those affected do well and how many do not.

Many people (as many as one in three) with autism spectrum disorders show severe symptom aggravation around the time of adolescence. About half of this proportion actually deteriorates, and may never again attain the level of functioning they had reached before puberty.

Prognostic factors

It has long been recognized that IQ above 70 and some communicative speech at early school age are the strongest predictors of a relatively better outcome in autism. An associated severe medical disorder and the presence of epilepsy, particularly if of early childhood onset, tend to predict a worse outcome. It is likely that an early diagnosis will help increase the odds for a positive outcome.

SUGGESTED READING

T. Attwood, *Asperger's Syndrome: A Guide for Parents and Professionals.* (London and Philadelphia: Jessica Kingsley Publishers, 1998).

S. Baron-Cohen & P. Bolton (eds.), *Autism: The Facts.* (Oxford: Oxford University Press, 1993).

D. Cohen & F. R. Volkmar, *Handbook of Autism and Pervasive Developmental Disorders.* (New York: Chichester, Wiley, 1997).

U. Frith, *Autism. Explaining the Enigma. 2nd Edn.* (Oxford: Blackwell Publishing, 2003).

C. Gillberg, *A Guide to Asperger Syndrome.* (Cambridge: Cambridge University Press, 2002).

C. Gillberg & M. Coleman, *The Biology of the Autistic Syndromes. 3rd edn.* (London: Cambridge University Press, 2000).

P. Howlin, Prognosis in autism: do specialist treatments affect long-term outcome? *European Child and Adolescent Psychiatry,* **6** (1997), 55–72.

L. Wing, Autistic spectrum disorders. *British Medical Journal,* **312** (1996), 327–8.

Appendix

Diagnostic instruments in the public domain

Questionnaires

The Autistic Behavior Checklist (ABC) (Krug *et al.*, 1980) is a 57-item symptom scale for completion by somebody who knows the child well. It has been well psychometrically validated and is useful for evaluating the symptom load in autism. Symptoms are given weighted scores (0, 1, 2, 3, 4) depending on specificity for autism. There are five subscales ('social', 'speech–language', 'behaviour', 'perception', and 'other'). Total scores of 70 and above are almost always indicative of autism or atypical autism. However, in children with other disabilities one would have to consider the possibility of autism even in those who score in the 45 to 69 range (Nordin & Gillberg, 1996). This scale is not appropriate for children with normal or superior IQ. It takes about 30 minutes to complete.

The Asperger Syndrome and Autism Spectrum Screening Questionnaire (ASSQ) (Ehlers & Gillberg, 1993, Ehlers *et al.*, 1999; Posserud *et al.*, 2005) is a 27-item screening scale for completion by teachers or parents. Symptoms are scored as 0, 1, 2 (normal, possibly deviant, definitely deviant). It was developed with a particular view to locate high-functioning cases of autism and Asperger syndrome in the general population of school-age children. It has good-excellent psychometric data to support it. In clinical practice a score of about 20 or above indicates a very high risk of an autism spectrum disorder. This scale is appropriate for those with an IQ in the near normal or normal range and is less well suited for those with mental retardation. It takes under 10 minutes to complete.

The Asperger Syndrome and Autism Spectrum Screening Questionnaire (ASSQ)

Name of the child . . . . Date of birth . . . .

Name of rater . . . . Date of rating . . . .

This child stands out as different from other children of his/her age in the following way:

	No	Somewhat	Yes
1. is old-fashioned or precocious	[ ]	[ ]	[ ]
2. is regarded as an 'eccentric professor' by the other children	[ ]	[ ]	[ ]
3. lives somewhat in a world of his/her own with restricted idiosyncratic intellectual interests	[ ]	[ ]	[ ]
4. accumulates facts on certain subjects (good rote memory) but does not really understand the meaning	[ ]	[ ]	[ ]
5. has a literal understanding of ambiguous and metaphorical language	[ ]	[ ]	[ ]
6. has a deviant style of communication with a formal, fussy, old-fashioned or 'robotlike' language	[ ]	[ ]	[ ]
7. invents idiosyncratic words and expressions	[ ]	[ ]	[ ]
8. has a different voice or speech	[ ]	[ ]	[ ]
9. expresses sounds involuntarily; clears throat, grunts, smacks, cries or screams	[ ]	[ ]	[ ]
10. is surprisingly good at some things and surprisingly poor at others	[ ]	[ ]	[ ]
11. uses languages freely but fails to make adjustment to fit social contexts or the needs of different listeners	[ ]	[ ]	[ ]
12. lacks empathy	[ ]	[ ]	[ ]
13. makes naive and embarrassing remarks	[ ]	[ ]	[ ]
14. has a deviant style of gaze	[ ]	[ ]	[ ]
15. wishes to be sociable but fails to make relationships with peers	[ ]	[ ]	[ ]
16. can be with other children but only on his/her terms	[ ]	[ ]	[ ]
17. lacks best friend	[ ]	[ ]	[ ]
18. lacks common sense	[ ]	[ ]	[ ]
19. is poor at games: no idea of cooperating in a team, scores 'own' goals	[ ]	[ ]	[ ]
20. has clumsy, ill coordinated, ungainly, awkward movements or gestures	[ ]	[ ]	[ ]
21. has involuntary face or body movements	[ ]	[ ]	[ ]
22. has difficulties in completing simple daily activities because of compulsory repetition of certain actions or thoughts	[ ]	[ ]	[ ]
23. has special routines: insists on no change	[ ]	[ ]	[ ]
24. shows idiosyncratic attachment to objects	[ ]	[ ]	[ ]
25. is bullied by other children	[ ]	[ ]	[ ]
26. has markedly unusual facial expression	[ ]	[ ]	[ ]
27. has markedly unusual posture	[ ]	[ ]	[ ]

Specify reasons other than above:

© 1993 Ehlers, S. & Gillberg, C.

The Childhood Autism Rating Scale – Revised (CARS-R) (Schopler *et al.*, 1988) is a mixture of a rating scale, brief interview and observation schedule. Some information from somebody who knows the child well is usually necessary, but somebody knowledgeable about autism may be able to fill out the scale after spending time with the child. It is the best validated of all autism instruments and has been used in dozens of studies across the globe. It provides a good measure of the severity of autism. Scores are in the 15–60 range and there is a cut-off for suspected autism at 30, with severe autism starting at 36.

There are a number of other scales/questionnaires, but they have not been psychometrically validated to the extent that the mentioned instruments have been.

Diagnostic interviews

The DIagnosis of Social and COmmunication Disorders (DISCO) (Wing *et al.*, 2002) is a structured/semi-structured comprehensive investigator-based interview for clinical and research purposes. It is intended for completion by a clinician well versed in the nature of the core problems associated with autism. It has excellent psychometric data to support its use in autism spectrum disorders (not just core autism). It has the additional asset of covering developmental issues and symptoms of most of the comorbidities encountered in autism spectrum disorders. It takes 2–4 hours to complete, and requires prior training. It provides clinical and research algorithm diagnoses within the full autism spectrum and is equally relevant for low- and high-functioning cases. It can also be used in the work-up of adult individuals with suspected autism spectrum disorders.

The Autism Diagnostic Interview – Revised (ADI-R) (Lord *et al.*, 1994) is a semistructured investigator-based interview developed for research. It has excellent psychometric data to support its use in childhood autism, but not in other autism spectrum disorder variants. It is the most widely used diagnostic instrument for autism in research. However, it is not really appropriate for clinical work with individuals in the upper intellectual levels, and it provides little or no information about the co-morbidities. Like the DISCO, it takes 2–4 hours to complete and requires prior training.

The Asperger Syndrome and Autism Spectrum Disorder Diagnostic Interview (ASDI) (Gillberg *et al.*, 2001) is a structured, investigator-based interview developed for use in research and clinical practice. Preliminary studies suggest good-excellent psychometric properties and good validity for autism spectrum disorders. It takes about 30–45 minutes to complete and will provide a good basis for suggesting a preliminary diagnosis of autism/Asperger syndrome in individuals with near normal, normal, or superior IQ.

Asperger Syndrome Diagnostic Interview (ASDI)

Name of individual rated:

Date of birth:

Age at examination:

Name of informant and relation to individual rated:

Rater:

Date of interview:

This interview is intended for clinicians well acquainted with Asperger syndrome and other disorders in the autism spectrum, even though there is no requirement for 'expertise'. The interview is investigator-based, i.e. the rater is expected to score each item only after determining that he/she has elicited sufficient information for a qualified rating to be made. This means that all the 20 areas listed need to be probed into in some detail. Examples of behaviours should be provided by the informant before a rating is assigned. The questions should, if at all possible, be read to the informant as they are written, but may occasionally be slightly re-worded in order to assure that the relevant area of functioning has been adequately covered.

Scores: $0 =$ does not apply, $1 =$ applies to some degree or very much

---

Area 1: Severe impairments in reciprocal social interaction (extreme egocentricity)

1. Does he/she exhibit considerable difficulties interacting with peers?   0   1

   If so, in what way?_____

2. Does he/she exhibit a low degree of concern or a seeming lack of interest in   0   1
   making friends or interacting with peers?

   If so, specify_____

3. Does he/she have problems appreciating social cues, i.e. does he/she fail to note   0   1
   changes in the social conversation/interaction or to take account of such changes
   in his/her ongoing interaction with other people?

   If so, describe_____

4. Does he/she exhibit socially or emotionally inappropriate behaviours?   0   1

   If so, in what way(s)?_____

   (Two or more scores of 1 = criterion met)

Area 2: All absorbing narrow interest pattern(s)

5. Is there a pattern of interest or a specific interest which takes up so much of   0   1
   his/her time that time for other activities is clearly restricted?

   If there is, comment_____

6. Is there a repetitive quality to his/her interest patterns/specific interest   0   1

    If so, specify_____

7. Are his/her interest patterns based more on rote memory than on true meaning?   0   1

    (One or more scores of 1 = criterion met)

Area 3: Imposition of routines, rituals and interests

8. Does he/she try to introduce and impose routines, rituals or interests on   0   1
    himself/herself in such a way as to produce problems for himself?

    If so, in what way?_____

9. Does he/she try to introduce and impose routines, rituals or interests on   0   1
    himself/herself in such a way as to produce problems for others?

    If so, describe_____

    (One or more scores of 1 = criterion met)

Area 4: Speech and language peculiarities

10. Was his/her language development delayed?   0   1

    If so, comment_____

11. Is his/her language 'superficially perfect' regardless of whether or not there are   0   1
    comprehension problems or other speech-language problems?

    If so, comment_____

12. Is his/her language formal, pedantic or 'overly adult'?   0   1

    If so, describe_____

13. Is there any characteristic about his voice (pitch, volume, quality, intonation,   0   1
    word stress, 'prosody', etc.) which you find peculiar or unusual?

    If so, in what way?_____

14. Are there any comprehension problems (including misinterpretations of   0   1
    literal/implied meanings)?

    If so, what kind of problems?_____

    (Three or more scores of 1 = criterion met)

Area 5: Non-verbal communication problems

15. Does he/she make limited use of gestures?   0   1

    If so, comment_____

16. Is his/her body language awkward, gauche, clumsy, strange or unusual?   0   1

    If so, comment_____

17. Are his/her facial expressions limited to a rather small repertoire?   0   1

    If so, describe_____

18. Is his/her general expression (including facial) sometimes inappropriate?   0   1

    If so, describe_____

19. Is his/her gaze stiff, strange, peculiar, abnormal or odd?   0   1

    If so, characterize_____

    (One or more scores of 1 = criterion met)

Area 6: Motor clumsiness

20. Has he/she been noted to perform poorly on neurodevelopmental examinations   0   1
    either in the past or in connection with the present interview?

    Comment_____

    (Score of 1 = criterion met)

    © 2001 Autism. SAGE Publications

Observation schedules/rating scales

The Autism Diagnostic Observation Schedule (ADOS) and Pre-Linguistic ADOS (PL-ADOS) (Lord *et al.*, 1989, 1994, DiLavore *et al.*, 1995) are psychometrically well-validated systematic observational schedules for rating autism-typical behaviours during structured interaction with the child. The scales are excellent for research purposes. However, they may 'overdiagnose' autism in children with hypoactivity (such as the 22q11 deletion syndrome) and may 'underdiagnose' the condition in those people with autism spectrum disorders who do much better in a structured test setting than in free-play situations.

Clinical checklists

Using the DSM-IV or ICD-10 symptom checklists for childhood autism will provide a good basis for considering an autism diagnosis in the first place. A similar Gillberg checklist for Asperger syndrome will be helpful in determining whether or not an individual might be in need of further assessment with a view to diagnosing that disorder. It has to be kept in mind that no final diagnosis can ever be made on the basis of just the information obtained on going over a checklist of this kind.

Medical work-up

The medical work-up required in autism is different from case to case. An individual decision has to be made by the expert child neuropsychiatrist, child neurologist or developmental paediatrician well acquainted with the various medical disorders known to be associated with autism spectrum disorders.

Psychological tests

A wide variety of psychological tests may prove to be useful in the work-up of individuals with autism spectrum disorders. One of the Wechsler scales is often appropriate, but with non-verbal individuals or when IQ is in the 50-and-below-range, then other tests may have to be used (Leiter 1997, Raven *et al.*, 1986, Griffiths, 1970). The Vineland Adaptive Behaviour Scales (Sparrow *et al.*, 1984) is an excellent tool for assessing the degree of overall social adaptation in various domains. It is useful across the board of intellectual functioning in autism spectrum disorders.

REFERENCES

Berument, S. K., Rutter, M., Lord, C., Pickles, A. & Bailey, A. (1999). Autism screening questionnaire: diagnostic validity. *British Journal of Psychiatry*, **175**, 444–51.

DiLavore, P. C., Lord, C. & Rutter, M. (1995). The pre-linguistic autism diagnostic observation schedule. *Journal of Autism and Developmental Disorder*, **25**, 355–79.

Ehlers, S. & Gillberg, C. (1993). The epidemiology of Asperger syndrome. A total population study. *Journal of Child Psychology and Psychiatry*, **34**, 1327–50.

Ehlers, S., Gillberg, C. & Wing, L. (1999). A screening questionnaire for Asperger syndrome and other high-functioning autism spectrum disorders in school age children. *Journal of Autism and Developmental Disorders*, **29**, 129–41.

Gillberg, C., Rastam, M. & Wentz, E. (2001). The Asperger Syndrome (and high-functioning autism) Diagnostic Interview (ASDI): a preliminary study of a new structured clinical interview. *Autism*, **5**, 57–66.

Griffiths, R. (1970). *The Abilities of Young Children. A Study in Mental Measurement.* London: University of London Press.

Krug, D. A., Arick, I. & Almond, P. (1980). Behavior checklist for identifying severely handicapped individuals with high levels of autistic behavior. *Journal of Child Psychology and Psychiatry*, **21**, 221–9.

Lord, C., Rutter, M., Goode, S. *et al.* (1989). Autism diagnostic observation schedule: a standardized observation of communicative and social behavior. *Journal of Autism and Developmental Disorder*, **19**, 185–212.

Lord, C., Rutter, M. & Le Couteur, A. (1994). Autism Diagnostic Interview – Revised: a revised version of a diagnostic interview for caregivers of individuals with possible pervasive developmental disorders. *Journal of Autism Developmental Disorders*, **24**, 659–85.

Nordin, V. & Gillberg, C. (1996). Autism spectrum disorders in children with physical or mental disability or both. Part II: Screening aspects. *Developmental Medicine and Child Neurology*, **38**, 314–24.

Posserud, M. B., Steijnen, M., Verhoeven, S., Lundervold, A., Stormark, K. M. & Gillberg, C. (2005). Factor analysis of the Autism Spectrum Screening Questionnaire.

Raven, J. C., Court, J. H. & Raven, J. (1986). *Coloured Progressive Matrices.*

Roid, G. H. & Miller, L. J. (1997). *Leiter International Performance Scale – Revised.* Wood Dale, IL: Stoeling Co.

Schopler, E., Reichler, R. J. & Renner, B. R. (1988). *The Childhood Autism Rating Scale (CARS).* Revised edn. Los Angeles: Western Psychological Services, Inc.

Sparrow, S. S., Balla, D. A. & Cicchetti, D. V. (1984). *The Vineland Adaptive Behavior Scales.* Circle Pines, MN: American Guidance Service.

Wing, L., Leekam, S. R., Libby, S. J., Gould, J. & Larcombe, M. (2002). The Diagnostic Interview for Social and Communication Disorders: background, inter-rater reliability and clinical use. *Journal of Child Psychology and Psychiatry*, **43**, 307–25.

17

Hyperkinetic disorders

Eric Taylor

Department of Child and Adolescent Psychiatry, Institute of Psychiatry, London, UK

Introduction

Many children show traits of behaving in an impulsive, inattentive and restless fashion. These behaviours, when not severe, need not constitute a problem. When extreme, however, they present a risk for the psychological development of the individual. Severe levels of 'hyperactivity' (the combination of impulsiveness, restlessness and overactivity) make children more likely to develop an antisocial adjustment, and more likely to show various aspects of personality dysfunction in later adolescence and adult life. Children's hyperactivity can also be very unpleasant for the caregivers. Both teachers and parents can find it hard to live with a hyperactive child, and their tolerance and ability to cope may determine whether it is presented as a problem. Children with hyperactivity rarely ask for help themselves, and are often not aware of a problem. The presentation to the clinician is therefore a complex blend of the skills and tolerance of adults surrounding the child and the qualities of the children themselves. They constitute the commonest reason for referral to child mental health or behavioural paediatric services in many countries. Effective physical and psychological treatments are available, and the management needs to be long term. Hyperactive behaviour problems therefore make up a large part of the work of most community mental health services for children.

Definition and classification

ICD 10 criteria

The ICD-10 definition of hyperkinetic disorder is based upon the simultaneous presence of all three main behavioural problems: attention deficit, overactivity and impulsiveness. They need to be present in more than one situation – for instance,

A Clinician's Handbook of Child and Adolescent Psychiatry, ed. Christopher Gillberg,
Richard Harrington and Hans-Christoph Steinhausen. Published by Cambridge University Press.
© Cambridge University Press 2005.

at school as well as at home, or in observation at the clinic as well as at school. They need to be at a level that is out of keeping with the child's development – not just chronological age, but mental development as well. The problems also need to have been present from an early age – before the age of 7 years by definition and in practice usually even earlier.

There are also a number of exclusion criteria – mostly, the presence of other disorders that could themselves be causes of hyperactive behaviour. The commonest in practice are autism spectrum disorders (see Gillberg, this volume) and affective disorders, especially anxiety (see Ollendick, this volume). The rationale for these exclusion criteria is disputed, because the nature of co-morbidity is not yet fully understood. It may turn out that the simultaneous presence of (for example) hyperactivity and autism spectrum indicates that two disorders truly are present – in which case the diagnostic criteria will need to change.

DSM IV criteria

The DSM IV category is called Attention Deficit/Hyperactivity Disorder (ADHD). The criteria are based upon the same list of behaviours as those that characterize the ICD-10 definition of hyperkinetic disorder. There are a few slight differences in wording of the items, but they are clearly intended to refer to the same general pattern. The rules for making a diagnosis from these items are, however, quite different.

- Unlike ICD-10, DSM-IV does not require that all three key behavioural difficulties should be present. Rather, impulsiveness/hyperactivity or inattentiveness can be grounds for the diagnosis even in the absence of the other. Indeed, the subdivisions within ADHD are 'inattentive' 'impulsive/overactive' and 'combined'. The ICD-10 criteria are therefore only met for cases falling within the 'combined' category of DSM-IV.
- The requirements for pervasiveness across situations in the DSM-IV are less stringent. Rather than criteria having to be met in more than one situation, there is only the requirement that some impairment should be present in more than one situation – and the impairment may be based on a sub-set of symptoms.
- The exclusion criteria applying to the co-existent presence of other disorders are less stringent. Instead of the requirement that autism and affective disorders should be absent, the criterion is that the symptomatology should not be better explained by another syndrome. This often leads to multiple diagnoses in DSM-IV terminology.

Clinical applicability

The practical consequence of these differences in definitions is that the ICD-10 category of hyperkinetic disorder is a severe sub-group of ADHD. Research on the hyperkinetic disorder sub-group has indicated that it is particularly likely to be associated with a marked response to stimulant medication, a poor response to behavioural treatment alone, and a high clustering of other neurodevelopmental anomalies such as delays in language and motor development. On the other hand, genetic evidence, such as the analysis of large twin studies, has suggested that the degree of heritability is very similar at the extreme level (hyperkinetic disorder), the moderate level (ADHD), and the minor levels of hyperactive behaviour within the non-referred population of children. No separate aetiological pathway has yet been established at any level of severity.

Clinicians therefore find it useful to use the concepts of both schemes. A broad notion of ADHD is helpful in the screening and initial detection of cases. However, the diagnostic and assessment work should not stop at the point where ADHD is recognized; but go on to a wider range of strengths and weaknesses (see below). One outcome of the full assessment will be a sub-categorization into whether the child also falls into the hyperkinetic disorder sub-group. The management schemes to be outlined are somewhat different for those who do and do not meet the more rigorous criteria.

Another outcome of a full assessment will be a description of the problems shown by people with impairment attributable to ADHD but who fall short of the full criteria for hyperkinetic disorder. Several distinctions need to be made, even though current scientific evidence does not allow for clear conclusions about whether valid subtypes are present or whether there is variation of expression within a single broader disorder.

The first distinction is of the type of problem shown: inattentive or overactive–impulsive.

- Attention deficit without overactivity often presents as a failure of academic progress. Children are not disruptive or overactive; they may be dreamy and even somewhat inert; but they are often muddled and disorganized in the classroom and find it hard to persist. Cognitive deficits are usually present, but are not primarily a specific attention problem: rather, they are at risk for a variety of changes including working memory problems, spatial skills and delays of language development; motor coordination is often poor. The variety of cognitive problems is often, but not necessarily, reflected in a low IQ.
- Overactivity without inattention seems to show a lower heritability than the other forms of ADHD; conduct problems are more likely to develop than in the purely inattentive form.
- Many referred children present with both: mixed type.

A second form of heterogeneity is in the contextual expression: whether it is predominantly at home or at school.

- School-predominant problems tend to appear later, only after school entry, and to be associated with academic problems such as specific disorders of reading.

• Home-predominant problems show fewer cognitive difficulties of any type and are more likely to be linked to family adversity.

Epidemiology

Prevalence rates

Several studies converge on a point prevalence for hyperkinetic disorder of about 1.5% in the primary school age population – which is the age at which the problem is most likely to be referred for specialist attention. In the UK, the rates are similar in studies stemming from the 1970s and 1990s – a period during which the recognition of the disorder has changed greatly. The administrative prevalence – the rate at which the disorders are in practice recognized – varies vary greatly between different European countries, from approximately zero to nearly 0.5 per cent.

Attention deficit without hyperactivity has received less research attention, but is troublesome for something like another 1 per cent of the school-age population.

The prevalence of the broader category of ADHD is, obviously, higher. The estimates vary from about 4 per cent to 19 per cent but the usual figures adopted are those of the DSM IV estimates of 3–5 per cent. The exact figures found in studies probably depend more upon the cut-off that is chosen than in any major differences between populations. Hyperactive behaviour is distributed continuously in the population, and the exact cut-off taken is somewhat arbitrary. In some populations – for instance, the Chinese population in Hong Kong – careful diagnostic measures have suggested that there may be a lower prevalence of disorder than in Europe. Interestingly, however, the apparent prevalence taken from rating scales was higher in Hong Kong than in western populations – illustrating the extent to which the disorder is socially defined and influenced by the concern that adults feel for these behaviours in different cultural settings.

Sex ratios

Studies in the general population have suggested that hyperactive behaviour is commoner in boys than in girls, with a ratio of about 2.5 to 1. In clinical populations, however, the sex ratio is much greater and figures of 4 to 1 are common in ADHD clinics, with some reporting sex ratios as high as 9 to 1. It seems probable that girls have some protection against the development of hyperkinetic disorders, but that, when disorders do develop, girls are less likely than boys to be referred for help.

Implications for clinical practice

The key implication is that the rates of disorder – even of the severe form of hyperkinetic disorder – are much higher than the figures for the disorders that are recognized in practice. There is a large reservoir of unmet need.

Clinical picture

Main features and symptoms

- Inattentiveness refers to a set of behaviours, not to the psychological processes that are indexed by tests of attention. The difference is fundamental, but sometimes forgotten: it is not possible to diagnose inattentive behaviour by cognitive tests, and the cognitive deficits that are seen in inattentive children often have little to do with the processes recognized by experimental psychologists as 'attention'. Several behaviours are involved, which may have different origins and different consequences.

- Forgetfulness often refers to the breaking off of a complex train of activities before it is completed.

- A lack of close attention to detail is also prominent: their productions in school are slapdash and their completion of the ordinary tasks of life is incomplete and neglectful.

- Distractibility is often described, indicating that the children are orienting to many features of the environment that are not regarded as task-relevant by adults. They make many changes of activity in a defined time. This orienting can be a personal style rather than incapacity, and indeed experimental analyses of test performance have suggested that irrelevant information does not worsen the performance of hyperactive children any more than would be the case for non-hyperactive children.

- Overactivity refers to an excess of movements, especially in situations that expect calm. The best way to identify a child with restless overactivity is not on the football field: in situations expecting high activity, a child with hyperkinetic disorder will not stand out from other children in this respect. (They may well stand out for other reasons, such as the disorganization and diffuseness of their activity.) Rather, situations such as the classroom, family visits or mealtimes – when children can ordinarily modulate their activity to a calmer level – will distinguish the hyperactive child from others. Excessive movement can still be detected even when the child is asleep. It seems to follow that overactivity cannot be reduced to inattentiveness or lack of compliance, but is a cardinal feature in its own right.

- 'Impulsiveness' means acting without reflecting. The exact behaviours that constitute this style vary a good deal. Both ICD10 and DSM-IV emphasize behaviour changes seen in the classroom. In this context, impulsive children may be acting out of turn, interrupting other children and blurting out an answer before the question is finished or understood. In relationships with peers, they may be thoughtless and insensitive to the feelings of others, they may intrude their own ideas about how a game should be played upon others, and they may neglect the usual practice of observing the activities of others before joining them. In the family, impulsive behaviours often involve thoughtless rule breaking. They appear as oppositional, not because they are deliberately defying rules, but because they are following their own concerns heedless of the household. Quarrels with other children in the house, and frequent tempers when thwarted, can also be testimony to the over-rapid decision making of impulsive children. Outside the home, they may get into dangerous situations, or into trouble with authorities, because of thoughtlessness. They are accident prone, and often frequent attenders in accident and emergency departments. They are sometimes in trouble because they have been the 'fall guys' for a group of offending children.

All these problems are sometimes shown by perfectly normal children. It is the extent, severity, and consistency of the behaviours in individual children that lead to their diagnostic identification. Clinical recognition therefore needs to be based upon experience of what is expected of children at different ages and at different developmental levels. Inexperienced parents or teachers may wrongly identify ordinary childish high spirits as evidence of hyperactive behaviour.

Subjectively, children with hyperactivity do not usually describe their problems in these terms. Occasionally, an older or more intelligent child may have recognized that 'my thoughts are in a muddle' or 'I can't keep myself still'. More commonly, however, the children's perception of the world is of one in which they are in trouble for most of the time but do not understand why. They are often the recipients of aggression from other children – sometimes in retaliation for previous events which the subject has forgotten. Measurements of family atmosphere have indicated that children with hyperkinetic disorder often live in a family atmosphere of hostility and criticism. The atmosphere may have been initiated by the child's actions, but once it has developed, it has its own influence upon later psychological development.

Differential diagnosis and co-morbidity

Most children with hyperkinetic disorder show evidence of other problems too (see Box 17.1). It is important to recognize them, because they may determine the course, indicate possible reasons for the development of hyperactivity, and call for treatment. They are seldom exactly 'co-morbid', in the sense of representing the presence of a different disease with a different aetiology; rather, they should usually be seen either as risk factors for the development of hyperactivity or as the result of the operation of risk factors similar to those that gave rise to the hyperkinetic disorder. 'ADHD' and 'hyperkinetic disorder' are descriptive categories, not explanatory, so the presence of a known cause does not mean that ADHD is absent. A child with a specific cause for behavioural problems – such as fragile-X or gross neglect – should still be recognized as showing ADHD. The causative problems are on a different diagnostic axis.

> ### Box 17.1. Problems often coexisting with hyperkinetic disorders
>
> Oppositional and conduct disorders
> Autism spectrum disorders
> Emotional disturbances (anxiety and depression)
> Bipolar disorder
> Tics and Tourette disorder
> Attachment disorders
> Psychosocial adversity
> Other medical illnesses
> Mental retardation
> Specific learning disorders
> Developmental coordination disorders

Other forms of disruptive behaviour

Clinicians need to distinguish between a child who has arrived at an anti-social adjustment because of hyperkinetic disorder and one who has followed different pathways into an anti-social adjustment. Oppositional and conduct disorders are very commonly co-morbid with hyperactivity; when this is the case, then the hyperactivity has usually come first and can be considered as the initiating problem. Other children, however, develop oppositional and conduct disorders without evidence of hyperactivity at all. Such children are frequently free of neurocognitive disabilities, and their onset of problems is later. The key aspect of differential diagnosis is the recognition of the presence or absence of inattentive and impulsive behaviour. The anti-social behaviour that is found in non-hyperactive conduct disorder is often motivated by emotions of protest, anger or despair; it is often associated with serious adversities in the psychological environment – rejection at home, over-authoritarian discipline or an inability to adjust to the social and learning demands of the school situation.

Autism spectrum disorders

Hyperkinetic disorder can co-exist with features of autism. There are several possible reasons.
- The first, and commonest, is that both behavioural patterns are present independently, but share an aetiological factor – such as a diffuse brain disorder.
- The second is that a child with autism may present a rather different pattern of overactivity – one in which motoric restlessness is associated with stereotypies and perseveration upon idiosyncratic concerns, rather than with the impulsive and frequently changing behaviours of hyperkinetic disorder. ICD-10 includes a

separate category of 'hyperkinetic disorder with stereotypies' to convey the flavour of this pattern, and to emphasize that it should be classified with the pervasive developmental disorders.

- Third, the overactivity may arise from complications of the autism: drugs that have been given for the treatment of the autism or related problems may give rise to adverse behavioural consequences.

The distinction between these different patterns calls for some diagnostic sophistication. The key element to establish is whether or not the classic symptoms of autistic disorders are present (see Gillberg, this volume). In clear-cut cases little difficulty arises, and the exclusion criteria built into ICD-10 mean that the diagnosis of autism receives priority. Many cases, however, are less well defined.

- The social difficulties of children with hyperkinetic disorder – isolation because of peer rejection, social incompetence because of not taking time to work out what is best to do – may masquerade as the more profound disability of children with autism. In such cases, it can be helpful to witness the social interactions of children at close hand. Children with hyperkinetic disorder only may be disinhibited in their manner, but they are not socially oblivious and their verbal understanding of social interactions (when they take sufficient time to think about them), is not necessarily impaired.

- The attention problems of children with hyperkinetic disorder can sometimes result in perseveration. They may become occupied with repetitive activities in a way that can give rise to suspicions of autism. In the pure hyperkinetic disorder, however, the preoccupations are not unsociable, they are not bizarre, and they frequently take the form of changing and exciting activities – for example, playing video games for hours on end. This perseveration is not a sign of good concentration; but it may well be present without the bizarre and preoccupied qualities of the play of autistic children.

- Language problems can be present in hyperkinetic as well as in autistic children, but will usually take a different form. The commonest communication difficulties in hyperkinesis are those of an expressive semantic type of language disorder. If a hyperactive child shows a receptive language disorder as well then this should give grounds for serious consideration of the possibility of autism.

Autism can be overlooked in children with hyperactivity, and may be unmasked when medication is successful in treating the hyperactivity. The chaotic and disorganized style of hyperkinesis may make it harder for the diagnostician to discern the more specific abnormalities of autistic communicative impairment.

When typical patterns of hyperkinetic disorder and autism are both present, then (pace ICD-10) it is clinically most convenient to regard them as co-existing disorders. The response to medication supports this – the prescription of stimulant medication may well have a dual effect in improving hyperactivity yet worsening autistic preoccupations.

Anxiety and depression

The agitation of anxious or depressed children may make them overactive, and their preoccupation with worries may make them appear inattentive in the classroom. Nevertheless, the distinction between the two can usually be made by the presence or the absence of disorganized and impulsive traits of behaviour anxiety and hyperactivity. Both problems may be present together, and it may then be difficult to disentangle which has taken priority: whether the adverse circumstances that the child's hyperactivity has produced is making the child worried and unhappy about this life situation; whether the apparent hyperactivity is a manifestation of anxiety; or whether there are risk factors in common such as major psychosocial stress. The anamnaestic account of life history is often most helpful in determining which problem has come first. When emotional problems and hyperactivity are present together, then treatment often requires nice judgements and specialist management is indicated. Adverse reactions by other people at home or at school may need to be detected and put right. Stimulant medication is not contraindicated in the presence of depression, but it can induce a depressed state and a second-line drug may need to be substituted. In the presence of anxiety, stimulants are less effective in routine practice; but the MTA study (see below) indicated that very carefully crafted medication with detailed monitoring of dosage could indeed be superior to intensive psychosocial therapy.

Bipolar disorder

The symptoms of overactivity, distractibility and impulsively unwise behaviour are characteristic of mania as well as of hyperactivity. A full manic picture can indeed be seen in childhood, though it is not common. The distinction is usually fairly simple: mania, rather than hyperactivity, is suggested by an episodic course and by an affect of elation and grandiosity. A family history of bipolar disorder can be a hint in the same direction, but should not be overinterpreted, because a parent with bipolar disorder may have been inaccessible to the child and thus contribute to states of inattentiveness and demanding behaviour through an environmental route.

Some authorities have advocated a great broadening of the category of mania in childhood, but this is not generally accepted. The relaxation of criteria increases cases by allowing in people with a continuous (rather than episodic) course, and with a mood of irritability rather than euphoria; and by including brief episodes of emotional upset rather than persistent mood changes over several weeks. This probably leads to a confusion with the volatile and rapidly changing mood states that are an integral part of the altered self-regulation found in many hyperactive children. When a child with hyperkinetic disorder becomes persistently depressed, then the reasons for it (notably, emotional stresses) should be sought with even higher priority than the exhibition of mood stabilizers.

Tourette disorder

Hyperactive behaviour is a common association of Tourette disorder (TD) (See Rothenberger, this volume). Clinical opinion, and scientific evidence, vary about the reason for this association. Family studies are conflicting about whether the linkage between the two is attributable to common genetic influences. Clinically, the salient features of hyperactive behaviour in children with TD are often the impulsiveness and restlessness, rather than inattention and disorganization. Neuropsychologically, test results have suggested that there may be cognitive differences between the two disorders. The picture is complicated, because hyperactivity may be the initial presentation in a child whose TD will appear only later (and sometimes be misinterpreted as an adverse reaction to stimulants). It is quite possible to overlook TD in the initial presentation of hyperkinetic disorder. The tics are often not very salient and the pathognomonic features, such as vocal tics, may not yet have appeared.

Multiple and minor tics may be misinterpreted as the restlessness of ADHD, or as fidgetiness, if the repetitive quality of the tics is not appreciated. In cases of doubt, it can be valuable to videotape sequences of the child's behaviour. Review may well indicate the repetitiveness that is a hallmark of tics.

When both problems are present together, then it is usually best to make a dual diagnosis. The two aspects of the child's disorder will need separate planning, and the sometimes adverse effect of stimulants upon tics will lead to management problems that may well call for a specialist opinion.

Attachment disorders

The disinhibited behaviour that is seen in some forms of attachment disorder (see Wolkind, this volume) can resemble the overactive and unreserved quality of hyperkinetic disorder. The distinction lies in recognizing the early disruptions of parenting, the shallow and 'promiscuous' quality of social interaction, and the early history of clinging behaviour that characterize the disinhibited form of attachment disorder.

Medical disorders

A number of physical disorders affecting the brain can produce the symptoms of hyperkinetic disorder. Since hyperkinetic disorder is a behavioural rather than an explanatory category, these are not alternatives to the diagnosis; but problems that should be recognized on a separate axis. The commonest such problems detected in a clinic for hyperactive disorders have been: epilepsy, hearing disability, fetal alcohol syndrome, chromosomal disorders (including Fragile X), Williams syndrome, Sanfillipo syndrome (which may present with hyperactivity before other physical stigmata are obvious), lead intoxication and other diffuse disorders affecting the brain such as tuberous sclerosis.

Learning and motor disability

- General intellectual impairment, as evidenced by a low IQ, is often associated with hyperactive behaviour, especially the inattentive component. This is sometimes because insufficient allowance is made for the fact that a child with developmental delay will be functioning at a lower level of attentional ability and self-control than a child of greater maturity. There is no generally established doctrine about how to make this judgement. A useful clinical rule of thumb is to determine the probable mental age of the child, consider what would be expected, in the control of attention activity and impulse, for a normal child whose chronological age is equivalent to that mental age, and make judgements of abnormality accordingly.

- Specific learning disabilities can also be encountered. These can take many different forms and there is no unique pattern of psychological test disturbance. Problems of working memory and attention are so frequent in hyperkinetic disorder that they do not call for an alternative diagnosis, and they may be solely responsible for poor academic learning. They cannot, however, always be assumed to be the sole cause. Specific problems in reading, numerical ability, and the expression of thoughts on paper can also be found. A child with academic problems should therefore receive a psychologist's assessment with psychometric tests, because the educational interventions needed may be wider than the correction of attention and memory.

- Developmental coordination disorder is also very common, perhaps in as many as half of children with hyperkinetic disorder. Within groups of children with ADHD, motor problems may cluster together with symptoms of inattentiveness, and this has led some clinical researchers to propose a subdivision of ADHD, 'Deficits in attention, motor control and perception' (DAMP). It is possible that the underlying neurocognitive problems are similar to some of those found experimentally in ADHD – poor timing and poorly sustained response readiness could underlie both. However, until research clarifies whether a valid subtype is present, and what its relation is to motor problems in children without ADHD, the ICD-10 approach is to recognize developmental coordination disorder when it is present and to classify it on a different axis, of specific disturbances of development. This avoids the trap of incoordination being used as diagnostic evidence for the presence of hyperkinetic disorder. These motor problems, even if transient, may have a considerable impact on development by impairing socially valued activities such as sport.

Diagnostic instruments

Rating scales

A wide variety of parent and teacher rating scales is available. In general, instruments developed for the specific purpose of assessing ADHD are more accurate than general-purpose psychopathological instruments. The sensitivity and specificity of such instruments often appear to be very good yet the classification obtained can be inadequate. Measures such as Conners' rating scales show an effect size for hyperkinetic children, compared to normal controls, of around three standard deviations; and this probably corresponds roughly to a 95 per cent level of sensitivity and specificity.

While this sounds very impressive, it is not really good enough for clinical practice. The difference in base rates implies that non-hyperactive children, although they show a much lower rate of hyperactivity as detected by rating scales, will still be wrongly identified as ADHD so often that they will outnumber the true cases. Causes of false positives include raters without sufficient appreciation of the developmental norms for that age, raters who bring qualities of their relationship with the child to bear on making their rating of behaviour, and contrast effects in which children are implicitly rated against other members of the family, or other members of the sub-culture.

In short, rating scales should be seen as valuable in screening, in group studies in which children are identified for research purposes, and for following the course of treatment when the raters remain constant throughout. They are not suitable on their own for the diagnostic identification of an individual child: too much of the variance in their scores is associated with the rater and with the situation in which the behaviour is rated, rather than the child's behaviour *per se*. Box 17.2 (Suggested rating scales) lists some of the best-established.

Detailed clinical interview with the parent (or other caregiver) is the most valuable single measure. In this context it is possible to go, beyond the request for a rating of whether a child's impulsiveness is abnormal, to the descriptions of the behaviour on which that description is based. The interviewer can then apply a clinically informed judgement as to whether that level of behaviour is in fact abnormal for the child. Box 17.3 (Diagnostic psychiatric interviews) lists some research interviews that may be useful in detailed and specialist practice, but are all quite time-consuming.

Observations of the child's behaviour are especially valuable in younger children. It may be possible to witness directly the overactivity, the disinclination to wait and the choice of immediate rather than delayed gratification. These can often be seen directly in younger children, for example by setting up a waiting situation in which the children will have a larger reward if they refrain from grabbing an immediate one. By the time of school entry, however, much of this overt behaviour will be modified – at least in the artificial circumstances of clinic assessment. The novelty of the situation, the focused adult attention and the structured nature of the situation all militate against hyperactivity being readily observable. The diagnosis should therefore not be dismissed for the sole reason that the child appears

---

Box 17.2. Suggested rating scales

- The Conners' Teacher and Parent Rating Scales – Revised (Conners, C. K. (1997). Conners' Rating Scales: Revised Technical Manual. Multi Health systems, North Tonawanda, New York) provide several subscales related to hyperactivity, inattentiveness and other problems. They show reasonably high test-retest reliability ($r = 0.63$–0.71) and internal consistency and provide sex- and age-specific norms. Research supports the concurrent validity of the scales in separating groups of hyperactive and normal children.
- The Rutter A(2) Parent and B(2) Teacher Scales have been revised into the Strengths and Difficulties Questionnaire (Goodman, 1997) which provides not only a brief (5-item) hyperactivity scale but also an overall measure of deviance and of the impact of symptoms on functioning. Test-retest reliability for parents is 0.73 and for teachers 0.74.
- The ADHD Rating Scale (DuPaul, 1990) for parent or teachers, allows economical assessment of the 14 symptoms of the DSM-III-R criteria.
- A Child Attention Problems scale was developed by Edelbrock (Barkley, 1991), based on items selected from Achenbach's Child Behavior Check List, to assess medication effects. Normative data are available and the scale is quite sensitive to stimulant drug effects, but further psychometric data need to be investigated.
- A German language Inattention, Hyperactivity and Impulsivity Checklist for Parents and Teachers (IHI/PT-Checklist) is presented by Doepfner *et al.* (1997) Therapieprogramm fuer Kinder mit hyperkinetischen Stoerungen (THOP). Weinheim: Psychologie Verlags Union (German version).

---

well controlled during assessment. Nevertheless, when abnormality is seen, then clinical observation is invaluable for detecting its pattern, its antecedents, and its consequences. Box 17.4 (Direct observational measures) describes some formal schemes.

When there is doubt about the diagnosis after the initial clinical assessment of a child, then it may be necessary to make observations in naturalistic settings by a visit to the school or the home. These visits are expensive in professional time, but can demonstrate the presence and nature of key problems. The consequences of the diagnosis, such as long term medication, are so serious that it is worth considerable investment of time and effort to be clear about the initial formulation.

Clinical checklists can be scientifically valid ways of recording clinical assessments systematically; for example the reliability and factor structure of the Maudsley Hospital Item Sheet have been reported as robust. HYPESCHEME (Curran *et al.*, 2001) can be completed from standardized measures or from systematic clinical

Box 17.3. Diagnostic psychiatric interviews

Questionnaires are not sufficient for individual diagnosis; they rely upon the respondents' judgement of what level of symptomatology constitutes a problem and tend to overestimate behavioural problems. Structured interviewing of parents has the advantage over questionnaires that possible ambiguity over symptom content and severity may be overcome by establishing better rapport between the respondent's and the interviewer's concepts of disturbed behaviour. In addition they allow documentation of the context, age of onset and chronicity of the problems. Most interview schedules have been developed to assess a wide range of psychopathological symptoms, including behaviour disorders.

- The Diagnostic Interview Schedule for Children (DISC) is a highly structured interview eliciting scores on symptom scales and incorporating algorithms to operationalize DSM-IV criteria for the major child psychiatric categories (Shaffer, D., Fisher, P., Piacentini, J. *et al.* (1996). *Journal of the American Academy of Child and Adolescent Psychiatry*). Test–retest reliability is reasonably good, with correlations of 0.7 to 0.8. Criterion validity has been assessed; there is a moderately good prediction of clinical assessments by a psychiatrist.
- The Schedule for Affective Disorders and Schizophrenia for school-age children (K-SADS) samples questions covering DSM-IV diagnoses; it requires extensive training and familiarity with research diagnostic criteria if the interviewer is to combine information from both parent and child into one diagnostic rating (Ambrosini, P. J. (2000). Historical development and present status of the schedule for affective disorders and schizophrenia for school-age children (K-SADS). *Journal of the American Academy of Child Psychiatry*, **39** (1), 49–58).
- The Child and Adolescent Psychiatric Assessment (CAPA) (Angold, A. & Costello, E J. (2000). The Child and Adolescent Psychiatric Assessment (CAPA). *Journal of the American Academy of Child and Adolescent Psychiatry*, **39**, 39–48) is a semistructured and investigator-based interview, existing in a survey form and a clinical form, for both of which considerable investigator training is needed. It is lengthy to administer, but provides detailed and comprehensive assessment of most forms of psychopathology.
- The Parental Account of Children's Symptoms (PACS) (Taylor, E. A., Schachar, R., Thorley, G. *et al.* (1986). Conduct disorder and hyperactivity: I. Separation of hyperactivity and antisocial conduct in British child psychiatric patients. *British Journal of Psychiatry*, **149**, 760–7) centres mainly around the hyperkinetic syndrome. It is a standardized, investigator-based interview in which parents are asked, not for their ratings of problems, but for detailed descriptions of what their child has done in specified situations over the previous week. The interviewers are trained to make their own ratings on scales of frequency and

severity of behaviours in that week and over the past year. Scales of hyperactivity, defiance, and emotional disorder are derived. The internal consistency is satisfactory (Crohnbach's alpha = 0.89 for hyperactivity) and inter-rater reliability is around 0.9.

- A German-language interview (Clinical Interview for Attention Deficit and Disruptive Behaviour Disorders, CIAD) is provided by Doepfner *et al.* (Doepfner, M., Schuermann, S. & Froelich, K. (1997). Therapieprogramm für Kinder mit hyperkinetetischen Störungen (THOP). Weinhein: Psychologie Verlags Union (In German).

Box 17.4. Direct observational measures

Behavioural ratings can be obtained in children's natural settings. Various recording schemes have been developed for research purposes, and reviewed by Luk (1985). Some are based in classrooms such as the Schachar *et al.* (1986) classroom observation scheme. They are especially relevant for high-frequency behaviours such as hyperactivity and have been shown to discriminate between hyperactive and normal children. However, these measures are quite expensive to apply and coding systems have therefore been developed for use in laboratory settings, such as those by Luk *et al.* (1987) and Dienske *et al.* (1985), and Barkley's ADHD Behavior Coding System (Barkley, 1991). The Groeningen Behaviour Observation Scale is generally applicable, e.g. in laboratory situations (Kalverboer, 1990). All direct observational measures imply the limitation that they record behaviour over a very restricted time period, that may or may not be representative of the child's usual behaviour.

---

assessments using a provided glossary; and computer algorithms then generate ICD-10 and DSM-IV diagnoses.

Psychological tests should not be seen as diagnostic instruments. The diagnosis is behavioural, not cognitive; and a normal test performance does not exclude the diagnosis. Few children with hyperkinetic disorder obtain abnormal scores on all tests of attention; but most obtain an abnormal score on at least one. Knowledge of tests related to attention and impulse control is a useful resource in the analysis of the child's behaviour (see Box 17.5, Psychological tests). The mechanical application of a test 'battery' is not, however, recommended. Individual children show a wide range of profiles of strengths and weaknesses. A skilled psychologist, however, can use the tests to confirm or disconfirm hypotheses about the reasons for altered learning or altered behaviour in individual children, and suggest the targets for therapy or education.

Box 17.5

Psychological testing is described by Sergeant and Taylor (2002). Standardized psychological tests of intellectual abilities (such as the Wechsler Intelligence Scales or Screening Instrument) are usually needed to interpret more specific tests of cognitive function.

- Continuous Performance Tests are available commercially in automated form (e.g. Conners, 2000). They are rather nonspecific in that errors can arise from many types of impairment, such as reduced speed of processing, as well as impulsive responding; but analysis of different patterns of error may give useful insights.
- Many tests of executive function are available (Shallice, 1982, Welsh *et al.*, 1990). A widely used set of executive function tests is provided in the CANTAB system (Robbins *et al.*, 1998) and there are some normative data. Planning and organization abilitites are included in the Behavioural Assessment of Dysexecutive Syndrome (Wilson *et al.*, 1996).
- The Tests of Everyday Attention for Children (TEACH) (Robinson *et al.*) have been widely used in studies of children and present tests based on cognitive theory in an accessible form. Tests of the ability to inhibit responses – conceptually, an important aspect of the development of impulsiveness – are in the experimental literature as 'stop', 'go–no go' and 'delay' tests. A computerized test battery – The Maudsley Assessment of Response Suppression (MARS) (Rubia *et al.*, 2001) – presents them, together with tests of the impact of reward, in an automated form. Older, pencil-and-paper tests such as the Matching Familiar Figures Test (MFFT) (Cairns & Cammock, 1978) or the Stroop (Cohen & Servan-Schreiber, 1992) also operationalize aspects of inhibition and are more convenient for clinical practice.

Licensed in many countries
  Methylphenidate
    'Ritalin'
    'Equasym'
    'Ritalin-SR' (sustained release, wax matrix, flat profile through day)
    'Concerta' (phased release, pharmacokinetic profile rising through day)
  Dexamfetamine
    'Dexedrine'
Licensed in USA but few other places
  Other longer-acting stimulants
    'Adderall', 'Metadate', Atomoxetine
Not licensed, but some evidence from randomized clinical trials (RCTs)
  Imipramine
  Bupropion

Clonidine

Nicotine patches

Not licensed, no RCT, but some expert recommendation

Moclobemide

Guanfacine

Venlafaxine

Modafinil

Risperidone

Not recommended

Pemoline (liver toxicity); Desipramine (cardiac problems)

Assessment

Even after the diagnosis of hyperkinetic disorder has been established, there is much assessment still to do.

- The strengths and weaknesses of family life and atmosphere should be judged; and an evaluation obtained of the extent to which the schooling is in keeping with the child's abilities and dispositions.

- A neurological examination, with emphasis on sensory motor co-ordination, is valuable in establishing the presence or absence of co-morbid developmental co-ordination disorder; and in giving clues to any of the other physical problems (see above) that may give rise to the hyperkinetic disorder.

- Hearing should always be assessed: Auditory inattention is, not surprisingly, a marked feature of children with non-obvious hearing impairment.

- A psychometric evaluation is useful, and will provide a good yield of clues for the analysis of an individual child's predicament. However, qualified psychologists are in short supply in many parts of the world, and if this is the case then the time available for testing is best employed on those children where there are indeed problems of school adjustment. When psychologists are not available at all, then estimates of developmental level can be obtained by the account of others (e.g. from the Vineland Developmental Scales) and by the direct assessment of children using tools such as the Wechsler Screening Instrument, Raven's Progressive Matrices test, and picture vocabulary tests – which do not carry the absolute requirement that they must be administered by a trained psychologist.

- Chromosomal screens are often ordered, but the cost effectiveness of this procedure is limited by the relatively low yield. My own practice is to reserve this for children who show other developmental delays.

- Electro-encephalography is not required unless there is clinical suspicion of epilepsy or a degenerative disorder: it brings a high yield of non-specific immaturities, such as abnormalities of rhythm, but these do not clarify the cause or make useful predictions about treatment response or future course.

• Other neurological investigations, such as brain imaging, are not routinely indicated. There is research evidence for structural and functional abnormalities of the brain, but the abnormalities are subtle, and there is too much overlap with the normal population for them to be useful in the individual case. They are required only if the history or examination has suggested possibilities (for example, of progressive or acquired brain disease) that need to be investigated further.

Aetiology

Genetic influences are known to be strong. A succession of comparisons between monozygotic and dizygotic twins has indicated heritabilities in the region of 70 per cent to 90 per cent. This is a high level of genetic influence, but it falls short of demonstrating that it amounts to an inherited illness. In present knowledge, the genetic effects do not seem to be bringing about a specific disorder of either hyperkinesis or ADHD. Rather, the genes act across the whole range of hyperactivity in the population, including the minor levels that are not associated with impairment. What is inherited, therefore, appears to be a trait rather than an illness. Furthermore, different components of the symptom complex may have somewhat different genetic determinants. Heritability is higher for hyperactive behaviour when it is combined with inattentiveness; impulsive behaviour in children who can concentrate well may have stronger environmental influences. Hyperactive behaviours at home and at school are multiply determined: some genetic influences are associated with a tendency to hyperactive behaviour in both settings, some only with one.

The presence of strong genetic influences in no way implies that environmental influences do not matter. In many analyses of twin studies, the interaction between the environment and the genetic constitution comes out as a contribution to heritability so that subtler effects of the environment can be missed. The environment in which children live can be associated in several ways with the genetic effects.

• First, there can be a passive correlation between genes and environment: parents make the environment of the child as well as transmitting their genes, so several aspects of the child's environment can be shaped by the continuing hyperactivity of the parents. Hyperactivity in the parents may contribute to making them antisocial; and it is known in other contexts that antisocial parents provide environments characterized by harsh and inconsistent reactions to children; and that these reactions are associated with the presence and persistence of antisocial behaviour in the children.

• Secondly, there may be an active (or evocative) correlation between the genes and the environment: the children alter the behaviour of the parents and consequently the environment in which they live. Good evidence of this comes from the effect of medication upon children in placebo-controlled trials; when medication reduces hyperactive behaviour in the children, then there is also a significant effect upon the expressed emotion shown by parents towards the children. Parental negativity and coercion are influenced by altering the child.

- The third way in which the environment may be important is through interactive effect with the genes: the expression of genes is different in different environments. In adoptive studies, for example, the risk for disruptive behaviour is increased if biological parents show a similar problem, and increased if adoptive parents do so; but the risk is greatly and disproportionately increased if both adoptive and biological parents show the same risk factors. The expression of the genetic endowment of the child is altered by the environment that is provided by the adoptive parents.

In counselling parents, therefore, it is not desirable to convey a crudely biological notion of a genetic illness whose manifestation has nothing to do with environmental influences. To the contrary, many environmental associations with ADHD are known, and need to be enquired about in a full assessment.

- In the pre-natal environment these associations include exposure to maternal alcohol drinking and cigarette smoking. Hyperactive behaviour is a common association of fetal alcohol syndrome, yet the presence of this risk factor is all too seldom detected even when it is there.
- Lead exposure, both in utero and in childhood is an association of hyperactive behaviour (which could be the result of a prior association with reduced IQ). Pre-natal exposure to certain drugs, including benzodiazepines and anti-convulsants, also predict later hyperactive behaviour.
- The role of birth trauma should not be exaggerated. Severe brain damage, usually of a kind causing neurological signs at the time, can cause organic syndromes including hyperactivity. In some very low birthweight children, malacic lesions in frontal lobes may be an antecedent of hyperactivity. In mild degrees of birth injury, however, one should be cautious about attributing hyperactive behaviour to an abnormal delivery. The association between birth weight and intelligence, for example, is present throughout the IQ range and not only when there is an abnormality. The association is likely to be mediated by other factors, such as social adversity and poor maternal (or grandmaternal) nutrition that contribute to both.
- In the early environment, major disruptions of attachment – such as those seen in children in depriving institutions – are a known association of hyperactive behaviour and are likely to be a causative influence. Brain injury at this time usually has diffuse rather than specific effects on mental development.
- Factors in the psychological environment can also be important in determining the course of children with hyperactivity. An antisocial outcome, for example, is more likely if children are rejected by their families, or their peers.

- Factors in children's diet may exert an influence on behaviour: probably not a direct toxic effect of certain foods (such as additives) on behaviour; but rather an idiosyncratic reaction of some children to certain foods. The commonest foods incriminated in double-blind trials have included wheat flour, cow's milk and citrus fruits and many other 'natural' substances as well as synthetic colourings and preservatives. Parents are often sophisticated about this, and indeed the one factor that predicts whether children will respond well to an elimination diet is whether the parents have already noticed a relationship between behaviour and specific foods. Most parents coming to clinics will already have experimented effectively. If there are clinical reasons for thinking that this approach can be taken further, then a dietician should be enlisted in the therapy. The most conclusive way of determining children's reactions is for them to adopt a *few food* diet for an assessment period, and add in, one at a time, the foods that are likely to be responsible.

The ways in which genetic and environmental factors can alter behaviour are being researched intensively: there are important clues, but few conclusions that are stable enough to yield useful counselling. Some of the specific changes in DNA are being identified. At the time of writing, two genetic variants – in the dopamine (4) receptor and the dopamine transporter molecules – have been robustly associated with ADHD. Even so, some competent studies have failed to find their presence: a likely explanation is that there is heterogeneity within the population. Meta-analysis has indicated that both these DNA changes are associated with ADHD at a very high level of significance; but the effect size is small. It is doubtful whether either of the genes can account for as much as 5 per cent of the variance in hyperactivity. The clinician should remember, in giving advice, that most children with DNA variants do not have ADHD; and most children with ADHD do not have any of the known DNA variants.

Both of the known genes are in the dopamine system. This may well be because that is where investigators have looked, rather than because it is the only system to be involved. The known effects of stimulants in reducing hyperactivity and in altering dopamine transmission have directed investigators towards examining genes within that system as key candidates. It seems probable that a main action of the stimulants is the inhibition of the dopamine transporter, with the consequence of increasing the amount of dopamine that is present in the synaptic cleft, and therefore enhancing the signal that is carried from one nerve to another.

There is probably some anatomical as well as biochemical localization of the disorder in the brain. Structural studies using magnetic resonance imaging have agreed that the brain size is often reduced in children with hyperkinetic disorder, and that certain structures (especially those in the frontal lobes and striatum) are altered disproportionately. These structures are of particular importance because in normal individuals they are activated during the performance of tests that involve the inhibition of a response.

At the neuropsychological level of analysis children with hyperkinetic disorder have a variety of impairments of test performance. One of the most constant findings is that their reaction times are slow and variable. This may reflect their being unprepared for a response when the time comes to produce it. Other cognitive changes include lowered IQ, poor performance on executive function tests such as planning, reduced waiting for delayed rewards, reduced ability to stop a response once it has been initiated, or to produce a response only after a wait, reduction in shifting attention rapidly and effectively from one source of information to another, poor performance on tests involving careful and detailed scanning of pictures, and low scores on tests involving the detection of infrequently occurring stimuli. Nobody yet knows how far these abnormal test performances reflect incapacity or a motivational change in carrying out the tests. Few of them (except the slow and variable reaction times) are known to be genetically associated with hyperkinetic disorder or ADHD, and none are known to be specific to hyperkinetic disorder, in the sense that they fail to show abnormalities in all other disorders.

Treatment

Clinical management

There is a substantial evidence base about the treatment of children with severe levels of hyperactivity. Most of the trials have been carried out in children diagnosed as ADHD; but in many of the trials the requirements for pervasiveness of disorder and absence of co-morbid conditions will mean that children approximate to the hyperkinetic disorder subtype. It is securely established that stimulants, such as methylphenidate, dexamfetamine and pemoline, are more effective than placebo in reducing hyperactive behaviour; and also that behaviour therapy is more effective than contrast conditions such as waiting lists.

The application of this evidence base to individual children is not straightforward. The fact that hyperactive behaviour is continuously distributed in the population makes judgement necessary about what level should be present before treatment is given. The need for differential diagnosis means that several other possible disorders have to be borne in mind. The frequency of association with co-morbid conditions and with physical and psychological stresses implies that a specialist assessment is necessary. The simple recognition of ADHD does not call only or necessarily for medication. The assessment needs to be rich enough that other key problems should be detected if they are present. For this reason, good practice involves a specialist assessment before therapy is begun.

- Children are often brought reluctantly into the treatment setting. They know that something is going wrong, but they do not know what and are often inclined to weight the unfairness of their environment more strongly than their contribution to the way that others treat them. Nevertheless, it is important that they should understand and become willing and responsible collaborators in the treatment process. If, for example, medication is given coercively, then it is not likely that their compliance will be good enough, or extended for long enough, to modify the natural history of disorder. Responsive discussions with them are an important way of bringing this about.
- Parents will often come with strongly formed attitudes towards the problems of hyperkinetic disorder and its treatment, sometimes deriving from misleading information in public media. They may be over estimating the value of medication and disinclined to consider anything else; or fearful or even resentful of the possible role of medication in achieving social control of their children. If referral has been initiated by the school, then they may be reluctant attenders themselves. If they are coming with predominantly home-based problems, then the situation may well have escalated to a level where the family relationships have become poisoned.
- Schools are often involved in referrals, and their attitudes too will vary greatly. Some may have required the child and parents to attend as a condition of continued placement in that school. Others may be so suspicious of what are perceived as crassly biological attitudes in the medical profession that they may give misleadingly positive impressions of a child's development in order to avoid medication.

The public controversies over the disorder and its treatment may therefore have created an attitude towards therapy that will need modifying before therapy can proceed. Education and counselling about the disorder should be extended for as long as is needed. The combination of informative but succinct handouts with a chance for individual discussion and questioning is usually the most effective. For many parents, group discussions are useful in listening to contrasting attitudes and hearing others ask questions that they may be reluctant to ask themselves. All these procedures can also help in managing family guilt. For many parents, the ill-regulated behaviour of their children will have been perceived by them and others as a parenting failure. The opposite perception – that the condition is wholly genetic and physical – may come as a substantial relief. It is important, however, to avoid nihilism about non-physical treatments. There is much that can be done by families, teachers, and the children themselves that can modify the outcome.

Treatment algorithms

The initial phase, as outlined above, is one of education, building up a treatment alliance and consulting with interested parties such as schools. The main specific treatments – stimulant medication and behaviour therapy – can then be deployed in a way that is consonant with family attitudes and the severity of the child's predicament.

One large-scale trial in the USA – the MTA study – has focused on the comparison of the two kinds of treatment. Children were allocated randomly either to careful medication management, to intensive behaviourally oriented psychosocial therapy, to a combination of the two, or to a simple referral back to community agencies (which usually resulted in medication). The main conclusions were that careful medication is more powerful than behaviour treatment, and considerably more effective than routine medication in the community. There were many advantages in adding medication to behaviour therapy; but relatively few to adding behaviour therapy to medication. The superiority of careful medication to behaviour therapy was all the more striking in that the behaviour therapy provision was much more intensive and prolonged than could be achieved by any community service. Combined therapy had some benefits: for example, the control of aggressive behaviour at home, improving the overall sense of satisfaction of parents and achieving 'normalization' (the reduction of problems to a level where none was rated as more than minor). These improvements are real, but would probably not justify the very high costs of the full treatment package in this research-based form.

It does not follow that medication is always the first choice in treatment. Though behavioural therapy may be less effective, it is still helpful for many children. The costs of a short course of parent training are comparable to those of medication; the outcome may be somewhat less favourable in terms of symptom reduction, but has the advantage of carrying very little physical hazard.

A reanalysis of the MTA study has assessed whether its conclusions apply to hyperkinetic disorder. The answer is that they do: the superiority of medication to behaviour therapy is greater in hyperkinetic disorder than in other types of ADHD, and the effects of behaviour therapy appear to be less. Most children whose problems are severe enough to get a diagnosis of hyperkinetic disorder will need medication. Family attitudes should of course be respected; but if a trial of psychological treatment has not produced substantial improvement within a few weeks, then medication should be advised.

For children at lesser degrees of severity – those who show ADHD but not hyperkinetic disorder – the choice of initial therapy is more evenly balanced. In these milder cases there are options about which treatment to start with. Decisions will depend on the analysis of the individual child, the strengths and weaknesses of their school and classroom environment, the severity of disturbance of peer relationships, and the preferences of the families. It is quite reasonable to start with either therapy, in the knowledge that one will proceed to the other should the response be suboptimal.

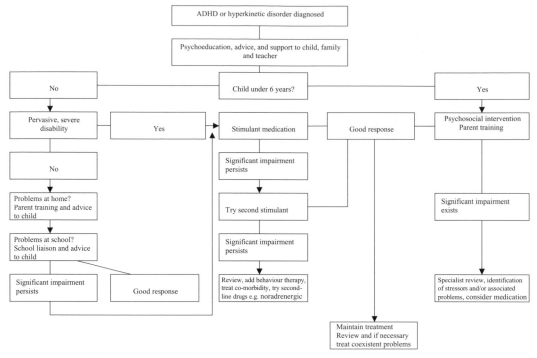

Fig. 17.1.   Initial treatment of children with activity/attention problems.

Children who show attention deficit without hyperactivity may also present suitable targets for stimulant medication. Research evidence is rather scanty but tends to favour the idea that stimulants are useful, often in lower doses than are required for the control of overactive and impulsive behaviour. Certainly inattentiveness is improved in children with mixed types of ADHD, and indeed poor scores on attention tests predict a good response to methylphenidate within mixed groups of children with ADHD. Care needs to be taken in the inattentive subgroup: first, that the degree of impairment is sufficient to justify the hazards of medication; and, second, that the inattentiveness is indeed a specific problem and not just an expected part of a more global pattern of mental retardation.

The need to have a second line of therapy for some children should particularly be stressed when behaviour therapy has been chosen as the first option. It is not rational to prolong any kind of psychological therapy in the face of suboptimal improvements and there should not be undue delay in proceeding to medication for those children whose behaviour is still holding back their development in school, and their social relationships. Figure 17.1 illustrates the treatment algorithm that embodies these principles.

Psychological interventions

The principles of behavioural intervention do not differ greatly from those used in therapy of other behavioural problems in childhood. As ever, the emphasis should be on the identification of specifically and operationally described problems; on the analysis of the contingencies that affect them; on the enhancement of adult attending to the child; and on the teaching to adults of techniques of effective instruction. Parent training approaches are relevant and group as well as individual approaches are sensible. However, trials of behaviour therapy for oppositional problems suggest that severe levels of hyperactive behaviour tend to predict a poor outcome, so some specific aspects of therapy deserve emphasis. Very rapid contingencies need to be applied. Children with hyperkinetic disorder can be seen as inhabiting a brief time perspective: the consequences of their actions do not have much impact if they are delayed. The children are often the recipients rather than the instigators of violence from other children – but other children's rejection of them may well be based upon provocative behaviour that happened sufficiently long before that the child with hyperactivity has forgotten it.

Several consequences follow.

- There is a particular need for speed in the delivery of rewards or response cost. Parents, for example, may need to make much more use of timers – so that after a set period, in which the target has been met, the bell rings and a reward such as a token is administered within a few seconds.

- There needs to be particular attention to explaining to the child which of their behaviours has earned the reward, or loss of reward.

- Rewards may lose their effect rather quickly. Star charts may work well for a couple of weeks but then fade. This is perhaps to be expected from the psychological findings, and indeed from findings in animals with hypodopaminergic states. Rewards need to be novel. From the beginning of a conditioning programme, rewards should be varied from time to time, and some novelty should always be present in the system.

- The use of self-management and self-instruction strategies have particular importance in hyperkinetic children. Their frequent failure to understand the relationship between their actions and the way that other people treat them means that verbal links need to be made, at first passively (in explaining to them) and later on more actively – by encouraging them to verbalize and to write down the reasons for cooperating with the programme and the targets they are setting for themselves. Trials have indicated that cognitive therapy alone is not a good way of treating hyperactivity in the short term; but experience suggests that in the long term the active engagement of the child in therapy makes a great difference to whether it will in fact be effective.

- In the classroom, token economies and backup with rapid and changing rewards are just as relevant as in the home. Several other suggestions in classroom management can be made with backing from the nature of impulsiveness and from small-scale clinical trials. The classroom organization should ensure proximity of the child to the teacher. It is all too easy, and very common, for a hyperactive child to be segregated from others at the back of the classroom. The result of this is likely to be an increase in disruptive and inattentive behaviour. In experimental psychological investigations, as well as in real life, the involvement of an adult can diminish or remove the impairments of psychological test performance.
- Transitions between activities in the classroom are also an opportunity for good management. It is at these times that hyperactive children are particularly likely to lose the thread of activity, to wander into different activities, and to become disruptive. If they change with the rest of the class, then the attendant disruption will make them more confused. If they move activities after the rest of the class, then the interregnum between activities can allow them time to misbehave and start a vicious cycle of confrontation. It is best practice for the target child to move individually to a new activity before the rest of the class, after which the others catch up. Classrooms may also need to modify their organization to allow hyperactive children to learn in short chunks and to let off their energy from time to time. This may mean some creativeness in organization: for instance they may be used as messengers and errand runners.
- A classroom aide (an unqualified person who can give individual attention to the child) is a common provision. This can be helpful, but usually only if the activity of the aide is focused. If their involvement is confined to restraining the child from misbehaviour, then they will quickly be perceived as an unwelcome and stigmatizing intrusion. It is however feasible for them to learn simple techniques of behaviour therapy, especially the administration of a token economy, and they can be very helpful in offering advice on what is productive and unproductive in making relationships with other children. These kinds of interventions, to be effective, need to be given rapidly and in naturalistic settings; so the advice of a school worker may be more useful than a formal social skills group in an artificial setting.

Appendix 17.1 (Some useful treatment manuals) lists suggested resources for exporting interventions to natural settings.

Pharmacotherapy

Central nervous stimulants, such as methylphenidate and dexamfetamine are the most generally applicable of all drugs in the treatment of hyperkinetic disorder. Both of these drugs, in spite of neuropharmacological differences, have similar effects on the behaviour of children; they reduce hyperactive behaviour, they enhance performance on several kinds of psychological tests, and they increase task attentiveness. Other helpful effects probably depend upon the level to which hyperactivity is reduced: relationships with other children are improved, family relationships become marked by greater acceptance and less hostility, and productivity in school work rises.

Box 17.7 (Available drugs) illustrates the range of drugs that are used. Initial medication should be as a trial, and methylphenidate is usually the first choice. The treatment should be discussed and explained before it is started; and in the early stages of treatment the family (and preferably the teacher) will need a quick and ready access to the prescriber to report progress and any adverse effects. The effect lasts only for a few hours: Three daily doses are recommended, but practical considerations may dictate a twice daily regime. The dosage should begin at a low level (0.2 mg per kilogram per dose) and be increased in the light of response. The *dosage* should be increased until either a good result is achieved, or adverse effects appear, or a ceiling of 0.7 mg per kilogram per dose is achieved – whichever comes first. If titration of methylphenidate does not produce a good response, then dexamfetamine (dose is half that of methylphenidate) should be given.

Longer-acting preparations of methylphenidate may also be used from the start of therapy. They are somewhat more expensive, but carry many advantages if the effect is long enough to make additional doses at school unnecessary. This makes the treatment more private, avoids stigma at school, and therefore improves compliance. From the school's point of view, it is hard to overstate the advantage that comes if dispensing a controlled medication is no longer on the list of school responsibilities. OROS-methylphenidate (Concerta) is the only such preparation to be widely available outside North America at present; an initial dose of 18 mg daily can be increased at intervals of 1 week up to 54 mg daily. If it is not effective, then immediate-release methylphenidate should be tried in repeated doses, titrated according to the response.

Monitoring should be carried out using rating scales of behaviours, (such as the abbreviated Conners' scale), completed regularly and systematically in different settings. When a therapeutic response is achieved, or when it is apparent that the treatment is not being effective then the child should be reviewed in person at the clinic. The reason for this is that some adverse effects – such as lack of spontaneity, depression and excessive perseveration – may not be adequately reported and need to be detected by personal observation. Physical monitoring should include plotting height and weight along standardized growth curves and examining the child in case any tics have appeared. The commonest adverse effects, usually elicited by questioning, are: insomnia, appetite disturbance, stomach aches, headaches and sensation of dizziness. Most of these adverse effects are dose related and transient and can be managed symptomatically.

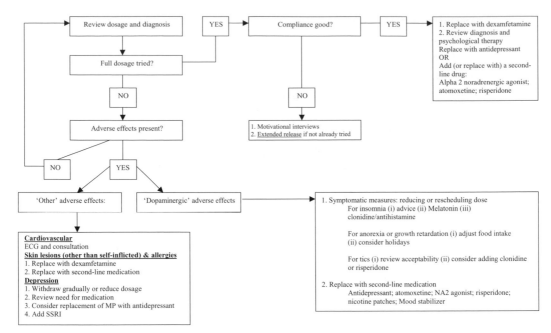

Fig. 17.2.   Treatment for ADHD refractory to methylphenidate.

- Insomnia has often been present before medication; sleep hygiene and behavioural approaches should be employed. It should be remembered that, while methylphenidate is capable of producing sleeplessness, it can also reduce insomnia, by easing children's transitions into sleep. Both reducing the dose and giving a later dose can be tried as a response to sleep difficulties.
- Poor growth in height or weight can occur and is probably due to appetite suppression. The child may need an altered balance of food during the day, with encouragement to a good breakfast (before the medication has taken effect) and permission for 'grazing' in the evenings – which parents often resist, but can result in an adequate food intake being maintained. Insomnia is sometimes due to hunger so food should be accessible to the child in the evenings. Reduction of dosage may be necessary to maintain eating. When a growth problem is a serious difficulty, then a 6-week holiday from the drug usually allows a catch-up growth. If it does, the holidays can be repeated; if it does not, then physical examination is needed in case growth failure has a different cause.

A lack of response to stimulant medication may stem from many causes and management is summarized in Fig. 17.2.

- The commonest reason is probably a failure to take the medicine. Children often find it unwelcome and stigmatizing. Adolescents often experience it as coercion by adult authority. Both issues are best tackled by developing the young person into an intelligent user. Education should be directed to the child at least as much as to family and school. If the prescriber listens to their concerns and adjusts medication accordingly, then the patient can become a partner in therapy. It is sometimes useful to get them to involve a trusted adult or friend to help in self-monitoring. Lack of insight is characteristic, and can lead to children underestimating the impact of medication.

- Another reason for non-compliance – unwelcome comments and attention from teachers and peers – can often be avoided by using an extended release preparation to avoid the need for repeated day-time doses. When adverse effects have led to limited compliance, then symptomatic management (see above) or dose reduction will usually suffice. When it does not, then second line drugs are indicated.

- One common mistake is to abandon stimulants prematurely in favour of second-line drugs. Some children need doses at the bottom of the range, some at the top, and fine-tuning dosage with monitoring by rating scales will increase the response rate. Only after this process should one judge that the disorder is refractory to stimulants. Full review is then indicated.

- It may be that further knowledge of the case will lead to recognition of another problem, such as pervasive developmental disorder or Tourette disorder; or a co-morbid condition such as an anxiety disorder. If so, then more selective drugs without dopaminergic actions are a logical choice. Anti-depressants such as imipramine or bupropion have reasonable trial evidence for superiority to placebo; and others such as venlafaxine and moclobemide have anecdotal evidence in support. Even more selective drugs may be able to control ADHD without adverse effects. Guanfacine, an alpha2 noradrenergic agonist, has been valuable in open trials. Atomoxetine, a selective inhibitor of the pre-synaptic noradrenaline transporter, has sound trial evidence and is licensed for both children and adults in the USA.

- Mood stabilizers such as valproate should be considered when a bi-polar element is present. Neuroleptic drugs can also reduce hyperactivity, probably through different mechanisms. Haloperidol is the best studied neuroleptic in controlled trials, but it is unacceptably toxic. Risperidone seems to be the most valuable in practice. Its metabolic effects, however, mean that it should be a drug of late resort. It is used most often for the combination of gross overactivity with aggression, and especially with children in the spectrum of autism.

The trial evidence so far has not given a rationale for how long therapy should continue. When drugs are needed, they are usually needed over a period of several years. Indeed, it is all too common for teenagers to stop medication prematurely and suffer deterioration in social and academic function as a result. In the absence of accepted consensus, individual trials should be carried out. Periodically – perhaps every 2 years – drug treatment should be gradually discontinued and functioning assessed after being off medication for two weeks. If problems return, the drug should be reinstated. I do not, however, routinely recommend holidays from or weekends off medication. In general, the purpose of such holidays is only to assess response or manage growth suppression (see above). Sometimes, however, families will prefer to use the medication only to cover schooldays. This can be sensible and cautious, but should alert the prescriber to a possible adverse effect of medication such as depression, social withdrawal or the suppression of spontaneity.

Outcome

In the follow-up of clinically referred samples, it is clear that hyperactivity can be highly persistent over time and can impair development. Several studies have followed clinically diagnosed school children with attention deficit-hyperactivity disorders over periods of 4 to 14 years; all have found that they show, by comparison with normal controls, a much higher rate of disruptive behaviour disorders at follow-up.

The risk is not only present for people referred to clinics. Longitudinal population studies have shown that hyperactive behaviour is a risk for several kinds of adolescent maladjustment. However, the degree of hyperactivity is not the only risk in children with ADHD; and therefore the reduction of hyperactivity should not be the only therapeutic goal. Indeed, it seems that the risk of ADHD is not only, or even most importantly, for adult ADHD, but for a range of problems in social adjustment. Lack of friends, work and constructive leisure activities are prominent in the adolescent outcome. Antisocial activities, including diagnosable conduct disorder, and motor accidents are also a worrying outcome; worrying, because they indicate that not only the person with ADHD but also the people around and the whole of society are the losers.

Management is long term. It is often complicated by co-morbidity and the presence of similar problems in caring relatives. All these impose a considerable challenge to service organization. The immediate challenge to clinicians is to achieve results as good as those in the best practice of research studies. The longer-term challenge is to develop the psychosocial and physical therapies that will allow a higher proportion of affected children to reach a good adult adjustment.

SUGGESTED READING

P. Hill & E. Taylor, An auditable protocol for attention deficit/hyperactivity disorder. *Archives of Diseases in Childhood*, **84** (2001), 404–9.

MTA, A 14-month randomized clinical trial of treatment strategies for attention-deficit/hyperactivity disorder. The MTA Cooperative Group. Multimodal Treatment Study of Children with ADHD. *Archives of General Psychiatry*, **56** (1999), 1073–86.

R. Schachar & R. Tannock, Syndromes of hyperactivity and attention deficit. *Child and Adolescent Psychiatry: Modern Approaches*, 4th edn (Oxford: Blackwell Publishing, 2002), pp. 399–418.

J. M. Swanson, J. A. Sergeant, E. Taylor, E. J. S. Sonuga-Barke, P. J. Jensen & D. P. Cantwell, Attention-deficit hyperactivity disorder and hyperkinetic disorder. *The Lancet*, **351** (9100) (1998), 429–33.

E. Taylor, Developmental neuropsychopatology of attention deficit and impulsiveness. *Development and Psychopathology*, **11** (1999), 607–28.

E. Taylor, J. Sergeant, M. Doepfner *et al.*, Clinical guidelines for hyperkinetic disorder. *European Child and Adolescent Psychiatry*, **7** (1998), 184–200.

Appendix. Assessment instruments

Questionnaires

Appendix 17.1.

Some useful treatment manuals

R. A. Barkley, *Defiant Children. A Clinician's Manual for Parent Training.* (New York: Guilford, 1987).

M. A. Bash & B. W. Camp, *Think Aloud. Classroom Program Grades 3–4.* (Champaign, Ill.: Research Press, 1985).

L. Braswell & M. L. Bloomquist, *Cognitive Behavioral Therapy with ADHD Children.* (New York: Guilford, 1991).

M. Dopfner, S. Schurmann & J. Frolich, *Das Therapieprogramm fur Kinder mit hyperkinetischem und oppositionellem Problemverhalten (THOP).* (Weinheim: Psychologie-Verlags-Union, 1996).

G. J. DuPaul & G. Stoner, *ADHD in the Schools. Assessment and Intervention Strategies.* (New York: Guilford, 1994).

P. C. Kendall & L. Braswell, *Cognitive-Behavioral Therapy for Impulsive Children.* (New York: Guilford, 1985).

G. W. Lauth & P. F. Schlottke, *Training mit aufmerksamkeitsgestorten Kindern.* (Weinheim: Psychologie Verlagsunion, 1993).

A. L. Robin & S. L. Foster, *Negotiating Parent–Adolescent Conflict.* (New York: Guilford, 1989).

J. Swanson, *School-based Assessments and Interventions for ADD Students.* (Irvine: K.C. Publishing, 1992).

Appendix 17.2. References for assessment measures

Questionnaires

Clinical Checklist for Hyperkinetic Disorders/ADHD (CCHD)

M. Doepfner, S. Schuermann & J. Froelich, *Therapieprogramm für Kinder mit hyperkinetischen Störungen (THOP).* (Weinheim: Psychologie Verlags Union (German version), 1997).

Conners' rating scales

C. K. Conners, *Conners' Rating Scales: Revised Technical Manual.* (New York: Multi-Health Systems, 1997).

Home situations questionnaire

R. A. Barkley, Attention-deficit Hyperactivity Disorder. A Clinical Workbook. (New York: Guilford Press, 1991).

Inattention, hyperactivity and impulsivity checklist for adolescents (IHI/A-Checklist)

M. Doepfner, S. Schuermann & J. Froelich, *Therapieprogramm für Kinder mit hyperkinetischen Störungen (THOP).* (Weinheim: Psychologie Verlags Union (German version), 1997).

Inattention, hyperactivity and impulsivity checklist for parents and teachers (IHI/PT-Checklist):

M. Doepfner, S. Schuermann & J. Froelich, *Therapieprogramm für Kinder mit hyperkinetischen Störungen (THOP).* (Weinheim: Psychologie Verlags Union (German version), 1997).

Interviews

Clinical interview for attention deficit and disruptive behaviour disorders (CIAD)

M. Doepfner, S. Schuermann & J. Froelich, *Therapieprogramm für Kinder mit hyperkinetischen Störungen (THOP).* (Weinheim: Psychologie Verlags Union (German version), 1997).

Diagnostic interview schedule for children–parent interview (DISC-P)

D. Shaffer, P. Fisher & M. K. Dulcan, The NIMH Diagnostic Interview Schedule for Children Version 2.3 (DISC-2.3): description, acceptability, prevalence rates, and performance in the MECA Study. Methods for the epidemiology of child and adolescent mental disorders study. *Journal of the American Academy of Child and Adolescent Psychiatry*, **35** (1996), 865–77.

Parental account of children's symptoms (PACS)

E. A. Taylor, R. Schachar, G. Thorley & M. Wieselberg, Conduct disorder and hyperactivity: I. Seperation of hyperactivity and antisocial conduct in British child psychiatric patients. *British Journal of Psychiatry*, **149** (1986), 760–7.

Observations

Observation in the clinic

S.-L. Luk, G. Thorley & E. Taylor, Gross overactivity: a study by direct observation. *Journal of Psychopathology and Behavioral Assessment*, **9** (1987), 173–82.

Groeningen behaviour observation scale

A. F. Kalverboer (ed.), *Developmental Biopsychology.* (Ann Arbor: University of Michigan Press, 1990).

Neuropsychological assessment

Continuous performance tests (CPT)

C. K. Conners, *Conners Continuous Performance Test II*. (Hurstpierpoint, UK: International Psychology Services, 2000).

Matching familiar figures test (MFFT)

E. Cairns & T. Cammock, Development of a more reliable version of the matching familiar figures test. *Developmental Psychology*, **11** (1978), 244–8.

Stroop

J. D. Cohen & D. Servan-Schreiber, *Psychological Review*, **99** (1992), 45–77.

TEACH (Test of everyday attention for children)

T. Manly, V. Anderson, I. Nimmo-Smith, A. Turner, P. Watson & I. H. Robertson, The differential assessment of children's attention: the Test of Everyday Attention for Children (TEA-Ch), normative sample and ADHD performance. *Journal of Child Psychology and Psychiatry*, **42** (2001), 1065–81.

Tower of Hanoi

M. C. Welsh, S. Pennington, Ozonoff, B. Rouse & E. R. B. McCabe (1990), *Child Development*, **61** (1990), 1697–713.

Tower of London

T. Shallice, *Philosophical Transactions of the Royal Society of London, Biology*, **298**, 199–209.

Wisconsin Card Sort Test

D. Grant & E. Berg, *The Wisconsin Card Sort Test: Directions for Administration and Scoring*. (Odessa: Psychological Assessment Resources, 1948).

18

Conduct disorders

Stephen Scott

Department of Child and Adolescent Psychiatry, Institute of Psychiatry, London, UK

Introduction

Conduct disorder is the commonest psychiatric disorder of childhood across the world, and the commonest reason for referral to child and adolescent mental health services. Unlike most disorders, it is entirely defined in terms of the individual's relationship with other people and society. There is a persistent pattern of antisocial behaviour whereby the individual repeatedly breaks social rules and carries out aggressive acts that disturb other people. This persistent tendency typically starts young – aged 2–4 years – and carries on until at least middle age. Thus a substantial proportion of children and adolescents with conduct disorder grow up to be antisocial adults, leading impoverished and destructive lifestyles; a significant minority will develop antisocial personality disorder (psychopathy). The personal impact and cost to society is high, since many domains of living are affected, and many professionals and agencies get involved in managing the sequelae. These include police and the criminal justice system, teachers and the educational system, social workers and housing agencies, and unemployment and benefit payment offices.

Two paradoxes are apparent in society's response to affected individuals. First, despite overwhelming evidence that this is a lifelong affliction, the moment an individual wakes up on the morning of their 18th birthday, they no longer have a psychiatric problem (there is no category of conduct disorder in adulthood). Instead, they are frequently just seen as a nuisance and bad, or sometimes even plain evil. Secondly, despite the wide array of public organizations affected, and the enormous economic cost to them, few agencies other than mental health services have systematic, proven remedies. Health services do not have a strong financial interest in investing in effective services for conduct disorder (and often don't), since they do not have to bear the brunt of the later long-term cost. This chapter

A Clinician's Handbook of Child and Adolescent Psychiatry, ed. Christopher Gillberg,
Richard Harrington and Hans-Christoph Steinhausen. Published by Cambridge University Press.
© Cambridge University Press 2005.

aims to show how to assess affected children, how to implement effective remedies, and what characteristics a preventive programme should have.

Classification

The ICD-10 classification has an overall category for conduct disorders, F91. As will be seen, it is divided into oppositional defiant disorder which mainly affects younger children, and conduct disorder which affects older children and teenagers. They are both variants of antisocial behaviour, so many clinicians call both conduct disorder. The ICD-10 Clinical Descriptions and Diagnostic Guidelines state:

> Examples of the behaviours on which the diagnosis is based include the following: excessive levels of fighting or bullying; cruelty to animals or other people; severe destructiveness to property; firesetting; stealing; repeated lying; truancy from school and running away from home; unusually frequent and severe temper tantrums; defiant provocative behaviour; and persistent severe disobedience. Any one of these categories, if marked, is sufficient for the diagnosis, but isolated dissocial acts are not.

An enduring pattern of behaviour should be present, but no time frame is given and there is no impairment or impact criterion stated.

The ICD-10 Diagnostic Criteria for Research differ, giving more detail which is useful to tighten up case definition in studies, but can be over-restrictive in clinical practice, as discussed below. The research criteria require symptoms to have been present for at least 6 months, and the introductory rubric indicates that impact upon others (in terms of violation of their basic rights), but not impairment of the child, should contribute to the diagnosis. The research criteria take a menu-driven approach whereby a certain number of symptoms have to be present. Fifteen behaviours are listed to consider for the diagnosis of conduct disorder, which usually but not exclusively apply to older children and teenagers. They are shown in Table 18.1.

Where there are sufficient symptoms of a co-morbid disorder to meet diagnostic criteria, the ICD-10 system discourages the application of a second diagnosis, and instead offers a single, combined category. There are two major kinds: mixed disorders of conduct and emotions, of which Depressive Conduct Disorder (F92.0) is the best researched; and Hyperkinetic Conduct Disorder (F90.1). There is only modest evidence to suggest these combined conditions may differ somewhat from their constituent elements.

The DSM-IV system follows the ICD-10 research criteria very closely and does not have separate clinical guidelines. The same 15 behaviours are given for the diagnosis of Conduct Disorder 312.8, with almost identical wording. As for ICD-10, 3 symptoms need to be present for diagnosis. Severity, and childhood or adolescent onset are specified in the same way. However, unlike ICD-10, there

Table 18.1. ICD-10 research diagnostic criteria for conduct disorder

Symptoms must have been present for at least 6 months, and impact upon others (in terms of violation of their basic rights), but not impairment of the child, can contribute to the diagnosis. Three Symptoms from this list have to be present, one for at least 6 months. Fifteen behaviours are listed, and can be grouped into four classes.

Aggression to people and animals
- often lies or breaks promises to obtain goods or favours or to avoid obligations
- frequently initiates physical fights (this does not include fights with siblings)
- has used a weapon that can cause serious physical harm to others (e.g. bat, brick, broken bottle, knife, gun)
- often stays out after dark despite parenting prohibition (beginning before 13 years of age)
- exhibits physical cruelty to other people (e.g. ties up, cuts or burns a victim)
- exhibits physical cruelty to animals;

Destruction of property
- deliberately destroys the property of others (other than by fire-setting)
- deliberately sets fires with a risk or intention of causing serious damage

Deceitfulness or theft
- steals objects of non-trivial value without confronting the victim, either within the home or outside (e.g. shoplifting, burglary, forgery)

Serious violations of rules
- is frequently truant from school, beginning before 13 years of age
- has run away from parental or parental surrogate home at least twice or has run away once for more than a single night (this does not include leaving to avoid physical or sexual abuse)
- commits a crime involving confrontation with the victim (including purse-snatching extortion, mugging)
- forces another person into sexual activity
- frequently bullies others (e.g. deliberate infliction of pain or hurt, including persistent intimidation, tormenting, or molestation)
- breaks into someone else's house, building or car.

There are three subtypes: conduct disorder confined to the family context (F91.0), unsocialized conduct disorder (F91.1, where the young person has no friends and is rejected by peers), and socialized conduct disorder (F91.2, where peer relationships are normal). It is recommended that age of onset be specified, with childhood onset type manifesting before age 10, and adolescent onset type after. Severity should be categorized as mild, moderate, or *severe* according to number of symptoms *or* impact on others, e.g. causing severe physical injury; vandalism; theft.

is no division into socialized/unsocialized, or family context only types, and there *is* a requirement for the behaviour to cause clinically significant impairment in social or academic functioning. Co-morbidity in DSM-IV is handled by giving as many separate diagnoses as necessary, rather than by having single, combined categories.

Table 18.2. ICD-10 research criteria for oppositional-defiant type of conduct disorder

To make a diagnosis of the oppositional-defiant type of conduct disorder (F91.3), four symptoms from *either* this list of eight symptoms *or* the 'main' conduct disorder 15-symptom list (see Table 18.1) have to be present, but no more than two from the latter. Unlike the 'main' variant, there is an impairment criterion: the symptoms must be amaladaptive and inconsistent with the developmental level (p161).

- has unusually frequent or severe temper tantrums for his or her developmental level
- often argues with adults
- often actively refuses adults' requests or defies rules
- often, apparently deliberately, does things that annoy other people
- often blames others for his or her own mistakes or misbehaviour
- is often 'touchy' or easily annoyed by others
- is often angry or resentful
- is often spiteful or vindictive

In DSM-IV, Oppositional Defiant Disorder is classified as a separate disorder on its own, and not as a subtype of conduct disorder. Diagnosis requires four symptoms from a list of eight behaviours which are the same as for ICD-10 (see Table 18.2), but unlike ICD-10, all four have to be from the oppositional list, and none may come from the main conduct disorder list. It is doubtful whether oppositional defiant disorder differs substantially from conduct disorder in older children in any associated characteristics, and the value of designating it as a separate disorder is arguable. In this article, the term conduct disorder will henceforth be used as it is in ICD-10, to refer to all variants; oppositional defiant disorder is included in this as a specific subtype.

Clinical applicability

In general, the clinical applicability of both ICD-10 and DSM-IV schemes is high. Making a diagnosis of conduct disorder is usually straightforward since parents readily volunteer the symptoms, although it is essential to obtain an independent report from school so as not to overlook behaviour in that context. Sometimes the diagnosis may be inappropriate since antisocial behaviour may arise as part of other disorders such as autism or mania, or not be severe enough to warrant a diagnosis. More commonly the diagnosis is correct but co-morbid conditions are missed. When using the ICD-10 clinical guidelines there are few cases one sees whom one feels ought to have the diagnosis but do not fit criteria, and vice versa few whom one feels do not have a problem but who meet criteria.

However, when using ICD-10 research criteria, or the very similar regular DSM-IV criteria, there is a problem because adolescent girls with significant problems can easily miss a diagnosis. Thus a teenager who is out all night with a criminal gang, taking narcotic drugs, highly sexually promiscuous and consequently pregnant and HIV positive, and repeatedly committing credit card fraud would nonetheless not qualify for a diagnosis of conduct disorder using ICD research criteria or DSM-IV. She would only meet two criteria (staying out against parental wishes, fraud), not three; she would, however, meet ICD 10 clinical guideline criteria. Too many of the ICD research and DSM criteria (see table 19.1) are typically carried out by boys only, e.g. forcing someone to have sex, using a weapon, breaking into a house. Such biased criteria can disadvantage disturbed girls by excluding them from research on causes and treatment.

Likewise with oppositional defiant disorder, the research criteria may be too tight to include a child who easily meets clinical criteria, and would benefit from treatment. Consider, for example, a 6-year old who hits other children every day until they bleed, is so aggressive and disobedient in class that he has been expelled from school, but seems not to be in control of himself. He only meets three ICD research or DSM criteria (argues with adults, easily annoyed, often angry) and so misses a diagnosis for which four are required; he easily meets clinical guideline criteria.

Epidemiology

Prevalence

The prevalence of oppositional-defiant type of conduct disorder in pre-school children has been found to be from 4 to 9 per cent. In school age children, oppositional–defiant type disorder is found in 6–12 per cent, whereas the more severe main conduct disorder type is less frequent, occurring in 2–4 per cent. In adolescents the rate of oppositional disorders has been rated as being as high as 15 per cent, and that of full conduct disorder 6–12 per cent. When including an impairment criterion, the British Office of National Statistics survey in 2000 found an overall prevalence of 5 per cent for all conduct disorders after interviewing 10 000 children and young people.

Early and adolescent onset patterns

There are major differences between early and adolescent onset. Those with an early onset display defiant and aggressive behaviour before the age of 8, but it typically begins around 3 years of age. They go on to accrue increasingly antisocial behaviours as they grow older. However, not all young children with this early onset pattern of problems progress to more severe difficulties later in childhood. Only about half persist; the remainder improve. Compared to the adolescent onset group, the early onset children already at 3 show a more difficult temperament (restlessness, inattention, negativity, irritability, etc.). At school age this group have cognitive, language and motor deficits, reading difficulties, adverse family contexts and poor parenting. By 18 they have fewer friends and feel socially alienated, victimized, and are callous and suspicious. They continue behaving antisocially as adults. This pattern of antisocial behaviour has been described as early onset-lifetime persistent.

Commoner by about 3 to 1 are the adolescent onset group who have not shown significant antisocial behaviour earlier in their lives. Moreover, by their early 20s they have reduced their level of antisocial behaviour to less than half the level of the early onset group. This group has been described as adolescence limited, although they may not completely stop in adulthood – further studies will answer this. The overall rate of arrests and convictions is somewhat lower than the childhood onset type, there are more girls (about 2:1 instead of 4:1 for childhood onset). Their behaviour tends to be less aggressive and violent, less impulsive, they have fewer cognitive and neuropsychological deficits, tend to come from less dysfunctional family environments, and tend to have more adaptive social qualities. Crucially, the adolescent onset group are more likely to stop offending in early adulthood than the early onset group. There is only a small group of individuals who commence persistent antisocial activity in adulthood, less than 10 per cent of the total.

Changes over time

There have not been surveys in the same locations using the same methods in different decades to say reliably whether conduct disorder is becoming commoner. However, there is better information about officially reported crime and self-reported criminal acts. Whilst crime reflects only one subset of antisocial behaviours, there is a strong overlap with adolescent conduct disorder as it covers non-aggressive acts such as theft, drug taking, and deception, and aggressive acts such as fighting and mugging. From 1945 to 1985 crimes committed by all ages increased greatly in Western and industrialized countries, by factor of over 20 (Spain and Canada), 10–15 (Sweden and Norway), and 1–6 (Australia, England, France, Germany, Italy, the USA). All the available evidence suggests that the juvenile component has risen in a similar way. Specific studies of conduct disorder across cohorts also suggest a rise over the last 40 years.

Gender

Conduct disorder is commoner in boys at all ages, but the ratio of boys to girls depends on the type. In childhood, for oppositionality, boys outnumber girls by around 4 to one. In adolescence the ratio narrows to around 2 to one. However, for DSM IV conduct disorder, which includes several violent offences, the ratio is up to 10 to one. Definitions that include abuse of drugs and precocious sexual activity show a greater proportion of girls.

Socioeconomic status

Conduct disorder is three to four times commoner in children who are in socio-economically deprived families with low income, or who receive state benefits or welfare, or who live in a poor neighbourhood. Each of these indices overlap considerably, and is a marker for many of the aetiological factors discussed below.

Area

Rates found in surveys carried out in westernized countries such as Britain, the USA, France, New Zealand, and Canada have found very similar rates when comparable methods have been used. Surveys in other locations such as Hong Kong and South America have found lower prevalences. Within countries, many but not all studies have found increased rates in urban compared to rural locations.

Implications for clinical practice

The epidemiological findings lead to a number of implications for organizing a clinical service. The high prevalence and high cost to society mean that planning for effective and accessible services should be notably cost effective. This, in turn, means that health planners need to get other agencies such as justice, education and social services to join in providing services. This then carries the implication that senior psychiatrists and psychologists should be spending as much time training up others to provide effective assessment and treatment, as they do in providing it directly themselves. Currently, in Europe and the USA, only 15–25 per cent children and adolescents with conduct disorder receive specialist help. This proportion is the lowest for any child psychiatric disorder – for example in contrast nearly 100 per cent of psychotic adolescents are seen by a specialist.

The preponderance in disadvantaged social groups means that services need to be easily accessible and attractive to those living in the areas under stressful conditions. Studies show that, to get good attendance and low dropout, several practical measures help, such as transport subsidies, child care for younger siblings during appointments, evening appointments and good quality refreshments. Providing non-stigmatizing services also increases uptake, for example by holding parent training classes in schools or community centres, or delivering them through health visitors or community nurses.

Clinical picture

Main features and symptoms

The type of behaviour seen will depend on the age and gender of the individual.

Younger children, say from 3 to 7 years of age, usually present with:

- general defiance of adults' wishes
- disobedience of instructions
- angry outbursts with temper tantrums
- physical aggression to people especially siblings and peers
- destruction of property
- arguing
- blaming others for things that have gone wrong and
- a tendency to annoy and provoke others.

In middle childhood, say from 8 to 11, the above features are often present but as the child grows older, stronger, and spends more time out of the home, other behaviours are seen. They include:

- swearing
- lying about what they have been doing
- stealing of others' belongings outside the home
- persistent breaking of rules, physical fights
- bullying of other children
- cruelty to animals and
- setting of fires.

In adolescence, say from 12 to 17, more antisocial behaviours are often added:

- cruelty and hurting of other people
- assault
- robbery using force
- vandalism
- breaking and entering houses
- stealing from cars
- driving and taking away cars without permission
- running away from home
- truanting from school
- extensive use of narcotic drugs.

Girls are less likely to be physically aggressive and engage in criminal behaviour, but more likely to show non-physical antisocial behaviours. These include:

- spitefulness
- emotional bullying (such as excluding children from groups, spreading rumours so others are rejected by their peers)
- frequent unprotected sex leading to sexually transmitted diseases and pregnancy
- drug abuse
- running away from home and
- truancy from school.

For boys and girls, no single behaviour carries special significance. The outlook is determined by the frequency and intensity of antisocial behaviours, the variety of types, the number of settings in which they occur, and their persistence. The main settings where antisocial behaviour in children and adolescents is manifested are home, school and in public. For general populations of children, agreement about the presence of antisocial behaviour at home and at school is low – the correlation between parent and teacher ratings on the same measures is only 0.2 to 0.3. There are many children who are perceived to be mildly or moderately antisocial at home but well behaved at school, and vice versa. However, for more severe antisocial behaviour, there are usually manifestations both at home and at school. Concerns about antisocial behaviour in public occur more commonly in adolescents and often lead to police involvement.

The duration of symptoms is another important consideration. Many children go through phases of becoming more defiant and argumentative for a few weeks or months. Sometimes, this may be a reaction to a change in circumstances such as settling into a new school, adjusting to a new step-parent, or losing a friend or loved one. Only when difficult behaviour has been present for say 6 months or more is it likely to indicate substantial problems.

The impact of enduring problems may however be substantial. At home the child often is subject to high levels of criticism and hostility, and sometimes made a scapegoat for a catalogue of family misfortunes. Frequent punishments and physical abuse are not uncommon. The whole family atmosphere is often soured and siblings also affected. Maternal depression is often present, and families who are unable to cope may, as a last resort, give up the child to be cared for by the local authority. At school, teachers may take a range of measures to attempt to control the child and protect the other pupils, including sending the child out of the class, sometimes culminating in permanent exclusion from the school. This may lead to reduced opportunity to learn subjects on the curriculum and poor examination results. The child typically has few if any friends, who get fed up with their aggressive behaviour. This often leads to exclusion from many group activities, games and trips, so restricting the child's quality of life and experiences.

On leaving school, the lack of social skills, low level of qualifications and presence of a police record make it harder to gain employment. The experience of rejection and failure at home, at school and with peers usually leads to a negative self-image and low self-esteem, but is not usually described by the young person as actively distressing. In later adolescence, intimate sexual relationships tend to be made with other young people who are also antisocial, and are frequently disruptive and violent.

Differential diagnosis

Here it is necessary to distinguish between the conditions listed below that are not conduct disorder but that may mimic it (differential diagnosis) and conditions that are discussed under assessment that may co-occur, but that do not rule out the diagnosis (co-morbidity). The differential diagnosis includes the following.

Hyperkinetic syndrome/Attention deficit hyperactivity disorder

These are the names given by ICD-10 and DSM-IV, respectively, for similar conditions. For convenience the term hyperactivity will be used here. The condition is characterized by impulsivity, inattention and motor overactivity. Any of these three sets of symptoms can be misconstrued as antisocial, particularly impulsivity which is also present in conduct disorder. However, none of the symptoms of conduct disorder is a part of hyperactivity, so excluding conduct disorder should not be difficult. A frequently made error, however, is to miss co-morbid hyperactivity when conduct disorder is definitely present. So much emphasis is placed on the irritating antisocial behaviour by parents and teachers that the clinician can easily fail to enquire properly about motor restless and inattention, which can be attributed to 'naughtiness'; if present, the diagnosis of hyperkinetic conduct disorder should be made.

Adjustment reaction to an external stressor, with or without post-traumatic stress disorder

This can be diagnosed when onset occurs soon after exposure to an identifiable psychosocial stressor such as divorce, bereavement, trauma, abuse or adoption. The onset should be within 1 month for ICD-10, and 3 months for DSM-IV, and symptoms should not persist for more than 6 months after the cessation of the stress or its sequelae. Post-traumatic stress disorder should also be considered and may present as part of the picture following persecution or abuse.

Affective disorders

Depression can present with irritability and oppositional symptoms but unlike typical conduct disorder mood is usually clearly low and in adolescence there may be vegetative features; also more severe conduct problems are absent. Early manic depressive disorder can be harder to distinguish, as there is often considerable defiance and irritability combined with disregard for rules, and behaviour which violates the rights of others. Sometimes, the mania only becomes obvious years later, but in retrospect was clearly driving the antisocial conduct. The greater risk, however, is to miss depressive symptoms in young people with definite conduct disorder. Low self-esteem is the norm in conduct disorder, as is a lack of friends or constructive pastimes. Therefore, it is easy to overlook more pronounced depressive symptoms, particularly as they are usually not complained of by the young person. If present, a diagnosis of depressive conduct disorder should be made. Systematic surveys reveal that around a third of children with conduct disorder have depressive or other emotional symptoms severe enough to warrant a diagnosis.

Autistic spectrum disorders

These are often accompanied by marked tantrums or destructiveness, which may be the reason for seeking a referral. Enquiring about other symptoms of autistic spectrum disorders should reveal their presence. With the increasing recognition of Asperger's syndrome and similar traits short of full-blown autism, a significant minority of children with conduct symptoms are proving to have more or less subtle deficits in social understanding.

Dissocial/antisocial personality disorder

In ICD-10 it is suggested a person should be 17 or older before dissocial personality is considered. Since at age 18 most diagnoses specific to childhood and adolescence no longer apply, in practice there is seldom difficulty. In DSM-IV conduct disorder can be diagnosed over 18 so there is potential overlap. A difference in emphasis is the severity and pervasiveness of the symptoms of those with personality disorder, whereby all the individual's relationships are affected by the behaviour pattern, and the individual's beliefs about his antisocial behaviour are characterized by callousness and lack of remorse.

Subcultural deviance

Some youths are antisocial and commit crimes but are not particularly aggressive or defiant. They are well adjusted within a deviant peer culture that approves of recreational drug use, shoplifting, etc. In some localities a third or more teenage males fit this description and would meet ICD-10 diagnostic guidelines for socialized conduct disorder. Some clinicians are unhappy to label such a large proportion of the population with a psychiatric disorder. Using DSM-IV criteria would preclude the diagnosis for most youths like this due to the requirement for significant impairment.

Diagnostic instruments

Standardized questionnaires and interviews are seldom necessary to make the diagnosis, which is usually straightforward. They can be very helpful, however, in detecting comorbidity. For example, the Strengths and Difficulties Questionnaire (SDQ) is brief, and just as effective at detecting hyperactivity as much longer alternatives; it should be filled in by both the teacher and the parent, and the young person if over 11 years old (the SDQ is reproduced in Appendix 18.1).

Assessment

Co-morbidity

In addition to characterizing the nature of the conduct disorder, the history and examination need to consider commonly occurring co-morbid conditions:

depression and hyperactivity as discussed above. Brain disorders and schizophrenia may also lead to conduct disorder, but their other features should be elicitable. Specific and general learning disabilites are common, and require psychometric testing as discussed below.

History

A thorough history should be taken from the parent. A detailed account of a typical school-day in the week and a weekend day is often revealing. Particular areas to enquire about include:

- the precise antecedents of the main behaviour complained of, and the response of all concerned
- the difference between the referred child and his siblings, so that one can try to answer why this particular child is affected
- the reaction of the parents to the child's antisocial behaviour: do they use sensible strategies consistently, or are they unduly harsh and erratic?
- the extent to which normal pleasant shared activities occur, such as playing games together, talking enjoyably at mealtimes – they have often ceased
- which behaviours the parents praise the child for – specific examples should be elicited – there may be few or none
- what the child is good at – what possible sources of self-esteem are there to build on, such as being good at football, knowledge of wild animals, etc.
- what are the parents' beliefs about the child and why they behave this way – do they, for example, believe it is due to genetic or brain factors, or to some traumatic event?
- whether either parent was conduct disordered as a child, or has been criminal or alcoholic
- the quality of the child's friendships, including any bullying
- questioning the father if he attends should be approached with a view to understanding and sympathizing with his experience – it is all too easy to 'take sides' with the mother when she appears to bear the brunt of the problem; this may lead to the father dropping out of sessions
- speaking with a sibling on their own is almost always useful. It may confirm the story and reveal gross favouritism, or reveal abusive punishments ('then Dad hits him with the brush'); or turn up unexpected or dubious characters ('he's sent to sleep at "Uncle Jack's" on Thursdays').

Observation of parent–child interaction

This is invaluable. This can be done when the family are seen together at the initial stage of the consultation. More will be revealed if the parent and child are also asked to play together for 10 minutes with an interactive toy; with adolescents, they can be invited to discuss a 'hot' topic with their parents such as keeping the bedroom tidy, coming home on time, etc.

Dimensions to look for in the parent include attachment-related behaviours such as:

- warmth
- ability to detect and respond sensitively to the child's cues and needs
- mutual enjoyment of the joint activity
- use of language that labels and acknowledges the child's emotional state ('you're frustrated by that puzzle').

ability to set limits as shown by:

- clear commands that spell out the desired behaviour ('keep the sand in the box' as opposed to 'don't be messy')
- following through with immediate consequences if not obeyed (taking the bucket from the child since they are still spilling sand)
- specific praise for compliance ('well done, for careful, tidy work with the sand')
- calm, non-abusive discipline strategies.

ability to promote positive aspects of child behaviour and character seen through:

- commenting positively on desired behaviours such as constructive play, calmly stated opinions, child's showing understanding of another person's point of view
- facilitation of a practical task such as building a model, or facilitation of expressing a point of view in a discussion
- helping the child solve a problem in a non-intrusive way that respects and promotes the child's autonomy. Dimensions to look for in the child include enjoyment, speed to get angry, affection demonstrated towards parent, sadness or withdrawal, self-confidence in activity or discussion.

Mental state examination

The child should always be seen on their own for at least 20 minutes. Mental state examination may reveal some evasiveness about the difficult behaviour, but appreciation of the child's strengths and demonstration of understanding, by the interviewer can go a long way in building trust. Many children will then reveal considerable sadness and sometimes frank depression; in that case asking the child to fill in a Child Depression Inventory or similar instrument is helpful in assessment and as a baseline for treatment. Asking about activities at home often reveals a barren life with few positive experiences. Interests and activities should be searched for so that these can be developed as part of the treatment plan. Relationships with siblings and friends may be poor, with the child feeling unloved in comparison to brothers and sisters. Children should always be asked about how parents punish them – some frankly abusive practices may be revealed.

Physical examination should be carried out, looking for dysmorphic features, usually most evident in the face and hands. In our clinic about 5 per cent of children with conduct disorder have clear dysmorphic features, although only half of these fit into a named syndrome; when they do, the child may exhibit typical features of the behavioural phenotype. Neurological examination may reveal clumsiness or dyspraxia in up to 20 per cent, which often responds to training from occupational therapists. The child's height and weight percentiles should always be recorded; failing growth that is reversed by being taken into public care may prove to be crucial evidence of neglect or abuse in court proceedings. Head circumference measurement may reveal previously undetected microcephaly. No medical tests are usually necessary, although chromosomal examination should be undertaken if dysmorphic features are found.

Cognitive assessment with a short form of an IQ test (such as the Wechsler Intelligence Scale for Children) and a reading test (such as the Wechsler Objective Reading Dimensions) is desirable if academic performance is subaverage. Fully a third of children with conduct disorder also have specific reading retardation, defined as having a reading level two standard deviations below that predicted by the person's IQ. While this may in part be due to lack of adequate schooling, there is good evidence that the cognitive deficits often precede the behavioural problems. General learning disability (mental retardation) is often missed in children with conduct disorder unless IQ testing, is carried out. The rates of conduct disorder and challenging behaviours rise several-fold as IQ gets below 70; vice versa they are far less common in those with high IQs. During testing, the child can be observed for symptoms of hyperactivity and inattention. If present, and confirmed by school and home accounts, then this will confirm the hyperkinetic syndrome or ADHD; but if they are absent, this does not rule out the diagnosis at all, since many hyperkinetic children can do well during testing since it involves frequent presentation of novel stimuli and repeated specific feedback in a one-to-one situation.

Cognitive testing also can reveal that a child's approach to tasks would benefit from intervention, for example in organizing their written work. If the child's IQ is found to be below 70, medical investigations to screen for causes of generalized learning disability should be carried out, including chromosomal analysis with specific testing for fragile X, biochemical tests for inborn errors of metabolism, thyroid function tests, blood lead levels, syphilis serology and HIV if indicated. An MRI scan may pick up previously undetected brain pathology, so is probably worthwhile if feasible. Our own series of reviewing results of medical investigations in 500 children with generalized learning disability found that brain imaging uncovered significant specific structural changes in 20 per cent.

A report from the school followed by a phone call or visit is essential. The letter requesting the report should ask for information about behaviour in school, academic performance, strategies that have been found to help, peer relationships and parental involvement; a questionnaire such as the SDQ should be filled in by the class teacher. An example of the SDQ is given in Appendix 18.1. Observation of the child in class may reveal marked motor overactivity and inattention, few social skills, or/and unresponsive, critical teaching style; observation in the playground may reveal social isolation or bullying.

Formulation

Finally, the information gathered from the history, examination, investigations and observations should be synthesized into a clear formulation. This should emphasize the child's story and viewpoint over the lifespan (it is easy to underplay this due to the strong emotions and irritation aroused in carers), identify predisposing, precipitating and perpetuating factors for the problem, and protective strengths that can be built on in the treatment plan. The formulation can be an exciting high point of the assessment where differing explanations for what has happened are considered and the current best hypothesis to explain the information is worked out. Taking 15 minutes to step back and write down a formulation over and above an account of the information gathered is time very well spent, and can help ensure major features of the story are not overlooked at the next visit.

Aetiology

As for any psychiatric disorder, both genetic and environmental factors contribute. Whilst in the last 20 years genetic factors and non-shared (unique) environment have become recognized as major determinants for most disorders, for conduct disorder family style, particularly parenting, is much more of a major cause, together with temperamental factors including hyperactivity and IQ.

Genetics

Twin studies: conduct disorder clusters in families

Until the 1980s most twin studies of antisocial behaviour showed a high concordance for monozygotic pairs at around 70–80 per cent, but also high concordance for dizygotic pairs at around 60–70 per cent, suggesting a major shared familial influence, a moderate unique environmental contribution for the individual, and only a limited genetic component. However, the subjects were mostly in their late teens, when the adolescent onset type outnumber the early onset type by about 3 to 1. More recent twin studies with subtype conduct problems suggest that, in older adolescents with pure conduct problems, family environment indeed has the overwhelming effect, but in younger conduct disordered children with co-morbid hyperactivity and other problems, genetic influences predominate.

Adoption studies

French and American adoption studies show two to three times higher rates of criminality in adolescence in infants adopted into lower SES families. Danish and Swedish adoption studies have confirmed the effect of the SES on the rearing environment, but have also investigated the adoptee's genetic potential for antisocial behaviour, as indicated by the birth parent's criminality. These studies show a marked genetic effect as well as the environmental one. What appears to be particularly damaging is the combination of a genetic predisposition plus an adverse upbringing, which interact to give a high rate of antisocial activity. Adoption studies are likely to underplay the importance of adverse environments, since adoption agencies select out prospective adoptive families who are notably dysfunctional and disadvantaged.

Genetic influences play a stronger role in the development of adult antisocial personality and criminality than in adolescent antisocial behaviour, due in part to the greater proportion of early onset types in this group. Cytogenetic and molecular genetic studies have not yet identified specific conditions associated with antisocial behaviour, except for the XYY karyotype where affected individuals show about three times the rate of criminal behaviour than controls or individuals with other chromosomal anomalies such as XXY, even allowing for their reduced IQ.

Family environment

Parent-child interaction patterns

Fine-grained analysis by Patterson has shown that the moment-to-moment responses of parents towards children have a powerful effect on their behaviour, called the coercive parenting style. In families with a conduct disordered child, the children are likely to be ignored when they are behaving reasonably, but criticized and shouted at when they are misbehaving. The consequence is that, to gain attention, they have to behave badly. What is perhaps surprising is that, for these children who receive very little positive attention, they are prepared to elicit often unpleasant and frankly hostile reactions from their parents rather than be ignored. In contrast, children who receive a reasonable amount of positive attention within the family tend to avoid behaving in a way which elicits negative attention. All this can be summarized as the attention rule, which states that children will behave in whatever way necessary to gain a reasonable amount of attention.

Other behaviours by parents unwittingly can raise the probability of disruptive behaviour in the child. Giving up insisting something the child finds unpleasant is carried out (e.g. tidying up the toys) unintentionally rewards the child for whining and refusing to do it, thus making the behaviour more likely next time a request is made (negative reinforcement). Giving in to demands and tantrums for what the child wants has similar effects (positive reinforcement for negative behaviour).

Most emphasis in social learning theory has been on the harmful effect of negative behaviour. However, other research has made it clear that the presence of positive parental behaviour is equally important. Children with antisocial behaviour are ignored for a lot of the time by their parents, who do not respond to their overtures to join in activities, nor praise them when they are behaving well. Not only does this make quiet prosocial activity less likely, but also no models are provided for the child to learn social skills such as turn-taking, negotiating skills, etc.

The implications of the impact of the immediate interaction patterns on child antisocial behaviour are far-reaching. Rather than the child being seen as innately aggressive or with an antisocial type of personality which is unchangeable, he can be viewed as responding to the immediate context he is in. Therefore, changing the context offers the possibility of changing the behaviour of the child. This allows some therapeutic optimism if the response contingencies around the child can be altered, and has led to the development of effective treatments.

Parenting practices

CD is strongly associated with harsh, erratic discipline, hostility directed at the child, lack of warmth and poor supervision. Follow-up and intervention studies show that these factors have a causal role in initiating and maintaining the child's disorder, and are not only a reaction to the child's behaviour. However, there is also good evidence that children with conduct problems elicit harsh negative parenting; both processes are operative. In adolescence, supervision becomes a major factor, with parents of antisocial youths typically not knowing where they are for several hours in the day and at night. Discord between parents is also associated with persistent antisocial behaviour. The association of conduct disorder with large family size, and with broken homes (divorce, single parenthood, adoption) seems chiefly to be mediated by parenting practices and the previous characteristics of the individuals, rather than by the impact of a large family or broken home in themselves.

Psychiatric disorder in parents

Depression features commonly in mothers; alcoholism, drug abuse and psychoses are not infrequent in parents of children with severe conduct disorder. These disorders exert their effects in childhood through the quality of interaction and parenting practices, and by affecting the inherited characteristics of the child. There is no specific child psychiatric disorder which is commoner, but conduct problems are more frequent as are emotional disorders. Children of depressed mothers may have impaired cognitive and social development.

Criminality of father

As an environmental influence, this is important and may be mediated through parent–child interactions and parenting practices as described above, plus an anti-social set of values and living in a deprived neighbourhood. It also represents an increased genetic risk.

Physical and sexual abuse

Either can lead to the emergence of conduct problems in girls or boys who were previously free of such problems. Physical aggression from the father is associated with more than doubling of rates of conduct disorder and quadrupling of rates of antisocial personality disorder. Sexual and physical abuse are associated with a wide range of poor outcomes. The exact ascertainment of their effect is difficult since they are usually associated with multiple other risk factors such as poor parenting and rejection, as well as genetic predisposition.

Pre- and perinatal risk factors

These have no or an extremely weak influence on antisocial behaviour. There is more evidence that prenatal in utero exposure to alcohol and cocaine can impair brain development and lead to impulsivity and lower IQ, and hence antisocial behaviour.

Environment beyond the family

School

The quality of school organization has been shown to affect rates of antisocial behaviour independently of home background. Poorly organized, unfriendly schools with low staff morale, high staff turnover and poor contact with parents have higher rates of conduct disorder even when catchment area characteristics have been allowed for.

Peer influences

Conduct disorder is more likely in children who associate with friends who have an antisocial attitude, value aggression, and commit destructive and rule-breaking acts. Associating with deviant peers increases conduct problems independently of the individual's level of aggression. In adolescence, quite a lot of antisocial behaviour is carried out with peers, sometimes in gangs. Together, conduct-disordered youths laugh and approve talk about antisocial activities and do not respond to talk about ordinary topics, so reinforcing the values put on delinquent acts. If children are rejected by their peers, the chance of later conduct problems is increased. This seems to apply particularly to early-onset conduct disorder. Treatments that put antisocial youths together in groups should be avoided since they often increase the level of antisocial behaviour.

Alcohol and drugs

Many of the risk factors which lead to alcohol and drug abuse are similar to those for antisocial behaviour. However, the relationship is more than just a passive over-lap. Antisocial behaviour increases the chances of substance abuse, and vice versa. Longitudinal surveys show that antisocial behaviour in childhood and adolescence increase the risk of later alcohol and drug related problems, which peak in the 20s. ('Problems' refers to regular hard drug or heavy alcohol use, with psychosocial impairment or medical complications as a result. This differs from occasional or 'recreational' use of marijuana or hallucinogens, which is far more widespread, or alcohol use without impairment.) With alcohol, heavy drinking increases the chance of crime as it causes disinhibition and is associated with a range of disorderly and violent offences. With drugs, there is an increase in theft and non-violent offences to get money to buy drugs; those who deal in drugs may use violent methods to protect their business.

Neighbourhood

Conduct problems are associated with overcrowding, poor housing, and poor neighbourhoods. How much these factors are causal or simply markers for other family or socioeconomic variables is unclear. Multivariate analyses suggest that, when factors such as poor parenting and maternal depression are accounted for, neighbourhood and poverty effects are not large. However, it is plausible that stress-ful living conditions with few amenities for children and many other demands on parents impair their ability to bring up their children constructively and respon-sively. Also, areas where there are closer relationships between neighbours with high perceived social cohesion by residents and informal social controls have less antisocial behaviour. Moving out of a deprived area reduces rates of antisocial behaviour.

Child characteristics

Temperament and personality

Infants with temperaments classified as 'difficult' at 3 are more likely to be referred for aggressive problems later on. The dimensions involved are behavioural impul-sivity (lack of restraint), short attention span and motor restlessness. Although not occurring at a clinical level, these are precisely the constituents of the hyperkinetic syndrome; together with the trait of negative emotionality (irritability, anger and bad moods) they have a clear modest effect in predicting later antisocial behaviour of the early onset type. Social anxiety on the other hand is protective.

Thinking style

Significant cognitive attributional bias has been shown in aggressive children and youths. They are more likely to perceive neutral acts by others as hostile, and are more likely to believe conflicts can be resolved satisfactorily by aggression. As the individual gets more disliked and rejected by his peers, the opportunity for seeing things this way increases. By late teenage these youths can have a highly suspicious attitude, and be quick to perceive disrespect from others and sometimes react explosively. Social skills are lacking. Emotional processes in antisocial children have been little studied, although self-esteem is often low and co-existent misery common. Youths with conduct disorder have been shown to plan their lives less than controls, so that they are more driven by events than in control of them.

IQ

Early-onset lifetime persistent children have IQs 8–10 points below controls. The relationship with antisocial behaviour weakens after allowing for social class but is still present, although it only accounts for a few percent of the variance. It is not just the effect of missing schooling, since it is present before children go to school. Much of the association can be accounted for by the association with hyperactivity. It seems likely that low IQ alone does not confer much increased risk of antisocial behaviour, but in the presence of adverse parenting and other risks it has an interactive effect.

Physiological characteristics

Physique has little influence on antisocial propensity. The relationship between testosterone (and other androgens) and antisocial behaviour is complex. Levels vary with age, type of antisocial behaviour and social rejection, so that no straight-forward conclusion can be drawn; certainly to date no obvious relationship has been shown between higher levels and more aggression. Serotonin is being investigated since reduced levels have been associated with suicidal, impulsive and aggressive behaviour in adults. However, samples have to be got through lumbar puncture so studies are usually on small incarcerated samples, where reduced levels of metabolites have been found in aggressive adults. Serotonin blood levels were reduced (effect size 0.5 standard deviation) in antisocial young adults in the Dunedin longitudinal study, but the relation of blood to brain levels has yet to be clarified. The same study recently revealed an increased risk for antisocial outcomes in individuals who were maltreated, but only if they did not have the genotype linked to monoamine oxidase A; put another way, there was a gene–environment interaction whereby maltreated individuals were less likely to become violent if they had the gene that confers high levels of MAOA expression.

Autonomic arousal however has shown a consistent albeit modest association with persistent antisocial behaviour in young people. Their pulse rates are lower, their skin conductance is less, as is their adrenaline and cortisol excretion. Some have postulated this leads to less anxiety when taking risks, others see it as part of a wider picture of decreased central nervous system inhibition. With all these physiological substrates and mechanisms, the direction of effect is unlikely to be only biology driving behaviour; equally, confrontative situations, social dominance, peer rejection and self-esteem are likely to influence physiological parameters.

Treatment

Clinical management and treatment setting

Engagement of the family is particularly important for this group of children and families as dropout from treatment is high, at around 30–40 per cent. Practical measures such as assisting with transport, providing childcare, holding sessions in the evening or at other times to suit the family will all help. Many of the parents of children with conduct disorder may themselves have difficulty with authority and officialdom and be very sensitive to criticism. Therefore, the approach is more likely to succeed if it is respectful of their point of view, does not offer overly prescriptive solutions, and does not directly criticize parenting style. Practical homework tasks increase changes, as do problem-solving telephone calls from the therapist between sessions.

Parenting interventions may need to go beyond skill development to address more distal factors which prevent change. For example, drug or alcohol abuse in either parent, maternal depression, and a violent relationship with the partner are all common. The algorithm in Fig. 18.3 below lists some of the difficulties that commonly occur in parents, and gives evidence-based interventions to address these. Additionally, assistance in claiming welfare and benefits and help with financial planning may reduce stress from debts.

A multimodal approach is likely to get larger changes. Therefore, involving the school in treatment by visiting and offering strategies for managing the child in class is usually helpful, as is advocating for extra tuition where necessary. If the school seems unable to cope despite extra resources, consideration should be given to moving the child to a different school, which specializes in the management of behavioural difficulties. Avoiding antisocial peers and building self-esteem may be helped by getting the child to attend after-school clubs and holiday activities.

Where parents are not coping or a damaging abusive relationship is detected, it may be necessary to liaise with the social services department to arrange respite for the parents or a spell of foster care. It is important during this time to work with the

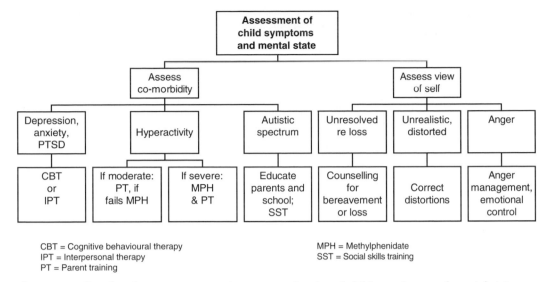

CBT = Cognitive behavioural therapy
IPT = Interpersonal therapy
PT = Parent training

MPH = Methylphenidate
SST = Social skills training

Fig. 18.1.   Flowchart for assessment and treatment planning of child symptoms and mental state.

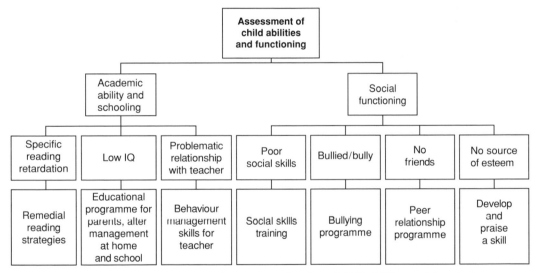

Fig. 18.2.   Flowchart for assessment and treatment planning of child abilities and functioning.

family to increase their skills so the child can return to the family. Where there is permanent breakdown, long-term fostering or adoption may be recommended. There is no evidence that inpatient admissions lead to gains that are maintained after the child is returned to their family, so this costly course of action is not recommended.

Treatment algorithms and decision trees

Figures 18.1 and 18.2 show possible outcomes of child assessment, with recommended treatment. As well as uncovering any co-morbidity and treating it

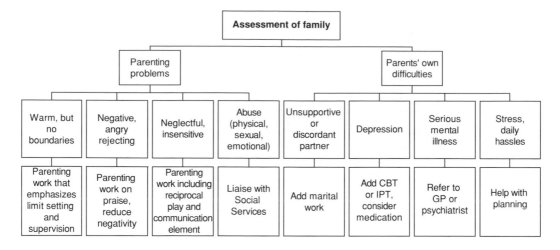

CBT = Cognitive behavioural therapy

IPT = Interpersonal therapy

GP = General practitioner/family doctor

Fig. 18.3.   Flowchart for assessment and treatment planning.

accordingly, it is important to assess the child's subjective experience. Not infrequently there are fears, or feelings of grief that are unknown or belittled by the parents. Exploring these sensitively and helping the parents face up to them and respond appropriately often helps to improve antisocial behaviour too. Assessing abilities both in school and outside is crucial. There is only limited gain to the child or young person if the antisocial behaviour reduces, but they continue to have no skills, no friends and low esteem; these conditions also make relapse more likely. Improving these aspects of psychosocial functioning is often under emphasized in treatment planning.

Figure 18.3 shows possible outcomes of the family assessment, with recommended treatment. Careful assessment of parental functioning is especially important in conduct disorder as it is such a major determinant of the problem, and such an effective and rewarding means of treatment. Direct observation of parenting is strongly recommended, as described in the assessment section above. Seeing the parents alone is necessary to elicit as frank an account as possible of their own views, difficulties, support systems and strengths.

Psychological interventions

Proven psychosocial interventions include those which singly or in combination address:

- parenting skills
- family functioning
- child interpersonal skills

- difficulties at school
- peer group influences.

Currently, there is a trend of changing clinical practice, away from individual *ad hoc* treatments to gradual introduction of systematic programmes that have evidence for their effectiveness. The latter consistently outperform 'usual treatment' in head to head comparisons in regular clinical settings. They are therefore to be encouraged, but persuading managers and clinicians to adopt them is likely to prove a slow process until effective outcomes are more highly prized, and evidence-based practice is insisted upon by politicians, managers, and most of all the families themselves. The children and young people do not deserve to be fobbed off with inferior interventions that are less likely to improve their life chances.

Parenting skills

Here, programmes are designed to improve parenting skills and the quality of the parent-child relationship. There are scores of randomized controlled trials showing these programmes are effective for children up to about 10 years old. They address the parenting practices identified in research as contributing to conduct problems. Typically, they include five elements.

Promoting play and a positive relationship

In order to cut into the cycle of defiant behaviour and recriminations, it is important to instil some positive experiences for both sides and begin to mend the relationship. Teaching parents the techniques of how to play in a constructive and non-hostile way with their children helps them recognize their needs and respond sensitively. The children in turn begin to like and respect their parents more, and become more secure in the relationship.

Praise and rewards for sociable behaviour

Parents are helped to reformulate difficult behaviour in terms of the positive behaviour they wish to see, so that they encourage wanted behaviour rather than criticize unwanted behaviour. For example, instead of shouting at the child not to run, they would praise him whenever he walks quietly; then he will do it more often. Through hundreds of such prosaic daily interactions, child behaviour can be substantially modified. Yet some parents find it hard to praise, and fail to recognize positive behaviour when it happens, with the result that it become less frequent.

Clear rules and clear commands

Rules need to be explicit and constant; commands need to be firm and brief. Thus shouting at a child to stop being naughty doesn't tell him what he should do, whereas, for example, telling him to play quietly gives a clear instruction which makes compliance easier.

Consistent and calm consequences for unwanted behaviour

Disobedience and aggression need to be responded to firmly and calmly, by for example putting the child in a room for a few minutes. This method of 'time out from positive reinforcement' sounds simple but requires considerable skill to administer effectively. More minor annoying behaviours such as whining and shouting often respond to being ignored, but again parents often find this hard to achieve in practice.

Reorganizing the child's day to prevent trouble

There are often trouble spots in the day which will respond to fairly simple measures. For example, putting siblings in different rooms to prevent fights on getting home from school, banning TV in the morning until the child is dressed, and so on.

Treatment can be given individually to the parent and child which enables live feedback in light of the parent's progress and the child's response. Alternatively, group treatments with parents alone have been shown to be equally effective. Trials show that behavioural parenting programmes are effective in reducing child anti-social behaviour in the short term, with moderate to large effect sizes of 0.5 to 0.8 standard deviations, and there is little loss of effect at 1 or 3 year follow up. Parenting skills interventions are chiefly used with younger children, although there is evidence for their successful use with delinquent boys.

Family functioning

Functional family therapy, multisystemic therapy, and treatment foster care aim to change a range of difficulties which impede effective functioning of teenagers with conduct disorder.

Functional family therapy addresses family processes that need to be improved, such as better communication between parent and young person, reducing inter-parental inconsistency, tightening up on supervision and monitoring, and negotiating rules and the sanctions to be applied for breaking them. Functional family therapy has been shown to reduce reoffending rates by around 50 per cent. Other varieties of family therapy have not been subjected to controlled trials for young people with conduct disorder or delinquency, so cannot be evaluated for their efficacy.

Multisystemic therapy was developed by Henggeler and colleagues in the USA. The young person's and family's needs are assessed in their own context at home and in their relations with other systems such as school and peers. Following the assessment, proven methods of intervention are used to address difficulties and promote strengths. Multisystemic therapy differs from most types of family therapy such as the Milan or systemic approach as usually practised in a number of regards. First, treatment is delivered in the situation where the young lives, e.g. at home. Secondly, the therapist has a low caseload (4–6 families) and the team is available

24 hours a day. Thirdly, the therapist is responsible for ensuring appointments are kept and for making change happen – families cannot be blamed for failing to attend or 'not being ready' to change. Fourthly, regular written feedback on progress towards goals from multiple sources is gathered by the therapist and acted upon. Fifthly, there is a manual for the therapeutic approach and adherence is checked weekly by the supervisor. Several randomized controlled trials attest to the effectiveness, with reoffending rates typically cut by half and time spent in psychiatric hospitalization reduced further.

Treatment foster care is another way to improve the quality of encouragement and supervision that teenagers with conduct disorder receive. The young person lives with a foster family specially trained in effective techniques; sometimes it is ordered as an alternative to jail. While the young person is living with the specially trained foster carers, the family of origin are trained in effective methods. Outcome studies following return to the birth family show useful reductions in rates of reoffending.

Child interpersonal skills

Most of the programmes to improve child interpersonal skills derive from cognitive behaviour therapy. Three of the most effective are Kendall's Self-Instructional Training, Lochman's Anger Coping Program, and Greenberg's Promoting Alternative Thinking Strategies (PATHS). These and other programmes have in common training the young persons to:

- slow down impulsive responses to challenging situations by stopping and thinking
- recognize their own level of physiological arousal, and their own emotional state
- recognize and define problems
- develop several alternative responses
- choose the best alternative based on anticipation of consequences
- reinforce themselves for use of this approach.

Over the longer term they aim to increase positive social behaviour by teaching the young person to:

- learn skills to make and sustain friendships
- develop social interaction skills such as turn-taking and sharing
- express viewpoints in appropriate ways and listen to others.

Typically, given alone, treatment gains with interpersonal skills training are good within the treatment setting, but only generalize slightly to 'real-life' situations such as the school playground. However, when they are part of a more comprehensive programme which has those outside the young person reinforcing the approach, they add to outcome gains.

Functioning at school

Difficulties at school can be divided into learning problems and disruptive behaviour. There are proven programmes to deal with specific learning problems for example specific reading retardation, such as reading recovery. However, few of the programmes have been specifically evaluated for their ability to improve outcome in children with conduct disorder, although trials are in progress. Pre-school education programmes for high risk populations have been shown to reduce arrest rates and improve employment in adulthood.

There are several schemes for improving classroom behaviour, which vary from those which stress improved communication such as 'circle time', and those which work on behavioural principles such as the 'good behaviour game' or are part of a multimodal package. Many of these schemes have been shown to improve classroom behaviour, and some specifically target children with conduct disorder. At the level of the individual teacher with a particularly disruptive child, two or three sessions spent imparting and refining basic behavioural management techniques can lead to substantial improvement in classroom behaviour and learning.

Peer group influences

A few interventions have aimed to reduce the bad influence of deviant peers. However, a number attempted this through group work with other conduct disordered youths, but outcome studies showed a worsening of antisocial behaviour. In modern treatments therefore, either youths are seen individually where an element is to try to steer them away from deviant peers, or the work is in small groups (say 3–5 youths) where the therapist can control the content of sessions. Some interventions place youths with conduct disorder in groups with well-functioning youths, and this has led to favourable outcomes.

Other interventions

In addition to removal from home and changing schools, there is some evidence that moving house to a better neighbourhood reduces conduct disorder, as does increasing family income. In the Great Smoky Mountains study in the USA, an Indian reservation community introduced a casino and so was able to pay every family $6000 per year. The rate of conduct disorder reduced significantly. This is not to recommend widespread introduction of casinos, which may encourage harmful gambling behaviour and bring criminal elements to an area, but rather, represents a reasonably unconfounded way of estimating the impact of poverty.

Pharmacotherapy

There is no convincing evidence that medication has any specific effects on conduct disorder. Extreme irritability just might be part of a manic illness and so respond to

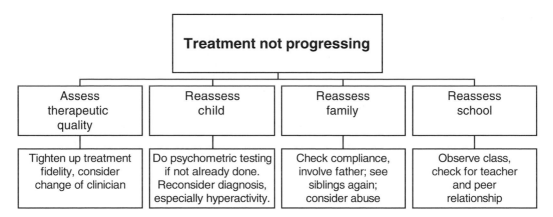

Fig. 18.4.   Flowchart for when treatment does not progress.

lithium, anticonvulsant or mood stabilizing drugs, but in the absence of clear other features confirming the diagnosis of a manic illness medication should not be given. Neuroleptics can, unsurprisingly, have a sedative effect and are not infrequently used for challenging behaviours in children and adolescents with mental retardation, but several studies show that, if psychosocial management is better, this usage declines or stops.

Where there is co-morbid hyperactivity in addition to conduct disorder, several studies attest to a large (effect size of 0.8 standard deviations or greater) reduction in both overt and covert antisocial behaviour, both at home and at school. However, the impact on long-term outcome is unstudied.

Monitoring and evaluation of treatment

If this reveals that treatment is not progressing, a number of possible causes and remedies should be considered. These are set out in Fig. 18.4. There is nearly always an understandable cause for failure of treatment progression. From the outset, treatment is unlikely to work if an evidence based programme or a similar approach is not being taken. Then, commonly it is because the parents are not being seen often enough or with sufficient clarity and specificity of instruction with repeated practice opportunities under supervision through role play. If, however, there is convincing evidence that the family is changing the contingencies around the child and the way he is being parented and encouraged, then mental retardation, hyperactivity and child abuse outside the family should be reconsidered. Likewise, if there is no improvement in school, a visit to determine what is going on both inside the classroom and on the playground should reveal what is happening, and if the environment has changed but the child has not, a similar re-evaluation is in order.

Prevention

Conduct disorder should offer good opportunities for prevention since:
• it can be detected early reasonably well
• early intervention is more effective than later
• there are a number of effective interventions.

In the USA, pre-school education programmes for disadvantaged children have been evaluated in terms of adult outcomes. The best known is the Perry/Highscope project, where 2–4 year olds received intensive nursery education half-time for 2 years. Aged 27, the individual fared better than controls on several psychosocial outcomes, including a third of the number of arrests for criminal offences, better jobs, higher income, and more stable marriages. Another effective preventive programme was begun even earlier in life, the Elmira project, where nurses visited others at risk during the early months of life. Follow-up into adulthood again showed a good reduction in antisocial behaviour, and gains in quality of life. However, other preventive programmes have had smaller effects, and it is emerging that it is crucial to use evidence-based programmes and implement them faithfully and with high quality: chopping and changing the programmes in an attempt to be flexible has not been associated with good results.

In the UK, our own team developed a 26-week parenting intervention called supporting parents on kids' education (SPOKES). It is delivered in schools to parents of 5- and 6-year-old children showing antisocial behaviour who are therefore at risk of developing conduct disorder. In the first term, parents are offered a behaviourally based programme using principles similar to those outlined above. In the second term they are offered specific techniques on how to support their children learn to read. A randomized controlled trial showed substantial reductions in antisocial behaviour and hyperactivity, and a gain in reading age of 7 months. Follow-up studies are under way to see whether the results are enduring and lead to the avoidance of an antisocial lifestyle.

In the USA a number of comprehensive interventions based on up-to-date empirical findings are being carried out. Perhaps the best known is families and schools together (FASTrack). Here the most antisocial 10 per cent of 5–6-year olds in schools in disadvantaged areas were selected, as judged by teacher and parent reports. They were then offered intervention which was given for a whole year in the first instance and comprised:
• weekly parent training in groups with videotapes
• an interpersonal skills training programme for the whole class
• academic tutoring twice a week
• home visits from the parent trainer
• a pairing programme with sociable peers from the class.

Table 18.3. Long-term outcome in adulthood of individuals with conduct disorder in childhood

Antisocial behaviour	Higher rates of violent and non-violent crimes, e.g. mugging, grievous bodily harm; theft, car crimes, fraud
Psychiatric problems	Increased rates of antisocial personality, alcohol and drug abuse, anxiety, depression and somatic complaints, episodes of deliberate self-harm and completed suicide, time in psychiatric hospitals
Education and training	Poorer examination results, more truancy and early school leaving, fewer vocational qualifications
Work	More unemployment, jobs held for shorter time, jobs low status and income, increased claiming of benefits and welfare
Social network	Few if any significant friends, low involvement with relatives, neighbours, clubs and organizations
Intimate relationships	Increased rate of short lived, violent cohabiting relationships; partners often also antisocial
Children	Increased rates of child abuse, conduct problems in offspring, children taken into care
Health	More medical problems, earlier death

Almost 1000 children were randomized to receive this condition or controls, and the project has cost over $50 million. However, so far, preliminary reports of outcome have been limited, with no improvement of antisocial behaviour at home on questionnaire measures and modest improvements in the classroom. There are a number of possible reasons for the smaller effects compared to those obtained in trials with clinically referred populations. The motivation of families may be less as they don't perceive they have a problem; starting levels of antisocial behaviour are lower, so there is not so far to go to reach normal levels; and keeping up the quality of the intervention across several sites is harder. It remains to be seen whether longer term effects will be greater.

Outcome

Short- and long-term sequelae

Of those with early onset conduct disorder (starting before age 8 years), about half persist with serious problems into adulthood. Of those with adolescent onset, the great majority (over 85%) desist in their antisocial behaviour by their early 20s. As can be seen from Table 18.3, not only are there substantially increased rates of antisocial acts, but the general psychosocial functioning of children with conduct

Table 18.4. Predictors of poor outcome for conduct disorder

Onset	Early onset of severe problems, before age 8
Phenomenology	Antisocial acts which are severe, frequent, and varied
Co-morbidity	Hyperactivity and attention problems
Intelligence	Lower IQ
Family history	Parental criminality; parental alcoholism
Parenting	Harsh, inconsistent parenting, with high criticism, low warmth, low involvement and low supervision
Wider environment	Low income family in poor neighbourhood with ineffective schools

disorder grown up is strikingly poor. For most of the characteristics shown in Table 18.3, the increased rates compared to controls is at least double for community cases who were never referred, and three to four times for referred children.

Prognostic factors

Prediction of outcome is fairly reliable, with models that include all factors explaining about 50 per cent of the variance. Many of the factors which predict poor outcome are associated with early onset; they are listed in Table 18.4. Interestingly, girls who have conduct disorder do no better than boys.

To detect protective factors, children who do well despite adverse risk factors have been studied. These so-called 'resilient' children, however, have been shown to have lower levels of risk factors, for example, a boy with antisocial behaviour and low IQ living in a rough neighbourhood but living with supportive, concerned parents. Protective factors are mostly the opposite end of the spectrum of the same risk factor, thus, for example, good parenting and high IQ are protective. None the less there are factors which are associated with resilience independent of known adverse influences. These include a good relationship with at least one adult, who does not necessarily have to be the parent; a sense of pride and self-esteem; and skills or competencies.

The path from childhood conduct disorder to poor adult outcome is neither inevitable nor linear. Different sets of influences impinge as the individual grows up and shape the life course. Many of these can accentuate problems. Thus a toddler with an irritable temperament and short attention span may not learn good social skills if he is raised in a family lacking them, and where he can only get his way by behaving antisocially and grasping for what he needs. At school he may fall in with a deviant crowd of peers, where violence and other antisocial acts are talked up and give him a sense of esteem. His generally poor academic ability and difficult behaviour in class may lead him to truant increasingly, which in turn makes him fall further behind.

He may then leave school with no qualifications and fail to find a job, and resort to drugs. To fund his drug habit, he may resort to crime, and once convicted, find it even harder to get a job. From this example, it can be seen that adverse experiences do not only arise passively and independently of the young person's behaviour; rather, the behaviour predisposes them to end up in risky and damaging environments. Consequently, the number of adverse life events experienced is greatly increased. The path from early hyperactivity into later conduct disorder is also not inevitable. In the presence of a warm supportive family atmosphere it is far less likely than if the parents are highly critical and hostile. Other influences can, however, steer the individual away from an antisocial path. For example, being separated from a deviant peer group; marrying to a non-deviant partner; moving away from a poor neighbourhood; military service which imparts skills (but not harsh boot camps, which have been shown to be ineffective in reducing offending).

In summary, much is known about the causes of conduct disorder, and there are many effective interventions available. The challenge is to make these more universally available, and to deliver them with quality and fidelity so the life chances of the young people improve.

SUGGESTED READING

Helpful books

M. B. Bloomquist & S. V. Schnell, *Helping Children with Aggression and Conduct Problems.* (New York: Guilford Press, 2002).

J. Durlak, *School-based Prevention Programs for Children and Adolescents.* (Thousand Oaks, California: Sage, 1995).

J. Hill & B. Maughan, *Conduct Disorders in Childhood and Adolescence.* (Cambridge: Cambridge University Press, 2001).

G. R. Patterson & M. S. Forgatch, *Parents and Adolescents Living Together.* (Eugene, OR: Castalia, 1987).

M. Rutter, H. Giller, & A. Hagell, *Antisocial Behavior by Young People.* (Cambridge: Cambridge University Press, 1998).

Seminal articles

M. T. Greenberg, C. A. Kusche, E. T. Cooke, & J. P. Quamma, Promoting emotional competence in school-aged children: the effects of the PATHS curriculum. *Developmental Psychopathology*, **7** (1995), 117–36.

S. W. Henggeler, Multisystemic therapy: an overview of clinical procedures, outcomes and policy implications. *Child Psychology and Psychiatry Review*, **4** (1999), 2–10.

A. Kazdin, Psychosocial treatments for conduct disorder in children. *Journal of Child Psychology and Psychiatry*, **38** (1997), 161–78.

P. C. Kendall & L. Braswell, *Cognitive-behavioral Therapy for Impulsive Children*, 2nd edn. (New York: Guilford Press, 1993).

J. E. Lochman & L. A. Lenhart, Anger coping intervention for aggressive children: conceptual models and outcome effects. *Clinical Psychology Review*, **13** (1993), 785–805.

T. Moffitt, A. Caspi, N. Dickson, P. Silva, & W. Stanton, Childhood-onset versus adolescent-onset antisocial conduct problems in males: natural history from ages 3 to 18 years. *Development and Psychopathology*, **8** (1996), 399–424.

D. Olds & H. Kitzman, Review of research on home visitation for pregnant women and parents of young children. *Future of Children*, **3** (1999), 53–92.

R. Sampson, S. Raudenbush, & F. Earls, Neighborhoods and violent crime: a multilevel study of collective efficacy. *Science*, **277** (1997), 918–24.

L. J. Schweinhart, H. V. Barnes, & D. P. Weikart, *The HighScope/Perry Preschool Study through age 27*. (Ypsilanti, MI: HighScope Educational Foundation, 1993).

S. Scott, Q. Spender, M. Doolan, B. Jacobs, & H. Aspland, Multicentre controlled trail of parenting groups for child antisocial behaviour in clinical practice. *British Medical Journal*, **323** (2001), 194–7.

C. Webster-Stratton, T. Hollinsworth, & M. Kolpacoff, The long-term effectiveness and clinical significance of three cost-effective training programs for families with conduct problem children. *Journal of Consulting and Clinical Psychology*, **57** (1989), 550–3.

Appendix 18.1. Strengths and difficulties questionnaire

For each item, please mark the box for 'not true', 'somewhat true' or 'certainly true'. It would help us if you answered all items as best you can even if you are not absolutely certain or the item seems daft! Please give your answers on the basis of the child's behaviour over the last 6 months.

Child's Name..   Male/Female

Date of Birth..

	Not true	Somewhat true	Certainly true
Considerate of other people's feelings	☐	☐	☐
Restless, overactive, cannot stay still for long	☐	☐	☐
Often complains of headaches, stomach aches or sickness	☐	☐	☐
Shares readily with other children (treats, toys, pencils, etc.)	☐	☐	☐
Often has temper tantrums or hot tempers	☐	☐	☐
Rather solitary, tends to play alone	☐	☐	☐
Generally obedient, usually does what adults request	☐	☐	☐
Many worries, often seems worried	☐	☐	☐

Helpful if someone is hurt, upset or feeling ill	☐	☐	☐
Constantly fidgeting or squirming	☐	☐	☐
Has at least one good friend	☐	☐	☐
Often fights with other children or bullies them	☐	☐	☐
Often unhappy, down-hearted or tearful	☐	☐	☐
Generally liked by other children	☐	☐	☐
Easily distracted, concentration wanders	☐	☐	☐
Nervous or clingy in new situations, easily loses confidence	☐	☐	☐
Kind to younger children	☐	☐	☐
Often lies or cheats	☐	☐	☐
Picked on or bullied by other children	☐	☐	☐
Often volunteers to help others (parents, teachers, other children)	☐	☐	☐
Thinks things out before acting	☐	☐	☐
Steals from home, school or elsewhere	☐	☐	☐
Gets on better with adults than with other children	☐	☐	☐
Many fears, easily scared	☐	☐	☐
Sees tasks through to the end, good attention span	☐	☐	☐

Do you have any other comments or concerns?

Overall, do you think that your child has difficulties in one or more of the following areas: emotions, concentration, behaviour or being able to get on with other people?

No	Yes – minor difficulties	Yes – definite difficulties	Yes – severe difficulties
☐	☐	☐	☐

If you have answered 'Yes', please answer the following questions about these difficulties:

• How long have these difficulties been present?

Less than a month	1–5 months	6–12 months	Over a year
☐	☐	☐	☐

• Do the difficulties upset or distress your child?

Not at all	Only a little	Quite a lot	A great deal
☐	☐	☐	☐

- Do the difficulties interfere with your child's everday life in the following areas?

	Not at all	Only a little	Quite a lot	A great deal
Home life	☐	☐	☐	☐
Friendships	☐	☐	☐	☐
Classroom learning	☐	☐	☐	☐
Leisure activities	☐	☐	☐	☐

- Do the difficulties put a burden on you or the family as a whole?

Not at all	Only a little	Quite a lot	A great deal
☐	☐	☐	☐

Signature...   Date..............
Mother/Father/Other (please specify:)

Thank you very much for your help

19

Elective mutism

Hans-Christoph Steinhausen

Department of Child and Adolescent Psychiatry, University of Zurich, Switzerland

Introduction

The term 'elective mutism' was originally coined in 1934 by the Swiss pioneer of child psychiatry, Moritz Tramer. However, it is assumed that the German physician, Kussmaul, was the first to describe three cases in 1877 under the term 'aphasia voluntaria'. Whereas the ICD-10 stuck to the original term 'elective mutism', the DSM-IV has slightly changed the term to 'selective mutism'. Both the original designation and the fact that the ICD-10 as the dominant European scheme of classification uses 'elective mutism' as the descriptor are the reasons why this chapter follows this term.

Children with elective mutism are rarely seen in clinical practice, although it may be assumed that there are some more in the general population who will either be referred rather late or perhaps never for assessment and intervention. Consequently, a large body of clinical knowledge rests on case reports or descriptions of small series of children with a few exceptions of studies based on more extended series of patients.

Definition and classification

According to the ICD-10, the following four criteria lead to the diagnosis of elective mutism:

- marked and consistent selectivity in speaking, i.e. failure to speak in social situations
- a normal or near-normal level of language comprehension
- a level of competence in language expression that would be sufficient for social communications, and
- demonstrable evidence that the child could and did speak normally or almost normally in some situations.

A Clinician's Handbook of Child and Adolescent Psychiatry, ed. Christopher Gillberg,
Richard Harrington and Hans-Christoph Steinhausen. Published by Cambridge University Press.
© Cambridge University Press 2005.

The DSM-IV criteria are largely comparable. In addition to the above-mentioned ICD-10 criteria, it is mentioned that the disturbance interferes with educational and occupational achievement or with social communication. Furthermore, DSM-IV criteria include some aspects of differential diagnosis by stating that the disturbance is not better accounted for by a communication disorder (e.g. stuttering) and does not occur exclusively during the course of a pervasive developmental disorder, schizophrenia, or other psychotic disorder.

The ICD-10 set of criteria seems to fully match the expectations of clinical applicability whereas the two additional criteria of DSM-IV are questionable because of violating some basic rules of classification of disorders. First, the interference with educational and occupational achievement is a true but nonspecific consequence of elective mutism because it also applies to many other psychiatric disorders. Secondly, the incomplete list of differential diagnoses may not be used as a defining criterion.

Epidemiology

There are only very few studies that tried to obtain prevalence rates of elective mutism in children in the general population. Generalization of findings is limited due to inherent methodological shortcomings including limited age range, small catchment areas lacking full psychiatric assessment or a combination of these factors. From these studies it seems prudent to expect prevalence rates clearly below 1 per cent of the child population with a range between 0.02 to 0.7 per cent. The prevalence rate may be slightly higher in the early school years and may show considerable regional or cultural variation.

From the few epidemiological studies, there is also no clear gender effect due to the very small number of cases. In the largest clinical series of 100 cases by the author there was an excess of females with a 1:1.6 ratio. Both in this series and also in other smaller samples, an increased proportion of migrant children has been observed. There is no indication that any social class is linked specifically to elective mutism.

Both clinical experience and limited epidemiological findings converge by indicating that elective mutism is a relatively rare clinical phenomenon. Thus, it cannot be expected that many child and adolescent psychiatrists share a solid expertise of the disorder's clinical phenomena.

Clinical picture

Main features and symptoms

The main feature of elective mutism is the selectivity in speaking. In contrast to total mutism with the child not speaking at all (an even rarer phenomenon than elective mutism), the child with elective mutism does not speak in certain social surroundings whereas he or she speaks without hesitation in other environments. Most typically, the child with elective mutism will not speak outside the home (i.e. at school or to a stranger) whereas he or she will have unrestricted communication in the family. In the author's series of 100 cases nearly 90 per cent of the patients followed this pattern whereas between 34 and 42 per cent of the children did not speak to other children – either in general or to specific children. The least common phenomenon is the child not speaking within the family or refusing to speak to certain family members. In the author's series there were only 2–13 per cent of children who followed this less frequent pattern.

At least in clinical cases there is a high proportion of children with elective mutism who show a variety of abnormalities of early history and development; pre-morbid speech and language disorder including predominantly expressive language and articulation disorders are very common (up to 40%) and more than two-thirds of these children may show pre-morbid behavioural abnormalities of various types including relationship problems, anxiety, sleep and eating disorders whereas disruptive disorders are relatively rare.

The onset of the disorder most typically starts around the age of 3–4 years. In most cases the onset is insidious rather than sudden with only a minority of children reacting to a significant life event. A few children with elective mutism may react to trauma, loss of a significant person or intrafamilial burden or crisis.

In addition to the main features of elective mutism there may be other co-morbid symptoms. Whereas almost all children with elective mutism present shyness and inhibition, many of these children show additional anxiety symptoms or disorders other than reluctance to speak. Thus, almost all children with selective mutism will also meet diagnostic criteria for social phobia or social anxiety disorder in childhood whereas a smaller proportion will also qualify for other anxiety disorders. In the author's series only two-thirds qualified for anxiety and slightly more than one-third for depression in terms of symptoms or syndromes. Only a minority of up to 20 per cent exhibited disruptive symptoms including opposition-defiance, aggression or hyperactivity. Elimination disorders are also quite common (up to a third) as are sleeping and eating disorders (20–30 %) whereas tics and obsessive-compulsive disorders are less frequent. Besides the very frequent association with speech and language delays, some children also show motor development delay or pervasive developmental disorders including Asperger syndrome.

Differential diagnoses

There are various other psychiatric disorders that have to be considered for differential diagnoses including some that might also present as a co-morbid disorder:

• anxiety disorders, predominantly social phobia and social anxiety disorders
• post-traumatic stress disorders and adjustment disorders

Table 19.1. Multidimensional assessment of children with elective mutism

- Core symptoms
  - Age and type of onset (insidious vs sudden)
  - To whom and where does the child speak (family, relatives, school, neighbourhood, public)
  - Language expression and comprehension
  - Social interaction skills (participation, friendships, familiar vs foreign settings)
- Co-morbid symptoms
  - Anxiety disorders, social phobia and anxiety disorders
  - Depressive episodes, dysthymia
  - Elimination disorders
  - Obsessive-compulsive disorders
  - Other co-existing symptoms
- History
  - Pre-morbid personality and temperament (shyness, inhibition, anxiety)
  - Pre-morbid behavioural abnormalities
  - Family history (shyness, speech and language disorders, mutism, anxiety disorder, other psychiatric disorders, bilingualism, migration)
  - Recent major and minor life events and traumas
- Medical assessment
  - Developmental and medical history
  - Physical and neurological examination
  - Speech and language history and examination (delay, fluency and complexity, expression and comprehension, speech quality, bilingualism, standardized language tests)
  - Audiological history (otitis media, hearing problems) and examination
- Cognitive and academic functioning
  - Standardized tests of cognitive skills and achievement
  - Teacher reports and grades
- Personality assessment
  - Standardized questionnaires for behavioural and emotional functioning
  - Anxiety and depression scales

- depressive episodes or disorders, specifically dysthymia
- developmental disorders including speech and language disorders, mental retardation, autism and rare disintegrative disorders
- schizophrenic psychoses, most specifically catatonia
- dissociative disorders and states and
- rare neurological conditions including aphasia and profound loss of hearing.

Assessment

As for most psychiatric disorders in children and adolescents the assessment has to be multidimensional. Table 19.1 presents an outline of the various levels and contents. In elective mutism the clinical interview has to be predominantly performed with the parent because the child will not speak to the clinician. However, as in other conditions, the observation of the child's behaviour will supplement findings coming from the interview with the parent.

There are no widely used specific diagnostic instruments in terms of interviews or questionnaires for elective mutism. The core symptoms may be examined in an unstructured fashion that is guided by the outline in Table 19.1 or the interview module as set out in the Appendix to this chapter. Likewise, the assessment of co-morbid symptoms in ordinary clinical practice will be guided predominantly by clinical expertise and skills. However, some clinicians might find structured interviews like the DISC-IV, CAPA or K-SADS useful if these forms are available to them.

While taking the history, the clinician must focus on the pre-morbid personality and temperament with most children with elective mutism showing shy and inhibited and anxious behaviour throughout their lifetime. Their vulnerability is also signalled by various pre-morbid abnormalities and a high load of abnormalities in the family history. These families often contain members with various speech and language disorders and abnormalities including taciturnity, reluctance to speak and sometimes also mutism. The family history may also reveal similar temperamental features in a parent or other psychiatric disorders in the relatives. In some children with elective mutism a bilingual family or environment due to migration forms a specific risk factor. For the relatively small group of children with a sudden onset of elective mutism, an analysis of the circumstances in terms of major life events or traumas is mandatory.

The medical assessment follows the general schedule and further specific recommendations. Both differential diagnosis and the assessment of co-morbid symptoms require a sound assessment of speech and language disorders including phonology, expressive and receptive language, and standardized testing (see Chapter 14). This may necessitate additional consultation with a speech and language specialist as does the requirement for an audiological examination in order to exclude hearing problems.

In order to exclude reduced performance due to developmental delay or learning disability, cognitive and academic functioning should be assessed by use of standardized tests. Non-verbal tests like Raven's coloured progressive matrices, the performance section of the WISC-III or various culture-fair tests are suitable for the non-speaking child. A teacher report not only provides information on the child's grades and achievement but may also help in getting more insight into the child's behaviour at school. The contact with the teacher is only the first step in order to plan and perform interventions.

Finally, personality assessment may be useful in adding information to the clinical picture as obtained from other sources. Broadband questionnaires based on cross-informant syndromes like the child behaviour checklist (CBCL) for parents, the youth self-report (YSR) for older children and adolescents, and the teacher report form (TRF) may provide information specifically on the internalizing problems that are captured by these instruments. The shy and inhibited behaviour is reflected in various temperament questionnaires specifically for younger children. Furthermore, various anxiety and depression scales may be used.

Aetiology

In the past, aetiological explanations have relied strongly on psychodynamic assumptions dealing with the relevance of impaired parent–child relationships with overprotective mothers and remote fathers, unresolved conflicts or reactions to trauma like sexual abuse, divorce or death of a parent or even frequent moves. With the decline of psychodynamic theory as a solid explanation of aetiology and pathogenesis, only little room is left for these assumptions both for the genesis of elective mutism and child and adolescent psychiatric disorders in general.

Current theory on the aetiology of child and adolescent psychiatric disorders is guided by a multidimensional model with some interacting factors also in elective mutism. Figure 19.1 presents a scheme of the various components of such a model. There is clear evidence that, among predisposing factors in most children with elective mutism, there is a temperament of shyness, inhibition and anxiety that paves the way for the development of not only reluctance to speak but perhaps also to the phenomenologically similar disorders of social phobia and anxiety disorder. In addition, one has also to assume that in a sizeable number of affected children a biological, brain-related vulnerability factor is operating. This assumption is generated by the frequent overlap with pre-existing or co-morbid developmental delays most particularly in the field of speech and language disorders. Furthermore, a family study by the author has also shown that the personality trait of taciturnity is significantly more frequent in first-, second- and third-degree families and that mutism may be found more frequently in families of affected children. Thus there is some evidence for the assumption that genetic factors may play a role in the aetiology of elective mutism. Similarily, other psychiatric disorders in the family and especially anxiety disorder may play a role.

Among various psychosocial factors serving as precipitating events two stand out as being relatively specific and frequent in the history of children with elective mutism, namely, bilingualism and migration. These typically intertwined factors may act as a further trigger of elective mutism in certain vulnerable children. Furthermore, trauma and major life events like sexual abuse, divorce or death of a caretaker may play a role in symptom development of some children with elective mutism. In some cases developmental challenges like entry into kindergarten or school may also have a triggering function.

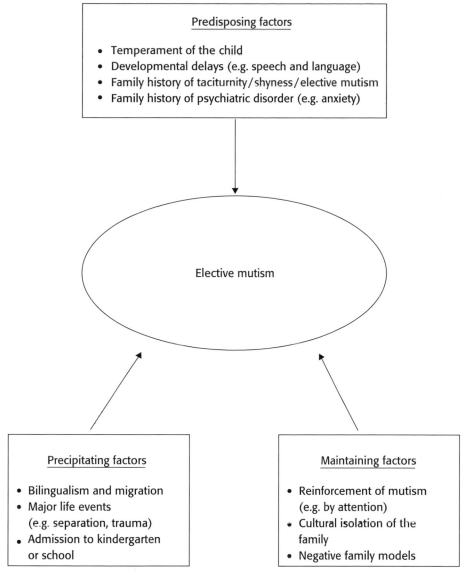

Fig. 19.1.   Multidimensional aetiological model of elective mutism.

Finally, a third group of aetiologically relevant characteristics serve as main-taining factors. They include the increased attention that the child gets by his or her symptom, inappropriate interventions, and other ways that serve to reinforce mutism. Further perpetuating factors include the cultural isolation of families with different ethnic and linguistic background and negative models that are provided by family members who themselves speak very little.

Treatment

Children with elective mutism require experienced therapists due to the nature of the symptoms and the refractory course over many years in some cases. The available treatment literature is of limited use only because most reports are based on case descriptions or very small sample sizes and almost no controlled conditions. As with other disorders, a wide variety of interventions have been used over decades focusing predominantly on psychodynamic approaches, speech therapy, behavioural techniques and less frequently on family therapy. Only recently, pharmacotherapy has been tried in a controlled way. A very helpful resource manual is listed among suggested readings at the end of this chapter.

Clinical management and treatment setting

Current clinical practice should follow the principle of multimodal treatment with components centering around the child, additional interventions addressing issues of the parents and families and incorporating the social environment, most particularly the school from an ecological point of view. Thus, the treatment has to be intensive and requires more than a short-term perspective. Typically, treatment will be performed on an outpatient basis with short (weekly) intervals. Inpatient admission may be needed only rarely, e.g. if a major trauma like sexual abuse or maltreatment require protection of the child.

Psychological interventions

Given the scant evidence on the effectiveness of psychological interventions in a disorder that is difficult to treat, this section will first describe interventions that seem less efficacious and then go over to more promising approaches. First, there is no clear and convincing evidence that psychodynamic or client-centred psychotherapy is efficacious so that long-term play therapy with the silent child will not lead to any demonstrable effects as regards the core symptoms of elective mutism. Even the inclusion of a confident of the child like a sibling or a peer to whom the child normally speaks may help to overcome the reluctance to speak in the treatment sessions.

Similarly, there is no strong evidence that family therapy based on the assumption that dysfunctional patterns are responsible for the child's symptom, in general, is of major help when treating elective mutism. However, the family should be involved in the treatment plan for two reasons. First, the family is essential in helping to generalize any treatment gains in individual treatment sessions and, secondly, the family needs to be specifically addressed and involved when there is evidence that sexual abuse by or major psychopathology of a family member is contributing to the child's symptoms.

A third intervention that has been tried repeatedly with elective mutism is speech therapy. Due to the frequent overlap with various forms of speech delay and deficits there is an assumption that correction of these deficits might help to also overcome the associated reluctance to speak. Interventions focusing on articulation and language training require the inclusion of some basic principles of all psychotherapeutic interventions, namely, the installation of a treatment alliance and some cooperation of the child. Given the lack of solid clinical evidence that speech therapy works in all children with elective mutism, it may be used only in a subgroup of children with minor severity of elective mutism and a strong underpinning by speech and language disorders.

Currently, the best thorough limited evidence that psychological interventions can be efficient and helpful comes from clinical experience with cognitive behaviour therapy. Elements of behaviour modification may be helpful in individual treatment with the child and in family and school-based interventions. The main principles in treating the core symptoms are reinforcement, stimulus fading, shaping and self-modelling.

Reinforcement has to be used in two ways. First, verbal behaviour in each occurring situation in which the child normally would not speak has to be positively reinforced. In the treatment session speaking may be rewarded initially by material reinforcers (e.g. candies, ice-cream, etc.) and later by social reinforcers only (e.g. praise). Secondly, reinforcement for staying mute has to be extinguished. These situations arise typically in the public (e.g. in a store or a restaurant) when other family members speak for the child. Thus, the use of reinforcement means both its application for speaking and its absence for the inappropriate mute behaviour.

The second principle of stimulus fading starts with very simple goals and then gradually increases the difficulty of the task. This may pertain to the length of communication (e.g. starting with 'Yes' or 'No' or saying 'Hello' and proceeding to more extended communications) or the complexity of the social situation in terms of the number of people being present in the environment. An example is given in Box 19.1.

In some children with elective mutism, particularly in those who have accompanying speech and language problems, shaping may be indicated. Shaping builds on the principle that complex behaviours should be broken down into basic components and gradually built up. Thus, with the mute child, mouth movements, non-verbal utterances, simple words and finally sentences and more complex communication should be developed gradually and reinforced until normal speech is achieved. This process may be supported by self-modelling in terms of exposing the child to audio or videotaped recordings of his or her communication. Later phases of treatment may also profit from role-playing and social skills programmes in order to address the social phobia that may be concomitant with elective mutism.

Box 19.1. Example of stimulus fading in an electively mute child

Step 1: Free communication at home with a parent.
Step 2: Free communication in the office with a parent.
         The door is closed and the therapist is absent.
Step 3: Free communication in the office with a parent.
         The door is open and the therapist is visible, but not in the room.
Step 4: Free communication in the office with a parent.
         The therapist is in the room, sitting at his desk but not involved in the communication.
Step 5: Free communication in the office with a parent.
         The therapist is joining the dyad without communication.
Step 6: Free communication in the office with a parent.
         The therapist starts communicating with a few phrases like 'How are you?'

Consecutive steps increase the verbal communication between therapist and child. At the same time verbal communication and presence of the parent is faded out in similar step-by-step approaches.

The principles of reinforcement and stimulus fading also apply to family and school-based interventions. Although most children with elective mutism frankly speak at home and do not speak outside the family, there is a minority of those who do not speak to certain family members. Unless there is not the situation of an abusing family member that may require other interventions, there are similar goals as for the school environment. One of the major goals that needs to be communicated to both the family and the school is that the child should not be forced to speak because of increasing the anxiety. All goals dealing with a modification of the behaviours should be introduced gradually and reinforced positively and with increasing verbal communication assistance should be gradually faded out.

In order to implement these principles and to overcome the child's reluctance to speak at school the guidelines as set out in Table 19.2 should be followed. With any child suffering from elective mutism these guidelines are essential due to the fact that the child is predominantly experiencing major stress at school. Thus a close cooperation with the teachers may not only reduce the stress for the child but also help the uninformed teacher to assist the child and to cooperate with the treatment plan. In some instances it may even be necessary to implement a school-based intervention as the prime intervention because the child is not willing or able to participate in individual treatment in the clinician's office. Thus, the clinician will be forced to restrict his efforts to mediated intervention only. In addition to teachers, peers or siblings also may be used as potent mediators of the intervention.

Table 19.2. Guidelines for school-based interventions in elective mutism

General principles
- Also the child with elective mutism has the right to an education; thus it should be kept in school and in regular classrooms.
- Accept the child as having a disorder in need of extra treatment and not as being oppositional-defiant.
- The child should not be forced to speak; alternative means of communication should be accepted.
- There should be a very close cooperation with the family and any treating clinician.
- Participation in an intervention programme should imply a gradual progress from simple to more complex goals.
- Communicate understanding of the child's behaviour and specific conditions to the entire class.

Specific goals
- Provide favourable conditions for social interaction by selecting small classes and groups including appropriate peers in and out of school.
- Depending on the stage and goal of the intervention accept and promote non-verbal communication by use of gestures, audiotaped homework, cards, etc.
- Increase verbal communication by starting with simple demands like greeting the teacher in the morning and when leaving school and progressing to more complex goals.
- Use positive reinforcement for communicative and interactive behaviour, specifically for speech.
- Implement specific speech and language training by speech therapists at school if indicated by expert assessment.

Pharmacotherapy

Because of the phenomenological similarity of elective mutism to social phobia, there have been a few investigations evaluating drugs that are used for the treatment of patients suffering from social phobia. The limited evidence shows that various selective serotonin reuptake inhibitors (SSRIs) may improve ratings of mutism and anxiety. However, a certain proportion of children may remain symptomatic; the duration and properly individualized doses for treatment are yet unknown. In addition, there is no knowledge whether or not a combination with the most promising intervention, i.e. behaviour modification, leads to better results.

Monitoring and evaluation of treatment

Progress of treatment rests on direct observation of communicative skills during treatment sessions and in the child's environment. Thus, monitoring by the therapist, the parents, and the school are essential. Direct counts of verbal communications may rarely be possible under ordinary clinical and social situations but simple rating scales may be easily constructed for the individual child's behaviour. More detailed and structured instruments are not available. However, it may be useful to follow the principle of multilevel evaluation by including broadband questionnaires like the Child Behaviour Checklist (CBCL) or narrow-band scales dealing specifically with anxiety symptoms. Feedback should be regularly obtained from the school by teacher reports or direct communication and from any ongoing speech and language therapy.

Information of patients and parents

As in each child psychiatric disorder, the patient and parents need a clear and easily understandable explanation of all assessment results, treatment plan, process of intervention and evaluation. It should be emphasized that currently we still do not know all details of the complex origins of the disorder but – at least in the majority of cases – no one including the child and the family members are to blame for the disorder. There are good chances to help the child in overcoming elective mutism and to prevent impairment of personal and social development.

Problematic issues

The basic principles of behaviour modification may be successfully implemented in individual treatment of the child in the clinician's office. The applicability of these principles rests on the basic understanding of the guardian and hopefully, also the child that the suffering of the child and the impediment of normal development are sufficient reasons to ask for treatment. The described principles work in the majority of children with elective mutism as long as the child shows the slightest form of cooperation that is required for treatment of elective mutism. Thus, the treating clinician will have to start with the simplest demands, e.g. non-verbal behaviour like nodding before going over to 'Yes' and 'No' answers.

However, if these very small amounts of cooperation are absent, the situation is more complicated. The inclusion of 'therapeutic pressure' as described in at least one treatment programme has to get the parents' or guardians' consent. The procedure rests on the availability of the therapist for an extended period (i.e. several hours) and the demand that the child may leave the room only after fulfilling a certain goal. This may be a single word in the first session and be gradually extended to several words and the like in further sessions.

There may be two problems with this approach. First, even this small amount of pressure may not be acceptable to parents or treating clinicians because of ethical or other concerns. From a behavioural point of view, the procedure may also be counterproductive because clearly negative reinforcement is operating. The child may only respond to the demand of the therapist in order to escape from a stressful and unpleasant situation. Thus, in these instances there is also a strong need for the implementation of positive reinforcement in terms of praise of even the slightest progress.

Outcome

Due to its low prevalence elective mutism has also not been studied extensively in terms of course and prognostic factors. The few observations from several decades are based mostly on single cases or small series of patients and most of them are based on insufficiently structured follow-up assessments. From these early follow-up studies, one can get the impression that almost all patients improve over time with a wide variety of intervention. A recent follow-up study by the author and his associates also points to improvement in terms of reluctance to speak over lifetime in almost all cases seen in young adulthood. However, a large proportion of young adults with former elective mutism still fulfil criteria for social phobia. Nothing is known as to the long-term effects of intervention.

SUGGESTED READING

S. P. Dow, B. C. Sonies, D. Scheib, S. E. Moss & H. L. Leonhard, Practical guidelines for the assessment and treatment of selective mutism. *Journal of the American Academy of Child and Adolescent Psychiatry*, **34** (1995), 836–46.

E. S. Dummitt, R. G. Klein, N. K. Tranger, B. Asche, J. Martin & J. A. Fairbanks, Systematic assessment of 50 children with selective mutism. *Journal of the American Academy of Child and Adolescent Psychiatry*, **36** (1997), 653–60.

N. H. Hadley, *Elective Mutism: A Handbook for Educators, Counselors and Health Care Professionals*. (Dordrecht–Boston–London: Kluwer Academic Publishers, 1994).

M. Johnson & A. Wintgens, *The Selective Mutism Resource Manual*. (Bicester, Oxon UK: Speechmark Publishing Ltd, 2001).

H. Kristensen, Selective mutism and comorbidity with developmental disorder/delay, anxiety disorder, and elimination disorder. *Journal of the American Academy of Child and Adolescent Psychiatry*, **39** (2000), 249–56.

H.-C. Steinhausen & R. Adamek, The family history of children with elective mutism: a research report. *European Child and Adolescent Psychiatry*, **6** (1997), 107–11.

H.-C. Steinhausen & C. Juzi, Elective mutism: an analysis of 100 cases. *Journal of the American Academy of Child and Adolescent Psychiatry*, **35** (1996), 606–14.

Appendix 19.1. Interview schedule for the assessment of children with selective mutism (H.-C. Steinhausen, 2001; modified after Hadley, 1994)

1. Onset and setting of mutism

1-1. How old was . . . . when you first noticed his/her electively mute behaviour? (Sudden vs. insidious onset)

1-2. Where or with whom does . . . . elect to be silent?

1-3. Has . . . . ever said why he/she does not talk in /at / to . . . .?

1-4. Do you believe there has been any event that may have led to the onset of the mutism (major life events, traumas)?

1-5. Can you identify the last time he/she spoke in school / kindergarden?

1-6. If 'yes', I wonder if you can tell me about the last time he/she spoke in school/ kindergarden?

1-7. In your opinion what purpose does the silence have for . . . .?

2. Play and social behaviour

2-1. Have your ever observed . . . . playing with other children?

2-2. If 'yes', in your estimation how often does . . . . play with other children during the course of a week?

2-3. Does . . . . speak to his/her peers during play?

2-4. If 'no', has . . . . ever told you why he/she does not talk to his peers during play?

2-5. Do you have an opinion about why . . . . does talk to other students during play at school?

3. Development and reactions

3-1. How would you describe . . . .'s language development?

3-2. Did . . . . need to be encouraged to speak when he/she first started talking?

3-3. Has . . . .'s teacher ever expressed concern to you about his/her mutism?

3-4. If 'yes', what did the teacher say or do to get . . . . to speak?

3-5. What was your reaction when you discovered that . . . . does not speak in . . . .?

3-6. Have you or a family member tried to get . . . . to speak in . . . .?

4. Communication within the family

4-1. Does . . . . talk at home?

4-2. How would you describe . . . .'s behaviour at home?

4-3. To whom does . . . . not speak in the family?

4-4. How would you describe . . . .'s talking at home? (Quality and type of any speech and language abnormality)

4-5. Does . . . . verbally protest when another person calls him/her names?

4-6. Does . . . . verbally protest when another person takes something which belongs to him/her?

4-7. Does . . . . verbally protest when another person strikes him/her?

4-8. Have you attempted to get . . . . to talk in the target setting?

4-9. If 'yes', what have you done to get . . . . to talk outside of the home?

4-10. Did . . . . ever say what would have to happen for him/her to begin to speak in the target setting?

4-11. If 'yes', what did . . . . say would have to happen for him/her to talk?

5. Family and the community

5-1. Check the following statements which describe the verbal behaviour of . . . . in the presence of visitors to your home. Does he/she:
   (a) greet relatives
   (b) greet friends
   (c) greet strangers
   (d) answer questions directed to him/her by relatives
   (e) answer questions directed to him/her by friends
   (f) answer questions directed to him/her by strangers
   (g) initiate conversation with relatives
   (h) initiate conversation with friends
   (i) initiate conversation with strangers

5-2. What does . . . . typically do when a stranger visits the home?

5-3. Does . . . . take part in any activities outside the home?

5-4. Is there anyone in . . . .'s immediate family who could be described as quiet to the point where he/she rarely speaks?

5-5. Is a language other than English spoken in . . . .'s home? (bilingualism)

6. Telephone use

6-1. If asked to answer the telephone with whom will he/she speak? (family members, relatives, other)

6-2. Will . . . . answer the telephone?

6-3. Will . . . . make a telephone call on his/her own?

6-4.   If 'yes', who does he/she call?

7. Communication in the target setting

7-1.   How does . . . . indicate that he/she wants something when in a setting in which he/she does not speak?

7-2.   Does . . . . respond with gestures if instructed to do so?

7-3.   If 'yes', can you identify the gestures which he/she typically uses?

7-4.   Does . . . . exhibit eye contact when you are talking to him/her?

7-5.   How do other people react to . . . .'s silence?

7-6.   Have you tried to get . . . . to talk in the target setting?

7-7.   If 'yes', what have you done to get . . . . to talk in the target setting?

7-8.   What does the teacher say or do to get . . . . to talk at school?

8. Treatment by professionals

8-1.   Has . . . . received professional help for his/her speech refusal?

8-2.   What made you refer . . . . for treatment?

8-3.   Which sort of treatment did . . . . receive?

8-4.   Did you play a part in the professional treatment?

8-5.   If 'yes', would you like to tell me about your participation?

8-6.   How long did the treatment last?

8-7.   How frequent were the treatment sessions?

8-8.   Was the professional treatment helpful to your child?

20

Attachment and disorders of attachment

Patricia Hughes[1] and Martin Newman[2]

[1]Department of Psychiatry, St George's Hospital Medical School, London, UK
[2]William Harvey Clinic, London, UK

Introduction

The modern story of attachment began soon after World War II, when John Bowlby (1907–1990) and Rene Spitz (1887–1974) independently began to document the fate of children separated from their parents, reared from infancy in orphanages, or placed in traumatic circumstances in institutions where care might be efficient but impersonal. What they found is familiar to us now: listless, apathetic children who had not had personal attention from an interested adult, and disinhibited, over-friendly children who made shallow relationships with any adult who passed through their world. John Bowlby's contribution to our understanding of child development was his perception that 'mother love' had evolutionary value, and that some behaviours that young children show with their parents might be biologically determined to support survival. Bowlby was no biological determinist, however, and fully recognized the importance of the quality of parental care and the potentially harmful effects of its loss early in life. His theory of attachment proposed that the need for safety is an organizing system in the psychosocial development of children, and that this is different and separate from the need for food or sex. The theory posits both innate characteristics, determined by evolution, and a continuing effect of the experienced environment on the developing child.

Two strands have run through the work that has followed Bowlby's original ideas, developmental and clinical. Developmental research has investigated both low risk populations, in which family circumstances are relatively stable and comfortable, and where child care is generally good, and high risk populations, who experience adverse circumstances of various kinds, and where the mother may have difficulty in providing optimal care for her child. Assessment of attachment in research groups generally assumes a relatively intact infant–parent relationship, and the feasibility

A Clinician's Handbook of Child and Adolescent Psychiatry, ed. Christopher Gillberg,
Richard Harrington and Hans-Christoph Steinhausen. Published by Cambridge University Press.
© Cambridge University Press 2005.

of assessing the infant–parent attachment pattern. In contrast, the clinical diagnosis of attachment disorder as defined in ICD and DSM describes children who have usually suffered extreme disadvantage, either from severe neglect or maltreatment at the hands of their parents, or from having been reared in institutions or multiple foster placements. Some of these children do not have a preferred attachment figure, though some may show attachment behaviour towards a maltreating parent.

Most children seen in child psychiatry or psychology services attend with their families. The majority have not suffered severe deprivation or maltreatment, and while they do not show the full range of criteria for attachment disorder (as defined by ICD or DSM classifications), they frequently demonstrate some of the features of sub-optimal attachment behaviours that have been identified in the research setting.

Attachment disorders were first included in the ICD-9 in 1975 and in DSM-III in 1980. In the revised editions of ICD-10 (1992) and DSM-IV (1994) the diagnostic criteria were somewhat refined. Although there is agreement that children who suffer maltreatment or who are reared in institutions are at greatly increased risk of showing a variety of behavioural problems, the diagnosis of reactive attachment disorder, in particular, has attracted a good deal of criticism, even in ICD-10 itself: '. . . there is continuing uncertainty regarding the diagnostic criteria to be applied, the boundaries of the syndrome, and whether the syndrome constitutes a valid nosological entity.' Meanwhile, developmental researchers have published cross-sectional and longitudinal studies of children whose attachment pattern is assessed in infancy or early childhood, and have begun to identify, more precisely, markers of vulnerability to future pathology in the early attachment relationship. One pattern in particular, the 'disorganized' category of infant attachment has been shown to be a predictor of subsequent behavioural and psychological problems.

In order to understand both the nature of what is meant by attachment behaviour, and the ways that young children manifest problems in this area, we will briefly outline the theory of attachment and summarize the research assessment of young children, including the developmental criteria for secure, insecure and disorganized attachment. We then outline the criteria for ICD and DSM diagnoses, and the assessment and treatment of attachment disorders.

The concept of attachment

According to Bowlby, the attachment system is designed to promote safety, thus attachment behaviour in young children is that which promotes proximity or contact with a person who offers protection. The attachment figure also provides a 'secure base' from which the infant can explore. Fear may activate the attachment system, so that the child immediately seeks a source of safety, namely an attachment figure. Secure children have confidence that the caregiver will respond appropriately when they signal their need for contact. Insecure children are less confident that the caregiver will give an appropriate or reliable response to a distress signal, and have learned strategies to deal this. Children whose attachment pattern is designated 'disorganized' show behaviour which is contradictory in terms of seeking the protection of a caregiver, and where there is evidence of breakdown of one of the three secure or insecure patterns.

The development of attachment behaviour in young children

During the early months of life, the infant signals his needs in various ways, by crying, suckling and grasping, and later by clinging and following behaviours. Although he will recognize familiar adults from early in his postnatal life, and will show preference for caregivers from 8 weeks or so, he is generally willing to accept contact and interaction from a variety of adults. In the second half of the first year, however, the infant begins to show some wariness around unfamiliar adults, and will more overtly use familiar caregivers for comfort. With repeated experiences of having his attachment needs aroused and met by a particular caregiver, his attachment behaviour will be shaped to maximize contact with that caregiver.

Attachment figures are people who have had substantial input in terms of play and comfort. Bowlby used the term 'monotropy' to describe the concept of a child having one highly preferred primary attachment figure, but a hierarchy of a limited number of other attachment relationships with other people, including the second parent, grandparents, siblings and other carers.

Bowlby hypothesized that as the human infant matures and develops motor skills which allow independent activity, and the cognitive ability to mentally represent experience, the attachment relationship becomes a prototype for a mental 'working model' which potentially guides behaviour in other relevant relationships. As the ability to mentally represent relationships increases, there is less need for the child to be in physical proximity to an attachment figure. With continuing maturity beyond infancy, the capacity to 'mentalize' continues, and the child comes to understand that other people may see things from a different perspective and have different experiences (the development of 'theory of mind').

Thompson (1999) has suggested that four inter-related representational systems are encompassed within the conscious and unconscious features of working models:

- social expectations of the attributes of caregivers and partners, established in the first year and subsequently elaborated
- event representations, with general and specific memories of attachment-related experiences retained in long-term memory from the third year

- autobiographical memories by which specific events are connected conceptually because of their relation to a continuing personal narrative and developing self-understanding from the fourth year
- understanding of other people and their thoughts, motives and intentions, which allows understanding of attachment and affiliative partners and the nature of relationships (theory of mind).

Research assessment of child attachment

By the age of 1 year, a child has had experience of how each caregiver is likely to respond to his attachment needs and will have developed a characteristic strategy for dealing with each attachment relationship, in order either to maximize contact, or to minimize anxiety with a relatively unresponsive or unpredictable caregiver.

The strange situation procedure

A variety of standardized research procedures have been used to evaluate infant and child attachment behaviour with a caregiver. The longest established and best validated of these is the Ainsworth Strange Situation Procedure, valid for infants between 12 and 20 months of age. This 20-minute procedure is intended to arouse the infant's attachment needs by stressing him with two brief separations from and reunions with his caregiver. Caregiver and infant are video recorded throughout, and infant behaviour examined in a frame by frame analysis, using standardized criteria. Infant attachment behaviour is categorized in two ways: first, whether secure or insecure, and secondly the degree to which disorganization of one of the three secure or insecure categories dominates the picture. On the basis of the child's behaviour during the procedure, he is allocated a classification of secure, insecure avoidant, insecure ambivalent or disorganized in his attachment to that caregiver (see Tables 20.1 and 20.2). The strange situation assesses the quality of a relationship: a child may be secure with one parent/caregiver and insecure with the other, disorganized with one and organized with the other.

Secure/insecure behaviour is classified as secure (B), avoidant-insecure (A) or ambivalent-insecure (C). Each of these patterns represents a coherent strategy which the infant uses to deal with the infant–caregiver relationship. Table 20.1 outlines the characteristic behaviour of each secure and insecure category of children in the strange situation procedure.

The disorganized (D) category was identified later than the three secure/insecure categories. Review of 'hard to classify' infants showed that the infants' strategies for dealing with attachment needs collapsed under stress, with breakdown of a consistent strategy (Main & Solomon, 1986, 1990). The term 'disorganization' was coined to indicate disruption of one of the secure-insecure patterns. Behaviours rated as disorganized take place in the presence of the caregiver and appear to lack

Table 20.1. Infant secure and insecure behaviours in the strange situation procedure

Secure infants (B classification)
- Secure infants explore the playroom with interest, and generally show good concentration and curiousity with toys
- They may or may not be upset by the separation: being upset is not an index of security, and is more proably related to temperament
- They are pleased to see the parent upon reunion
- They show no, or almost no, anger towards the parent
- If upset by separation, the secure child will seek proximity and contact on the parent's return, will use her for comfort and return to play quickly. If not upset, the child will greet the parent warmly and will usually seek contact over the following few minutes
- About 65% infants in European and US populations are classified as secure with a parent

Avoidant–insecure infants (A classification)
- Avoidant insecure infants explore the playroom with apparent confidence, but the quality of their play generally shows lower concentration than secure children
- They typically ignore the parent's departure
- On the parent's return they show little interest or warmth, may avoid eye contact and do not seek proximity.
- When the parent returns, their attention may remain on the toys or playroom rather than the parent.
- About 25% of infants in European and US populations are classified as avoidant–insecure with a parent.

Ambivalent–insecure infants (C classification)
- Ambivalent–insecure infants are usually wary of exploration in an unfamiliar playroom, even in the presence of the parent
- They are usually very upset by separation
- Upon the parent's return, they urgently seek proximity but show both clinging and anger to the parent
- They are not readily comforted, and are slow to settle and to return to play
- About 10% of infants in European and US populations are classified as ambivalent–insecure with a parent.

an observable goal, intention or explanation, as shown in Table 20.2. Disorganized behaviours are scored on an assessment of the infant's behaviour in the presence of the caregiver throughout the procedure, and if the overall score is above a cut-off point, a primary category of D is allocated. A secondary category to designate the underlying secure / insecure disrupted pattern is always allocated: D/A, D/B, D/C.

Any child may be angry and hard to settle when tired or stressed, and an observation of angry or negative behaviour with a parent should not be misinterpreted. The classifications are valid only when assessed in the standardized procedure, and coded by researchers trained in the coding process. The strange situation procedure is thus unlikely to be of practical use in routine clinical practice. However, clinicians may observe the absence of characteristic secure behaviours of a child

Table 20.2. Indices of disorganized attachment in the strange situation

Behaviours rated as disorganized (D classification) take place *in the presence of the caregiver* during the strange situation procedure and appear to lack an observable goal, intention or explanation. They include:

- Sequential display of contradictory behaviours, such as strong attachment behaviour suddenly followed by, or together with, avoidance, freezing or dazed behaviour
- Simultaneous display of contradictory behaviours, such as strong avoidance with strong contact seeking, distress or anger
- Undirected, misdirected, incomplete and interrupted movements and expressions – for example, extensive expressions of distress/crying accompanied by simultaneous movement away from, rather than toward, the mother
- Stereotypies, asymmetrical movements, mistimed movements and anomalous postures, such as stumbling for no apparent reason and only when the parent is present.
- Freezing, stilling and slowed 'underwater' movements and expressions
- Direct indices of apprehension regarding the parent, such as hunched shoulders or fearful facial expressions
- Direct indices of disorganization and disorientation such as disoriented wandering, confused or dazed expressions or multiple rapid changes in affect
- About 14% of children in non-clinical populations show a disorganized pattern of attachment behaviour. This is always awarded with a secondary secure/insecure classification.

with a caregiver, or may note the presence of some of the indices of anxiety, seen in insecure or disorganized attachment.

Predictive validity of infant attachment research categories

Most studies report that infants classed as secure have advantage in later social competence and co-operation. While a few studies show no significant association between security and better social development, no study shows advantage to children classified as insecure or disorganized in infancy. The further from the early assessment, the less clear are associations between early secure classification and harmonious parent–child relationship. Short-term follow-up in the second year has shown that securely attached children demonstrate greater enthusiasm, compliance and positive affect, and less frustration and aggression during shared tasks with their mothers. However, it is likely that this assessment is relational: mothers of secure children were also observed to be more supportive, sensitive and helpful to the children than the mothers of children classified as insecure. Reports from age 5 to 10 find a weaker association between early security and harmonious parent–child relationship, though any advantage found is in the direction of children designated secure in infancy.

In later peer relationships, secure children also appear to be advantaged. Siblings securely attached to their parents play more harmoniously together than insecurely attached siblings, and at 3–5 years, secure children socialize more competently and are better liked by peers, though this finding has not been consistently replicated. Children secure in infancy are less dependent on teachers, and though they make less bids for attention, their claims are more likely to be successful than children who were classified as insecure. At the age of ten, some studies find that secure children are more socially competent, some find no significant association.

Studies published before the D category was identified found an inconsistent pattern of association between avoidant classification and aggressive behaviour. The discovery of the D category showed that avoidant behaviour was often displayed in combination with disorganized behaviour and the disorganized component predicted later aggression whether or not the disorganization was associated with avoidant classification. There is now evidence from both cross-sectional and longitudinal investigations that disorganized infant attachment predicts controlling, coercive or caretaking behaviour towards the parent in middle childhood. Assessment of the play of these children has found characteristic themes of catastrophes, violent fantasies, helplessness or extreme inhibition. In addition, children who show disorganized attachment with their mothers have been shown to possess fewer concrete and formal operational skills compared with children who show an organized attachment pattern. In peer relationships, disorganized children appear less competent in play quality and conflict resolution. Van IJzendoorn's metanalysis of relevant studies concluded that the predictive validity of disorganized behaviour is established in terms of problematic stress management, an elevated risk of externalizing problem behaviours at 6 years, and a tendency for disorganized infants to show dissociative behaviour later in life.

Despite the links between D classification and subsequent behavioural problems, disorganized attachment is not a diagnosis, and is not included in ICD-10 or DSM-IV. There is an asymmetrical relationship between the category and behavioural pathology. Although D behaviour in infancy is a vulnerability factor for later adverse development, some children who were D in infancy develop without significant subsequent behavioural problems. On the other hand, a large proportion of children with identified behavioural or clinical problems show the disorganized pattern of attachment in infancy, or currently show controlling/coercive/caregiving behaviour with the caregiver. In addition, children who are abused or neglected are likely to show this pattern, and may continue to do so even when good alternative care is instituted.

Parental behaviour in secure and insecure dyads

Attachment categories are validated further by correlation with observation of infant parent behaviour in the home. Ainsworth's detailed observations of infant and mother interaction (before the D category was identified) found that infants rated avoidant or ambivalent in the strange situation were more overtly angry and non-compliant and cried more at home than infants rated as secure, and that mothers of insecure infants were less sensitive to their infants' needs, more interfering with the children's activities and less accessible to their infants' bids for attention than mothers of secure infants. Most subsequent observational studies of maternal sensitivity to infant signals have confirmed Ainsworth's original observations about the association between maternal sensitivity and infant security.

Parent–infant interaction between disorganized dyads

Disorganization of a coherent attachment pattern is prominent among maltreated children, but also occurs in children who have not been abused. It has been suggested that the affect between parent and disorganized infant included fear, either infant fear of the parent, or parental fear of the infant. This leads to conflict between the infant's wish for proximity and apprehension that contact might be damaging. Home observational studies have confirmed that frightened or frightening parental behaviour is associated with infant disorganization. In later childhood, parenting of coercive/controlling children is characterized by helplessness and sometimes fear of the child, although this may alternate with parental aggression or hostility.

Parental factors associated with disorganized attachment behaviour

About 14 per cent of infants in middle class non-clinical groups, and 24 per cent in disadvantaged groups show a primary classification of disorganized attachment. Among children who have been maltreated, about 80 per cent of infants are classified as disorganized. There is evidence that disorganized attachment is associated with specific parental psychological conditions or social problems including child maltreatment, parental major depressive disorder, parental bipolar disorder, anxiety disorder, low income and chronic depression, and high parental alcohol intake.

In families where the parent has not suffered serious mental illness or social disadvantage, infant D classification is associated with parental experience of trauma or loss of an attachment figure which is unresolved, as measured by the adult attachment interview.

Short-term stability of attachment categories

Stability of three-way (secure/insecure) classification has been found to be between 50 per cent and 96 per cent with assessments between 2 and 6 months apart. In general, higher stability is found in more socially advantaged samples, where circumstances are likely to be stable. Meta-analysis of the D classification of nine samples with gaps between 2 and 60 months estimated stability of D classification to be strong ($r = 0.34$).

Attachment beyond infancy

Attachment to particular others is a human need throughout life and is not confined to infancy. The essential feature of a secure attachment is that the other has an ability to recognize and respond appropriately to the individual's state of mind and emotional needs. Children at all stages form new and continuing attachments, and adults are often deeply attached to a partner and certain other adults. Children's ability to form new attachments is important for children who are placed in long-term fostering or who are adopted. Adoption from adverse circumstances to loving families is usually highly successful during the first four years of life (although extreme deprivation may have enduring effects after 2 years). Though children who have been subjected to ill treatment, deprivation or institutional rearing beyond four years of age may have some continuing social difficulties, many late adoptions are successful, and certainly have better outcome than either continuing institutional care or a return to a biological family where care is poor.

Can infant temperament account for infant secure/insecure behaviour?

The weight of evidence indicates that attachment patterns relate mainly to parental mental representations of attachment and by implication to aspects of parental behaviour towards the infant, rather than to infant temperament. First, attachment behaviour has been found repeatedly to be specific to a relationship, so that a child may be secure with one parent and insecure or disorganized with the other. Secondly, the infant's attachment classification with a parent at 12 months can be predicted with about 75 per cent confidence during the pregnancy from evaluation of the parent's representation of attachment using the adult attachment interview. Thirdly, the attachment behaviour with the primary caregiver in infancy is more predictive of subsequent psycho-social development than that with other caregivers, even when the caregiver is not biologically related. Finally, measures of infant temperament have predicted distress in response to separation, but have not predicted whether the infant is secure or insecure.

Research assessment of attachment in older children

Modifications of the strange situation procedure have been developed for use with pre-school children for whom the classifications are secure, insecure avoidant, insecure ambivalent and controlling/caregiving with the caregiver. These later assessments are less well validated than the strange situation.

Disorders of attachment

ICD 10 includes two categories of Disorder of Attachment: Reactive Attachment Disorder (RAD) and Disinhibited Attachment Disorder (DAD). Criteria for

Table 20.3. Diagnostic guidelines for attachment disorder, ICD-10

Reactive attachment disorder of childhood
1. An abnormal pattern of relationship with caregivers
2. Develops before the age of 5 years
3. Involves maladaptive features not ordinarily seen in normal children
4. Persistent, yet reactive to sufficiently marked changes in patterns of rearing

Young children show strongly contradictory social responses that may be evident at parting or reunion. Infants may respond to caregivers with a mixture of approach, avoidance and resistance to comforting. There may be apparent misery, lack of emotional responsiveness, withdrawal reactions and/or aggressive responses to their own or others' distress. Fearfulness and hypervigilance may occur. Though most children show interest in peer interactions, social play is impeded by negative emotional responses. This disorder may be accompanied by failure to thrive, and impaired physical growth, which should be coded according to the appropriate somatic category.

Disinhibited attachment disorder of childhood
1. Unusual degree of diffuseness in selective attachments during the first 5 years
2. And general clinging behaviour in infancy
3. And/or indiscriminately friendly, attention-seeking behaviour in early or middle childhood
4. Usually difficulty in forming close peer relationships
5. May be associated emotional or behavioural disturbance
6. In most cases a clear history of rearing in the first years that involved marked discontinuities in caregivers or multiple changes in family placements

attachment disorders are similar in DSM-IV, though nomenclature is slightly different. ICD-10 category Reactive Attachment Disorder is equivalent to DSM-IV's RAD Inhibited Type, and ICD-10 category Disinhibited Attachment Disorder is equivalent to DSM-IV's RAD Disinhibited Type. The diagnostic guidelines for ICD-10 diagnoses are outlined in Table 20.3, and for DSM-IV in Table 20.4.

Problems with current ICD and DMS nosology

1. The criteria for ICD and DSM attachment disorder categories focus on social relationships in general, rather than on the attachment relationship and its specific consequences.
2. Attachment disorders have been defined narrowly as associated with severe deprivation and maltreatment. It has been suggested that the disorders as presently described might be more accurately designated 'maltreatment disorders'. It is possible for a child to have a highly unsatisfactory but stable relationship with a caregiver who does not neglect or overtly maltreat the child.
3. Attachment and attachment disorders are by their nature relational and do not fit comfortably into nosological systems that characterize the disorder as person centred.

Table 20.4. Diagnostic guidelines for attachment disorder, DSM-IV

Reactive attachment disorder of infancy or early childhood

A. Markedly disturbed and developmentally inappropriate social relatedness in most contexts, beginning before age 5 years, as evidenced by either (1) or (2)

    (1) Inhibited type.   Persistent failure to initiate or respond in a developmentally appropriate fashion to most social interactions, as manifest by excessively inhibited, hypervigilant, or highly ambivalent and contradictory responses (e.g. the child may respond to caregivers with a mixture of approach, avoidance, and resistance to comforting, or may exhibit frozen watchfulness).

    (2) Disinhibited type.   Diffuse attachments as manifest by indiscriminate sociability with marked inability to exhibit appropriate selective attachments (e.g. excessive familiarity with relative strangers or lack of selectivity in choice of attachment figures).

B. The disturbance in Criterion A is not accounted for solely by developmental delay (as in mental retardation) and does not meet criteria for a pervasive developmental disorder.

C. Pathogenic care as evidenced by at least one of the following:

    (1) persistent disregard of the child's basic emotional needs for comfort, stimulation, and affection

    (2) persistent disregard of the child's basic physical needs

    (3) repeated changes of primary caregiver that prevent formation of stable attachments (e.g. frequent changes in foster care)

D. There is a presumption that the care in Criterion C is responsible for the disturbed behaviour in Criterion A.

4. There is lack of clarity in criteria regarding the severity of the symptoms included in RAD and in the co-morbidity of attachment difficulties with other disorders.

5. The validity of the age cut of 5 years has not been demonstrated.

6. There is no standardized or widely accepted protocol to validate the diagnosis. Criteria are needed to evaluate severity as well as quality of the child's interactions with different people and across different settings.

Validation of the ICD and DSM categories of attachment disorder

Despite the criticism of the ICD-10 and DSM-IV criteria, the validity of the two diagnostic categories, inhibited/emotionally withdrawn and disinhibited/indiscriminate patterns, has been demonstrated using DSM-IV criteria to show that these diagnoses can be reliably identified and there is some preliminary evidence for their validity.

Alternative nosology

A further nosology of attachment disorders that encompasses a more comprehensive range of the problems of attachment seen in clinical practice is outlined in Table 20.5. This divides attachment disorders into three broad categories:

Table 20.5. Alternative nosology of attachment disorders (Zeanah, Mammen, and Lieberman, 1993)

Disorders of non–attachment

Infants with a disorder of non-attachment do not show reliable preference for a caregiver

The predominant affect may range from emotional withdrawal to indiscriminate sociability

Two subtypes can be distinguished:

Type I
- Emotional withdrawal
- Constriction of affect
- Little evidence of spontaneous pleasure either in social interaction or in exploration of the environment

Type II
- Indiscriminate sociability
- Shallow affect
- Overly bright smiles, phoney laughter
- Superficial expressions of affection
- Separation protest absent or expressed in relation to many people including strangers

Disorders of non-attachment are seen in institutionalized children, and in children who have experienced frequent moves of care and mediocre foster care

Disordered attachments

The child shows a clear preference for a caregiver

The preference is characterized by intense and pervasive conflict due to anger, fear, anxiety of other negative emotions

Negative emotions may not be expressed directly, but masked by defences such as avoidance, transformation of affect, fighting, inhibition, and precocious competence in self-care

When children become capable of autonomous locomotion from about 10 months, disordered attachments tend to be manifested in distortions of secure base behaviour. There are pronounced and persistent alterations in the balance between attachment and exploratory behaviours, prompted by the child's fear of the mother or uncertainty about her availability. Three categories are described

Disordered attachment with inhibition
- Distinguished from non-attachment by the clear preference for the attachment figure
- Either inordinately lengthy periods of proximity and contact, or pronounced avoidance of the attachment figure and hypervigilance
- Marked curtailment of exploration
- Does not approach, touch or manipulate objects
- Social interaction with unfamiliar persons absent or perfunctory
- Restriction of affect, predominance of sober affect tinged with hypervigilance and fear

Disordered attachment with self-endangerment
- Reckless, accident prone and aggressive behaviours in the context of attachment
- Consistent failure to use mother for social monitoring

Table 20.5. (cont.)

- In unfamiliar settings, child darts from mother, repeatedly moves away without tracking mother's whereabouts, fails to heed mother's calls
- When hurt, tends to ignore or rebuff mother
- Aggression may be turned to self, with hitting, biting or headbanging
- Toddlers who show this pattern also manifest anxiety: separation protest, hypervigilance alternating with darting away, prolonged temper tantrums, etc.

Disordered attachment with role reversal
- Precocious competence in self-care
- Toddlers may seem unusually competent in keeping track of parent and restoring proximity
- Excessively solicitous to caregiver
- Sensitive to caregiver's mood, age inappropriate amounts of caregiving behaviour
- May alternat with angry, punitive or controlling behaviour

Disrupted attachment disorder: bereavement/grief reaction
This category is based on the premise that loss of the primary attachment figure is inherently pathogenic in infancy because the child does not yet have the cognitive and emotional resources to cope adaptively with the loss. Severe and prolonged distress is not inevitable, especially if a substitute primary attachment figure is available.

Reactions may include:
- Crying, calling and searching for the absent attachment figure
- Refusal to accept alternative comfort
- Emotional withdrawal
- Lethargy, sad facial expression and lack of interest in age appropriate activities
- Eating and sleeping may be disrupted
- There may be regression in developmental milestones, e.g. reverting to baby-talk
- There may be either apparent indifference or extreme sensitivity to reminders of the absent figure

1. Disorders of non-attachment in children who lack an attachment figure
2. Disordered attachment in children who have an attachment figure
3. Disrupted attachment of children who have lost an attachment figure

This nosology has the considerable advantage in that it derives from the reality of the situations that will be seen by the clinician and gives some meaning to the child's behaviour. Both this classification system and the conventional ones will recognize the attachment problems of a child who has never had opportunity to form a stable attachment. However, this extends the classification of the 'reactive attachment disorder' to include children who may not have been severely maltreated, but whose primary attachments are clearly poor. This alternative nosology allows classification of relationships according to quality, type and degree of psychopathology, and additionally, it is congruent with current research on attachment.

Reactive attachment disorder (RAD) (ICD-10)

Definition and classification (ICD-10)

RAD is characterized by persistent abnormalities in child's pattern of social relationships, which are associated with emotional disturbances and reactive to changes in environmental circumstances.

Main features:

- persistent, abnormal pattern of relationships with caregivers
- develops before 5 years
- strongly contradictory or ambivalent social responses to caregivers
- arises in context of severe parental neglect or ill treatment.

Epidemiology

Data are not available to determine prevalence or incidence of RAD: there are no epidemiological studies that examine the prevalence, incidence or natural course of RAD. Such information as we have at present is based on clinical description of cases. The lack of data has been suggested to be due to changes in diagnostic criteria and to lack of familiarity with the disorder among clinicians. Concern has been expressed that the condition is over-diagnosed and may be used loosely as a blanket term to describe almost any disordered behaviour shown by children who have been maltreated or neglected. It has been proposed that estimates of prevalence can be derived from available statistics on child maltreatment. However, there are two problems in doing this. First, data on child abuse is itself not very reliable; secondly some maltreated children do not show behavioural problems, either RAD or other, and behaviour problems are not specific to RAD.

Clinical picture

Main features and symptoms

The cluster of behaviours is common in children who have suffered neglect and abuse of various kinds. The overall clinical picture is one of a fearful attitude to adults, with withdrawal from contact, and socially maladaptive behaviours which extend across different social situations, and there is an overall inhibition of the attachment system at times when attachment behaviours are ordinarily activated.

Characteristically the child shows a picture of inhibition, fear and hypervigilance, sometimes described as 'frozen watchfulness', which does not respond to comforting from the caregiver or others. There is marked emotional disturbance which is evident as apathy, misery, lack of emotional responsiveness and withdrawal reactions, such as huddling on the floor.

There are strongly contradictory social responses that may be most evident at times of parting and reunions. The child may approach the caregiver with averted gaze, look away strongly while being held, or respond to the caregiver with a mixture of approach and avoidance. Though the child may show interest in peers, social play is inhibited by negative emotional responses, and the child may show aggression in the face of their own or others' distress. Some children show a failure to thrive physically, and impaired physical growth.

Differential diagnosis

The condition should be differentiated from pervasive developmental disorders (PDD).

1. RAD is strongly associated with previous abusive or neglectful care, while PDD is not.
2. The abnormal pattern of social responsiveness seen in children with RAD remits to a considerable extent if they are placed in a nurturing adoptive or long-term foster family. This does not happen in children with PDD.
3. Though children with RAD may show impaired language development, they do not show the abnormal qualities of communication characteristic of autism.
4. Autistic children, but not children with RAD, frequently have persistent and severe cognitive deficits that do not respond significantly to environmental change.
5. Persistently restricted, repetitive and stereotyped patterns of behaviour, interests and activities are a feature of childhood autism, but not RAD.

Co-morbidity

Children who have suffered severe abuse or neglect may show a range of symptoms, including autistic-like patterns and attention-hyperactivity, and disinhibited social behaviours, in addition to the symptom cluster characteristic of inhibited reactive attachment disorder. This lack of specificity invites the question of whether this can be considered a specific disorder of attachment, or whether another explanation of the multiple problems presented by these children might be more useful.

Relationship between RAD and disorganized attachment

Although the diagnosis of RAD encompasses more than the relationship with caregivers or attachment figures, there are striking similarities in the criteria for disorganized attachment with a caregiver and the relationship with the caregiver which is observed in RAD. The relationship is skew: and many children who show some signs of disorganization of attachment are not clinically disturbed, while it is probable that all who fulfil the criteria for RAD will be classified as disorganized with one or both parents. We think it likely that D behaviour is encompassed in the larger picture of RAD.

Aetiology

Social factors

A history of ill-treatment or neglect is usual when a diagnosis of RAD is made.

Familial factors

The understanding of how infant disorganization of attachment develops may help illuminate the process by which a child develops the behaviours characteristic of RAD. Although the disorganized category is a research one, most maltreated children fall into this group. In addition, the specific behaviours which lead to a classification as disorganized are similar to those used to allocate the diagnosis of RAD in a clinical setting, and a child who shows fear and marked approach-avoidance to the caregiver is likely to fall into both classifications. An assumption that there is overlap between the categories may help us understand the phenomena observed in RAD.

Soon after the D category was identified, researchers noted that fear was often observable between parent and child when the relationship was disorganized. We would expect that a child who has been abused by its parent will show fear. For this child, having the same person as a source of protection and of threat is inherently confusing, and so a simultaneous show of approach and avoidance is understandable. However, it is more surprising to find that some mothers show fear and helpless behaviour with the child. Mothers who have themselves suffered abuse at the hands of an attachment figure, or who have suffered the traumatic loss of an attachment figure, and who are unresolved in relation to the abuse or loss are more likely to have a child who shows disorganization of attachment. It is plausible that the child evokes attachment related thoughts or memories, that this causes the mother to show unexplained fear, and that this unexplained state is inherently frightening to the child.

A psychodynamic explanation is that the mother has often herself been severely deprived, and that caring for a vulnerable child stimulates her own unmet needs and related anger, which she cannot cope with, but which she attributes to her child. She then feels helpless to meet the enormous need that she perceives, and fearful that the child will retaliate when she fails. The child has a confusing experience of his ordinary need for care being perceived as demanding and aggressive, and of his being seen as a source of fear for his mother.

Biological factors

Although the quality of care is the strongest aetiological factor in the development of attachment disorders, biological factors may be important either in vulnerability to development of adverse attachment patterns, or in maintaining problem behaviours.

1. There is some association between irritability in the neonatal period and later insecurity, though this is modified by quality of social resources for the family. However, it suggests that infant characteristics may potentiate inadequate caregiving when caregivers themselves are also stressed.

2. Research in non-human primates and in rats shows that severe deprivation in the early months of life may have permanent effects on the developing brain, and that affect regulation in particular may be impaired in these animals. Infant monkeys subjected to prolonged isolation show severe difficulty in social behaviours, and depressive-like reactions to later isolation.

3. Salivary cortisol levels appear to be higher in disorganized infants than in other infants during and after the strange situation procedure. It has been suggested that D infants are repeatedly subjected to a problem which they cannot solve (whether to approach or avoid the caregiver) and thus lack an effective strategy to deal with stress, which results in higher and more enduring levels of stress hormones.

Disinhibited attachment disorder (ICD-10)

Definition and classification

DAD is generally seen only in children who have had extended periods of institutional care or who have been in multiple foster placements. It is characterized by a pattern of forming multiple, shallow relationships, and corresponding difficulty in discriminating between caregivers who offer stable support and affection and those with whom the relationship is relatively superficial.

Main features

- unusual degree of diffuseness in selective attachments during the first 5 years
- generally clinging behaviour in infancy
- and/or indiscriminately friendly, attention seeking behaviour in early or middle childhood
- usually difficulty in forming close peer relationships
- may be associated emotional or behavioural disturbance
- history of institutional rearing and/or frequent changes of caregiver.

Epidemiology

As with RAD (inhibited/withdrawn type) there are a lack of systematic data on the prevalence of the disorder as defined by the ICD-10 and DSM-IV. There are some data, however, describing the socially diffuse and disinhibited behaviours shown by children who have been institutionalized. This suggests that over a third of young children in long-term placements in institutions show the indiscriminate pattern of social behaviour that is characteristic of DAD.

Longitudinal research with children adopted from Romanian orphanages into families in the UK and Canada, show that there is marked improvement among previously institutionalized children, but that even after several years have elapsed, a small number of children (4% in the UK study) show a significant degree of indiscriminate sociability, and a further 15 per cent show mild signs at some time. In both studies, vulnerability to the symptoms of DAD was related to the length of time that the child had spent in the institution.

An earlier longitudinal study of children adopted from institutions before 4 years, showed that at age 16, though overly friendly behaviour had lessened, some children still showed significant peer-relationship problems. These included being adult-orientated, having more difficulties in peer relations, not having a best friend, not turning to peers for support and being less selective in choosing friends. These findings were strong enough to suggest a kind of ex-institutional syndrome of problematic peer relatedness.

Clinical picture

There is over-arousal of attachment behaviour with little discrimination, resulting in multiple superficial relationships. This indiscriminate behaviour leads to a lack of selectivity in choosing those from whom to seek comfort, support and nurturance. The over-friendliness with relatively unfamiliar adults has been designated 'indiscriminate sociability'. The child may make shallow attachments to adults or peers, but will drop the relationship when the 'attachment figure' disappoints. Caregivers may describe their own subjective sense that the child is only superficially attached to them.

Main features and symptoms

This pattern of behaviours arises in the first 5 years of life, and once established, shows a tendency to persist. In early childhood the child usually shows clinging, and diffuse, non-selectively focused attachment behaviour. By around 4 years, the diffuse attachments remain but clinging is replaced by attention-seeking and by indiscriminately friendly behaviour.

In middle and later childhood, children whose care situation has improved may have developed selective attachments, but may continue to show attention-seeking behaviour, and may have continuing difficulties with peer interaction.

Differential diagnosis

The condition should be differentiated from attention deficit hyperactivity disorder (ADHD), from Asperger syndrome and hospitalism in children.

Children with a diagnosis of ADHD may show disinhibition in social relationships and attention-seeking behaviours which may be confused with the over-
friendly and attention-seeking of children with DAD. However, children with
ADHD also show impaired attention, restlessness and impulsive actions which
are not characteristic of DAD.

Children suffering from Asperger syndrome show a lack of sensitivity to social
cues and inappropriate responses to the emotions of others, which must be differentiated from the social disinhibition of DAD. Generally, however, children with
Asperger syndrome are not over-friendly and do not demonstrate attention-seeking
behaviour. In addition, they do not have either the history of deprivation characteristic of the attachment disorders, nor a history of early clinging behaviour.

Hospitalism occurs in children who experience the stress life event of an illness
requiring hospital treatment, and who in this context may be liable to attention-
seeking and aggressive behaviours. The problem is specific to the stress of being in
hospital, and is usually distinguished easily from the longer-standing problem of
DAD.

Co-morbidity

Children who have experienced institutionalization show a range of symptoms,
including autistic-like patterns and attention-hyperactivity, and may simultaneously show symptoms of reactive attachment disorder.

Aetiology

As DAD was first identified in institutionalized children, it has been assumed that
institutional rearing is a cause of the syndrome. Early researchers, including Bowlby,
suspected that the problem was in part a lack of personal interest from caregivers,
and also a lack of continuity of care. Subsequent findings have questioned the
latter supposition, as the syndrome is found even in institutions where high staff
turnover is not a problem, but the assumption of deprivation inherent in a lack of
specific interest in the child remains. In poorly staffed institutions this lack may be
augmented by a limited quantity of attention, as well as impersonal quality.

Assessment of attachment disorders

History taking may be compromised by the fact that the child may not be brought
for assessment by a caregiver who has known him over a long period, either because
he has been removed from the care of maltreating parents, or because he is in the
care of foster or adoptive parents having previously been in long term placement
in an institution. Children with disinhibited attachment disorder are unlikely to
be brought for assessment and treatment until placed in long-term foster care or

adopted, when the problem of forming attachment to the new parents becomes a relevant issue.

Diagnosis and assessment

Assessment is based on a focused history and a systematic observation of child–caregiver interaction. A detailed history will allow the clinician to identify obstacles to the development of normal attachment patterns, and may include physical or emotional unavailability of caregivers because of illness or addiction, or extended separation for any reason.

It is also important to exclude other causes which might account for the reported behaviours, in particular, any developmental disability. History taking may be compromised by the fact that the child may not be brought for assessment by a caregiver who has known him over a long period. A history of maltreatment or neglect is usual, though not a requirement for the ICD-10 diagnosis.

If the child can be seen with his usual caregiver, then the following behaviours should be observed and evaluated:

- the style of showing affection and seeking comfort from the caregiver: a lack of affectionate exchange between child and caregiver is cause for concern
- the degree of co-operation between child and caregiver
- inability to seek support from the caregiver
- excessive dependence and clinging to the caregiver
- overt fear or apprehension towards the caregiver
- failure to check back or to use the caregiver as a secure exploratory base.

Other sources of information

Other information will usually be collected:

- review of information held in files and other records
- discussions with professionals who have already met the family
- interviews with parents and children
- direct observations of parents and children.

Examination of files

Files may contain a great deal of information, but this is insufficient to establish a diagnosis. Information from files needs to be interpreted, looking for patterns in behaviour, relationships, and parenting. A history of abuse or neglect, or critical incidents such as illnesses, injuries and accidents should be noted. Factors relating to the parents, including absences from home, drug or alcohol misuse, mental or physical illness should be noted. The parents' own childhood experiences and any history of abuse or disruption during childhood may be relevant.

Information from other agencies

Many agencies may become involved with certain families, and it is important that there is adequate communication between professionals in the different agencies. Close liaison and face-to-face meetings between professionals will usually help in deciding how to coordinate care of the child and family. Though confidentiality and disclosure must be respected, where a child may be at risk, appropriate disclosures are sanctioned.

Interviews

The parents' or caregivers' view of the problem, and of factors which may have contributed to difficulties with the child are important. The parents' current situation and family and childhood history may be relevant and useful. Parents should be asked about their expectations of themselves as parents, and their expectations of their child. Attitudes to discipline may be important in families where abuse is suspected. Children should be interviewed in an age-appropriate manner, listening to what they say and exploring their experiences and feelings.

Observations of parents and children

Observation includes assessment of the home and physical environment, of both verbal and non-verbal behaviours of parents and children at home, and of parental consistency, sensitivity and availability. It is often useful to observe children in other settings such as school. There should be careful distinction between behaviour actually observed, and conclusions that the observer draws from those observations.

Treatment of attachment disorders

Treatment within the family

Interventions within the family seek to modify the quality of interaction between children and their social environment, which includes parents, family, peers and other adults.

A number of common features run through all interventions of children who show signs of disordered attachment. These include:

- establishing a therapeutic alliance with a child and with parents, with a sympathetic, non-blaming approach to understanding the family difficulties
- consideration of the expectations or internal working models that parents use in their interactions with their children
- efforts to increase the sensitivity, availability and responsiveness of parents
- efforts to increase self-esteem, social empathy, reflectiveness, and a sense of efficacy of parents.

Parent focused interventions

These are intended to reduce parental stress, improve self-esteem and allow parents to be more available and responsive to their children's needs. Parents are more likely to cooperate if they feel that the practitioner has an empathic understanding of their views, and this forms the basis for establishing a therapeutic alliance.

- Practical help with finance, housing, advocacy or other advice may be essential for some families
- Training in generic problem solving skills
- On-going support from community and self-help groups
- Some couples may benefit from joint counselling to improve their sensitivity and responsiveness to each other.

Child focused interventions

The aim of child focused interventions:

- to raise children's self-esteem
- to increase their competence socially, emotionally and behaviourally
- to improve their emotional understanding of themselves and of others.

Techniques include play therapy, music therapy, psychotherapy, including cognitive behaviour therapy, drama therapy and group work. Children may benefit from opportunities to recognize and name feelings, think about motivations and actions, to reflect on past and present relationships, and to consider the interactions between relationships, feelings and behaviours. For example, self-esteem may be improved when a child successfully accomplishes a task, perhaps one involving their attachment figure.

A child's ability to affect and influence the world around them, to believe that they can make a difference and they have some control over what happens increases their sense of self-efficacy, a known resilience factor. Professionals should be aware of places and people who could potentially provide children with such positive experiences. Success at school in sports, music and practical skills as well as academic matters is likely to increase self-efficacy. Children who are given or assume responsibility for important and valued activities at home or school have better outcomes. However, children who have been neglected and maltreated may avoid, resist, or feel anxious about new opportunities. Interventions may be aimed at helping them recognize such opportunities, and encourage them where they might normally refuse. Work with teachers, youth workers, school teachers and more skilled foster carers may be of help. Self-reflection, positive cognitive processing, metacognition and the ability to accept the reality of negative experiences may all act as protective mechanisms.

Parent–child interaction

Techniques may be directly aimed at the parent–child interactions, and are intended to help parents develop more effective parenting skills. These may include:

- changing parental perceptions and attributions of the children's behaviours
- learning to identify and respond to the child's needs for comfort, play and discipline appropriate to his age
- learning to be consistent and effective in limit-setting
- practising all these behaviours with the help of a therapist.

Many of the techniques used with parents and children separately may be used when both children and parents are present.

Pharmacological treatments

There is little place for pharmacological treatment of children who show disorder of attachment. However, if a parent or caregiver is depressed or otherwise suffering from mental illness, assessment and appropriate treatment may be instigated.

Removal from parental care

It is sometimes necessary to remove children from high-risk environments and place them in children's homes or other residential accommodation, or with foster-carers or adoptive parents. A parent may be unable to care for the child even with community support, because of mental illness, disability or substance misuse, a child may be in danger because of continuing physical or sexual abuse, or the parent may be absent, in hospital or prison, with no alternative care available.

In institutions, the development of a preferred attachment may be facilitated by providing a primary attachment figure for each child, in an attempt to minimize or prevent attachment difficulties/disorders. However, children raised even in well staffed institutions remain vulnerable to having greater difficulty with social relationships than home reared children.

Outcome

Non-clinical populations

Evidence of attachment insecurity in the absence of problem behaviours does not constitute a diagnosis, and it should be remembered that there is flexibility in attachment behaviour during childhood. Insecure, and even disorganized, attachment does not inevitably predict problems in development, and the most that might be claimed is that disorganization of attachment is a vulnerability factor. However, it has been shown that an educational booklet together with video feedback sessions is effective in improving maternal sensitivity in insecure dyads.

Family interventions

There is evidence from case studies that family interventions improve the quality of parent–child interaction. However, there is a lack of good quality systematic research into the course, epidemiology and response to treatment of attachment disorders within the family.

Adoption

Children who show the symptoms of RAD, if placed in good quality adoptive families are usually subsequently able to establish secure (or non-pathological insecure) relationships with their caregivers. Those who remain in institutional care, or who are returned to their biological parents, unless there is considerable change in family circumstances, are unlikely to do so. Recent adoptions of Romanian orphans who had spent several years in poor quality institutions, and who were placed in adoptive families in the UK and Canada have shown that vulnerability to disinhibited behaviours after adoption is in linear relationship with time spent in the institution.

While adoption before the age of 4 years is usually successful, adoption of older children has a higher risk of breakdown. Many of these children have experienced very poor quality care, and exhibit highly challenging behaviour with their adoptive families. While 2 per cent of children in the US are adopted, over a third of children in residential treatment centres are adopted children. Adopted children are twice as likely to display psychosocial problems later in life and two to three times more likely to develop conduct disorders than non-adopted children. This outcome is improved if support and training is provided for the adoptive family.

SUGGESTED READING

N. W. Boris & C. H. Zeanah, Clinical disturbances of attachment in infancy and early childhood. *Current Opinion in Pediatrics*, **10** (4) (1998), 365–8.

R. F. Hanson & E. G. Spratt, Reactive attachment disorder: what we know about the disorder and implications for treatment, *Child Maltreatment*, **5** (2) (2000), 137–45.

D. A. Hughes, Adopting children with attachment problems. *Child Welfare*, **78** (5) (1999), 541–60.

J. Cassidy & P. Shaver (eds.), *Handbook of Attachment*. (New York: Guilford Press, 1999).

A. F. Lieberman & C. H. Zeanah, Disorders of attachment in infancy. *Child and Adolescent Psychiatric Clinics of North America*, **3** (3) (1995), 571–87.

T. G. O'Connor, M. Rutter & the English and Romanian Adoptees Study team. Attachment disorder behaviour following early severe deprivation: extension and longitudinal follow-up. *Journal of the American Academy of Child and Adolescent Psychiatry*, **39** (6) (2000), 703–12.

J. Robertson & J. Robertson, *Young Children in Brief Separations*. (Film series). (London: Tavistock Institute of Human Relations, 1967–72).

M. Rutter & L. A. Sroufe, Developmental psychopathology: concepts and challenges. *Development and Psychopathology*, **12** (3) (2000), 265–96.

R. A. Thompson, Early attachment and later development. In *Handbook of Attachment*, ed. J. Cassidy & P. Shaver (New York: Guilford Press, 1999), pp. 287–318.

B. Tizard, *Adoption: A Second Chance.* (London: Open Books, 1977).

M. H. Van IJzendoorn, C. Schuengel & M. J. Bakermans-Kranenburg, Disorganized attachment in early childhood: meta-analysis of precursors, concomitants and sequelae. *Development and Psychopathology*, **11** (1999), 225–49.

S. L. Wilson, Attachment disorders: review and current status. *Journal of Psychology*, **135** (1) (2001), 37–51.

C. Zeanah, O. K. Mammen & A. F. Lieberman, Disorders of attachment. In *Handbook of Infant Mental Health*, ed. C. Zeanah (New York: Guilford Press, 1993), pp. 332–49.

C. H. Zeanah, Disturbances of attachment in young children adopted from institutions. *Journal of Developmental & Behavioral Pediatrics*, **21** (3) (2000), 230–6.

21

Tic disorders

Aribert Rothenberger and Tobias Banaschewski

Department of Child and Adolescent Psychiatry, University of Göttingen, Germany

Introduction

Usually, tic disorders have their onset around school entry and in many cases they develop into a complex neuropsychiatric disorder with a high variety of associated problems. Only about 15 per cent of cases remain with their tics only. On the other hand, there is a tendency of spontaneous remission of tics after adolescence. Hence, refined developmental psychopathological knowledge is necessary to diagnose and treat the patients in an adequate manner.

The interaction of tic expression with stress sensitivity and tic awareness is another point of practical relevance. Although the background of tic disorders has been the subject of ignorance and speculations for at least the past 300 years, today we accept genetic, neurodynamic and psychological factors as well as their interplay. All of these have to be assessed in each individual case concerning tic control.

Finally, knowledge of the short-term and long-term spontaneous temporal patterning of tics is important for the clinician, because it informs decisions about when to initiate anti-tic interventions, when to change drugs and when to be patient and simply provide close monitoring and support to the family to cope with the psychosocial problems.

Definition and classification

The main features of tic disorders are:
- motor and/or vocal tics (see Table 21.1)
- begin in proximal areas (head, face, neck)
- occurrence of tics many times a day (every day or intermittently; waxing and waning)
- duration of tics from 4 weeks to more than 1 year

A Clinician's Handbook of Child and Adolescent Psychiatry, ed. Christopher Gillberg,
Richard Harrington and Hans-Christoph Steinhausen. Published by Cambridge University Press.
© Cambridge University Press 2005.

Table 21.1. Examples for simple and complex motor and vocal tics

Tic symptom dimensions	Examples
Simple motor tics Sudden, brief, meaningless movements	Eye blinking, eye movements, grimacing, nose twitching, mouth movements, lip pouting, head jerks, shoulder shrugs, head jerks, abdominal tensing, kicks, finger movements, jaw snaps, rapid jerking of any part of the body
Complex motor tics Slower, longer, more 'purposeful' movements	Sustained 'looks', facial gestures, biting, touching objects or self, thrusting arms, throwing, banging, gestures with hands, gyrating and bending, dystonic postures, copropraxia (obscene gestures)
Simple phonic tics Sudden, meaningless sounds or noises	Throat clearing, coughing, sniffling, spitting, screeching, barking, grunting, gurgling, clacking, hissing, sucking, animal noises and countless other sounds
Complex phonic tics Sudden, more 'meaningful' utterances	Syllables, words, phrases, or statements such as 'Shut up', 'Stop that', 'Oh, okay', 'I've got to', 'Honey', 'What makes me do this?' 'How about it?' or 'Now you've seen it'; speech atypicalities (usually in rhythms, tone, accents, or intensity of speech); echo phenomena, including immediate repetition of one's own speech (palillalia) or another person's words or phrases (echolalia); and coprolalia (obscene, inappropriate, and aggressive words and statements)

Adapted from Leckman, J. F., King, R. A. & Cohen, D. J. Tics and tic disorders. In: Leckman *et al.*, eds. *Tourette's Syndrome – Tics, Obsessions, Compulsions: Developmental Psychopathology and Clinical Care.* New York: John Wiley, 1998; 23–42.

- suppressibility of some tics for a short period of time (after the age of 10 years)
- premonitory sensorimotor sensations before tics (after the age of 10 years)
- presence of tics also during sleep.

The definition of tics, their occurrence and duration as well as the sub-categories are shared by ICD-10 and DSM-IV (see Table 21.2 and 21.3). ICD-10 has an additional category ('other tic disorders'; F 95.8) and no clear criterion for onset. Since both major classification systems are about 10 years old, recent important main features on suppressibility, tic awareness and tics during sleep are either not mentioned or are referred to in a way that does not tally with the current knowledge base.

Epidemiology

Prevalence and incidence rates

Based on the analysis of different community surveys within the last 15 years, tics can be observed in about 10 per cent of elementary school children and in about

Table 21.2. Classification of tic disorders according to ICD-10

Diagnose	Criteria	ICD-10
Transient tic disorder	Duration of tics not longer than 10 months	F 95.0
Chronic motor or vocal tic disorder	Chronic motor *or* vocal tics for a period of more than one year	F 95.1
Tourette syndrome	Chronic motor *and* vocal tics for a period of more than one year	F 95.2
Other or not specified tic disorder	Does not fulfil the criteria of the other mentioned tic disorders	F 95.8/F 95.9

4–18 per cent of adolescents. The variability depends on the sample and the procedure chosen. Chronic tic disorders have a prevalence rate of about 3–4 per cent.

For Tourette syndrome (TS), prevalence rate findings seem to converge around
1 per cent (range: 0.05–3%). In children and adolescents the reported frequency
is clearly higher compared to adults. This reflects the tendency of a spontaneous
remission of symptoms. The rate for spontaneous remission (seen over years) is
about 50–70 per cent for simple/multiple tics, for TS between 3 and 40 per cent.
Follow-up studies of TS suggest that approximately one-third of children with TS
will be symptom free as adults. Another one-third will have only mild symptom
severity that does not require clinical attention. Adults who do have symptoms
severe enough to be referred (remember: there is an under reporting and
under-awareness even for severe tics in adults!) for clinical treatment therefore
are unusual representatives of all subjects who have lifetime diagnosis of TS.

Sex ratio and ethnicity

With a rate of 3–4.5:1, males are predominantly affected by tic disorders. There are
no differences in prevalence and incidence rates or for gender relationship in relation
to cultural and ethnical influences, but there are gender differences in relationship
to associated psychopathology. Females more often show self-injurious behaviour,
trichotillomania and sometimes more obsessive-compulsive behaviour in general,
while in males externalizing behaviour can be seen more often.

Implications for clinical practice

Tic disorders are more common in school children than was previously accepted.
The cases seen in the community may be milder in intensity and associated with a
less severe but qualitatively similar co-morbid psychopathology compared to young
people with tic disorders seen in clinics. Despite this, tic disorders may be a source of
stigma and decreased quality of life for the family. Thus, there is a need for vigilance

Table 21.3. Classification of tic disorders according to DSM-IV

I. Diagnostic criteria for Tourette disorder (DSM-IV 307.23)
   A. Both multiple motor and one or more vocal tics have been present at some time during the illness, although not necessarily concurrently.
   B. The tics occur many times a day (usually in bouts), nearly every day or intermittently throughout a period of more than 1 year; and during this period, there was never a tic-free period of more than 3 consecutive months.
   C. The disturbance causes marked distress or significant impairment in social, occupational, or other areas of functioning.
   D. Onset before age 18.
   E. The disturbance is not caused by the direct physiological effects of a substance (e.g. stimulants) or a general medical condition (e.g. Huntington's chorea or post-viral encephalitis).

II. Diagnostic criteria for chronic motor or vocal tic disorder (DSM-IV 307.22)
   A. Single or multiple motor or vocal tics, but not both, have been present at some time during the illness.
   B. The tics occur many times a day, nearly every day, or intermittently throughout a period of more than 1 year; and during this period there was never a tic-free interval of more than 3 months.
   C. The disturbance causes marked distress or significant impairment in social, occupational, or other areas of functioning.
   D. Onset before age 18.
   E. The disturbance is not caused by the direct physiological effects of a substance (e.g. stimulants) or a general medical condition (e.g. Huntington's chorea or post-viral encephalitis).
   F. Criteria have never been met for Tourette disorder.

III. Diagnostic criteria for transient tic disorder (DSM-IV 307.21)
   A. Single or multiple motor and/or vocal tics.
   B. The tics may occur many times a day, nearly every day for at least 4 weeks, but for no longer than 12 consecutive months.
   C. The disturbance causes marked distress or significant impairment in social, occupational, or other areas of functioning.
   D. Onset before age 18.
   E. Disturbance is not caused by the direct physiological effects of a substance (e.g. stimulants) or a general medical condition (e.g. Huntington's chorea or post-viral encephalitis).
   F. Criteria have never been met for Tourette's disorder or chronic motor or vocal tic disorder.

IV. Diagnostic criteria for tic disorder, not otherwise specified (DSM-IV 307.20)
   This category is for a tic disorder that does not meet criteria for a specific tic disorder. Examples include tics lasting less than 4 weeks or tics with an onset after 18 years of age.

Adapted from *Diagnostic and Statistical Manual of Mental Disorders*, 4th edn (DSM-IV). Copyright © 1994 American Psychiatric Association.

for tic disorders in school-age children, in primary care and in educational settings, so that children with potentially serious problems like TS with co-morbidity can be identified and assessed, and effective management packages can be formulated to address their needs where necessary.

Clinical picture

Main features and symptoms

The core psychopathological features of tic disorders are motor and vocal tics, which have to be present at some time during the illness. A tic is a sudden, rapid, recurrent, non-rhythmic, stereotyped motor movement or vocalization. Tics usually begin in proximal areas of the body (head, face and neck) and may be interpreted as isolated and disinhibited fragments of voluntary movements. They represent actions of functionally co-acting muscle groups in one or several parts of the body (either a few at the same time or sequentially in bouts). Tics are not goal orientated, seem to have no meaning, are suppressible for a short period of time and can be preceded or followed by sensory motor sensations. Tics vary over time, in form, intensity, frequency and complexity. They are either simple or complex, and they wax and wane.

In extreme cases tics can be obscene (e.g. copropraxia, coprolalia) or self-injurious (e.g. hitting with the fist against the head). Vocal tics vary from simple sniffing or throat clearing to speech fragments and short sentences. Some patients repeat movements (echopraxia) and speech of other people (echolalia) or own words (palilalia).

Sometimes there are premonitory sensory motor sensations before tics. The sensations can be described as diffuse inner tension and restlessness. They can be described as high sensitivity of inner pressure, urge and impulse towards movement activity. They can also be perceived as an itch and pain (or hoarseness). These kinds of inner feelings can also be focused within certain parts of the skin, muscles and joints.

Some patients report a certain sensation 'not just right' after a tic. These post-monitory urges can be very unpleasant and provoke the patient's action in the sense that he has to repeat the tics in a voluntary manner until he has the 'just right' feeling in his body. While the patients feel forced by their disorder, they can be angry and discouraged but they also register a short release of inner tension which may facilitate the voluntary repetition of a tic the next time.

Motor and vocal tics occur in bouts over the course of the day and change in severity over weeks and months. These episodes are characterized by stable inter-tic intervals, i.e. time between successive tics, of short duration, typically

0.5–1.0 seconds, on the other hand there can be dystonic tics, which have a longer duration. Over minutes to hours, bouts of tics happen in groups. Over the course of weeks to months, many episodes of tics arise. This periodic higher-order combination of tic bouts could be the basis of the well-known waxing and waning course of tic disorders. In uncomplicated cases, severity of motor and vocal tics peaks early in the second decade of life, with many patients showing a striking reduction in tic severity by age 19 or 20 years. However, the more severe cases of tic disorders (Tourette syndrome) may arise in adulthood.

A large range of auditory or visual cues can also prompt tics, but the nature of these cues is usually highly selective for individual patients – a cough, a particular word, an alignment of angles or specific shapes. Further, tics can increase during emotional activity (e.g. anxiety, anger, happiness). Also, stress and tiredness ('relaxing' from more controlled behaviour) or use of stimulants may increase tic frequency, while concentrated work, muscle relaxation, supine position as well as use of cannabis and alcohol may decrease tics. Tics usually do not interfere with intended and goal-directed voluntary movements. Tics can also be seen during sleep (lower frequency, lower intensity, less complexity).

Tic disorders seem to represent a continuum from transient tics or chronic motor/vocal tic disorders through to TS. Nevertheless, the categorization according to the major classification systems is helpful since tic disorders can be clearly categorized at the time point of assessment, which follows different medical and/or psychological treatment options.

Differential diagnoses and co-morbidity

Both medical illnesses and psychiatric disorders have to be considered for differential diagnosis. Although there does not exist a specific laboratory test or specific precursors for tic disorders, the diagnosis can be made with certainty by medical history, clinical investigation and neurological assessment and thus tic disorder can be clearly differentiated from other movement disorders (Table 21.4)

Medical illnesses and symptoms that have to be included are epilepsy, mannerism, restless legs syndrome, blepharospasm, torticollis, stereotypies, chorea, dystonia, myoclonus, tremor, athetosis, akathisia, ballismus (some probably in the framework of Wilson's disease, Sydenham's chorea, hyperthyreosis, encephalitis, head trauma, brain tumour and intoxications) (Table 21.5).

Psychiatric disorders have to be considered both for purposes of differential diagnosis and as co-morbid disorders. A variety of sensorimotor, cognitive, emotional and/or social behavioural problems can be observed. About 85 per cent of Tourette syndrome patients have associated neuropsychiatric problems. These are often responsible for any psychosocial impairment. Co-morbid problems can be found more frequently when there is a family history with tic disorders, early onset

Table 21.4. Differential diagnosis of tics

Classification	Differential diagnosis
Simple motor tics	
• Clonic	Myoclonus
	Myokymia
	Fasciculations/fibrillations
	Hemiballism
	Tremor
	Chorea
	Seizures
• Dystonic	Dystonia
	Athetosis
• Tonic	Muscle spasms and cramps
	(e.g. Blepharospasm, facial spasm)
Complex motor tics	Mannerism
	Stereotypies
	Restless legs syndrome
	Seizures
	Tardive dyskinesia
	Conversion disorder

Phenomenology of tics	Differential diagnosis
Abrupt onset	Myoclonus
	Chorea
	Hyperexplexia
	Paroxysmal dyskinesia
	Seizures
Sensory phenomenon	Akathisia
(urge → relief)	Restless legs syndrome
	Dystonia
Perceived as voluntary	Akathisia
Suppressibility	All hyperkinesias (but less then tics)
Decrease with distraction	Akathisia
	Psychogenic movements
Increase with stress	Most hyperkinesias
Increase with relaxation (after a period of stress)	Parkinsonian tremor
Multifocal, migrate	Chorea
	Myoclonus
Fluctuate spontaneously	Paroxysmal dyskinesias
	Seizures
Repetition (non-rhythmic)	Stereotypies
Present during sleep	Myoclonus (segmental)
	Periodic movements
	Painful legs/moving toes
	Other hyperkinesias
	Seizures

Origin → brain tumour, encephalitis, brain trauma, intoxication, immunreaction, vascular problems

Modified after Cohen, Jankovic & Goetz, 2001).

Table 21.5. Co-morbidity in Tourette syndrome

Co-morbidity	%
ADHD	60
OCB	32
OCD	27
Anger and control problems	26
LD	23
Mood disorder	20
Social skill problems	20
Anxiety disorder	18
Sleep disorder	16
OD/ODD	15
Coprolalia	14
Self-injurious behaviour	14
Stuttering	8
PDD	4.5
Mental retardation	3.9
Trichotillomania	2.7
TS only, no co-morbidity	12

After Freeman *et al.* (2000).

of tic disorders or a high severity of the symptomatology. Tics are occasionally associated with Asperger syndrome or conversion disorder. Many children with a tic disorder show non-fluent speech, including stuttering.

In about half of the cases with chronic tics or Tourette syndrome (TS) there is a hyperkinetic disorder (HD; attention deficit–hyperactivity disorder) that starts about 2 to 3 years before the tics and is still present when tics show some remission around later adolescence (Fig. 21.1). Patients with TS plus HD have a higher risk of psychopathology including emotional impulsivity, sleep problems, learning problems, dyslexia and dyscalculia, emotional problems and externalizing behaviour.

There is a very close relationship between obsessive-compulsive behaviour and tic disorders. About 30–60 per cent of TS patients suffer from obsessions and compulsions and about 30 per cent fulfil the diagnostic criteria of obsessive compulsive disorder (OCD). Obsessive-compulsive phenomena usually appear in early adolescence, i.e. several years after the beginning of the tics and at the time when obsessive-compulsive disorders without co-morbidity usually come into play (Fig. 21.1). Because of phenomenological similarities, it can often be difficult to differentiate between compulsions and complex tics. There is a symptom continuum

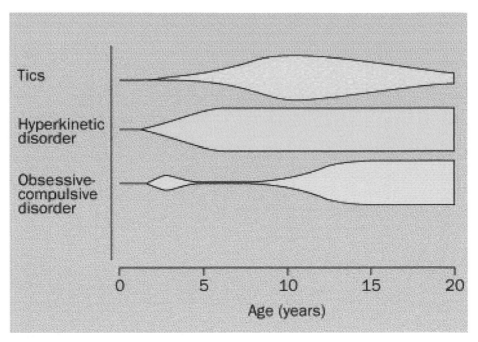

Fig. 21.1.
Age at which tics and co-existing disorders affect patients.
Width of bars shows schematically the amount the disorder affects a patient at a particular age (Leckman, 2002).

from tics to a mixture of tics/urges/obsessions/rituals/compulsions up to clearly diagnosable OCD. In tics there is a non-pleasant sensorimotor sensation whereas OCD is combined with an unpleasant cognitive–emotional/affect–logic state and with anxiety. Also, compulsions are rather related to the objective (to reduce inner tension) than to a related muscle group. Tics, on the other hand, have not the function to reduce anxiety. The closest relationship between OCD and TS can be seen in the 'just right' phenomenon. Some TS patients describe an inner urge and an internal struggle to control them. Other antecedent sensory events include generalized inner tension that can be relieved only by performance of a tic.

While in tic disorders obsessive compulsive behaviour shows a focus on sexual, aggressive and sensorimotor symptoms (including counting, touching, hoarding, tactile and visual symmetry), OCD patients without tics present more often with thoughts and images correlated to anxiety (e.g. contamination fears, controlling and washing). Coprolalia and self-injurious behaviour in TS patients are seen as an obsessive-compulsive behaviour.

Emotional disorders can be found in the medical history and at investigation. Separation anxiety, general anxiety, panic attacks, phobias and depressive symptoms as well as autistic and schizoid symptoms have been described. The emotional situation (stress, anxiety, fear but also happiness) can influence tic expression, but this appears to be the case in only about half of the patients. Emotional symptoms seem to be secondary to the chronic course and psychosocial difficulties during the tic disorder. Also, one has to remember, that treatment with neuroleptics may provoke depressive symptoms and school refusal.

Sleep disorders seem to be intrinsic to tic disorders. About 12–44 per cent of TS patients show difficulties falling asleep or staying asleep, bed-time separation anxiety and parasomnias such as sleep walking and night terror. Polysomnographic investigations have shown reduced sleep efficiency and tics during all sleep stages, which may lead to additional arousals. The reduced sleep efficiency may lead to drowsiness during the day and increased stress sensitivity leading to more frequent and more intense tics during the daytime. Sleep problems are more common in patients with a severe tic disorder, a family history of tics and associated neuropsy-chiatric problems.

Although usually of normal intelligence, about 50 per cent of children with TS show some learning problems (difficulties in visual perception and visuomotor integration, fine motor abilities, speech–language perception and speech fluency, dyslexia and dyscalculia). A close relationship with HD explains most of the learning problems.

Assessment

As with other disorders, tic disorders require a full psychiatric assessment of the history, development of symptoms, psychopathological features, and family functioning.

Diagnostic instruments like the Tourette Syndrome Symptom List (TSSL for tic observation by parents), and – for expert rating – the Tourette Syndrome Symptom Scale (TSSS; the latter two can be found in the Appendix), the Tourette Syndrome Global Scale (TSGS) and the Diagnostic Confidence Index (DCI) may be helpful in some respect. Questionnaires for co-morbid psychiatric conditions should also be included in the clinical assessment procedure. For a diagnostic flow chart, see Fig. 21.2. The following issues need to be considered specifically.

* The behavioural symptoms of tic disorders require a clinical interview with the parents and the patients. The most reliable information comes from the mother, who is highly sensitive concerning tics and often feels guilty and over-responsible. Children under 10 years of age are seldom aware of their tics. It is important to explore the type of tics (motor, vocal) and to find out the localization (proximal, distal), the frequency and intensity and the course (e.g. waxing and waning, intermittent remissions), as well as somatosensory sensations before or after a tic. Also, it is important to ask for subjective explanatory models, psychosocial burden and how the family dealt with the problems, how well they are informed

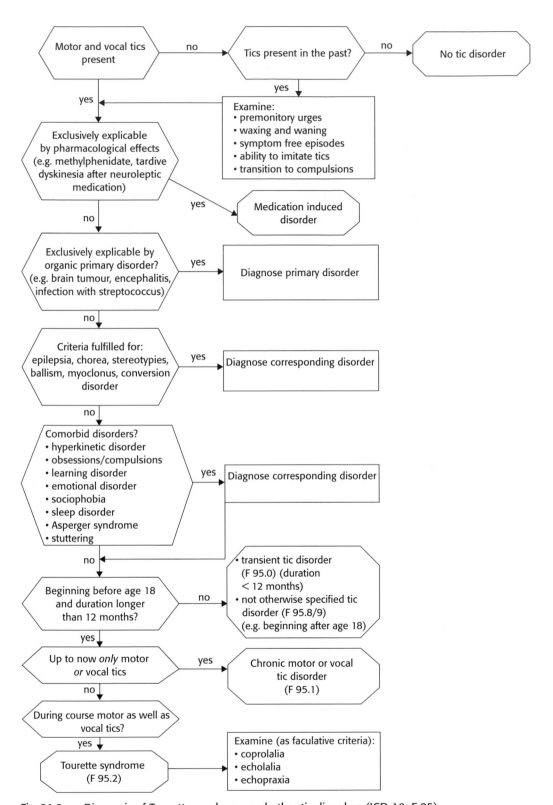

Fig. 21.2.   Diagnosis of Tourette syndrome and other tic disorders (ICD-10: F 95).

about the background of tic disorders and what interventions have been made so far.

- In addition to the defining criteria, significant other clinical symptoms (e.g. features of hyperkinetic disorder, anxiety/depression, obsessive-compulsive disorder) should also be addressed.

- Due to the variety of potential other medical disorders a careful physical assessment and follow-up medical assessments are mandatory.

- The physical examination should often include some laboratory investigations (EEG; MRI/CCT or blood tests for antibodies against *Streptococcus*, *Mycoplasma*, *Borrelia* and *borna* virus may occasionally be helpful for differential diagnosis or for rare aetiological explanations of tics).

- More important are psychological investigations with behavioural observations and neuropsychological testing. One has to bear in mind that, during testing, for the most part tics will not be observed other than during the breaks.

- Because of the involvement of the family, family functioning requires further interviewing and testing, especially the mother–child interaction is important (see above). The patient's mother feels not sure, but guilty, doubtful, unhappy and sad, because she thinks of educational problems, mental disorders and her own helplessness within the context of social expectations. This may hold for a long time in spite of being informed about tic disorders by psychoeducation and resolves mostly when the child has passed puberty and taken his own responsibility of his tic disorder. The family may contribute to diagnosis also by fulfilling the TSSL to support the expert in severity rating with the TSSS or the Tourette syndrome DCI or TSGS.

- As with other child and adolescent psychiatric disorders, all findings of the assessment should be integrated into the Multi-axial Classification System (MAS) as recommended by the WHO.

- Many patients and families often feel supported, understood and reassured by hearing a more or less detailed account of our understanding of the pathogenesis and natural history of tic disorders. Knowledge that their experience is similar to that of other families, and that many of the most puzzling features of the disorder are typical (such as waxing and waning, symptom variation, ability to suppress tics for a period of time, and premonitory urges) can be a great reassurance to families.

Aetiology

The pathophysiological background of tic disorders is determined mainly by neurobiological factors. Its complex development and picture (including associated symptoms, which in the case of tic disorders plus hyperkinetic disorder may reflect a separate entity) seems to be created by multiple determinants and risk factors and their interaction. Thus, environmental influences cannot be neglected.

Biological mechanisms

Genetic studies in twins and families provide compelling evidence that genetic factors are implicated in vertical transmission in families with vulnerability to TS and related disorders. At present, the nature of vulnerability genes that predispose individuals to develop the disorder are unknown. Many genes probably play a role. Clarity about the nature and normal expression of even a few of the susceptibility genes in TS is likely to provide a major step forward in understanding the pathogenesis of this disorder. Tic disorders and obsessive-compulsive disorders may be two alternative manifestations of the same genetic disposition. It seems that several vulnerability genes influence the development of tic disorders and other additional genes may be responsible for the expression of the severity of the tic symptomatology. Recent genetic studies report, that genes on chromosome 4, 8 and 11 may play a special role. Genetic variation at loci for dopamine receptors, dopamine transporters, various noradrenergic genes and few serotonergic genes seems to be unlikely to be a major source for vulnerability to tic disorders, but in concert these alleles could have an important cumulative effect.

Many epigenetic factors have been implicated in the pathogenesis of TS. For example, children with a low birth weight are more likely to have tics and hyperkinetic symptoms by age 6 years than controls. Further, androgenic steroids during critical periods of fetal development could play a role in the development of the syndrome. Some neuroendocrinological findings suggest that a subset of patients with tic disorders could be characterized by heightened reactivity of the hypothalamic–pituitary–adrenal axis and related noradrenergic sympathetic systems.

The past decade has seen the re-emergence of the hypothesis that post-infectious autoimmune mechanisms contribute to the pathogenesis of some cases of TS. Especially, Mycoplasma, Borrelia, and group-A β hemolytic streptococci (GABHS) are known to be a possible trigger of immune-mediated disease in genetically predisposed individuals (about 5–10%). Acute rheumatic fever is a delayed sequela of these bacteria, arising about 3 weeks after an inadequately treated infection of the upper respiratory tract. Rheumatic fever is characterized by inflammatory lesions of the joints, heart or central nervous system (Sydenham's chorea). This disorder and TS probably affect common anatomic areas – the basal ganglia of the brain and related cortical and thalamic sites. Some patients with Sydenham's chorea have motor and vocal tics and symptoms of obsessive-compulsive and attention deficit/hyperactivity disorder, suggesting that, at least in some instances, these disorders share a common cause. As in Sydenham's chorea, anti-neuronal antibodies have been reported to have arisen in the sera of some patients with TS. Paediatric autoimmune neuropsychiatric disorder associated with streptococcal infection (PANDAS) has been suggested to represent a distinct clinical entity and include cases of TS and OCD, in which a GABHS infection is likely to have preceded symptom onset. Although the importance of antibodies against neurones in relation to cause, and the association with previous GABHS infections, remains a topic of great debate, treatments based on these mechanisms are still experimental but show some promise. However, the diagnostic criteria for PANDAS are set at a very high threshold: abrupt onset or exacerbations of clinical symptoms, temporal relationship to infection, episodic course, prepubertal onset, positive throat culture for strep or elevated serum antibodies reflected by Anti-DNAse and ASO. It seems premature to apply testing and antibiotic or immune-modifying therapies routinely, if these criteria are not fulfilled.

In the recent years, studies with neuroimaging and neurophysiology have focused on the motor, sensorimotor, association, inhibitory and limbic (motivational and threat detection) neurocircuits that course through the basal ganglia. These circuits direct information from the cerebral cortex to the subcortex, and then back to specific regions of the cortex, thereby forming multiple cortical–subcortical loops. Hence, inhibitory problems in the cortico-striato-pallido-thalamico-cortical regulatory system seems to be the pathophysiological basis of tic disorders with a sensorimotor part responsible for tics while limbic affections are merely related to stress sensitivity and its interaction with tics. Neuroimaging and neurophysiological studies have shown that voluntary tic suppression involves activation of regions of the prefrontal cortex and caudate nucleus and bilateral activation of the putamen and the globus pallidus. Thus, the prefrontal cortical regions have a crucial role in expression of tic symptoms. While a high dopaminergic sensitivity in the basal ganglia leads to a disturbance of the subcortical automatic inhibition of spontaneously neuronal-triggered movements, the connections to the frontal cortex are used to suppress this unwanted activity voluntarily, which otherwise may lead to tics. Thus, voluntary frontal activation helps patients with tic disorders for a better self regulation of their unvoluntary tic behaviour. Automatic and controlled self-regulation of tics can be supported by a sound sleep (Fig. 21.3). Deficits in motor inhibition may lead to increased sensorimotor urges, coupled with an increased arousal level. Thus, children with tics show difficulties falling asleep and staying asleep. Finally, the reduced sleep efficiency exerts daytime sleepiness with stress vulnerability and increased risk for tics during daytime.

Psychosocial mechanisms

Possible psychosocial risk factors for genetic vulnerable individuals include severe psychosocial trauma, recurrent daily stresses (e.g. teasing by peers) or extreme

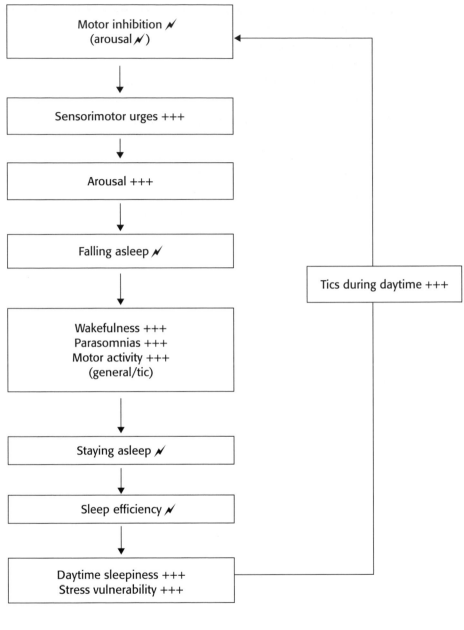

Legend: ↗ disturbed
           +++ increased

Fig. 21.3.   Neurodynamic model: tics and sleep behaviour.

emotional excitement, exposure to androgenic drugs and chronic intermittent use of cocaine and other psychostimulants.

Secondary and modulating factors of tic disorders include mainly factors which are associated with events of anxiety, emotional trauma and social meetings. This shows that psychosocial stress, which is interpreted subjectively as a burden and not as a chance, is important. On the other hand, relaxed and concentrative work may decrease tics, and a normal or very good stress resistance helps to cope successfully with the tic disorder and its associated problems. The subsets of these two groups seem to be half and half.

Secondary problems in parent–child interactions can be found in many of the families where mothers have difficulties to estimate their child's emotions adequately. The mothers feel guilty, responsible and punished by each tic of the child. Mothers need years to come to terms with competent coping with the tic disorder of their child (mostly around the ages of 13–15 years of the child). Family conflicts, tensions and problems in mother–father interaction can arise and lead to further complications of the family environment. Parents often are helpless as to how to educate their child. They tend to switch from one extreme to the other thus increasing the interactional difficulties of the families. This may lead to stress-related increase of tics and may finally be interpreted as the primary cause of the disorder. But, in fact, this reduces the compensatory abilities of the patients according to psychosocial stressors. Only a few patients use their tics voluntarily, to avoid critics and requirements (e.g. school and homework).

Children with tics tend to withdraw from social activities while being teased. Difficulties in contact with peers have more often the background of hyperkinetic disorder or obsessive-compulsive disorder than a recent tic symptomatology. Patients with tic disorders usually show age-appropriate leisure activities and hobbies and have basically good coping mechanisms. The possible protective factors include further informed and supportive home and school or occupational environment, maintenance of good sleep hygiene, regular physical exercise regimen, presence and use of special talents (e.g. exceptional social skills, athletic skills, musical abilities, academic gifts).

Treatment

Clinical management and treatment setting

Usually, a multi-modal treatment for tic disorders is indicated, either on an outpatient or an inpatient basis. Most cases can be guided as outpatients. Inpatient or day care treatment should be provided for one or more of the following indications:

- tic disorder of high severity and complexity
- complicated co-morbid conditions (e.g. multiple co-morbidities)
- unsuccessful outpatient treatment
- severe psychosocial complications.

Within the hierarchy of the treatment decisions (see Fig. 21.4), the multi-modal approach includes psychoeducational and supportive interventions within a context of a long-term relationship with the clinician who can help the patient, family and school to deal with the changing manifestations of the disorder through the years. One has also to take into consideration that stress can exacerbate tics. Therefore, therapeutic attention to difficulties in self-esteem, social coping, family issues and effects on tic severity and on anxiety and depression has to be taken into account. Patients' self-help groups and their supportive role of understanding and modelling of the coping behaviour of experienced families are recommended. Parents should be encouraged to build on their child's strengths behind the tic problem. With these steps, many uncomplicated cases of tic disorder can be successfully managed. When patients present with co-morbidities as well as with tic disorders, it depends on the psychosocial burden of the different aspects of the psychopathological problems, which disorder has to be treated first. To meet the biopsychosocial needs of the patients, their treatment should preferably take place in a child and adolescent psychiatric unit. The most helpful treatment approach is psychopharmacotherapy.

Pharmacotherapy

Although drug treatment is first line to reduce tics the vast majority of patients with tic disorders need not be given medication since they only have tics without psychosocial impairment and with good coping skills and medication seems not to influence the course of the disorder. There exists no perfect anti-tic drug. All helpful drugs can suppress tics but none can cure them. Drugs cannot be used effectively just when tics are at there worst and then taken off. Medication has to be planned for the long term, at least for 1 year, because with the natural waxing and waning pattern of tics it is often difficult to distinguish response to an intervention from spontaneous waning of symptoms. Thus it is usually best to avoid beginning or increasing drugs as soon as an exacerbation begins. In the case of the latter, a competent guidance of the family over weeks is important to see how the spontaneous course of the tics is. Only if tic symptomatology remains problematic, is starting of the medication, increasing of the medication or change of drugs indicated. Otherwise, unnecessary high dosages and side effects may be provoked. One should also have in mind that slow titration procedures and tapering out procedures have to be planned to avoid side effects and to find the optimal dosage that allows the child and the family to develop a better psychosocial situation and a constructive arrangement with the topic. The various drugs including dosages are shown in Table 21.6.

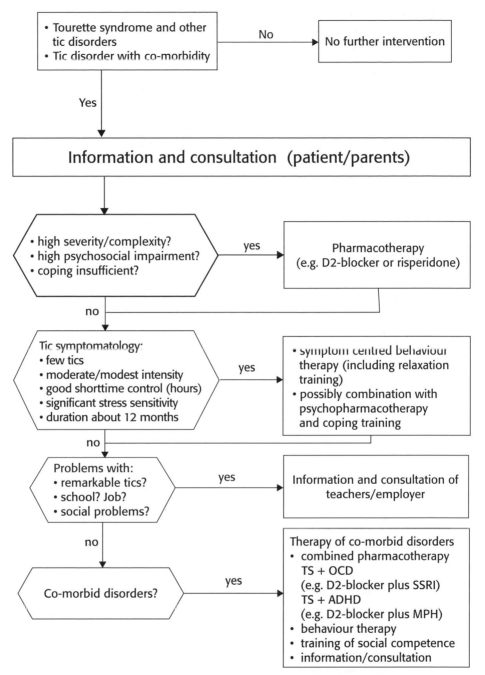

Fig. 21.4.   Treatment of Tourette syndrome and other tic disorders (ICD-10: F 95).

- Stereotactic brain surgery only in extreme TS with obsessive-compulsive disorder and self injurious behaviour otherwise not treatable.
- Experimental therapy (△9-tetrahydrocanabinal, immunomodulation, antibiotics in case of infection; botulinumtoxin) is practicable only in specialized centres.

Table 21.6. Medications used in treatment of TS and associated disorders

Medication	Indication(s)	Starting dose (mg)	Dose range (mg)	Laboratory tests and monitoring
SSRIs				
Fluoxetine	Depression* OCD*	2.5–5	2.5–60	None
Fluvoxamine	OCD*	12.5–25	25–200	None
Sertraline	OCD*	25	25–200	None
TCAs				
Clomipramine	OCD*	25	50–200	Plasma level, EKG
Imipramine	Anxiety*	10–25	20–450	Plasma level, EKG
Atypical antidepressants				
Bupropion	ADHD*	75	75–450	None
Stimulants				
Dextroamphetamine	ADHD*	2.5	2.5–30	Height, weight, hemodynamics
Methylphenidate	ADHD*	2.5	2.5–60	Height, weight, hemodynamics
Pemoline	ADHD*	18.75	18.75–112.5	(+) Liver function, height, weight
Beta-blockers				
Clonidine	ADHD**	0.05	0.1–0.3	Hemodynamics
Guanfacine	Tics**	0.5–1.0	1–4	Hemodynamics
Neuroleptics				
Tiapride	Tics*	2 mg/kg	2–10 mg/kg	Liver function blood count, weight
Sulpiride	Tics* OCD	2 mg/kg	2–10 mg/kg	Liver function blood count, weight
Risperidone	Tics DBD	0.25	2–4	Liver function blood count, weight
Pimozide	Tics*	0.5–1.0	1–6	Liver function neurologic exam blood count, weight
Haloperidol	Tics**	0.25–0.5	0.25–15	Liver function neurologic exam blood count, weight

*positive (efficacious) placebo-controlled studies.

**suggestive (or mixed) placebo-controlled studies.

(+), hepatotoxicity reported with treatment with pemoline.

SSRIs = selective serotonin re-uptake inhibitors.

TCAs = tricyclic antidepressants.

DBD: disruptive behaviour disorders.

The drugs of first choice to reduce tics are the D2-receptor antagonists such as tiapride, risperidone, pimozide (no longer available in many countries), haloperidol and sulpiride. Efficacy of these drugs is associated with their potency in blockade of post-synaptic dopamine 2 receptors. These substances are helpful in about 70–80 per cent of the patients and are able to reduce tics to a resting level of about 20–30 per cent. The benzamides, sulpiride and tiapride show fewer extrapyramidal motor side effects and a very low risk of tardive dyskinesias compared to pimozide and haloperidol. Sulpiride is able not only to reduce tics but also to improve obsessive compulsive symptoms, anxiety and depression. Although pimozide shows also an acceptable ratio of efficacy and safety on tics, one has to control for potential QTc changes and therefore baseline and follow-up in electrocardiography is recommended; this is true also for risperidone and ziprasidone, and haloperidol. The most typical dose related side effects of neuroleptics are sedation and dysphoria with *de novo* development of separation anxiety and school refusal; also weight gain plays an important role. One should also be familiar with potential cytochrome P450-related drug reactions, because fatal interactions have arisen with pimozide and erythromycin-related antibiotics. Further, combinations with, e.g. serotonin re-uptake inhibitors like fluvoxamine have to be taken into consideration. Drugs can also reduce nightly tics and improve the sleep efficiency.

In accordance with the neuromodulatory role of tonically active neurons in the striatum, other drugs are used to reduce tics. Guanfacin and clonidine are two alpha-2-adrenergic agents, which may be helpful in low dosage, which can be gradually increased. The main side effect of these two drugs in the recommended dose range is sedation, sometimes accompanied by irritability as well as cardiac arrhythmias with clonidine. Further, γ-aminic-acid modulating drugs like clonazepam and baclofen, tricyclic antidepressives (desipramine, clomipramine), cannabinoids and even dopamine agonists like pergolide and levodopa have been used to reduce tics. Unfortunately, some of the drugs may even increase tics. The use of botulinum toxin is rarely indicated and should be used only by specialized centres.

Co-existing tics and hyperkinetic symptoms should be treated only with tiapride, if hyperkinetic symptoms are mild. When moderately expressed, a combination of tiapride and methylphenidate may be helpful and in cases of severe hyperkinetic disorder with mild tics methylphenidate can be the drug of first choice. In a few patients with tic disorders, methylphenidate may exacerbate tics. But there are many others where there is no influence on tics and even tic reduction can be observed. In sum, there is no contraindication for the parallel use of tiapride and methylphenidate.

Researchers of one large-scale, double-blind, clinical trial reported recently, that the combination of clonidine and methylphenidate was most effective in treatment of children with both attention deficit/hyperactivity disorder and chronic tics. This study showed that these two drugs had differential effects with clonidine being most helpful in impulsivity and hyperactivity, and methylphenidate being most helpful for symptoms of inattention.

Co-existing obsessive-compulsive behaviour and anxiety with tic disorders allows a primary use of sulpiride which reduces tics, anxiety, depression and obsessive compulsive behaviour. Otherwise, a combination of tiapride, pimozide or risperidone with a serotonin re-uptake inhibitor or clomipramine is recommended.

The connection between GABHS infections and *PANDAS* remains controversial, and therefore antibiotic prophylaxis and ardous experimental treatments (plasma exchange or intravenous immunoglobulins) should be considered only with expert child psychiatric and paediatric consultation. At present, the main mandate for the clinician is to be vigilant in assessment of children with pharyngitis or those exposed to streptococcal infection.

Psychological interventions

The evidence basis for psychotherapy in tic disorders is small. Habit reversal and progressive muscle relaxation have some scientific support. Concerning problems with anxiety, depression and self-esteem as well as sociophobic behaviour additional psychological interventions might be helpful.

- First, there is good clinical evidence that supportive psychotherapy is an important component in the multimodal treatment of tic disorders. It has many similarities to the approach in other psychiatric disorders.
- A more specific and tic-related intervention is habit reversal training. Tic patients use spontaneously different strategies to reduce their tics voluntarily in order to gain a certain self-control over their tics for the daily life. The abilities to be aware of the premonitory sensorimotor sensations before a tic and the suppressibility of tics are important although the first is no prerequisite for the latter. Both phenomena increase with age, where the age around 10 years plays a critical role. If it is not possible for the patient to suppress the tic completely, he may try to integrate the tic movement within his usual behaviour (masking). Thus, the objective of the different behavioural therapies is (1) to use the self-regulatory mechanism of the patients as the starting point and (2) to train him for better self-control by modifying, optimizing, systematizing and automatizing the psychological procedure.

The basis of behavioural therapeutic planning is the functional behavioural analysis of the tic situation before a direct modification and reduction of tic symptomatology can be done by habit reversal, including awareness training of tic behaviour, response description, response detection, awareness of inner signs, awareness of external triggering situations, competing response practice. Other components

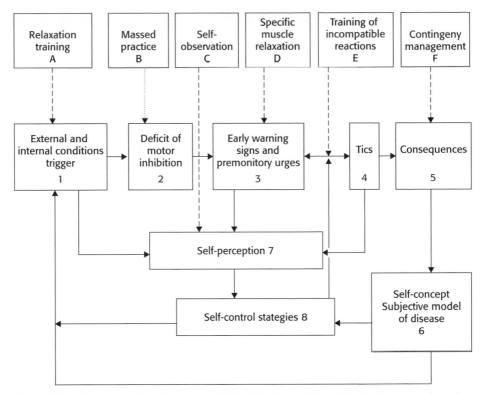

Fig. 21.5.   Connections between tic relevant variables (1–8) and hypothesized approaches for behaviour therapeutic techniques (A–F).

include relaxation training, increase in sustained motivation and adherence as well as generalization training. This intervention may be useful for a few patients, but systematic clinical trials have not been done.

Given a sequential process on the way towards the appearance of each single tic or a bout of tics (from external/internal trigger to behaviour), the consequences after the tic (reactions of others, self-perception and self-concept) are influencing self-control strategies close to the actual tic and feedback mechanisms related to the sequential process of tic appearance. Behavioural interventions can be guided by this model. Thus, relaxation training can reduce stress related to daytime vulnerability for tics, massed negative practice might increase inhibitory effects for some minutes, pre-tic sensorimotor phenomena may be used to focus on relaxation of the involved muscles or activate their antagonists, while contingency management for consequences has limited effect on tics (see Fig. 21.5).

Behavioural treatment of hyperkinetic disorder in children with tics is similar to that in hyperkinetic disorder only. This also holds true for tic-related obsessive compulsive disorder.

The success of psychological interventions depends on the compliance of the patients, because high motivation, self observation and self control abilities are necessary. This is difficult for children younger than 10 years as well as for adolescents. Therefore, a modification of sensorimotor premonitory sensations and tic specific relaxation of muscle groups (based on the approach of progressive muscle relaxation) may be an alternative to integrate tics in socially acceptable movements.

The combination of behavioural therapy and psychopharmacotherapy may be helpful to prepare and support behaviour therapy and stabilize its effects; on the other hand this combination may increase compliance for drug treatment and intensify pharmacological effects. Behaviour therapy may also allow to reduce drug dosage.

In sum, if reduction of tics is necessary, behaviour therapy is secondary to drug treatment and is an alternative only when drug treatment is contraindicated, shows no effect or if there is no compliance for pharmacotherapy. Psychodynamic psychotherapy cannot be recommended as a primary method to reduce tics. Training for social competences is in some cases useful as an anti-stress treatment. The behavioural therapeutic approach can also be used to treat associated problems at the psychopathological and the family interactional level.

Psychoeducational measures and rehabilitation

- Besides counselling (see above) some cases of very severe tic disorders (e.g. Tourette syndrome with multi-co-morbidity) may lead to psychosocial isolation of patients, and generate a degree of impediment of 50–80 per cent. Therefore, sometimes rehabilitation in special institutions is necessary.

Outcome

Systematic longitudinal observations into adulthood of patients with tic disorders are lacking. Therefore, no clear-cut statement can be given. Nevertheless, some crude assumptions can be made on the available empirical basis.

Although our evidence based empirical information is still small, we may assume that about 10–30 per cent of Tourette patients, who were seen as children, remain chronically impaired in adulthood. After 15 years about 45 per cent of TS patients are free from symptoms and the severity of tics decreases for about 60 per cent. At the same time, the psychosocial functioning increases and co-morbidities partly disappear. In conclusion, the long-term outcome of patients with tic disorders generally is relatively benign.

Usually, in all tic disorders there is reduction of tics during late adolescence and early adulthood with better social adaptation and an efficient use of self control and coping strategies. Thus, in most cases the use of tic-reducing drugs can be reduced from 60 per cent at the beginning to about 30 per cent in the long run. In about 70–80 per cent of children tics are ameliorated by adult age. Some patients still show mild tics during adulthood and a few patients have a severe Tourette syndrome with psychosocial impairment all life long (mainly influenced by co-morbid disorders like OCD). Although there is a high psychosocial burden coming from the symptoms and associated psychiatric problems, only a few cases show essential impairment in the areas of school, occupation and social interaction.

Risk factors contributing to a poor outcome include positive family history, pre- and perinatal problems, co-morbid psychiatric disorders, emotional problems, and vocal and highly complex peripheral tics. The severity of tics and the psychosocial situation of the family during childhood of the patient seem not to be important for the outcome of tics.

Factors of resilience include positive parent–child relationship and good peer relationship, high impulse control and affect regulation, superior cognitive abilities, well-developed coping abilities, psychosocial support and stress resistance.

Since coping with tics is a highly important factor for psychosocial functioning, all these factors contribute to a favourable development at school and in society, i.e. for a healthy life with cognitive, emotional, physical and social well-being.

SUGGESTED READING

T. Banaschewski, W. Woerner & A. Rothenberger (in press), Premonitory sensory phenomena and suppressibility of tics in Tourette Syndrome – developmental aspects in children. *Developmental Medicine and Child Neurology*, **45**, 700–3.

D. J. Cohen, J. Jankovic & C. G. Goetz, Tourette Syndrome. In *Advances in Neurology*. Vol. 85. (Baltimore: Williams & Wilkins, 2001).

R. Freeman, D. K. Fast, L. Burd, J. Kerbeshian, M. Robertson, P. Sandor & Tourette Syndrome International Database Consortium, An international perspective on Tourette Syndrome: selected findings from 3500 cases in 22 countries. *Developmental Medicine and Child Neurology*, **42** (2000), 436–47.

K. D. Gadow, Tics and psychiatric co-morbidity in children and adolescents. *Developmental Medicine and Child Neurology*, **44** (2002), 330–8.

P. J. Hoekstra, C. G. M. Kallenberg, J. Korf & R. B. Minderaa, Is Tourette's syndrome an autoimmune disease? *Molecular Psychiatry*, **7** (2002), 437–45.

T. Kostanecka-Endres, T. Banaschewski, J. Kinkelbur, *et al.*, Disturbed sleep in children with Tourette Syndrome – a polysomnographic study. *Journal of Psychosomatic Research*, **55** (2003), 23–9.

J. F. Leckman, Tourette's syndrome. *Lancet*, **360** (2002), 1577–86.

J. F. Leckman & D. J. Cohen (eds.), *Tourette's Syndrome, Tics, Obsessions, Compulsions: Developmental Psychopathology and Clinical Care.* (New York: John Wiley, 1999).

G. H. Moll, H. Heinrich & R. Rothenberger, Transcranial magnetic stimulation in child psychiatry – disturbed motor system excitability in hypermotoric syndromes. *Developmental Sciences*, **5** (2002), 381–91.

M. M. Robertson, Annotation: Gilles de la Tourette syndrome – an update. *Journal of Child Psychology and Psychiatry*, **4** (1994), 397–411.

M. M. Robertson, Tourette syndrome, associated conditions and the complexities of treatment. *Brain*, **123** (3) (2000), 425–62.

M. M. Robertson & J. S. Stern, Gilles de la Tourette Syndrome: symptomatic treatment based on evidence. *European Child and Adolescent Psychiatry*, **9** (Suppl. 1) (2000), 60–75.

T. J. Spencer, J. Biederman, S. Faraone *et al.*, Impact of tic disorders on ADHD and outcome across the life cycle: findings from a large group of adults with and without ADHD. *American Journal of Psychiatry*, **4** (2001), 611–17.

Tourette Syndrome Study Group, Treatment of ADHD in children with tics: a randomized controlled trial. *Neurology*, **58** (2002), 527–36.

J. Yordanova, C. Dumais-Huber, A. Rothenberger & W. Woerner, Frontocortical activity in children with comorbidity of tic disorder and attention deficit hyperactivity disorder. *Biological Psychiatry*, **41** (1997), 585–94.

Appendix 21.1. *Tourette Syndrome Symptom List (Revised – TSSL)*

Name of patient _____   ID _____

Date _____

Rate each symptom by putting the appropriate number in the box each day. (Use the reverse side for any detailed comments).

0 = Not at all or symptom free. 1 = Just a little. 2 = Pretty much.			3 = Very much. 4 = Extreme. 5 = Almost always.			Rater:	☐ Patient ☐ Father ☐ Mother ☐ Other		
Date	MON	TUE	WED	THU	FRI	SAT	SUN		
SIMPLE MOTOR 1. Eye blinking								SUM OF 1–11 MON - SUN	
2. Other facial tics									
3. Head jerks									
4. Shoulder jerks								# OF SYMPTOMS 1–11 MON - SUN	
5. Arm movements									
6. Finger or hand movements									
7. Stomach jerks									
8. Kicking leg movements									
9. Tense parts of body									
10. Other:									
11. Other:									

COMPLEX MOTOR 12. Touching part of body									SUM OF 12–22 MON - SUN
13. Touching other people									
14. Touching objects									
15. Can't start actions									
16. Hurts self									# OF SYMPTOMS 12–22 MON - SUN
17. Finger or hand tapping									
18. Hopping									
19. Picks at things (clothing, etc.)									
20. Copropraxia									
21. Other:									
22. Other:									
SIMPLE PHONIC 23. Noises									SUM OF 23–28 MON - SUN
24. Grunting									
25. Throat clearing									
26. Coughing									# OF SYMPTOMS 23–28 MON - SUN
27. Other:									
28. Other:									
COMPLEX PHONIC 29. Words									SUM OF 29–35 MON - SUN
30. Repeats own words/sentences									
31. Repeats others' speech									
32. Coprolalia (obscene words)									# OF SYMPTOMS 29–35 MON - SUN
33. Insults (lack of inhibition)									
34. Other:									
35. Other:									
BEHAVIOUR 36. Argumentative									SUM OF 36–41 MON - SUN
37. Poor frustration tolerance									
38. Anger, temper fits									
39. Provocative									# OF SYMPTOMS 36–41 MON - SUN
40. Other:									
41. Other.									

Appendix 21.2. *Shapiro TS Severity Scale*

RATINGS

TICS NOTICEABLE TO OTHERS	TICS ELICIT COMMENTS OR CURIOSITY	PATIENT CONSIDERED ODD OR BIZARRE	TICS INTERFERE WITH FUNCTIONING	INCAPACITATED, HOMEBOUND OR HOSPITALIZED	SUM OF RATINGS _____ GLOBAL SEVERITY RATING
no (0)	no (0)	no (0)	no (0)	no (0)	0) NONE = 0
very few (.5)	no (0)	no (0)	no (0)	no (0)	1) VERY MILD = 0 to < 1
some (1)	no (0)	no (0)	no (0)	no (0)	2) MILD = 1 to < 2
most (2)	possibly (0.5)	no (0)	no (0)	no (0)	3) MODERATE = 2 to < 4
all (3)	yes (1)	possibly (1)	occasionally (1)	no (0)	4) MARKED = 4 to < 6
all (3)	yes (1)	yes (2)	yes (2)	no (0)	5) SEVERE = 6 to 8
all (3)	yes (1)	yes (2)	yes (2)	yes (1)	6) VERY SEVERE = > 8

Variables

The TS Severity Scale yields seven variables that can be used for different clinical and research purposes: Tics Noticeable to Others; Tics Elicit Comments or Curiosity; Patient Considered Odd or Bizarre; Tics Interfere with Functioning; Incapacitated, Homebound or Hospitalized; Total Sum of Ratings; and Global Severity Rating.

Tics Noticeable to Others

0   Tics are not present.

0.5 Tics are infrequent or mild and usually are not noticed by employers, teachers, friends or strangers, although some family members or very close friends may be aware of the presence of tics. Symptoms can be diminished significantly or controlled completely in public places.

1   Same as above, except tics are noticed by most friends and occasionally by some employers, teachers, or strangers.

2   Same as above, except tics are noticed by many or most employers, teachers and strangers.

3   Same as above, except tics are noticed by all individuals.

Tics Elicit Comments or Curiosity

0   Tics are not present or are so infrequent and mild that they are not noticed and do not elicit comments and curiosity from employers, teachers, and friends, although they may be apparent to close family members.

0.5 Tics are more frequent and apparent and possibly elicit comments or curiosity by some individuals.

1   Tics are frequent and apparent and elicit comments or curiosity by all individuals.

Patient Considered Odd or Bizarre

0   Tics are not present or are infrequent and mild and other individuals would not consider the patient odd or bizarre.

1   Tics are more frequent, startling, or distort the appearance of the patient, and some observers consider the patient odd or bizarre.

2   Tics are frequent, startling, or distort the appearance of the patient, and most or all observers consider the patient odd or bizarre.

Tics Interfere with Functioning

0   Tics are absent or are present but do not interfere with academic, vocational, social, or psychological functioning and coordination.

1   Tics occasionally or somewhat interfere with academic, vocational, social, or psychological functioning or coordination.

2   Tics frequently, usually or always interfere with academic, vocational, social or psychological functioning or coordination.

Total Sum of Ratings

The Total Sum of Ratings is the sum of the ratings of the five factors listed above. The rater has the option of assigning half scores on all factors, e.g., 0.5 for ratings that fall between values.

Global Severity Rating

The Total Sum of Ratings is assigned a Global Severity Rating using the ranges (listed in parentheses) in the last column.

22

Elimination disorders: enuresis and encopresis

Alexander von Gontard

Department of Child and Adolescent Psychiatry, University of Hamburg, Germany

Introduction

Enuresis and encopresis are common disorders of childhood with a high spontaneous cure rate. They are therefore often considered to be 'developmental disorders'. They are associated with high emotional distress for children and parents, as well as with increased rates of co-morbid behavioural disorders. Especially in daytime wetting, somatic symptoms such as urinary tract infections often co-exist. Therefore, a detailed assessment of both somatic and psychological aspects is essential to ensure an optimal and specific treatment.

In addition, several distinct subtypes of elimination disorders have been identified, which differ according to their aetiology, pathophysiology and clinical features.

Enuresis

Definition and classification

The main features according to both the ICD-10 and DSM-IV classification schemes are:

- involuntary wetting at night or during daytime
- from the age of 5 years onwards
- after organic causes have been ruled out.

The differences between the two classifications systems regarding:

- the duration of the wetting, which is shorter in DSM-IV (3 months) than in ICD-10 (6 months)
- the frequency of wetting of two or more times per week or the alternative and less stringent criteria of high emotional stress according to DSM-IV; in contrast, children under 7 years need to wet two or more times per month, and those

A Clinician's Handbook of Child and Adolescent Psychiatry, ed. Christopher Gillberg,
Richard Harrington and Hans-Christoph Steinhausen. Published by Cambridge University Press.
© Cambridge University Press 2005.

Table 22.1. Diagnostic criteria for non-organic enuresis (F98.0) according to ICD-10 (research criteria)

A. The child's chronological and mental age is at least 5 years.

B. Involuntary or intentional voiding or urine into bed or clothes occurs at last twice a month aged under 7 years, and at least once a month in children aged 7 years or more.

C. The enuresis is not a consequence of epileptic attacks or of neurological incontinence, and not a direct consequence of structural abnormalities of the urinary tract or any other non-psychiatric medical condition.

D. There is no evidence of any other psychiatric disorder that meets the criteria for other ICD-10 categories.

E. Duration of the disorder is at least 3 months.

A fifth character may be used, if desired, for further specification:

F98.00 Nocturnal enuresis only

F98.01 Diurnal enuresis only

F98.02 Nocturnal and diurnal enuresis

over 7 years only once a month to be considered to have enuresis according to ICD-10.

In contrast to these two official classification schemes, voluntary wetting is often a reflection of severe psychopathology and should not be termed 'enuresis'. Also, any co-morbid psychiatric disturbance should be diagnosed separately and should not exclude the diagnosis of enuresis (as in ICD-10).

The main shortcomings of ICD-10 and DSM-IV is that they do not differentiate adequately between subtypes of wetting and thereby have not yet kept abreast with recent research on enuresis in the fields of child psychiatry, paediatrics and paediatric urology. Thus, the time of day when wetting occurs is the only criterion considered and therefore only nocturnal and/or diurnal subtypes are considered (see Tables 22.1 and 22.2).

Generally, it is useful first to differentiate between enuresis and urinary incontinence. True 'enuresis' is characterized by complete emptying of the bladder (though in the wrong place and time) in contrast to 'urinary incontinence' with evident signs of bladder dysfunction. Most children with night wetting do have true enuresis, while day wetting children have some form of urinary incontinence. Neurogenic and structural forms of urinary incontinence are rare, while functional forms predominate.

Among nocturnal enuresis, four main subtypes can be differentiated according to two main criteria: the length of the longest dry period in the past and the presence of daytime symptoms (see Table 22.3). If the maximal dry interval was less than 6 months, primary nocturnal enuresis is diagnosed; if it exceeds 6 months, secondary nocturnal enuresis. Monosymptomatic enuresis means that

Table 22.2. Diagnostic criteria for enuresis (307.6) according to DSM-IV

A. Repeated voiding of urine into bed or clothes (whether involuntary or intentional).

B. The behaviour is clinically significant as manifested by either a frequency of twice a week for at least 3 consecutive months or the presence of clinically significant distress or impairment in social, academic (occupational), or other important areas of functioning.

C. Chronological age is at least 5 years (or equivalent developmental level).

D. The behaviour is not due exclusively to the direct physiological effect of a substance (e.g. a diuretic) or a general medical condition (e.g. diabetes, spina bifida, a seizure disorder).

Specify type:
Nocturnal only
Diurnal only
Nocturnal and diurnal

Table 22.3. Classification of nocturnal enuresis

	Maximal dry interval <6 months	Maximal dry interval >6 months
	Primary nocturnal enuresis (PNE)	Secondary nocturnal enuresis (SNE)
No signs of bladder dysfunction* during daytime	Primary monosymptomatic nocturnal enuresis (PMNE)	Secondary monosymptomatic nocturnal enuresis (SMNE)**
Signs of bladder dysfunction* during daytime present	Primary non-monosymptomatic nocturnal enuresis (PNMNE)	Secondary non-monosymptomatic nocturnal enuresis (SNMNE)**

* Signs of urge, frequency, voiding postponement, dyscoordination, soiling – i.e. similar to children with functional urinary incontinence – but without daytime wetting.

** These subtypes have not been widely used so far, which is not very logical, as both mono- and non-monosymptomatic forms exist among secondary nocturnal enuresis too.

there are no other daytime signs suggestive of lower urinary tract dysfunction. In non-monosymptomatic nocturnal enuresis, children only wet at night, but do show signs such as urge and frequency, voiding postponement, intermittent micturition or constipation and encopresis.

The classification of daytime wetting is more complicated (see Table 22.4), but fortunately, each subtype has distinguishing main symptoms. The three most common syndromes of daytime wetting are:

• urge incontinence, characterized by urgency, frequency and voiding of small volumes of urine; it is caused by an overactivity of the bladder during the filling phase

• voiding postponement with a low voiding frequency and retention of urine in certain situations

Table 22.4. Classification of daytime wetting with main distinguishing symptoms

Type of daytime wetting	Main symptoms and features
Urge incontinence	Frequency with > seven voidings per day, small volumes, urge symptoms
Voiding postponement	Infrequent micturitions < times per day, postponement
Detrusor–sphincter dyscoordination	Straining to initiate and during micturition, interrupted stream of urine
Stress incontinence	Wetting during coughing, sneezing, small volumes
Giggle incontinence	Wetting during laughing, large volumes with complete emptying
Lazy-bladder syndrome	Interrupted stream, emptying of bladder possible only by straining

- detrusor–sphincter dyscoordination (also misleadingly named 'dysfunctional voiding') characterized by straining and intermittent micturition due to a paradoxical contraction of the urinary sphincter (instead of relaxation) during the voiding phase.

Rare forms include:

- stress incontinence with voiding due to increased intra-abdominal pressure (coughing, sneezing)
- giggle incontinence with complete emptying of the bladder induced by laughing
- lazy-bladder syndrome with retention of large volumes of urine and incomplete emptying due to decompensation of the bladder.

Epidemiology

Prevalence

The prevalence of nocturnal enuresis has been investigated in several longitudinal and transsectional epidemiological studies around the world. The rates are quite comparable from one country to another: thus, 15 per cent of the 5-, 10 per cent of the 7-year-old children, 1–2 per cent of adolescents and 0.3–1.7 per cent of adults are affected. The spontaneous cure rate is 14 per cent per year. The age of achieving complete dryness is not affected by toilet training or other psychosocial factors, but seems to follow a biologically determined pattern. Primary nocturnal enuresis is twice as common as secondary nocturnal enuresis. No reliable epidemiological data exist for mono- and non-monosymptomatic forms.

Day wetting is less common, 2–3 per cent of 7-year-old children and <1 per cent of adolescents are affected. Urge incontinence and voiding postponement are the most common forms, but again, reliable epidemiological data is lacking for the subtypes.

Sex ratios

One and a half to two times more males are affected by nocturnal enuresis, while the sex ratios for daytime wetting are reversed or equal (1.0 to 1.5 females to 1 male). Urge incontinence has the highest rate of affected girls.

Implications for practice

Due to secrecy and lack of exchange with others, many children and parents are not aware how common nocturnal enuresis and daytime wetting really are. This information, i.e. to know that many others are affected, can be a great emotional relief for many families.

Clinical picture

Main features and symptoms

The main symptom is, obviously, the involuntary wetting into the bed, clothing or diapers after the age of 5 years – irrespective of the amount of urine. As the specific symptoms differ greatly from one subtype to another, they have to be discussed separately.

Nocturnal enuresis

Children with primary nocturnal enuresis have never been dry for more than 6 months in a row. Children with SEN have been dry for longer than half a year – irrespective at what age and if the dry interval occurred spontaneously or was achieved by treatment. The relapse is often precipitated by adverse life events or co-morbid psychopathology.

In monosymptomatic nocturnal enuresis the voided urine volumes are large – the bed is often soaking wet. Many children show an increased urine production at night (polyuria). In addition, they are described as 'deep sleepers' by parents and have been shown to be more difficult to arouse than non-enuretics in standardized studies.

Children with non-monosymptomatic nocturnal enuresis show similar symptoms as children with functional urinary incontinence – except that they do not wet during the day (see Tables 22.3 and 22.4). Thus, many children have typical symptoms of detrusor instability (i.e. spontaneous contractions during the filling phase) including urgency and frequency during the day. At night, multiple wetting episodes are common – often detected by multiple activation of the bell during alarm treatment (see below). Other children have a reduced micturition frequency of only two to three times per day (voiding postponement) or have difficulties during voiding (dyscoordination). These symptoms are often overlooked by parents and clinicians, but have great therapeutical implications, as they have to be treated first. The most important instrument to adequately differentiate mono- from non-monosymptomatic enuresis are the 24-h (better 48-h) frequency/volume charts (see Appendix).

Daytime wetting

Children with urge incontinence (UI) have to empty their bladder more than seven times per day with unusually small volumes for their age (frequency). Often, they sense a sudden, imperative urge to void, which is counteracted by holding manoeuvres such as squatting, pressing their legs together, sitting on their heel or performing the so-called curtsey sign. The likelihood for wetting increases with tiredness and is thus more common in the afternoons and evenings. The wetted volumes are often small and not visible through the clothing. Perigenital dermatitis and urinary tract infections (UTIs) can co-exist and aggravate the wetting.

The most important sign of voiding postponement (VP) is a low micturition frequency of less than five times per day. Voiding is postponed in typical situations such as school, during play or watching TV. The fuller the bladder gets, the more the sense of (urgency) increases, which again is met with holding manoeuvres, i.e. contraction of the voluntary pelvic floor muscles. The voided volumes are larger, residual urine, vesico-ureteral refluxes and UTIs can develop.

Children with detrusor–sphincter dyscoordination (DSD) have difficulty initiating and maintaining the micturition due to the paradox contraction of the urethral sphincters instead of relaxation. Therefore, the most important clinical signs are straining and an interrupted stream of urine into several portions. The rate of medical complications is highest with this subtype with UTIs, reflux and even upper urinary tract pathology. Diagnosis and treatment at an early stage is therefore absolutely essential.

For the rare syndromes, children with stress incontinence wet small volumes of urine whenever the intraabdominal pressure is increased, for example during coughing and sneezing. In giggle incontinence, the clothing is visibly wet as a complete emptying of the bladder is initiated by laughing. And in the lazy-bladder syndrome, an enormous distension of the bladder, residual urine and incomplete emptying is typical – as the detrusor is decompensated.

Differential diagnosis

Medical illnesses have to be excluded, especially in day wetting children, in whom they are much more prevalent than in nocturnal enuretics. The organic causes of wetting include structural abnormalities such as posterior urethral valves, ectopic ureters, epi- and hypospadias and other malformations of the urinary tract. Neurogenic urinary incontinence is typical in spina bifida or the tethered-cord syndrome. The most common medical causes are UTIs, rarer causes to be considered are diabetes mellitus and insipidus.

Psychiatric co-morbidity

Many children (and parents) are distressed and bothered by the wetting. Seventy per cent of children can even state explicitly that they experience disadvantages through the wetting, like not being able to sleep over with friends, feeling isolated and being teased by friends. Their self-esteem is reduced, but returns to normal upon attaining dryness. Some parents feel guilty, others react with annoyance and anger, a minority even punishes their child. This so-called 'parental intolerance' is especially likely to arise when parents attribute their child's wetting to a voluntary, even hostile, act.

In contrast to these common, subclinical symptoms, most wetting children are not psychiatrically disturbed. The rate of psychiatric disorders is two to four times higher for the whole group of wetting children in epidemiological as well as clinical studies. This means that 20 per cent to 40 per cent of children show some form of co-morbid disorder – with substantial variation across subtypes. Thus, the rates are especially high among children with SNE and VP, low with PNE and UI. Children with monosymptomatic PNE have the lowest rate of co-morbid disorders – no higher than among non-wetting children.

Externalizing disorders predominate. There seems to be a specific co-morbidity of PNE and ADHD and of VP and conduct disorders. Emotional disorders are less common, but can co-exist with UI and SNE. The associations of wetting and co-morbid disorders are complex: obviously, disturbances can develop as a consequence of the wetting; both adverse life events, as well as co-morbid disorders can precede a relapse in SNE; the specific co-morbidity of PNE and ADHD is most likely due to neurobiological factors; and wetting and psychological factors can simply co-exist by chance and show no causal association.

Diagnostic instruments and assessment

Due to the increased co-morbidity for psychiatric disorders, at least a short screening for behavioural and emotional symptoms should be carried out – by history, observation, exploration and mental state examination. Some suggestions for relevant questions are found in Appendix 22.1. It is advisable to use general questionnaires such as the CBCL (Achenbach) routinely in every case. Only if indicated, should a full formal child psychiatric assessment and psychological testing be carried out. Basic child psychiatric approaches will not be dealt with in this context, instead the focus will be on the diagnosis of the specific type of wetting.

Table 22.5. Standard and extended assessment of wetting problem

Standard assessment
Sufficient for monosymptomatic nocturnal enuresis and for most other forms
History
Frequency/volume chart
Questionnaires
Physical examination
Sonography
Urinalysis

Extended assessment
Only if indicated
Urine bacteriology
Uroflowmetry
Paediatric and urological assessment: radiology, cystoscopy, urodynamic investigations, etc.

As shown in Table 22.5, a standard approach is sufficient for all cases of monosymptomatic nocturnal enuresis and for most other cases, as well. Only if indicated are further diagnostic measures needed – especially in day wetting children and in cases with non-monosymptomatic nocturnal enuresis.

- The most important step in the diagnosis of enuresis and urinary incontinence is a careful and detailed history. As this is such a vital part of the diagnostic process, a suggestion for history taking is shown in Appendix 22.1.
- The second most important instrument is the frequency/volume chart, as depicted in Appendix 22.2. Over 24 hours, if possible 48 hours (usually over the weekends), parents and children are asked to measure and document when and how much they void and drink, as well as observe other symptoms such as urge symptoms. This instrument is so essential, as daytime symptoms are often overlooked and therefore will not be picked up even in a detailed history. Only the information gained by direct measurement can differentiate between mono- and non-monosymptomatic NE, as well as between VP an UI. It should therefore never be omitted.
- Parental questionnaires are a useful adjunct to check and augment the information obtained in the history. An example of a widely-used questionnaire is shown in Appendix 22.3.
- A complete physical examination is mandatory, including the genital and anal area, the spine and the lower extremities. A neurological examination is advisable.
- There is some controversy regarding the use of sonography in nocturnal enuresis. Routine ultrasound will pick up malformations of the urinary tract, but is also essential to identify two functional parameters: residual urine (after voiding) and

hypertrophy of the bladder wall – both of which are common in urinary incontinence. Ultrasound should therefore always be performed at least in day wetting children and in those with non-monosymptomatic NE.

- An urinalysis with dip-sticks is usually sufficient as a screening procedure in most cases. If a urinary tract infection (UTI) is suspected, urine microscopy and bacteriology is mandatory.
- All other diagnostic steps are not needed routinely, but require special indication. Uroflowmetry (measurement of the urine stream), combined with an EMG of the pelvic floor is a non-invasive examination that can identify disturbances of the emptying phase of the bladder. It is absolutely indicated if DSD is suspected. Radiology (cysto-urogram) is indicated if urethral stenoses or vesico-urethral-refluxes are suspected. Rarely, a complete urological work-up is needed in functional urinary but is absolutely needed if an organic form of urinary incontinence is suspected.

Aetiology

Enuresis and functional urinary incontinence are 'psychophysiological' disorders with a complex interaction of somatic and psychological factors. As the relative contribution of each differs for each subtype, they have to be discussed separately.

Nocturnal enuresis

NE is a genetically determined maturational disorder of the central nervous system. The evidence for the genetic basis of this disorder is impressive: 60–80 per cent of children with enuresis have relatives who also wetted, only a third are sporadic cases. The concordance rate for monozygotic is higher than for dizygotic twins. Nearly half of the families follow an autosomal dominant mode of inheritance. Several chromosomal loci of interest have been identified by linkage studies.

Pathophysiologically, one contributing factor is an increased urine production at night (polyuria) associated with circadian variations of the antidiuretic hormone (arginine vasopressin) in subgroups of children. Two factors are essential, however, for wetting episodes to occur: children show a lack of arousal, i.e. they do not wake up when the bladder is full; and they have a lack of inhibition of the micturition reflex, i.e. they are not able to suppress the emptying of the bladder and sleep through the night. Both effects are mediated through centres of the brainstem.

In monosymptomatic NE only the CNS is affected – the function of the bladder is completely normal during day and night. In contrast, non-monosymptomatic NE forms do show additional signs of bladder dysfunction – the same as with day wetting children. The latter can be considered to represent variants of NE and functional urinary incontinence.

PNE is almost exclusively genetically determined. Psychosocial factors play a negligible role and the psychiatric co-morbidity is not increased. In SNE, the same genetic factors act as a disposition for a relapse that is precipitated by life events and psychiatric disorders. This disposition seems to persist life long: thus, former enuretics carry an eight-fold risk as adults to wet at night.

Daytime wetting

UI also has a clear genetic basis with higher rates of affected relatives and with first positive molecular linkage results. Pathophysiologically, it is a disturbance of the filling phase of the bladder. Instead of a continuous filling without major increase of the intravesical pressure, UI is characterized by repeated spontaneous contractions in partially filled bladder (this has led to the synonyms of 'overactive bladder' or 'detrusor instability'). These contractions lead to the sense of urge, which children try to control by using the voluntary muscles of the pelvic floor (holding manoeuvres). If they don't succeed or don't get to the toilet in time, wetting occurs. Emotional and behavioural symptoms can develop as a consequence of the wetting, but do not play a contributing role in the aetiology of UI.

In contrast, VP is an essentially psychogenic, acquired condition. The most common co-morbid disorder is ODD (oppositional defiant disorder). In fact, in many children the postponement of micturition and the retention of urine can be considered as a sub-symptom of a more general oppositional defiant conduct disorder. In others it represents an acquired habit that has persisted and can be reinforced by (negative) parental responses.

DSD, too, is an acquired syndrome characterized by the paradoxical contraction of the urethral sphincter during micturition. In some children, it can develop out of an UI by the excessive use of the pelvic floor. In others, it is an isolated symptom. And finally, in a subgroup it is associated with severe psychopathology, including severe depression, following sexual abuse and deprivation.

The aetiology of the rarer forms is summarized: stress incontinence occurs due to an insufficiency of the urethral sphincter. Giggle incontinence is a genetic syndrome with an overlap with cataplexy and narcolepsy: laughing induces a complete reflective emptying of the bladder in addition to postural symptoms. And finally, the lazy-bladder syndrome can be considered as the final stage of VP and DSD in which the detrusor muscles is decompensated.

Treatment

As evident from the heterogeneity of childhood wetting problems, an effective treatment relies on a detailed and exact diagnosis of the specific subtype, which again has to be discussed individually. However, a few general points have to be considered.

- Ineffective types of treatment should be discontinued.
- Any constipation and encopresis should be dealt with first.
- Oral fluids often have to be increased, as many children do not drink enough.
- Day-wetting and daytime symptoms need to be treated first.
- The treatment should always be symptom orientated and include cognitive-behavioural elements.
- Unspecific measures such as psycho-education, provision of information, emotional support, increasing motivation and alleviating anxiety and feelings of guilt are essential, i.e. a good therapeutical relationship with the child and parents.

Nocturnal enuresis

Thus, in NE ineffective measures such as waking, lifting, fluid restriction and non-indicated medication should be discontinued. The first step should be a baseline of 4 weeks: children are asked to document in a chart, which nights were dry and which were wet. Symbols such as sun and clouds are often used. If a marked decline of wet nights occurs, this simple method can be continued for longer than a month. If, however, the child wets every night with no sign of change, the charts should not be followed through for the entire month. Several studies have shown that charts are sufficient for 15–20 per cent of children to achieve dryness – all others will require more specific measures.

The most effective mode of treatment for NE is, without any doubt, alarm treatment. Many randomized controlled trials have demonstrated that 60–70 per cent of children will reach dryness with a high long-term stability. Children and parents do, however, need to be motivated. The two types of alarms – body-worn and bed-side alarms – are equally effective. The alarm needs to be applied every night for a maximum of 16 weeks. Parents and children are instructed to ensure that the child is awoken completely when the alarm sounds, goes to the toilet, voids the remaining urine, changes bed clothes and pyjama and resets the alarm. The course of alarm treatment should be documented by parents and regular follow-up visits should be arranged to enhance the compliance and tackle any arising problems.

If necessary, the effects of alarm treatment can be enhanced by operant behavioural techniques such as 'arousal training', a simple, but effective token system. If children turn off the alarm, get out of bed and to the toilet within 3 minutes, they receive two tokens. If they don't, they have to return a token. To reduce frustration in younger children, it is best only to give positive rewards.

In contrast, dry bed training (DBT) is a highly complex behavioural treatment including both reinforcing, as well as aversive elements. In recent meta-analyses, it was shown to be no more effective than alarm treatment alone. It should therefore be reserved for special groups, such as treatment-resistant adolescents with NE.

Pharmacotherapy is less effective than alarm treatment, but is indicated if short-term dryness is required (school outings, holidays), the family is not able or willing to perform alarm treatment, in chronic treatment-resistant cases (especially adolescents) or in combination with alarm-treatment. Only two substances have a proven anti-enuretic effect: desmopressin (or DDAVP: 1-deamino-8-D-arginine vasopressin) and tricyclic antidepressants such as imipramine.

DDAVP is an analogue of the antidiuretic hormone with proven antidiuretic and assumed CNS effects. In 70 per cent, dryness or a reduction of wet nights occurs, but the relapse rate is high after medication is stopped. Even after prolonged use, only a maximum of 18–38 per cent remain dry. Side effects are not common and usually benign, such as stomachaches and headaches. The only severe, though very rare, side effects are hyponatremia, convulsions and loss of consciousness, requiring intensive care treatment. No fatalities have been reported. Still, parents have to be informed and are advised not to let their children drink after DDAVP has been taken. The medication is given once a day in the evening. The dose has to be titrated individually. The dose of the preferred intranasal application ranges from 20 μg to 30 μg to a maximum of 40 μg. The comparable oral doses are 0.2 mg (one tablet) to 0.4 mg (two tablets). After a maximum of 3 months, a medication should be withdrawn to see if it is still needed. If a relapse occurs, it can be continued. Some evidence suggests that a gradual tapering off is associated with less relapse than sudden withdrawal.

The use of antidepressants in the treatment of NE (especially imipramine) has declined, even though they have similar success and relapse rates as DDAVP. The doses required are lower and the time of onset is shorter than in the treatment of depressive disorders. The doses should start with 10 mg or 25 mg once/day in the evening. They can be increased to the range of 1.0 to 2.5 mg/kg body weight/day – but these larger doses should be distributed three times over the day. Due to cardiac side effects (even fatalities under desmipramine, but not imipramine), tricyclics require close clinical monitoring, with blood count, other laboratory parameters and ECGs. Also, accidental poisoning has been reported repeatedly.

Daytime wetting

In day wetting children, any medical conditions such as UTIs should, of course, be tackled first. More than with nocturnal enuretics, children and parents need basic, cognitive information on the specific mechanisms involved, as many are not aware even of the anatomy and physiology of the lower urinary tract. Again, all ineffective measures should be stopped, especially any form of retention control training, as this can induce and chronify DSD by the excessive use of the pelvis floor muscles.

In UI, the main line of treatment is cognitive-behavioural with the aim of enhancing central awareness and control of bladder functions without the use of holding manoeuvres. Children are instructed to go to the toilet as soon as they sense an urge and document in a chart if their underpants were dry (symbol: flag) or wet (cloud). In about a third of all children with UI, this is sufficient leading first to a reduction of wet episodes and finally of the micturition frequency. In two-thirds of children, additional anticholinergic medication is needed. The standard medication is oxybutinin, starting with 0.3 mg/kg body weight/day in three doses to a maximum of 0.6 mg/kg body weight/day. The maximum doses should not exceed 15 mg/day. It should be introduced in small steps to minimize side effects, which include tachycardia, dry mouth, flushing and blurred vision. The side effects are reversible and dose dependent. If tolerated, oxybutinin is given over several months in combination with the behavioural training and then slowly discontinued. Alternative medications include propiverin (which is effective, but not available in many countries) and detrusitol (which has less side effects, but is not approved for use in children in some countries yet).

The treatment of VP again is behavioural-cognitive with the aim of increasing the micturition frequency to seven times a day – and thereby reducing the tendency of urine retention. Children are instructed to go to the toilet at regular intervals and to document this in a plan. Digital wrist-watches with alarm signal can act as useful reminders in older children. Because of the high rate of externalizing disorders, often other child psychiatric interventions such as stimulant medication (for ADHD), behavioural treatment (for ODD), individual and family treatment are needed.

DSD is treated most effectively by a visual and/or acoustic biofeedback using uroflow and pelvic-floor-EMG signals. The usually requires referral to special centres.

All of the rare forms require a multiprofessional approach, including paediatric urological expertise. Stress incontinence is treated behaviourally and pharmacologically, rarely operatively. Giggle incontinence can be treated behaviourally (with a conditioning programme) and with high-dose methylphenidate (due to the overlap with narcolepsy). And the lazy-bladder syndrome can require intermittent catherization in addition to training.

Outcome

The long-term outcome has been studied in detail for nocturnal enuresis – with 60–70 per cent of children achieving dryness with alarm treatment and 50–60 per cent remaining dry even long-term. The effectiveness of pharmacotherapy is less good. All interventions have to be compared with the spontaneous cure rate of 14 per cent per annum. Still, a small group of 1–2 per cent will persist into adolescence and 1 per cent even into adulthood.

The long-term effects of day wetting has not been studied as extensively as in NE. UI has the best over-all prognosis. The effects of biofeedback training for DSD

Table 22.6. Diagnostic criteria for Nonorganic encopresis (F98.1) according to ICD-10 (research criteria)

A. The child repeatedly passes feces in places that are inappropriate for the purpose (e.g., clothing, floor), either involuntarily or intentionally. (The disorder may involve overflow incontinence secondary to functional fecal retention.)

B. The child's chronological and mental age is at least 4 years.

C. There is at least one encopretic event per month.

D. Duration of the disorder is at least 6 months.

E. There is no organic condition that constitutes a sufficient cause for the encopretic event.

A fifth character may be used, if desired, for further specification:

F98.10 Failure to acquire physiological bowel control

F98.11 Adequate bowel control with normal feces deposited in inappropriate places

F98.12 Soiling associated with excessively fluid feces (such as with overflow)

Table 22.7. Diagnostic criteria for Encopresis according to DSM-IV

A. Repeated passage of feces into inappropriate places (e.g. clothing or floor) whether involuntary or intentional.

B. At least one such event a month for at least 3 months.

C. Chronological age is at least 4 years (or equivalent developmental level).

D. The behaviour is not due exclusively to the direct physiological effects of a substance (e.g., laxatives) or a general medical condition except through a mechanism involving constipation.

Code as follows:

787.6 With constipation and overflow incontinence

307.7 Without constipation and overflow incontinence

have been proven even in long-term follow-ups. The prognosis of VP depends very much on the co-morbid oppositional and defiant symptoms.

Encopresis

Definition and classification

The diagnostic criteria according to ICD-10 and DSM-IV are shown in Tables 22.6 and 22.7. The definitions are comparable: encopresis is diagnosed by

- involuntary or intentional soiling in inappropriate places
- at least once a month
- in a child 4 years or older
- after organic causes have been ruled out.

Again, the duration of the disorder differs, ICD-10 requiring 6 months and DSM-IV only 3 months (see Tables 22.6 and 22.7). Both classification systems define subtypes. The differentiation according to DSM-IV is more explicit, more relevant in daily practice and widely used in research: encopresis can occur with and without constipation and overflow incontinence. Constipation itself is not defined adequately in the classification systems. The two main features are either bowel emptying less than three times a week or – and this is an important addition – clinical signs of constipation such as abdominal pain, palpable masses, etc. In other words, some children pass stools every day, but still show retention of old stool masses and constipation.

Epidemiology

Prevalence

The prevalence of encopresis varies from one epidemiological study to the next, which implies that, in addition to biological factors, environmental influences such as the type and onset of toilet training have an effect on attaining continence. This seems to apply only for the toddler age, while the rate of soiling in older pre-school children is not affected by toilet training. In summary, 2–3 per cent of 4-year olds and 1–2 per cent of school-age children soil. It is rarely diagnosed in adolescents and adults, which does not necessarily mean that it does not occur, as the diagnosis of 'encopresis' is not used in adult medicine or psychiatry (being replaced by the umbrella term of 'fecal' or 'anal incontinence', which includes both functional and organic forms).

Primary and secondary (i.e. a relapse following a symptom-free interval of >6 months) forms are equally common. Soiling almost exclusively occurs during the daytime and only exceptionally at night. Three to four times more boys than girls are affected. No reliable epidemiological data for the subtypes with and without encopresis exist. In clinical studies, due to recruitment biases, encopresis with constipation is over-represented in departments of paediatric gastroenterology, while child psychiatric units are bound to see more children with encopresis without constipation.

Clinical picture

Main features and symptoms

The two subtypes differ greatly regarding clinical signs and symptoms and therefore have to be discussed separately. The two groups have been compared in clinical studies with great differences in their signs and symptoms (see Table 22.8).

Children with encopresis with constipation (i.e. retentive encopresis) defecate less often, they complain about abdominal pain and painful defecation. Abdominal

Table 22.8. Differences between encopresis with and without constipation (Benninga *et al.*, 1994)

	Encopresis with constipation $N = 111$	Encopresis without constipation $N = 50$
Boys	68%	86%
Age (mean)	8.0	9.0
Toilet trained	56%	69%
Age at which toilet training started (years)	1.5	2.0
Bowel movements/week (mean)	seldom (2×/week)	Often (7×/week)
Large amounts of stools	yes (61%)	No (0%)
Normal stools (consistency)	54%	82%
Daytime soiling	77%	68%
Episodes/week	7×/week	3,5×/week
Night time soiling	33%	6%
Episodes/week	seldom	seldom
Pain during defecation	50%	30%
Abdominal pain	41%	22%
No rectal sensation	18%	6%
Good appetite	58%	78%
Colon transit time	Long (62.4 h)	Normal (40.2 h)
Orocaecal transit time	No difference	No difference
Palpable abdominal mass	39%	0%
Palpable rectal mass	31%	0%
Normal defecation dynamics	41%**	54%**
Daytime urinary incontinence	12%	7%
Night time urinary incontinence	29%	10%
CBCL total score in the clinical range*	38.5%	44.2%
Laxative therapy	helpful	Not helpful, even worsening

* 10% in normative population (cut-off: 90th percentile).
** controls: 93%.

masses are palpable and the appetite is reduced. They soil large amounts of stool of hard consistency – mainly during the day and respond well to laxative treatment. Concomitant wetting during the day, as well as the night is common.

In contrast, children without constipation (i.e. non-retentive encopresis) go to the toilet more often, stools are of normal consistency and the encopretic episodes occur less often and almost always during the day. Pain is rare, abdominal masses are not palpable and the appetite is not reduced. Colon transit time and rectal sensitivity are normal. Treatment with laxatives is not helpful and can, in fact, lead to a worsening of the soiling. It is therefore, of great therapeutic importance to identify the specific subtype of encopresis.

Differential diagnosis

Organic forms of fecal incontinence have to be ruled out. These include gastrointestinal infections, as well as malformations of the GI tract. Stool retention and constipation can be induced by endocrinological factors (i.e. hypothyroidism), as well as by a wide variety of pharmacological agents. In rare cases, abdominal tumours have to be ruled out. The most important differential diagnosis is Hirschsprung's disease, a congenital aganglionosis of the colon. Symptoms usually present from birth with signs of GI obstruction, abdominal pain and stools of reduced diameter. Eighty per cent of cases are identified by the age of 4 years, i.e. the age at which encopresis can be diagnosed.

Co-morbidity

Encopresis has a high co-morbidity with other child psychiatric disorders, as well as with wetting problems.

Even in paediatric settings, the rate of clinically relevant behavioural symptom scores is in the range of 40 per cent – a four-fold increase compared to controls and the normative population. Externalizing disorders predominate, with ADHD being the most common single diagnosis. The rate of emotional disorders is also increased. Encopresis is also more common in children with mental retardation. The overall rate of disorders is the same for children with and without constipation.

Diagnostic instruments

Again, a thorough history is the most important step in the diagnostic process (see Table 22.9). Some of the important questions to ask are included in the interview for wetting problems (see Appendix 22.1). As soiling and wetting show such a high concurrence, one should always inquire if the child wets at night and/or during the day and specify the type of enuresis or urinary incontinence. Also, special parental questionnaires can be used to check the information provided in the history. Some of the important items are included in the parental questionnaire for wetting problems (Appendix 22.3).

The paediatric physical examination should always include the anal region and check for abdominal masses. There is some controversy regarding the importance of routine rectal examinations. They should never be omitted if organic forms of stool incontinence is suspected or in treatment-resistant cases. If an infection is suspected, stool bacteriology should be performed.

Table 22.9. Standard and extended assessment of encopresis

Standard assessment
Sufficient for most cases of encopresis
History
Questionnaires
Physical examination
Sonography

Extended assessment
Only if indicated
Stool bacteriology
Radiology: plain abdominal X-ray
Colon contrast X-ray
MRI of colon
Manometry
Endoscopy and biopsy

Abdominal sonography has become a very useful instrument to differentiate encopresis with and without constipation and retention. In the latter cases, retrovesical impressions and the enlargement of the rectum and sigmoid can be seen and measured. The course of laxative treatment can be followed and documented.

Plain abdominal X-rays and MRI of the colon are not indicated routinely, but should be considered in chronic cases that do not respond to usual treatment to rule out any underlying organic causes. Manometry, X-rays of the colon with contrast media and endoscopic biopsies are indicated if, for example, Hirschsprung's disease is suspected. Children should be referred to specialized centres in all of these cases.

Aetiology

Of the two subtypes, the aetiology and pathophysiology of encopresis with constipation has been studied in greater detail. Genetic factors seem to play a role. Twin studies have shown a much higher concordance rate for monozygotic compared to dizygotic twins. In addition, environmental factors clearly play a major role in activating a cascade of events leading to chronic stool retention. Thus, chronic constipation usually arises out of an acute constipation in infancy and at toddler age. It is often triggered by painful defecation (such as anal fissures, dermatitis, etc.) or by stressful life events (such as separation of parents, birth of sibling). Late and inconsequent toilet training can also be a contributing factor. Children, who insist on defecating into the diapers, but not the toilet (toilet refusal syndrome) are also at higher risk for constipation.

Independent of the type of trigger, an acute constipation can merge into a 'vicious circle' with increasing retention of stool up to extreme forms of mega-colon. In this process, stool masses accumulate, peristalsis and sensitivity dimin-ish, which again facilitates further stool retention. Newer, soft stools can seep in between the old, hard stool masses and induce soiling. Therefore, the term 'over-flow incontinence' is misleading – 'interflow incontinence' more aptly describes the situation.

Many of the somatic symptoms, such as variations of the secretion of gastroin-testinal hormones or the paradoxical contraction of the external sphincter are most likely to be secondary effects of this 'vicious circle'. Equally, dysfunctional intrafamilial interaction can at least partially be understood as a secondary effect of retention and soiling. In addition, the common symptoms of day and night wetting are most likely due to local factors such as retrovesical compression of the bladder neck and bladder by stool masses. Thus, treatment of the constipation alone can lead to dryness in some children.

Treatment

The basic treatment approaches are the same in both types of encopresis. In addition, children with constipation require an initial evacuation and laxative treatment – children without constipation do not. Therefore, the basic principles will be dis-cussed first.

- A careful diagnostic work-up should precede all therapeutic interventions.
- Treatment should be symptom-orientated with the aim of alleviating soiling (and constipation if present).
- Cognitive-behavioural approaches are more effective than insight-oriented, psychodynamic or child-centred approaches.
- Co-morbid psychiatric disturbances require separate diagnosis and treatment.
- Parents and children are often not aware of the associations of retention and soiling, for example, and need detailed information.
- Emotional support, continued guidance and a good therapeutic relationship are absolute prerequisites.
- A baseline without intervention can usually be skipped.
- The most important component is regular stool training: children are asked to go to the toilet (or are sent by their parents) three times a day after the main mealtimes (breakfast, lunch and supper), as the defecation reflexes are most active postprandially. They are instructed to sit in a relaxed position for 5–15 minutes. Legs should be apart and not be dangling down. The feet should have contact with the ground, otherwise a small foot stool should be provided. Children are allowed to engage in pleasant activity such as reading comics. A chart is used the document the course of the training. Of special interest are: if the child went

to the toilet voluntarily or had to be sent by the parents; if it had defecated or urinated; and if the clothing had been soiled. If necessary, this programme can be enhanced by a simple token system. Often, rewards are not required, especially if the child is involved in the documentation and can witness the progress being made.

• In addition, nutritional information and changes in the diet, introducing more fibres and a balance of nutrients can be helpful. Increasing the amount of oral fluids is equally important, as many children do not drink enough.

Encopresis with constipation – laxative treatment

Laxative treatment is necessary only in cases with proven constipation. It should never be performed in children without constipation – underlining again the importance of a good diagnosis. Also, laxative treatment alone is not effective and always needs to be combined with other behavioural interventions such as stool training. Two phases are usually necessary:

• an initial evacuation of stool masses with enemas. Phosphate enemas (in one-way plastic tubes) are usually used and well tolerated if children are prepared. There will be some discomfort with the first enema, so children should be instructed carefully. They should lie on their sides, legs pulled up, let the tube of the enema (cream can be used as a lubricant) be introduced and try to wait a few minutes before defecation. The masses can be enormous and clogged toilets have been reported. One should ensure that the enema is not retained, as phosphate intoxication through absorption can occur in younger children.

• maintenance period: Once the stool masses have been removed, a maintenance over many months is necessary to ensure that the retention does not recur and that the distended colon returns to normal size and function.

• In some children, regular enemas once or twice a week will continue to be necessary. In addition, oral laxatives need to be given, as well. Often, lactulose in liquid or powder form as a stool softener is sufficient and is well tolerated by most children. One to three teaspoons (or tablespoons) a day with the meals are sufficient. If the stools become too liquid, the dose is simply reduced. Recently, a new laxative (polyethylene glycol 3350) has shown promising results and may become the standard laxative in the future.

In some centres, biofeedback training using intrarectal pressures and perianal EMG signals have been performed. Recent randomized controlled trials have demonstrated that they are no more effective than the standard treatment. In one study, an intensive behavioural training alone was even more effective than if combined with biofeedback. Therefore, biofeedback can no longer be recommended as routine treatment for encopresis. It might have a place for the treatment-resistant cases or if special abnormalities of the defecation dynamics are present.

Outcome

Several long-term follow-up studies show that 58–76 per cent of children with encopresis remain free of symptoms, while a third merge into a chronic course with remaining symptoms of soiling. Risk and protective factors remain to be identified in the future.

SUGGESTED READING

Enuresis

R. J. Butler, *Nocturnal Enuresis – The Child's Experience.* (Oxford: Butterworth-Heinemann, 1994).

R. J. Butler, Annotation: night wetting in children: psychological perspectives. *Journal of Child Psychology and Psychiatry*, **39** (1998), 453–63.

A. von Gontard, Annotation: day and night wetting in children – a paediatric and child psychiatric perspective. *Journal of Child Psychology and Psychiatry*, **39** (1998), 439–51.

A. von Gontard, H. Schaumburg, E. Hollmann, H. Eiberg & S. Rittig, The genetics of enuresis – a review. *Journal of Urology*, **166** (2001), 2438–43.

A. von Gontard, *Einnässens im Kindesalter: Erscheinungsformen – Diagnostik – Therapie.* (Stuttgart: Thieme Verlag, 2001).

J. D. van Gool & G. A. de Jonge, Urge syndrome and urge incontinence. *Archives of Disease in Childhood*, **64** (1989), 1629–34.

K. Hjälmas, T. Arnold, W. Bower, *et al.*, Nocturnal enursis: an international evidence based mangement strategy. *Journal of Urology*, in press, 2003.

G. Läckgren, K. Hjälmas, J. van Gool, *et al.*, Nocturnal enuresis – a suggestion for a European treatment strategy. *Acta Paediatrica*, **88** (1999), 679–90.

R. H. Largo, L. Molinari, K. von Siebenthal & U. Wolfensberger, Does a profound change in toilet training affect development of bowel and bladder control? *Developmental Medicine and Child Neurology*, **38** (1996), 1106–16.

E. J. Mikkelsen, Enuresis and encopresis: ten years of progress. *Journal of the American Academy of Child and Adolescent Psychiatry*, **40** (2001), 1146–58.

M. W. Mellon & M. L. McGrath, Empirically supported treatments in pediatric psychology: nocturnal enuresis. *Journal of Pediatric Psychology*, **25** (2000), 193–214.

M. E. K. Moffat, Nocturnal enuresis: a review of the efficacy of treatments and practical advice for clinicians. *Developmental and Behavioral Pediatrics*, **18** (1997), 49–56.

T. Neveus, G. Läckgren, T. Tuvemo, J. Hetta, K. Hjälmas & A. Stenberg, Enuresis – background and treatment. *Scandinavian Journal of Urology and Nephrology*, Suppl. 206 (2000).

J. P. Norgaard, Pathophysiology of nocturnal enuresis. *Scandinavian Journal of Urology and Nephrology*, Suppl. 140 (1991).

Encopresis

M. A. Bennigna, H. A. Buller, H. S. Heymans, G. N. Tytgat & J. A. Taminiau, Is encopresis always the result of constipation? *Archives of Disease in Children*, **71** (1994), 186–93.

D. J. Cox, J. L. Sutphen, S. M. Borrowitz, B. Korvatchev & W. Ling, Contribution of behavior therapy and biofeedback to laxative therapy in the treatment of pediatric encopresis. *Annals of Behavioral Medicine*, **20** (1998), 70–6.

B. Felt, C. G. Wise, A. Olsen, P. Kochhar, S. Marcus & A. Coran, Guideline for the management of pediatric idiopathic constipation and soiling. *Archives of Pediatric and Adolescent Medicine*, **153** (1999), 380–5.

A. von Gontard, *Enkopresis: Erscheinungsformen – Diagnostik – Therapie.* (Stuttgart: Kohlhammer Verlag, 2003).

V. Loening-Baucke, Urinary incontinence and urinary tract infection and their resolution with treatment of chronic constipation of childhood. *Pediatrics*, **100** (1997), 228–32.

M. L. McGrath, M. W. Mellon & L. Murphy, Empirically supported treatments in pediatric psychology: constipation and encopresis. *Journal of Pediatric Psychology*, **25** (2000), 225–54.

Appendix 22.1. History of wetting problem and possible Co-morbid disorders

Presenting symptom:

General introduction: Do you know why you and your parents are here today?

Time of wetting: Is it because you wet the bed or because your pants are wet during the day?

Start with the most important symptom, i.e. night or daytime problems

Nocturnal wetting:

Frequency of wetting: Do you wet the bed every night or are there dry nights? How many nights per week is your bed wet (or dry)?

Amount of wetting: Is the bed damp or completely wet?

Depth of sleep: How deeply does your child sleep? Is it easy or difficult to wake him/her? What do you have to do to get you child awake? Does your child sometimes wake up at night to go to the toilet (nocturia)?

Dry intervals: What is the longest time period that your child has been completely dry (days, weeks, months)? How old was your child then? Were there events at the time of the relapse, which might have been of influence for your child to start wetting again?

Impact and distress: How is it for you when your bed is wet? Are you sad, annoyed, angry, ashamed- or do you feel it does not matter? Do you want to get dry? Are you willing to do something about it and put some effort into the therapy?

Social consequences: Have you been teased by somebody else about the wetting? Have you avoided sleeping over with friends or join in on outings with your school class?

Daytime wetting and micturition problems during the day

Frequency of wetting: Are your pants wet every day or do you also have dry days? How many days per week are your trousers wet? Does it happen that you wet during the day not once, but several times? How many times does it usually occur?

Amount of wetting::   Are the pants damp or really wet? Can the wet spot be seen through the clothing?

Timing during the day: Do you usually wet during the morning or in the afternoons (evenings)?

Frequency of micturition:	How often does your child go to the toilet during the day (3, 5, 10 or 20 times? Normal range: five to seven times per day)?
Voiding postponement:	Have you ever noticed that your child does not go to the toilet right away, but postpones the voiding as long as possible? In which situations does this happen most often (for example: in school, coming home from school, while playing, while watching TV or during other activities)?
Holding manoeuvres:	How do you notice that your child needs to go to the toilet? Does your child seem to be absent-minded? What exactly does your child do to postpone voiding? Have you ever noticed that your child crosses the legs, jumps from one leg to the next, holds the tummy or genitals, squats or sits on the heels?
Urge symptoms	Does it happen that your child feels a sudden and strong urge to go to the toilet (even though it goes to the toilet often)? For example, how long can you drive by car or go shopping, before your child has to go to the toilet? Do you have enough time to wait for the next cloakroom or do you have to stop right away to let your child void?
Dry intervals during the day:	When did your child get dry during the day? Is it still wetting during the day: what was the longest time period your child has ever been dry (days, weeks, months?). How old was your child then? Were there events at the time of the relapse, which might have been of influence for your child to start wetting again?
Problems with micturition:	Does your child have to strain at the beginning of micturition or does the urine come spontaneously? When voiding, is there one continuous stream or is the voiding interrupted? If it is interrupted, how many portions are there? And does your child have to strain to get it going again?
Urinary tract infections:	Does your child complain about pain during voiding? Does your child have to go the toilet more often than usual? How many urinary tract infections has your child had so far? When did the first infection occur? Has your child had infections with fever and pain in the kidney areas? Have the infections been treated with antibiotics? Has your child had an antibiotic long-term prophylaxis? Is it taking medication at the moment? Has your child had skin infections in the genital area (dermatitis)?
Medical complications:	Have there been other medical complications such as refluxes, operations, etc.?
Eating and drinking habits:	Please describe the eating habits of your child: Does your child prefer biscuits, white bread other low fibre food? How much and what does your child drink over the day?
Attributions:	What do you think is the cause of your child's wetting problem? Do you have any idea how it happened? Have you ever felt guilty about it? Have you ever blamed yourself about it? Have you ever been blamed by others? Do you think your child is doing it on purpose? Who is distressed the most about the wetting: you or your child? What do you think should change? What are your expectations? Are you and your child willing to cooperate actively?

Treatment trials

Previous therapy: What have you tried so far to get your child dry? Ineffective forms of
                         'treatment': fluid restriction, waking, holding, punishment, other
                         measures?; effective forms of treatment: charts and calendars, rewards,
                         alarm treatment, medication, which? (minirin, imipramine, others?). How
                         were the treatment trials conducted: please describe for how long with
                         which effects? Whom have you consulted for your child's wetting problem:
                         paediatrician, urologist, psychologist, psychiatrist, child guidance centres,
                         etc.? Which investigations have been performed so far?

Encopresis

Soiling: Does your child sometimes soil its underwear? How many times per week
                         does it happen? Are they large amounts or stool smearing? Does it happen
                         only during the day or also at night? How does your child react when it
                         soils? How old was your child when it became clean (stools in the toilet and
                         not in the diapers)? Have there been any relapses in the past?

Toilet habits: How often does your child have bowel movements per week? Does it
                         ever happen that your child does not have bowel movements for several
                         days in a row? Is your child constipated regularly? Is the elimination
                         of stools painful? Has there been blood on the stools? What have you done
                         so far?

Child psychiatric history

The child psychiatric history is divided into the presenting symptom(s), the personal and developmental
history and the family history. In most cases, parents and child are seen and asked together – this way
differing views can be assessed easily. In some cases, it is best to ask parents alone without the child (i.e.
marital conflicts, abuse, etc.). In others, it can be useful to see and talk to the child alone. Some children are
more open to talk about their problems when the parents are not present (less conflicts of loyalty towards the
parents).

Presenting symptom

At the end of the wetting history, it is useful to ask an open question regarding other problem areas.

Other behavioural problems: Are there other areas in your child's behaviour that you are worried about? –
                              please describe these in detail!

*As in the history of the wetting problem, each presenting symptom should be dealt with in turn. Following points
are useful to consider:*

Presenting symptom: Please describe the problem in your own words as detailed as possible! How
                         often does it occur? In which situations (at home, in school, with friends)?
                         How does your child react? How do you react? When did it begin? How has
                         it developed so far? Has it remained the same, got worse or diminished in
                         intensity, frequency, etc.? What have you done about it so far? Has the child
                         been presented, examined or treated for the problem? Where, by whom and
                         with what effect? What are your main worries? What would you like to

change? How do you think this could change? What do you expect from the presentation here?

It is also useful to ask a few general questions about possible problem domains that can occur in children and that might be missed by an open question. If parents should answer positively, each of the problems should be explored in detail.

Other problem areas

Externalizing problems:	Is your child restless, constantly in movement, too active for its age? Is your child distracted easily? How long can it concentrate on one thing? Are there certain situations that are especially difficult to sustain concentration – in school, for example? Does your child act impulsively, without thinking? Is your child sometimes aggressive – verbally, towards objects or people? How does your child react towards rules? Does it obey your rules? Or is it oppositional? How does your child react if you set limits and say no? Are there any special problem areas: homework, coming home too late, lying, stealing, etc.?
Internalizing problems:	Is your child sad, unhappy, withdrawn? Has your child lost interest in play, seeing other children? Does it find it difficult to get an activity going? Does your child worry. Are there problems with sleeping or eating? Are there fears and anxieties: towards certain objects or animals (phobias)? towards strangers, groups of children (social anxiety), when you go away (separation anxiety) or without apparent reason (generalized anxiety)? Has your child developed any peculiar habits, rituals or interests? Does it tend to repeat things in the same way?

Personal and developmental history

Pregnancy:	Was the pregnancy planned (desired?) or unexpected? What were your feelings during pregnancy? Were there any medical complications? Were there any events that you found stressful?
Birth	Was the delivery at the expected date, too early, too late? Was it a spontaneous birth? Were there any complications during or after birth? What was the birthweight of your child?
Infancy	Was your child breast-fed? For how long? If not, what were the reasons? Was your child a quiet, content or active baby (temperament)? Were there any problems with feeding, weight gain, sleeping, excessive crying?
Motor development	When did your child start sitting, standing, walking freely?
Speech and language	When did your child say its first words (and which were they)? When did your child say its first two-word sentences? Were there any problems with articulation, the way sentences were formed (expressive language) or with understanding (receptive language)?
Kindergarten	When did your child enter kindergarten? Did your child show problems staying there, i.e. separation? Were there any problems with other children or with the kindergarten teachers? If yes, please describe.

School	When did your child enter school? Which grade is it in now? What type of school? Did it have to repeat a grade? Does it like to go to school? If yes or no, please describe. What are the favourite subjects? What are the grades in the different subjects? Does your child have special problems with the teachers, with other children? – please describe.
Leisure time	What does your child do in its free time? What are favourite games and play (role playing, construction games, activity games, computer games, etc.)? Are there any planned activities? What are the interests and hobbies? Does it do any sports? Does your child have friends (how many and how intense)? Does your child spend its free time alone or with friends? What role does your child have in groups with other children of the same age?
Illnesses	What illnesses, operations, hospital treatment, accidents, allergies has your child had so far?
Family History	
Parents	Age, occupation (school training), illnesses. Marital relationship? Have you wetted as a child? How would you describe your relationship to your child?
Siblings	Age, biological sibs?, school-grade, illnesses and wetting problems. How would you describe the relationship of the brothers and sisters to each other? Are there especially close bonds or rivalries?
Other relatives	Other cases of wetting, other illnesses, especially psychiatric and nephrological

Regarding the problem of enuresis and urinary incontinence (as well as nocturia and micturition problems such as urge) we have made it a routine to draw a complete pedigree over three generations. Often, other relatives will be missed, unless one asks directly and explicitly if they have wetted in the past (or currently).

It is usually best to end the history by asking another open question like: is there anything else we might have missed or that you might feel to be of importance?

Appendix 22.2. Frequency/volume chart

24-hour Frequency/Volume Chart
Instructions:
Dear parents,
To be able to assess and treat the wetting problem of your child in the best possible way, we would appreciate your help and your observations.

Please fill out this chart on a day without school or kindergarten (weekend or holiday). Please document whenever your child goes to the toilet or when it wets. This should start on one morning and continue through to the next morning. **If possible, please fill out two charts on two days in a row, as this is even more reliable.**

Please talk to your child about it beforehand. You should not send your child to the toilet. Instead, he/she should tell you when he/she wants to go to the toilet and should empty the urine into a measuring cup. Please measure the amount of urine, record it with the time of day in the chart. You do not have to collect the urine, but can discard it afterwards.

If your child needs to strain to start getting the voiding going or if the stream is interrupted, please note this in the next column.

If your child wets his/her clothes, again please note the time and if they were wet or damp.

If your child feels a sudden urge to go to the toilet, please note this with the time in the next column.

If you observe that your child crosses his/her legs, squats or tries to hold back the urine in any other way, please note this (with the time) in the next column.

Finally, please measure and note the amount of fluids your child drinks during the day (with times).

Thank you very much for your help!

24-hour-frequency/volume chart

Name _____   Date of birth _____

Date _____

Time	Urine volume (ml)	Straining/ interrupted stream	Wetting: Damp/wet?	Urge	Comments/ observations	Drinking fluids (ml)

Appendix 22.3. Parental questionnaire

Parental questionnaire: enuresis/urinary incontinence (Beetz, von Gontard, Lettgen, 1994; translated and adapted by A. von Gontard, 2003)

Name: _____   Date of birth: _____

Date: _____

	YES	NO
Daytime wetting:		
Does your child wet his/her clothes during the day?	☐	☐
Has your child ever been dry during the day?	☐	☐

If yes, for how long? _____ (weeks/months/ years)

And at which age? _____ (years)

On how many days a week does your child

wet during daytime? _____ (days per week)

How many times a day does your child wet? _____(times per day)

	YES	NO
Is the clothing usually damp?	☐	☐
Is the clothing usually wet?	☐	☐
Does urine dribble constantly?	☐	☐
Does your child wet his/her clothes immediately after having gone to the toilet?	☐	☐
Does your child notice when he/she wets?	☐	☐

	YES	NO
Night-time wetting		
Does your child wet the bed (or diapers) during the night?	☐	☐
Has your child ever been dry during the night?	☐	☐

If yes, for how long? _____ (weeks/months/ years)

And at which age? _____ (years)

On how many nights a week does your child wet? _____(nights per week)

	YES	NO
Is the bed usually damp?	☐	☐
Is the bed usually wet?	☐	☐
Does your child wake up to go to the toilet?	☐	☐
Does your child wake up after wetting the bed?	☐	☐
Is your child a deep sleeper, i.e. difficult to wake up?	☐	☐
Has any other member of your family wetted (day or night)?	☐	☐

If yes, who? _____

	YES	NO
Toilet habits		

How many times a day does your child void? (on average) _____(times/day)

How long can your child manage without going to the toilet (during shopping, car

trips, etc.)? _____(hours)

	YES	NO
Does your child go to the toilet him/herself if he/she needs to?	☐	☐
Do you have to send your child to the toilet?	☐	☐
If your child wants to pee, does he/she have to strain at the beginning or during voiding?	☐	☐
When your child voids, is the stream interrupted?	☐	☐
Does your child hurry and not take enough time for voiding?	☐	☐

	YES	NO
Observable reactions		
Does your child feel a sudden urge to go to the toilet?	☐	☐
When your child needs to void, does he/she have to rush to the toilet immediately?	☐	☐
Does your child cross his/her legs, squat, sit on a heel, etc. to prevent wetting?	☐	☐
Does your child postpone going to the toilet as long as possible?	☐	☐

If, yes, in which situations (school, play, TV, etc.), Please specify _____

	YES	NO
Urinary tract infections		
Has your child ever had a urinary tract infection?	☐	☐
If yes, how many _____(times)		
Has your child had urinary tract infections with fever?	☐	☐
Has your child been treated for an illness of the urinary tract?	☐	☐

If yes, please specify _____

	YES	NO
Stool habits		
Does your child have daily bowel movements?	☐	☐
If not, how many times/ week? _____(times/week)		
Is your child regularly constipated?	☐	☐
Does your child soil his/her underwear (during the day)?	☐	☐
Does your child soil during sleep?	☐	☐
If yes, small amounts (smear)	☐	☐
Or large amounts (stool)	☐	☐
How often does your child soil? _____(times/week)_____(times/month)		
Has your child previously had complete bowel control?	☐	☐
If yes, at what age _____(years)		
And for how long _____(months/years)		
Does the soiling occur in special situations?	☐	☐

If yes, please specify _____

	YES	NO
Behaviour: wetting		
Is your child distressed by the wetting?	☐	☐
Are you distressed because of your child's wetting?	☐	☐
Has your child been teased because of the wetting?	☐	☐
Are there any things your child did not do (school outings, sleeping over with friends) because of the wetting?	☐	☐
Does your child wet more often in stressful times?	☐	☐
Is your child cooperative and motivated for treatment?	☐	☐
If your child had been dry before, do you see any event that might be associated with the relapse?	☐	☐

If yes, please specify _____

What in your opinion is the reason for the wetting?

Please specify _____

Behaviour: general   YES   NO

Does your child have difficulties in accepting rules?   ☐   ☐

Is your child restless, on the go, easily distracted?   ☐   ☐

Does your child have difficulty concentrating?   ☐   ☐

Is your child sometimes anxious?   ☐   ☐

Is your child sometimes sad, unhappy, withdrawn?   ☐   ☐

Does your child have problems in school?   ☐   ☐

If yes, please specify _____

Does your child have problems is other areas?

If yes, please specify _____

23

Physical and sexual abuse

Arnon Bentovim

The London Child and Family Consultation Service, Harley, St., London, UK

Introduction

There have been records of the abuse of children in many parts of the world. Historical records exist of unkempt, malnourished, rejected and abused children. However, the issue did not receive widespread attention medically until the publication of Kempe's seminal work, The Battered Child Syndrome in 1962. The term was coined to characterize the clinical manifestations of serious physical abuse in young children. It is now evident that child abuse is a global problem, which occurs in a variety of forms and is deeply rooted in cultural, economic and social practices. Kempe described the sequence of the ways in which societies begin to perceive and socially construct the different forms of abuse. He described the first observation of the severely physically abused child, followed by an awareness of the neglected child, then an awareness that children could be rejected and emotionally abused in their families, and in institutions, or could be induced into illness states by parents who themselves need support through the medical pathway. He also described the process of recognition of the extensive inappropriate sexual activities with children.

This chapter will look at the different phenomena of abusive actions against children, attempt to identify some unifying themes and how they influence the way that professionals act, and to define the role and tasks of child and adolescent psychiatrists. It is evident that the children who are subject to child abuse are subject to multiple and pervasive stressful effects, which have widespread negative effects on development, and affect all aspects of children's functioning. There is major impact on a child's emotional life, on his or her attachments, and the development of a sense of self in relationships.

The ultimate goal of intervention is prevention, and to ensure that children are wanted and cared for adequately, that they live in a context where their needs are

A Clinician's Handbook of Child and Adolescent Psychiatry, ed. Christopher Gillberg, Richard Harrington and Hans-Christoph Steinhausen. Published by Cambridge University Press. © Cambridge University Press 2005.

protected and they are exposed to as few risks to their development as possible. This will ensure that they achieve their potential and that the emotional and physical health of future generations are assured.

Definition and classification

To take a broad approach to understanding and defining child abuse, it is essential to account for the differing standards and expectation of parenting behaviour in a wide range of cultures. Because child abuse is essentially attributable to the adult's way of relating and treating the child, the cultural context in which the family is living has a responsibility for defining what is or what is not good enough care. There is a complex balance between cultural expectations that children's behaviour should be controlled, disciplined and fit with societal expectations and at the same time that they be given encouragement, stimulation, warmth and autonomy. Families interpret the different expectations of society in the light of their own history. Individuals both comply with family and cultural expectations, and may also rebel and follow more antisocial pathways.

Different cultures have different rules about what are acceptable parenting practices. Child-rearing beliefs diverge on which practices are abusive or neglectful. Generally, differences are more to do with emphasizing particular aspects of parental behaviour. In many cultures, however, there is general agreement that child abuse should not be allowed, and there is virtual unanimity where very harsh disciplinary practices and sexual abuse are concerned.

The WHO consultation on child abuse prevention drafted the following definition,

Child abuse or maltreatment constitutes all forms of physical and/or emotional ill-treatment, sexual abuse, neglect or negligent treatment or commercial or other exploitation resulting in actual or potential harm to the child's health, survival, development or dignity in the context of a relationship with those caring individuals who have responsibility, trust or power.

Some definitions focus on the behaviours or action of adults, whilst others focus on the degree of harm caused or potential for harm. It is evident that there is a complex relationship between the two. An understanding of the impact of negative parental behaviour can only be understood if an analysis is made of the nature of the child's environment, and the level of the child's resiliance or vulnerability. Satisfactory models to understand the phenomenon of child abuse rely on a broad based ecosystemic approach to the care of children. This attempts to look at a wide range of factors in the lives of children to understand what are the risks, and which the protective factors, and when interventions are required.

Specific definitions of forms of abuse include the following.

- *Physical abuse* is defined as those acts of commission, or omission by a care-giver which cause actual physical harm, or have the potential for harm. Physical abuse also includes the induction of illness states through the administration of medication or noxious substances.

- *Sexual abuse* is defined as those acts where a caregiver uses a child for sexual gratification. Acts range from exposure and witnessing sexual activities – none contact abuse, to forms of contact abuse, genital touching, mutual masturbation, attempts or actual intercourse. The essential issue is the child or young person not having the knowledge or maturation to be able to consent.

- *Emotional abuse* includes the failure of a caregiver to provide an appropriate and supportive environment including acts that have an adverse affect on the emotional health and development of a child. This includes inappropriate restriction, denigration, ridicule, threats and intimidation, discrimination or other non-physical forms of hostile treatment. Involvement in activities such as prostitution, anti-social activities, exposure to domestic violence or marital conflict, drug addiction or mental illness may also represent forms of emotional abuse depending on the nature of the child's role.

- *Neglect* refers to the failure of a parent to provide for the development of the child – where the parent is in a position to do so – including areas such as health, education and emotional development, nutrition, shelter and safe living conditions. Thus there is a distinction made between neglect from the circumstances of poverty, and neglect occurring when reasonable resources are available to the family or caregiver.

- *The harmful effects of child abuse.* It is the paediatrician's task to define the degree of physical harm and impact on a child's physical development. From a child and adolescent psychiatric perspective, it is helpful to focus on the issue of the nature of psychological harm done to the child. It is helpful to think of the harm of child abuse as being a 'compilation of significant events, both acute and longstanding, which interact with the child's ongoing development, and interrupt, alter or impair physical development and significantly psychological development. Being the victim of significant harm is likely therefore to have a profound effect on a child's view of themselves as a person, and on their future lives. The serious harm caused by the different forms of child abuse represents a major symptom of failure of adaptation by parents to their role, involving family and society.' Bentovim 1998.

Figure 23.1 describes each category of abuse in terms of severity. The implications of these different levels have implications for their effect on children's development, and also for the levels of intervention required.

Least severe	Moderate abuse	Severe abuse
Bruising, no fractures in an older child	Bruising in a baby, fractures not including head and neck	Fractures, multiple, over a period of time, different sites, particularly with fractures around the head and neck in a baby under 6 months.
Weight parallel rather than markedly below third centile	Growth failure, but not length, basically of weight	Severe non-organic failure to thrive with stunting in both length and weight
Mild degrees of neglect without major failure to care, and family chaos	Failure of care, moderate degrees of deprivation and neglect	Severe neglect, deprivation state, skin, hair changes, severe accidents due to poor supervision
Critical, scapegoating, confusing atmosphere, emotional disorder without major conduct problems	Rejection, privation but with tendencies towards conduct problems rather than frozen regression and retardation	Severe rejection resulting in pseudo-autistic regresses, states of frozen watchfulness, pseudo-retardation
Sexual exhibitionism	Sexual abuse, shorter duration, fondling and/or oral contact	Sexual abuse, longstanding, involving attempted or actual genital or anal intercourse, particularly in younger children associated with gross physical signs, major sexualized patterns.
	Fabrication of symptoms leading to investigation	Induction of illness of such severity that life is threatened, e.g. suffocation, attempted drowning

Fig. 23.1.   Levels of severity of abuse.

ICD-10 criteria and DSM-IV criteria

In ICD-10 classification of mental and behaviour disorders, child abuse is not seen as a psychiatric diagnosis as such, but would be recorded as an aspect of descriptors, e.g. included in the axis for cognitive impairment if this is related to abuse, or in the axis of physical illness if there has been fractures or growth failure, or in axis five to describe problems relating to the social environment, negative life events, problems related to upbringing and psychosocial circumstances and family history of mental and behavioural disorders, which may be relevant. In those cases where other disorders have developed as a result of exposure to abuse there may be the observation of an attachment disorder, an emotional disorder, or a conduct disorder.

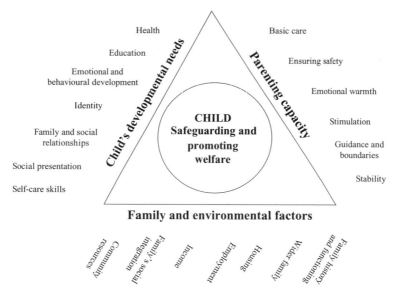

Fig. 23.2.   Assessment frameworks.

DSM-IV criteria do include a category of physical or sexual abuse of the child as a V code to be included in axis one, as well as being able to define other evidence of psychological harm, also under axis four, psychosocial and environmental problems. The global assessment of functioning, axis five, is also helpful, particularly for children who have been exposed to extensive stress. This includes the various areas of functioning, in educational contexts, the family and social contexts drawing attention to the level of functioning as a result of abuse. This gives useful information for assessment of intervention effects.

The ICD-10/DSM-IV criteria have a useful role. Although abuse syndromes are seen as an axis one diagnosis from the mental health perspective in DMS-IV, the fact that a system is available where it is possible to define the multiple negative contexts in a child's environment does give a broad view of the level of concerns focussed on the child.

A framework, which attempts to look systematically at the child's needs, the parenting capacities, and social and environmental factors (see Fig. 23.2) may well be a useful additional approach to classification. It frames a broad view of the child's needs from multiple perspectives.

Epidemiology

Estimates of the frequency of child abuse are usually derived from incidence or prevalence studies. Incidence levels refer to the number of new cases referred to professionals in a defined population over a specified period of time, usually a year. Prevalence refers to the proportion of the defined population affected by child abuse during a specified time period – usually childhood. It is now recognized that there are five levels of professional recognition or public awareness of child abuse and neglect.

- *Level one:* children who are reported to protective agencies such as social services, the police or non-government organizations whose task it is to monitor and to protect children.
- *Level two:* those children who are 'officially known' to a variety of agencies for reasons other than abuse and neglect, including involvement in matrimonial disputes, anti-social behaviour, e.g. delinquency, truancy. They are not regarded by the community as abused or neglected in the same way, but are often subject to family contexts of considerable stress.
- *Level three:* abused and neglected children known and of concern to other professionals such as schools, hospitals, medical practitioners, mental health agencies, but not reported as abused or neglected as such. In some contexts they are thought of as children 'in need'. The focus on other issues such as a parent's mental health, or marital violence may lead to a failure to consider the issue of child protection.
- *Level four:* are abused or neglected children recognized by neighbours, relatives, but who are not reported to a professional agency.
- *Level five:* children not recognized as abused or neglected by anyone, perhaps the individuals involved do not regard their behaviours or experiences as maltreatment. Situations have not yet come to the attention of outside observers who would recognize them as such.

Incidence studies are mainly concerned with reported and recorded cases of abuse to children: Level one children. However, many cases of child abuse do not come to the notice of reporting authorities, and prevalence studies attempt to find out these hidden cases by asking a sample of adults if they were abused during their childhood, for instance. The majority of child abuse prevalence studies have been on sexual abuse. The children who are most vulnerable to physical abuse and neglect occur in the youngest group, the 0- to 1-year olds. Adults recall of these abusive experiences is limited because of restricted memories of the first 3 to 4 years of their lives. The earliest recall for serious abuse is around $2\frac{1}{2}$ years.

Official reporting rates

Level one of the professional recognition continuum demonstrates a range of 2.6 children per 1000 suffering child maltreatment in the UK, 15 per 1000 in the USA, 5.8 per 1000 in Australia with a different proportion in each country of emotional abuse, neglect, physical abuse and sexual abuse.

Two incidence studies of Level One to Level Three have been carried out. An American study demonstrated that, when carrying out a far more detailed investigation of cases, a rate of 23.1 per 1000 children suffered maltreatment, yet only 9 per cent of those children were cases investigated by child protection services. Schools, hospitals, social services, mental health agencies who do not have official expectations to investigate child abuse concerns recognize seven times the number of child victims than did investigatory agencies. A similar study of child sexual abuse in Northern Ireland noted that approximately four times as many cases were discovered when a more extensive search for cases was made than those reported.

Incidence studies

Incidence studies attempting to ascertain cases at level four have been carried out through surveys in households in various parts of the world using the Conflict Tactics Scales. The level of abusive violence was ascertained through questions about punching, kicking, biting, hitting, beating up or using a knife or a gun on their child. A rate of 1 in every 10 American children were reported as being subject to severe physical violence, whereas only 1 in 7 of those children who were severely physically injured was reported. It is clear from these studies that harsh parental punishment is not confined to a few places or a single region of the world. There are frequent reports of hitting children with an object, or parts of the body other than the buttocks. Harsher forms of violence such as choking children, burning or threatening with knives or guns occur but less frequently.

Using children as reporters rather than adults it is evident that severe violence occurs in certain countries with very considerable frequency. Spanking is the most common disciplinary measures reported, but slapping the face or head is frequently used as a punishment. A substantial amount of harsh punishment also occurs in schools and other institutions at the hands of teachers and others responsible for the care of children.

Prevalence studies

Prevalance studies have mainly been confined to child sexual abuse. A percentage of adults and adolescents affected range from 6.8 to 54 per cent of women and girls, and 3 to 25 per cent of men and boys. A broad definition of sexual abuse not involving contact will ascertain many more cases than one involving only contact or penetrative acts. Recent studies of prevalence in the UK using computer-assisted safe interviewing indicate 7 per cent of young people report severe physical abuse, 16 per cent sexual abuse, in the US 22 per cent men, 19.5 per cent women report physical abuse, 14 per cent of men and 32 per cent of women sexual abuse.

There can be considerable biases in the recognition, reporting and registration or substantiation of cases depending on social class, ethnicity, perceived status and experience. Over time there has been a process of a rapid increase in reported cases, with greater recognition of abuse.

However, there has been a more recent decrease in the incidence of both physical and child sexual abuse in the US and the UK of around 30 per cent. Public education and a change in public attitudes towards violence in families has had an effect in reducing the incidence of physical and sexual abuse on children. Neglectful care, however, remains at a high level and has a more pervasive effect on family life, often associated with significant parental mental illness, domestic violence and substance abuse.

Implications for practice

The important factors to emerge from this overview of incidence prevalence and associated risk factors is that there is a large group of children who have been, or are being maltreated. Only a fraction are being reported to child protection practitioners. Fortunately, the majority of children are not abused or maltreated. An understanding of the underlying rate of the problem and characteristics of the population help in assessing the individual cases referred and the likelihood that maltreatment is present.

There has been a concern that a focus on child protection may take a priority over providing adequate childcare and that identifying cases takes up a great deal of energy. Taking a view that what needs to be assessed are the needs of the child and their family is preferable, making a distinction between those children who need protection, and those whose family need support. Child welfare legal systems need to balance the rights of children and families to be given every support to assist them, as well as the rights of children not to be subject to overwhelming levels of violence and abuse. Living in a climate of violence can lead to re-enactment of abuse in the next generation, and the inter-generational aspect of child abuse, although controversial, is an important explanatory model to understand the phenomenon.

A critical appraisal of strengths and difficulties risk and protective factors is required in the individual case, and an assessment of the communities needs based on an appraisal of the characteristics of community characteristics and resources. In a population of 10 million children, about 4 million will be vulnerable because of living in stressful circumstances, 300 000–400 000 will have a need for services and about 70 000–80 000 will need alternative care because of parental death, breakdown of family life, or because of abuse.

Clinical picture

Physical abuse

Physical abuse is usually presented either directly by a child, parent or an interested third party. Presentation is described in Box 23.1.

Box 23.1. Presentation of physical abuse

- Repetitive patterns of injury, parents using different hospitals to avoid detection.
- Injuries not consistent with the history, too many, too severe, the wrong kind, the wrong distribution, wrong age.
- A pattern of injury, which strongly suggests abuse, for example bruising to a young baby. Few reasonable explanations for the injuries. Multiple injuries may be observed following what is described as moderate fall. Severe head injuries in babies and toddlers, rib fractures; sub-dural hematoma and retinal haemorrhage associated with violent shaking, multiple cigarette burns; fractures in infants and toddlers are all characteristic of severe child abuse.
- The presence of other signs of abuse, e.g. neglect, failure to thrive, sexual abuse.
- Unusual behaviour in parents, e.g. delay in seeking medical advice, refusal to allow proper treatment or admission to hospital, unprovoked aggression towards staff.

Injuries may be discovered incidentally, for example a child being allowed to go to school or nursery, or to another person's care when injuries may be found and reported. In such situations parents often deny knowledge of the injury and no satisfactory explanations are given – although there may be a covert wish for discovery. This may be a way of drawing attention to overwhelming family stress, which cannot be openly acknowledged. The relevant features from the history are illustrated in Box 23.2.

Each of the particular forms of abuse, failure to thrive, physical abuse, and neglect has characteristic patterns. Different forms of abuse often present in the same family and present at different times in differing ways. The analogy of an iceberg with multiple impact points describes child abuse aptly. Poisoning, suffocation and Munchausen syndrome by Proxy are forms of dangerous physical abuse, which are not characterized by the loss of control, punitiveness and anger, associated with physical abuse, more a perception or a belief that the child has a physical illness. The parent has to convince the medical team that this is the case and does so by describing or inducing symptoms, requesting investigation or intervention. Behavioural difficulties may be interpreted as having physical causes. Whilst the child becomes the focus of medical attention, the parent gains the support and comfort of being the parent of a sick child, receiving care and support by proxy. Death may result from any of these forms of physical abuse, long-term physical or psychological harm.

Child sexual abuse occurs in a number of different contexts as illustrated in Box 23.3.

Box 23.2. Important features in the history of physical abuse

- A discrepant history which changes with the telling or who tells it. Details are vague or unclear. Exact details of time, place, persons and actions are required to clarify the presentation. There needs to be a comparison of accounts of various professionals, major differences needing explanations. Parents may not give the same story.
- An unreasonable delay in seeking help or care, especially following a fracture or serious burn or scald is a strong indicator of an abusive situation. Denial that a child is in pain, minimization of symptoms is common. A baby may be left tucked in a cot, only to be brought hours later when he refuses a feed or begins to have a seizure.
- Family crises need to be investigated. There may be a family crisis or a complicated home situation, which has precipitated, bereavements, break-ups of relationship, loss of job. This may be the context for loss of parental control. Stresses need to be revealed, and parents need to be listened to.
- Trigger factors are behaviour in the child which precipitated a parent's violence, inconsolable crying, difficult feeding or wetting, stealing or lying may all provoke an angry outburst on a stressed parents part.
- Parental history of abuse, parents' traumatic experiences, children are important but may be forgotten or repressed. A history of having grown up in care may be relevant.
- Unrealistic expectations of children are another important factor. Children expected to love, accept and validate the parents. When a child cries or will not take foods, he may be felt to be rejecting or punishing to an insecure parent. Obsessional and rigid patterns of child rearing may be expressed in other ways. Meticulously clean and tidy home may be present or contexts of severe neglect.
- Social isolation from friends, extended family and professionals is a common finding. As abuse escalates parents find it increasingly difficult to allow anyone into their lives for fear of discovery, and the isolation grows.
- Past history of high levels of parental anxiety, frequent admissions to hospitals in the first months of life, frequent accidents, behavioural difficulties, growth and development delays may all be sources of anxiety, the source of stress and the result of poor care.

Figure 23.3 illustrates the common patterns of presentation through disclosure, physical indicators, psychosomatic indicators, behavioural indicators at different developmental stages, association with learning or severe learning problems or social indicators.

> **Box 23.3. Different contexts when child sexual abuse occurs**
>
> 1. As an intrafamilial pattern of abuse, including abuse within nuclear and extended family. This may incorporate family friends, lodgers or close acquaintances with the knowledge of the family. Abuse within adoptive or foster families is also included.
> 2. Extra-familial includes abuse with adults frequently known to the child from a variety of sources including neighbours, family, friends, school friends, parents, as well as abuse within 'sex rings', either family or stranger led.
> 3. Institutional abuse includes abuse occurring within schools, residential children's establishments, day nurseries, holiday camps, for example cubs, brownies, boy scouts and other organizations both secular and religious.
> 4. Street or stranger abuse includes assaults on children in public places and child abduction.

The general impact of abuse on development

In a general view of the process of abusive action the negative interlocking aspects of relationships occur between parent and child within a social context. Associated with physical abuse and sexual abuse is a closely associated, emotionally abusive attitude towards the child. There is often an absence of a protector or potential protectors are neutralized. The perpetrator often feels overwhelmed by impulses to actions of a physically, sexually or emotionally abusive nature, which are felt to be overwhelming, and beyond control. The cause is often attributed to the victim, who in line with individual, family and cultural expectations is construed as responsible for the victimizer's feelings and intention. Actions on the victim's part to avoid abuse are interpreted as further cause for disinhibition of violent action or justification for further abuse. A process of silence or dissociation spreads to victim and victimizer and those who could potentially protect, and may lead to the delayed recognition of severe abusive patterns, or the maintenance of a context of secrecy and silence throughout childhood. There is a tendency for both victim and victimizer to minimize experiences, dismiss events, blame themselves or others. The repeated nature of violent actions, traumatic stressful effects come to organize the reality and the perceptions of those participating, including potential protectors, and professionals who become involved in the family situation. There is a pressure not to see, not to hear or not to speak so that identification becomes problematic and complex.

When considering the general effects on development it is helpful to consider three major areas of development within children and young people to understand the way in which the various forms of abuse impact. These areas also act as a focus for therapeutic work:

Presentation of child sexual abuse (adapted from Vizard & Tranter 1988)

1. Disclosure	By child or third party.
2. Physical indicators	Rectal or vaginal bleeding, pain on defecation Sexually transmitted disease (STD) Vulvovaginitis/vaginal discharge/'sore' Dysuria and frequency, urinary tract infections Physical abuse, note association of burns, pattern of injury, death Pregnancy
3. Psychosomatic indicators	Recurrent abdominal pain Headache, migraine Eating disorders, bulimic variety Encopresis Secondary Enuresis Total refusal syndrome
4. Behavioural indicators i) Pre-School	Sexually explicit play, 'excessive' masturbation, insertion of foreign bodies (girls), self-mutilation, withdrawn, poor appetite, sleep disturbance, clingy, delayed development, aggression.
ii) Middle years	Sexualized play, sexually explicit drawing or sexual precocity, self-mutilation, anxiety, depression, anger, poor school performance, mute.
iii) Teenagers	Sexually precocious, prostitution, anxiety, anger, aggression, depression, truancy, running away, solvent/alcohol/drug abuse, self-destructive behaviour, overdoses, self-mutilation, suicide.
5. Learning or severe learning problems. Physical handicap	May present with depression, disturbed (including aggressive) behaviour. Sexualized behaviour. Attempts at disclosure not understood. May be physical and psychosomatic indicators as above.
6. Social indicators	Concern by parent or third party, sibling, relative or friend of abused child. Known offender in close contact with child.

Fig. 23.3.   Common patterns of presentations.

- the regulation of emotion
- the development of attachments
- the developments of an adequate sense of self.

Although these three areas are considered separately, they reinforce each other, are intertwined and come to underpin the relationship models of the individual child and young person both within his family and within the social context. Overwhelming stress is a characteristic feature of physical and sexual abuse and there is an inter-related biological and psychological response. A child or young person living in a world invaded by fear and anxieties has its ways of relating, coloured and directed by such experiences. The greater the exposure to stressful factors, the more likely it is that extreme responses will be shown.

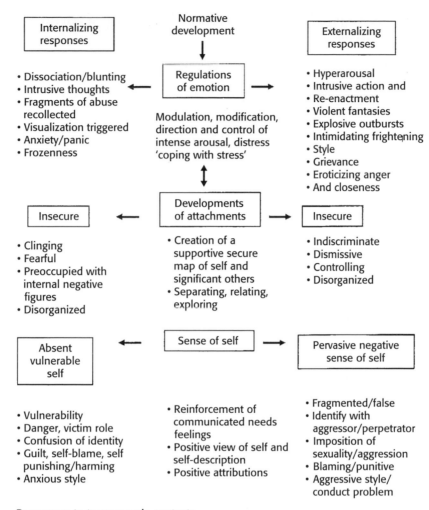

Fig. 23.4.   Responses to traumagenic contexts.

Figure 23.4 describes the traumatic effects of living in a context where the child is exposed to a cumulative set of abusive experiences. It is helpful to think of responses in each significant area as externalizing or internalizing, and the direction of responses is indicative of the coping mechanisms used – a general avoidant mode, or an active coping response.

Regulation of emotions

Internalizing emotional responses describe the sense of being overwhelmed and intruded upon. Blanking out, deleting, dissociating, blunting is the response. However there may be intrusive thoughts, fragments of abuse are recollected, flashbacks of intense overwhelming experiences occur. Anxiety, panic attacks, frozenness result. Avoidance of people, places and objects, which remind the child of abusive action, is a predominant mode of relating, or clinging to perceived 'safe' figures, including the abuser!

Externalizing responses represent the opposite. Instead of blunting, there is hyperarousal; instead of recollections or fragments of abuse, which feel thrust into mind, the impulse is towards intrusive action, re-enactment towards others who are forced to contain overwhelming emotions. Violent fantasies, explosive outbursts are seen, and an intimidating, frightening style of relating results. The emotional states that predominate are those to do with grievance. Anger may be eroticized in an intertwining of sexuality and anger. Closeness evokes overwhelming desires to intrude, attack, sexualize.

Effect on attachments

Aversive parenting evokes insecure patterns of the self and others. If relationships are sufficiently disrupted, attachments will be indiscriminate, the child seeking to attach himself or herself to any adult they meet. Response to a context of fear, anxiety and unpredictability can lead to a clinging, insecure attachment. Maintaining closeness and intensity is a mode of coping, leading to a preoccupation with internal negative experiences and figures. These responses are reinforced by the internalizing responses, augmented by intrusive fragments of recollected abuse, visualizations, flashbacks triggered. A process of disorganization takes over, switching from state to state as a result of feeling overwhelmed by uncontrollable emotional experiences as a consequence of living in a context of pervasive abuse.

Alternatively, coping may be dismissive, aversive in character, avoiding contact, or alternately attempting to take control. Again, this mode of relating, if linked with the externalizing emotional response of hyperarousal, intrusive action, explosive outbursts, comes to characterize the style of relating. Such patterns can become highly disorganized, switching from a clinging state of being preoccupied with internal figures, to a state of controlling, dismissive or indiscriminate ways of relating. The more extensive the abusive context, the more disorganized the attachment pattern.

The confluence of negative representational models of attachment figures and of the self, and the self in relationship to others, makes maltreated children extremely vulnerable to functioning maladaptively in peer relationships and school-related issues.

Sense of self

Children growing up in a climate of violence can develop a profound absence of self. In the internalizing mode, the image and presence of the abusive parents occupy psychological space. There is a sense of vulnerability, danger, identification with a victim role, intense confusion of identity and responsibility. The child believes if they are subject to anger, to rage, to punishment, then they must be an appropriate subject for such treatment. This results in guilt, self-blame, and a self-punitive harming style. Self-harm becomes a distraction, a way of distracting from emotional pain, and becomes a way of taking control to cause pain oneself. This gives an illusory sense of control over the environment rather than feeling like the passive vessel evoking anger in an inconsistent unpredictable way.

The sense of vulnerability, victim of self or absence of self is associated with blunted, dissociated affect, and a preoccupation characteristic of internalizing modes of coping with emotional attachments. Switching may be seen between the absent vulnerable sense of self to a state of invulnerability, from powerlessness to omnipotence. The pervasive negative sense of self can predispose to an identity with the aggressor, or the perpetrator. Sexuality and aggression may be imposed on others, a blaming, punitive, aggressive style may develop with fragmentation of self, the development of false selves, and a variety of different identifications, and borderline functioning.

Specific effects of abuse on development

Peer relationships

The two main effects of experiencing severe abuse on peer relationships are those of showing physical and verbal aggression, including responding with anger and aggression to friendly overtures and signs of distress in others. Other observations have been a high degree of withdrawal and avoidance of peer relationships. This seems to be an active strategy of avoidance, leading to increasing isolation. The experience of being maltreated thus leads children along different pathways to peer rejection and isolation.

Adaptation to school

The school environment exerts direct effects on educational achievement. Skills acquired in the elementary grades serve as a foundation for success in higher education, and future employment opportunities. Understanding of social relationships and emotional responsiveness also emerge out of the school environment. Adaptation to school, including integration into the peer group, acceptable classroom performance and orientation for achievement, is a process that is important for all children. The child's experience in the home provides an important foundation on which the transition to the school setting is built. Children who have been maltreated are at high risk for failure in school. A potentially positive experience could serve to reverse an early trajectory of maladaptation, but more often confirms the maltreated child's negative history and maladaptive relationship patterns.

Physically abused children prove to be aggressive, non compliant, acting out, and function more poorly on cognitive tasks. Neglected children have severe and variable school difficulties. They are often described as anxious, inattentive, unable to understand their work, lacking in initiative, heavily depending on teachers. They rarely express positive feelings or show a sense of humour. Sexually abused children are often unpopular, anxious, inattentive and unable to understand expectations. Such children have lower grades, they do not establish secure relationships, and are over-concerned with issues of security, due to an expectation of unresponsitivity and rejection from adults. All aspects of the school environment provide difficulties for maltreated children. Failure occurs very readily, although there are some children who appear to sink themselves into learning as an attempt to avoid having to think about home stresses.

Long-term mental and physical health

Disruptions in achieving developmental steps in earlier areas also have an implication for the child's functioning across his or her lifespan. Developmental liabilities may become enduring vulnerability factors, which increase the risk for the emergence of physical and mental health problems. Maltreated children have elevated levels of disturbance across a wide range of areas, rather than in any specific field. There are higher rates of diagnoses of attention deficit hyperactivity disorder, oppositional disorder and post-traumatic stress disorder, noted generally amongst maltreated children. There are links noted with borderline personality disorders, substance abuse, suicidal and self-injurious behaviour, somatizing disorders, anxiety, depression and dissociation and attachment disorders. Thus across childhood and into adulthood, maltreatment poses an increased risk for a wide range of disturbances in functioning. This in turn affects parental roles and adult functioning.

The harmful effects of physical abuse on development

Physical abuse usually occurs in the context of an abusive atmosphere within the home. High levels of punitiveness, unexpected pain and hurt, the misuses of power and authority involved in physical abuse also have major effects on the behavioural pattern of the child. Physically abused infants demonstrate high levels of negative feelings and little positive. Such feeling states persist, children are rated as over-active, distractible and aggressive.

There is a connection between the sense of powerlessness, resulting from invasion of the body, vulnerability, absence of protection and a repeated fear and helplessness. This can result in fear, anxiety and an inability to control events, along with learning difficulties, despair, depression and low sense of efficacy seen as 'frozen watchfulness'. This sense of helplessness may lead to the development of a need to control and dominate, to aggressive, abusive patterns, or the development of 'a shell' to ward off feelings about the other person.

Behaviours indicative of poor self-control have been described. They include distractibility, negative emotions, low enthusiasm and resistance to direction.

Within the school, patterns of behaviour may include attention seeking, extremely provocative behaviour to adults and bullying. Children are perceived as difficult to manage, less socially mature, rejected by peers, deficient in social skills and liable to commit violent criminal acts.

The harmful effect of emotional abuse

Emotional abuse may also be associated with emotional neglect and may take many forms. It can take the form of a lack of care of physical needs, a failure to provide consistent love and nurture, and also overt hostility and rejection. The long-term consequences on social, emotional and cognitive and behavioural development may be far-reaching and profound if the child is habitually subject to verbal harassment, or if a child is disparaged, criticized, threatened and ridiculed. The inversion of love by substituting rejection and withdrawal for affection, verbal and non-verbal is the epitome of emotional abuse and neglect.

Emotional or psychological abuse has been defined as the destruction of the child's competence to be able to function in social situations. Being denied appropriate contact with peers within or outside school, and being forced to take on a particular role in relation to parents, can therefore be seen as having a major destructive effect on the child's competence to function in social contexts. Qualitative dimensions have been described, including persistent, negative inaccurate attributions; emotional unavailability, unresponsiveness or neglect; failure to recognize individuality and boundary; inconsistent expectation and mis-socializations.

Parents can feel as if they are the abused children rather than vice versa. Children can be inducted into parental caretaking roles, and may not be encouraged to be involved in appropriate play, relationships with peers, and development of a true self. The extreme of the parental role occurs when there is incestuous abuse and the use of the child as a sexual partner whether by father or mother, inducting the male or female child into a parental or partner role inappropriately.

In marital breakdown one parent may use a child as partner against the other parent, and the attachment relationships are disrupted. There is a potential for the creation of a rejecting, resentful relationship. Blaming and faultfinding may undermine what may have been a good enough relationship. Accusations of abuse by the other parent can further undermine the potential for developing a secure attachment with parents, despite separations. Marital violence and exposure to violence can have a similar effect as being physically abused.

When parents have a psychiatric illness a major concern is the adult's involvement of the child in their psychotic process, such as a shared delusionary state or paranoid beliefs, as well as the accompanying neglect. Adaptation to parental lifestyles may also cause significant harm, e.g. where children become part of a parents' drug culture, prostitution or other antisocial activities, and become confused in terms of socialization into the appropriate moral views of what are appropriate societal values. The boundary between a lifestyle and sharing family beliefs vs being persuaded to use drugs, become prostituted, or involved in direct antisocial acts, may be a fine one, and depends on a comprehensive assessment of the child and family.

Harmful effects of physical neglect

Physical neglect comprises both a lack of both physical care taking and supervision, and a failure to fulfil the developmental needs of the child in terms of cognitive stimulation. Severe neglect is associated with major retardation of cognitive functioning and growth, poor hygiene, withdrawal and in extreme states a pseudo-autistic state, all of which can rapidly reverse in alternative care. These states are associated with the sense of parental hopelessness and helplessness, or poor quality institutional care. There is often a striking reversal of neglect when the child is in a different context. The question has to be asked whether a parent can be helped through his or her sense of helplessness towards a new ability to provide adequate stimulation to ensure growth and development rather than failure and deprivation. Professionals, like parents, may feel helpless and overwhelmed by large families living in very poor conditions, with very little social support.

The harmful effects of illness induction

In recent years there has been major concern about children who are actually induced into illness states by the administration of medications (non accidental poisoning) or are perceived and described as having symptoms which require investigation, particularly fits and faints: 'Munchausen syndrome by proxy'.

A number of reports of deliberate suffocation of children have been published. The commonest form is smothering in which a pillow or similar object is used to cause mechanical obstruction to the child's airways. The condition presents in infancy, either as an alleged apnoeic attack, or, in the most serious cases, an apparent cot death or sudden infant death syndrome (SIDS). There may be a substantially increased risk to siblings of the victim.

A deeply ambivalent parental view of the child is observed with an apparently close relationship between mother and child. On closer examination there is observed to be a deeply anxious form of attachment. The mother and a few fathers appear to construct an illness scenario together with doctors, who are keen to ensure that physical symptoms are fully investigated. There is a desire that the child should be cared for, and the fictitious illness investigated, yet at the same time there is a wish to maintain the illness state and continue putting the child at risk as a way of solving other major individual and family problems. Being in hospital, caring for a sick child, gives 'care by proxy' to the parent. Parents often have a history of prolonged contact with health agencies, 'seeking support' through illness states.

Unnecessary medical investigations may cause unnecessary pain and risk, and inappropriate treatments can have dangerous side effects. For a child to see his or herself as having a major handicapping condition or disability or take on an invalid role where there is a normal potential for health is also a cause of significant harm.

Child psychiatrists are currently being asked to diagnose children as requiring medication, or requiring investigation for autism or Apserger's syndrome. This may relate to the underlying dynamic noted in medical forms of illness induction where the parent is intolerant of children's behavioural difficulties and are seeking alternative physical explanations.

The harmful effects of sexual abuse

The traumatic effects of child sexual abuse can be summarized by stating that there are multiple affective, cognitive and behavioural effects and such effects persist. The earlier the disruptions occur, the more adversely subsequent phases of development may be affected.

The immediate post-traumatic stress disorders associated with sexual abuse are as follows:

– re-experiencing, where children were observed to talk about abuse, playing out abusive patterns
– flashbacks and nightmares
– indulging in inappropriate sexual activity
– memories occurring in places or with people and objects associated with the
– abuse and considered to be symbolic of them
– visualization, drawing, day dreaming their experiences
– avoidant responses associated with the avoidance of people, places and things associated with abuse.

Children are often fearful of going into particular houses or rooms, or of people who reminded the child of the abuser, perhaps of a particular gender, e.g. dislike of men or older people. Associated with this is an often extreme unwillingness to talk about abuse, and evidence of deletion – a 'hole' in the mind – a total lack of memory, including memories earlier than the abuse itself.

The children often complain of difficulties falling or staying asleep, associated with anxieties about going to sleep. Irritable aggressive behaviour may be noted, a reversal of the previous passive sense of having to be involved with abuse. Distractibility, difficulty in concentrating and a degree of hyperalertness shown by anxiety or being easily startled may be noted in a previously calm child.

Differential diagnoses

The diagnosis of physical or sexual abuse can be straightforward, but there can be considerable complexities. To make a diagnosis requires the putting together of the pieces of a jigsaw. Multidisciplinary assessments are required, a team working together, including a paediatrician to examine and interpret the physical symptoms and findings, a social worker to investigate and understand the social and family context; and a child and adolescent psychiatrist to assess the impact of any possible experiences on the child, to make an assessment of the parent and the family and provide a broad-based view to make an accurate diagnosis. Skilled police investigators may also be part of the team, the development of dedicated investigation teams provides a breadth of experience in making a diagnosis. There is a distinction between the initial phases making a diagnosis and later stages when a complex clinical picture needs to be put together, and decisions about possible intervention made. Child and adolescent psychiatrists often have a key role in the latter stages.

The diagnosis of physical abuse requires an understanding of the impact of various abusive situations, and to make a distinction between those injuries which are part of the everyday activities of childhood, e.g. accidents, falls, fights and sporting activities of children and those injuries which are caused by hitting, striking, shaking. The most concern arises with very young children who present with a particular pattern of bruising and injuries of different ages and stages, in particular locations which are characteristic of physical abuse, accompanied with finger marks, bite marks, burns which are consistent with physical injury. Given that children's response to physical abuse is silence, and parental denial, physical appearance is often the key to what has happened to the child. It is essential to establish the context of any injury, neglectful care can be associated with preventable accidents. The impulsive risk taking of a highly active hyperkinetic child can lead to injury which has to be distinguished from abusive actions.

The diagnosis of factitious illness by proxy or munchausen syndrome by proxy can be highly complex because of a presentation of forceful complaints that the child has episodes of fits, abdominal pain or hyper-active behaviour without physical evidence. Alternatively children are presented in various illness states, apnoeic attacks in early childhood, phases of unconsciousness, which may have been induced by giving medication, or substances such as salt, interference with life support mechanisms in hospital, wounds becoming unexpectedly infected.

To make a diagnosis requires an awareness of the possibility that the presentation may be induced by a parent. This requires a high level of careful observation and investigation of the possibility without prematurely revealing a concern. A parent who has indeed induced an illness state would be tempted to go to another hospital. Careful multi-disciplinary work can helpfully include a child and adolescent psychiatrist in observations of the child and parent to establish whether there is possible secondary gain for a parent in having a sick child. A child with a disability may be induced into a state of chronic invalidism if the parent is seeking support through the medical systems.

The diagnosis of sexual abuse can also be straightforward if a child makes a clear statement consistent with abuse, if there are supportive physical findings present, and if the alleged perpetrator takes responsibility for the act and provides a history which is consistent with the statement of the child. More often, the child's statement is contradictory, inconsistent and unclear, the physical findings are equivocal, and there is a high level of denial by the alleged perpetrator. To make a diagnosis requires a careful and skilled approach to each of the pieces of the jigsaw. Interviewing needs to rely on approaches which are open, builds on the account given by a child, and encourages a child-led approach rather than an approach which is led by the interviewer. Facilitation of the child's statement is helpful depending on the age and stage of the child. An approach which attempts to get the child to agree with the interviewer's suggestions can distort and lead to inaccuracies. Memories of abuse can reflect experiences to which a child has been subjected, but can also be developed falsely by pressure and belief by a parent who may be convinced that a partner is abusing a child sexually, or a therapist who is convinced presenting symptoms are accounted for by traumatic experiences. Traumatic experiences also distorts memories through the process of dissociation and defensive elaboration. A process of statement validity has been developed to assess the credibility of a statement, looking for details such as the recounting of elements of abusive experience which would be out of a child's knowledge. There may also be features which are consistent with children who have been induced into false beliefs that they have been abused through the use of language which reflects adult convictions, rather than the child's experience, and without affective responses.

The general assessment of a child is helpful to assess whether a traumatic process has occurred, observations of the child's general behaviour, response in the school or patterns of relationships with family members and with peers can provide a key piece of the diagnostic puzzle. Dissociated responses can give an appearance of a child who has not been traumatized, so that an accurate and broad-based assessment is required.

Child and adolescent psychiatrists are often asked to interview young people who it is alleged have behaved abusively. Open approaches to interviewing are essential, to point out to a young person that to have behaved abusively is dangerous, and that such a young person needs help, and the more open the young person is about their actions, the more likely it is that they will receive the help they require. Requests to give as full an account of what has been alleged against them is a helpful approach, to give the young person time to consider another child's statement, and to ask for details, and to elaborate any element which could give an indication of abusive action is a helpful approach. Exploration of young people's experiences of abuse is also necessary.

A knowledge of the thinking and feelings of children who are abused as well as those who abuse can help unlock experiences which the child or young person wishes to keep silent, or has been silenced by an adult abuser.

Making a diagnosis of sexual abuse in children who do not have language, have learning disability or are autistic is a highly complex process. Children with learning difficulties, speech and language delays are vulnerable to being abused as a potential perpetrator may feel that the child will not have the capacity to speak about their experience of abuse. Observations of a child's behaviour which has changed recently may trigger concerns, unexpected sexualization of behaviour is a possible indication, or unexpected severe regression of a child who is making good progress. Utterances may have an unusual sexual contact bearing in mind that conditions such as Gilles de la Tourette associated with swearing and sexualized language can also be another cause of inappropriate language.

The use of diagrams, dolls with explicit anatomical features, have been used to allow a young child to demonstrate sexualized behaviour that he or she would not be expected to be aware of. There has been concern that such aids to diagnosis may have a leading effect on children who may explore using such anatomically explicit dolls. Behaviour enacted, whether with dolls, or with other children and adults, may have a quality of response which is outside what would be expected for the age and stage of the child, and may be accompanied by sounds and physical responses which could not have been understood without experiences. Exposure to pornographic material may be used by some perpetrators as a way of grooming and inducing a child to take part in sexual activities. Inadvertent exposure can also be highly confusing, and can have an erotizing effect. To make a diagnosis requires an openness to the possibility that a child has been abused, despite a context which appears caring and concerned. Inappropriate conclusions and certainty of diagnosis should not be arrived at without adequate careful consideration and being aware an accurate diagnosis requires the pieces to fit together, rather than one piece providing certainty, and being aware of alternative explanations for unusual behaviour in vulnerable children.

Diagnostic instruments

In the Appendix an account is given of instruments, which have been commissioned, by the UK Department of Health to assist professionals in assessment of children in need and their families, including where children are in need of protection as well as in need of more general services. The home assessment provides an evidence-based approach to the assessment of the parenting environment, provided for the child by the principal caretaker. The family assessment provides a broad-based approach to carrying out an extensive assessment of the family context. Other instruments are available for more individual assessment, both in childhood and in adolescence to reinforce basic clinical approaches to interviewing.

Assessment

A key contribution to be made by child and adolescent psychiatrists is communicating with vulnerable children and carrying out extensive family assessments. Initial assessments of maltreated children or those who have been potentially significantly harmed are often carried out by police/social work teams, but more in-depth interviews are often required, both to understand further about the effect of abuse, and the extensiveness. There has been considerable controversy about the nature of in-depth interviews. The principal implications from research for practitioners undertaking such interviews with the child are as follows.

- A child's free account is preferable to answers obtained from specific questions because the account is likely to be fuller and more accurate.
- Direct questions should not be leading in type, repeated frequently or associated with any type of pressure from the professionals. They should be followed by open-ended questions, or invitations to a child to say more.
- Bias and pre-supposition should be avoided.
- Interviews should be planned in advance, enabling clear identification for the purpose of the interview.
- Children should be prepared for in-depth interviews so that they know what to expect and to involve them in the process.
- Interviews should have an introductory rapport-building phase. A flexibly employed structure to the session is useful.
- Interviews should be recorded carefully in the most appropriate ways.
- False or erroneous accounts can emanate from children, adult carers or from professional practice.
- It is essential to listen and understand a child.
- To convey genuine empathic concern.
- To convey the view that it is the child who is the expert, not the professional. It is helpful to work within an environment, which encourages critical view of practice. It is helpful to have a scheme which includes:
  - An introductory, rapport gaining phase which helps establish a working relationship, engages the child's interests, and places the child or young person at ease.

Box 23.4. Exploratory questions (from Jones, 2003)

- Has anybody done anything to you that upset you? (await response) Or made you unhappy?
- Has any person hurt you? (await answer) Or touched you in a way that you didn't like?
- Or touched you in a sexual way, or in a way that you didn't like?

A circular, permission-giving question can be useful in some circumstances. For example, in circumstances where the possibility of victimization or adversity is strong, yet the child appears to be reticent, a question like the following could be used:

- Some children talk about being upset or hurt in some way – has anything like this happened to you?

- The aim is to encourage a child freely to recall memories and perceptions of adverse experiences, to do so without introducing or suggesting any version of events that emanates from the practitioner. Often a single open-ended prompt is sufficient to enable the child to start talking freely about areas of concern.
- If not, there needs to be an enquiry into suspected adverse experiences which may link to the fact that children have spoken to someone about particular concerns, may have been found to have a physical condition which raises the possibility of maltreatment, or behaviour changes may have led to concern. A variety of probes and appropriate questions need to be developed to help explore the different abusive experiences which it is known children have been exposed to in general, or which is known specifically about the child who is being assessed (Box 23.4).

Once an assessment of the extensiveness of abuse perpetrated against the child has been established, it is essential to establish the family dimension.

- The degree of responsibility taken by the perpetrator of abuse needs to be assessed, and the fit between the perpetrator's explanation and the victim's account. Does this make sense; is it possible to draw together the strands of what has happened to be able to plan a rational approach to work?
- What is the attitude of the non-abusing caretaker, the degree of sympathy and belief in the victim's statement, the attitude towards the perpetrator, whether that perpetrator is a young person within the family context who has abused a younger child, or a partner of the parent? Is it possible for the parent to hold their own needs for a partner separate from the needs of the child? What is the general quality of parenting, e.g. the home assessment of responsivity, warmth, acceptance, organization of care?

- What is the relevant family history of parents as individuals, do they have a history of abuse themselves, their relationship history, the nature of present and past marital and parenting relationships with siblings and general family functioning.
- It is possible to assess the level of family health using instruments such as the family assessment (see Appendix). This examines family competence, the capacity to provide adequate care for children, the nature of discipline, the management of conflict and decision making. These basic functions are underpinned by characterological factors such as identity, sense of family togetherness, the quality of communication, listening, hearing, the alliances between family members both within the same generation and across generational boundaries. Assessments can be made both qualitatively and quantitatively, and a profile of family strengths and difficulties can be constructed. A variety of approaches should be used to stimulate family interaction, e.g. tasks and interviews, to help professionals make judgements, which then help to act as a focus for therapeutic work.
- It may well be that such family information can only be gathered through meetings with subsystems of the family. The absence of full knowledge and understanding of the extensiveness of abuse, responsibilities and protective capacities mean that it may not be appropriate to involve the abused child in family meetings at this stage. Motivation for help both by the child who has been victimized, and family members needs to be assessed at this stage, and the balance between protection and therapeutic work.

Aetiology

Factors increasing children's vulnerability

Vulnerability to child abuse whether physical, sexual or neglect depends in part on the child's age. Fatal cases are found largely amongst young infants. Young children are also at risk for non-physical abuse. Sexual abuse rates tend to rise in middle childhood and after the onset of puberty. Sexual abuse can also be directed at young children, by individuals with a strongly paedophilic orientation.

Girls are at higher risk than boys for infanticide, sexual abuse or neglect or forced prostitution. The majority of studies also show that the rates of sexual abuse are 1.5 to 3 times higher amongst girls than boys. Male children appear to be at greater risk of a receiving harsh physical punishment in many countries reflecting differences with respect to the role attributed to males and females. Premature infants, twins and handicapped children are also shown to be at increased risk for physical abuse and neglect. It may well be that low birthweight, prematurity, illness or physical or mental handicap may interfere with attachment processes and make a child more vulnerable to abuse, or additional demands for care strains the resources of carers who may already be coping with other significant life stresses.

Men tend to be more common perpetrators of life-threatening head injuries, severe fractures and other fatal injuries. In general terms, however, women may use more physical discipline than men, but not so severely as men. Sexual abuse of children, both female and male is predominantly perpetuated by men, studies showing that over 90 per cent of perpetrators are men.

Physically abusive parents are more likely to be young, single, poor and unemployed and have less education than non-abusing counterparts. Family size and overcrowding can also increase the risk, unstable family environments where composition of the household frequently changes is a feature of many situations where abuse occurs, particularly neglect.

Parents who are more likely to physically abuse children report feelings of low self-esteem, poor impulse control, mental health problems. They may display other antisocial behaviour. Neglectful parents have many of the same problems and have difficulty planning important life events, and managing the day to day aspects of providing adequate care. Such factors impact on the capacity to parent. When associated with disrupted social relationships, an inability to cope with stress and difficulty in accessing social support systems, small events such as crying or oppositional behaviour can evoke disproportionate responses. Such parents show greater irritation, annoyance in response to children's moods, less supportive affectionate attitudes. Parents are not playful and responsive, but tend to attribute hostile motives to their children as providing good reason to be punitive or sexual.

Parents maltreated as children are at higher risk of abusing their own children. However, risk factors are often linked and responsible for cumulative stress, a climate of violence and the perpetration of abusive action. Protective factors, e.g. one caring parent, a supportive extended family, active social support can ameliorate the impact of factors. Numerous studies have shown the strong association between poverty and child maltreatment, abuse being higher in communities with high levels of unemployment and concentrated poverty. Chronic poverty adversely affects children through its impact on parental behaviour and availability of community resources. Deteriorating physical and social infrastructure and few resources and amenities, also have an impact on the general well-being of families.

The availability of 'social capital', that is the degree of cohesion and solidarity in the community is also an important link factor. Children living in areas with less social investment are at greater risk of abuse and have a higher level of psychological or behavioural problems. Social networks and neighbourhood connections can act as protective factors.

Cultural values and economic forces shape the choices facing families and response to these forces. Inequality related to sex and income are also likely to relate to child maltreatment. The nature and availability of preventative mental healthcare, the early identification of cases of abuse and intervening at early stages can all play a part in prevention and the strength of the social welfare system provides a safety net.

Protective factors in sexual abuse

Children will not all suffer the same long-term effects. One of the more important factors which dictates the extent of significant harm is how much support the children receives from family members after a disclosure is made. A mother's belief in her child's statement concerning abuse reduces the ill effects on the child. Children feel less depressed and feel better about themselves when they know that they are believed and supported by the parent who should be most supportive. Paradoxically therefore in sexual abuse, the effects of abuse and the depth of harm depends both on the extent of abuse and the ability of the parent to respond with support and belief once that abuse has been disclosed.

Treatment

Clinical management

The clinical management of all forms of child abuse is a complex process. Figure 23.5 gives a transgenerational model of the process of abusive action. The upper level representing the family level, progressing to the interactional elements leading to abusive effects, the impact on development and the effect on longer-term mental health, partnering and parenting. Intervention is possible at any level – preventatively with an at-risk family situation, at the point of abusive action, or subsequently when behavioural manifestation occurs at various points of development.

The responsibility for management of such concerns on behalf of the community is usually best met in a social welfare agency set up through statutory guidance or laws which indicate how such matters should be investigated, and by whom. A number of different professionals need to be involved in the process. There needs to be guidance to help professionals from social welfare agencies, the police and health and education agencies to know how to act appropriately when there are concerns about abuse. It is evident from the many different forms of child abuse and significant harm present, that there is no one professional or groups of professionals who take the responsibility for identifying the presence of abuse. Questions need to be asked as a matter of urgency. Is a child in immediate danger? Does the child need to go to hospital? Can the child stay at or return home? Can the person against whom an allegation has been made be assisted or required to leave home

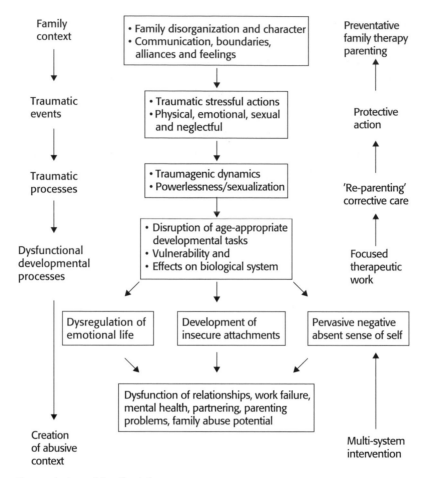

Fig. 23.5.   Transmission of family violence.

in order that the child can remain pending further investigation? Will placement with relatives be appropriate and safe? Is temporary accommodation appropriate? Is some form of emergency protection order needed? What services could or should be offered?

There are a number of professional structures which help achieve this goal.

Strategy discussions

These bring together professionals from health, social services and the police to discuss an initial concern. The aim is to rapidly gather information to help make a decision about provision of immediate protection, or whether a process of assessment is sufficient. A decision may be taken at this point that the injuries presenting are so severe and life threatening that a criminal investigation becomes necessary rather than a child protection enquiry pursuing a civil process.

A child protection conference

This gathers together the family and those professionals who can discuss concerns, make decisions about whether a child protection plan is required, and what services are required for the children and family. At this point child and adolescent psychiatrists may be involved. They may have been the professionals who have raised concerns, or more frequently because a mental health problem of a child and family requires assessment. Referral to a child and adolescent service may be one of the decisions made in terms of the services required for a child who has presented through this process.

A child protection plan

A child protection plan, is required, together with a setting up of a core group to monitor how this is best administered. A multi-disciplinary approach ensures both the safety of the child, and the appropriate provision of services, including therapeutic interventions, which may be indicated. It is important in this care planning approach that professional roles are defined, and responsibilities for setting the goals agreed and for appraising what progress has been made.

A family group conference

This may be set up as a result of concerns raised which brings together members of the family with an appropriate convenor to discuss the protective needs of the child, and how the family will help support and help itself.

Review conferences

These are a structure to assess the ongoing protection and work of the family. A decision can be made at this or an earlier point not to pursue further action. If it seems that the protective needs of the child are not being met proceedings may be required in a court to ensure that a child is provided with services or is adequately protected, particularly if it appears that a child is being harmed significantly and that the level of harm is continuing.

Core assessment

The core assessments are a structure, which lays down the criteria for more extensive assessments of children and families within the context of the framework for assessment of children and their families, and often requires a collaborative assessment from health and education. At this point child and adolescent psychiatrists may be requested to carry out more specialist assessments of the mental health needs of children in families, to assess the impact of parents on children's emotional development, and if the child has been significantly harmed or at risk of serious significant harm in the future. What interventions would be required for the child and family and are the parents able to accept therapeutic work?

Court proceedings

Depending on the severity of injury of the child, and the degree of complexity of the family context, a decision may need to be made about involving a court in reinforcing decisions. A child may need to be removed permanently from a parent. The court will need to be convinced that a child has been so severely significantly harmed, that parenting cannot be improved within the child's timeframe, and there will be a risk to the future health and wellbeing of the child. Child and adolescent psychiatrists have an important role in this context as expert witnesses who can comment on both the state of the child as a result of the abuse to which he has been exposed, and also comment on whether the family can change within the children's timeframe. A complex set of responses may follow, further therapeutic work, fostering or adoption.

Providing child and adolescent psychiatric services within the child protection field

From the flowchart it is evident that complex structures develop to ensure children are adequately protected. Ensuring the rights of a child to grow up safe from abuse and neglect, helped to meet their full potential, is an aim, which should be embodied in law. The rights of children need to be recognized. There is an inevitable conflict of view within the family and between professionals whether a child is being cared for adequately. There can be considerable debate about what constitutes adequate parenting, and whether a child is being cared for well enough or not. Attempts have been made to standardize both definitions of abuse, and to define the thresholds when professionals ought to interfere within the family, the limits of confidentiality, and what are appropriate legal processes to balance the child's needs and the parents' responsibilities.

Families should be supported to care for their children; action needs to be taken when significant harm is accruing. Defining that point is often where child and adolescent skills are required, particularly to look at the emotional component, a key aspect of every form of abuse, and when forms of abuse are present which cause emotional harm rather than physical harm.

This means by definition that the family is not commissioning the child and adolescent psychiatrist, with a request for help with a problem parents perceive. Other professionals perceive the problem not the family. The child and adolescent psychiatrist is working in a complex field. The client may well be the Social Services Department or the Court rather than the family. In such circumstances ordinary rules of confidentiality cannot apply. It is important to consider how best to meet with children and families, yet to ensure that the client, the Social Welfare Department or the Court, is part of the process, linking of a social worker within the assessment process itself is helpful or to ensure that the child and adolescent psychiatrist attends those relevant meetings where family/professional issues are being discussed, and where decisions are being made.

Therapeutic work

It is helpful to think of phases of therapeutic work:
- a phase of disclosure of abuse
- a phase of treatment when the child is safe
- a phase when rehabilitation of a seriously abused child is considered
- a phase if a longer term new family is required.

Stage 1: The phase of disclosure

This is often an extensive phase. Initial concerns have often meant that professionals have become involved, or brought together through a process of strategy meetings or case conferences, or core assessments. However, the full extent of abuse perpetrated against a child may not be known in detail, or aspects of family life which may include mental health issues have not been fully ascertained, or only come to light at a later date. The phase of disclosure includes the process of assessment and the making of and formulating the situation to decide on an appropriate plan of treatment, in the light of the prognosis for therapeutic work.

Stage 2: The phase of treatment in a context of safety

During this phase there needs to be work where the victim is separated from the abusive context, whether through providing the family with a protective context, e.g. a family centre, living with a protective parent/family member, the perpetrator living separately, or the child living in alternative care. A good deal of the work during this phase is inevitably focussed on the individual. Abuse focused therapeutic work for victims whether individually or within group contexts is required to repair attachments, to manage emotional disregulation, and develop a healing sense of self.

Disruptions of a child's attachment can be repaired through individual and group work. Individual therapists need to create a working alliance with the child or young person, to be consistent and reliably available and to create a sense of safety. Group work fosters cohesion, belonging and identity, provides a sense of safety in the group to reverse the fears inherent in family life and share support – substituting pleasure and playfulness for pain. Family work can foster the development of secure attachments both in the phase of separateness or as the situation moves to the next phase of rehabilitation. Connections may be made through a caring parent, sharing and comparing their own experiences in their family with the child's experience. It is important that family therapy techniques such as reframing negative behaviour and positive connotation (giving apparently negative behaviour a positive meaning) connect children with family scripts and the experiences that parents have had growing up themselves. The process of 'externalizing' distances abusive experiences from self and relationships, and strengthens and promotes bonds within the family with a protective parent. Later the sharing of experiences with the abusing parent which have been learnt from their own therapeutic work can help the child or young person feel part of the family context, rather than being blamed, excluded and scapegoated.

Therapeutic work with emotional dysregulation is aimed at reducing anxiety, developing a capacity to cope with emotional problems, and to be able to effectively process experiences of abuse by sharing and exposing them either with an individual therapist, the group contexts and eventually with family members. A variety of approaches are helpful to monitor arousal, and foster containment. To be involved in such work, a protective parent needs to be able to be open to the experiences of the child, to be able to listen and share, and contain what may have been an extreme sense of terror, fear and powerlessness at the hands of the abusive parent. The development of safe family care rituals to cope with sleeping difficulties is required, ways of coping with excitement, anger, sexualized behaviour, and a change of relationship style to avoid retraumatization.

For the child to develop a more satisfactory sense of themselves, he or she has to be helped to realize that what is defined as problematic, e.g. switching off angry oppositional behaviour, fear and avoidance are part of a survival strategy and a strength not a weakness. Family work needs to be absolutely clear about the origins of blame, to help the child understand the way in which the abuser attributes abusive action to the victim rather than taking responsibility themselves. Where rehabilitation is a possibility, family work requires a carefully planned apology and taking of responsibility for abusive action. This must be more than the often brief acknowledgement which is possible in the earlier phases of work.

Stage 3: Rehabilitation phase

Rehabilitation requires that parents confront their abusive behaviour. When both parents have taken part in abusive action they need to acknowledge the extensiveness of their abusive actions, to understand their origins of abuse, and the damaging effect on the child. The 'apology session' is a valuable component of part of a rehabilitation process. Questions the child has about what has happened to him or her can be put to the abusive parent. Responses can be worked out with the therapists, and a joint meeting established where responsibility could be taken and victims freed from their own sense of confusion and guilt and attribution of abuse to their own actions.

Intensive couple therapy may be required because of the secrecy, and often associated violence between parents, before meetings involving the victim and siblings can be initiated. Permanent family structures are required where protection is uppermost.

Research on outcome indicates that in severe physical abuse rehabilitation is not possible in about 30 per cent of cases because of a failure to progress through such a process. In child sexual abuse treatment in 9 per cent of children could be rehabilitated to the family, which included the abuser. 52 per cent could live with a protective parent, and again 37 per cent could not live with any family members because of rejection or disbelief and needed a new family context.

Stage 4: New family phase

When a child cannot return home, intensive family work with a new family context is required, planning long-term care, and preparation of a family for a child who has experienced extensive abuse. Sexually abused children may have a high level of sexual knowledge, may be prone to a sexual behavioural disorder and may have an aggressive or victimizing stance themselves. There needs to be planning of a protective context within the foster family, and careful consideration of the appropriate mode of contact with the original family. Work with the foster family or alternative adoptive family is essential to maintain an appropriate supportive stance, and to incorporate the victim into a new family context. Child and adolescent psychiatrists have a particular role in working with families who are attempting to provide care for these often disruptive but highly needy children.

Evidence of effectiveness of intervention

There have now been a number of controlled trials of therapeutic work with various forms of abuse, and reviews of effectiveness examining a number of studies have been carried out.

Child sexual abuse

In the field of sexual abuse it is essential to protect the child, increase social support available to the child and their family, and to treat psychological symptoms and behaviours associated with abuse. A team or core group approach and interdisciplinary working with mental health professionals is likely to be best suited to meet the many and varied needs of children and families.

Therapeutic approaches, particularly focused therapies based on cognitive behavioural models have been found to be effective ways of treating these symptoms. The focus of treatment needs to include symptoms of depression, anxiety and post-traumatic stress, dissociative or sexualized and other behavioural problems. Parental involvement improves the outcome leading to greater benefit for children. Non-directive, supportive approaches are not as effective empirically as cognitive-behavioural approaches. Group therapeutic approaches compares favourably with more individual psychodynamic approaches. However, no single approach has demonstrable benefit for all children who have been sexually abused.

Whilst cognitive behavioural approaches for instance are effective in some circumstances, one of the implications from treatment outcome studies is that flexibility within treatment programmes, or a range of available treatments is absolutely essential. There are a wide variety of psychological outcomes and consequences of sexual abuse which needs to be addressed in therapeutic work, as well as the variety of ages and special needs of child victims, particularly those who have begun to behave abusively. Using objective measures of outcome is helpful to assess the changing responses and states of children so that the issue of pursuing an effective approach can be followed.

Child physical abuse

A limited number of studies using a control approach to evaluate treatment approaches characterized by physical abuse have been carried out. Cognitive-behavioural treatment with all family members individually, or family therapy using an interactional/ecological model has been shown to be more effective than routine community management. A family therapy approach led to children reporting their parents being less violent towards them, and both approaches helped to reduce children's aggressive behaviour, family conflict and the transmission of an aggressive style from parent to child. Effective intervention requires a firm link between the care agency and the therapeutic team.

Multi-systemic therapy is a powerful model, which although used more frequently with conduct disordered young people is also effective in the child abuse field. It fits with the general approach advocated of stages of therapeutic work, understanding the fit between identified problems and the broader context, emphasizing positives and using strengths as levers for change. Services need to fit with the needs of the family. Responsible behaviour should be promoted, action-orientated approaches targeting well-defined problems, developmentally appropriate treatment goals and success being defined. Interventions need to be provided with intensity, positive reinforcement of small gains, and evaluated from multiple perspectives. Caregivers need to be empowered to promote change.

Outcome

Short-term effects

Each form of abuse has particular effects on development as described in early sections on attachments, on emotional regulation and sense of self. There are effects on physical and mental health, on adaptation to school, adaptation to social contexts, peer relationships and the capacity to make satisfactory sexual relationships.

Longer-term effects

The longer abuse continues, the more extensive it is, for example involving penetrative abuse, the older the child, and the greater the number of stages that abuse continues through, the more disturbed the child is likely to be, the more depressed and sad, and the greater their loss of self-esteem. Children who have suffered chronic long-term sexual abuse feel very negatively about themselves and all aspects of their relationships, and they have very high levels of distress.

Traumatic sexualization enlarges the traumatic effects described earlier and leads to a cycle of avoidance of anything to do with sexuality. Alternatively sexual pre-occupations occur and sexually inappropriate behaviour with other children and adults.

Girls follow a female 'mode' internalizing, blame themselves, attribute sexual abusive action to some aspect of themselves, often reinforced by the abuser who perceives the child's affection to be a sexual invitation. Thus a victim mode with compliant responses is more likely. There is a tendency to self-mutilation, self-harm and anxiety and depression.

Boys generally follow a male mode and externalize their responses, look for somebody else to blame and take over their negative self-representation. They find someone younger to abuse who reminds them of their own powerlessness. As a result they may develop an abusive, hostile, aggressive style of relating, with associated conduct disorders and substance abuse. Some girls may also follow this 'male' externalizing mode response.

Boys are more likely to adopt a sexually abusive orientation if they have been physically abused as well as sexually abused in their own families, if there is violence between the parents, if they have suffered disruptions of care and have been rejected by their family. An attitude of grievance is more likely to occur under these circumstances with the adoption of an abusive role in turn.

Being subject to penetration is a significantly traumatic effect that causes long-standing effects without adequate treatment even when emotional support has been offered to the child or young person.

One of the most worrying responses in older girls particularly those who have been abused are major depressive symptoms, poor self-esteem and self-worth, and self-injurious behaviour. There may be overdosing, wrist slashing, bulimic responses, re-enactment of abusive experiences, and gaining relief through hurt, suicidal attempts of self-starvation, 'total refusal syndromes' – withdrawal, refusal to eat, talk or walk.

A sense of betrayal and stigmatization is felt as a result of the threats, secrecy and self-justifying attitude of the abuser. Guilt and a low opinion of oneself, may lead to drug and alcohol abuse, promiscuous seeking of redeeming relationships, and clinging to unstable partners can all be responses to the victimization process. Problems of partnering and parenting follow.

Males show similar patterns, with more emphasis on abusive patterns, substance and alcohol misuse.

Prognostic factors

On the basis of the assessment of the child's needs, it is helpful to construct a prognosis. The elements include:

- the level of abuse perpetrated, and the extensiveness of traumatic damage caused to the child's physical and emotional health and the level of care that the child will require to recover the specific therapeutic work required and level of parental skill
- the degree of responsibility for the state of the child taken by the parents, and the capacity to provide the care the child requires
- the level of parental psychopathology and the motivation the parent has to undertake the necessary therapeutic work to reverse the personal attributes which have contributed to creating an abusive context and to ask whether issues such as drug addiction, mental health problems, parental violence are amenable to treatment within the child's timeframe, and whether the parent has the capacity to provide more adequate care within the child's timeframe
- the general attitude of the parents to the professional, whether there is a prospect of a reasonable collaborative approach, or a negative stance of denial
- the availability of settings for therapeutic work, whether this is on an outpatient day or residential basis.

A hopeful prognosis requires that parents take adequate responsibility for abusive action where appropriate, there is a protective capacity within the family, e.g. a non-abusive parent who recognizes that his or her partner has abused the child, and is prepared to protect the child over and above their relationship with their partner. There needs to be the possibility of a capacity for change in parents who have been abusive, with a willingness to work reasonably co-operatively with child care professionals, and to accept the need for change even if it is with the motivation of maintaining children within the family context rather than them being removed, or removed permanently. There needs to be the potential for the development of a reasonable attachment and relationship between the parents and children, a capacity to provide adequate care for the particular child or children. Appropriate therapeutic settings need to be available, whether on an outpatient basis, a day-care setting, or residential resource depending on the severity of abuse, the nature of family difficulties and strengths, and the nature of the task to be tackled to achieve a satisfactory outcome. The prognosis is hopeless for family work when none of these criteria is fulfilled. Where there is rejection of the child, a failure to take responsibility for the state of the child, the needs of parents take primacy over the needs of the children, a combative oppositional stance to professionals emerges, or psychopathology in parents, e.g. drug abuse, serious marital violence, or longstanding personality or intellectual problems which may not be amenable to therapeutic work, or where there is complete inability or unwillingness to accept that there are problems. In such situations family work has no place since the child will be persuaded to withdraw their statements or to become part of a process of maintenance of secrecy and denial.

Situations are of doubtful progress where professionals are not yet clear from the original work with the family whether the situation is hopeful or hopeless. There is uncertainty whether there is adequate taking of responsibility, whether parental pathology is changeable, whether there is going to be willingness to work with care authorities and therapeutic agencies, or whether resources will be available to meet the extensiveness of the problem. Further work needs to be suggested to help clarify the needs of the child and the capacity of the parents to provide adequate care.

A good deal of the approach to work will depend on the assessment of the child. Severely traumatized children may be re-traumatized through contacts with an abusive parent, even when a parent is taking responsibility for abusive action. The child may need a level of care beyond the parents' capacity, despite good motivation. Planning needs then to take place with the child individually, in groups or with a foster parent or protective parent before contact with abusive parents can be considered.

SUGGESTED READING

A. Bentovim, *Trauma Organised Systems, Physical and Sexual Abuse in Families*. (London: Karnac, 1995). (Also translated into German, Spanish and Czech).

A. Bentovim, Significant harm in context. In *Significant Harm, Its Management and Outcome*, ed. M. Adcock & R. White (London: Significant Publications, 1998).

A. Bentovim, Working with abusing families. In *The Child Protection Handbook*. 2nd edn, ed. K. Wilson & A. Jones. (Edinburgh: Bailliere Tindall, 2001).

A. Bentovim, Preventing sexually abused people from becoming abusers, and treating the victimisation experiences of young people who offend sexually. *Child Abuse and Neglect*, **26** (2002), 661–78.

A. Bentovim, A. Elton, J. Hildebrand, M. Tranter & E. Vizard, *Child Sexual Abuse within the Family, Assessment and Treatment*. (Bristol: John Wright, 1988).

A. Bentovim & L. Bingley Miller, *The Family Assessment of Family Competence*. (Brighton: Pavilion Press, 2001).

T. Brugha, P. Bebington, C. Tennant & J. Hurry, The list of threatening experiences: a subset of 12 life event categories with considerable long-term contextual threat. *Psychological Medicine*, **15** (1985), 189–94.

A. Cox & S. Walker, *The Home Inventory*. (Brighton: Pavilion Press, 2002).

S. Creighton, Recognising changes in incidence and prevalence. In *Early Prediction and Prevention of Child Abuse, A Handbook*, ed. K. Browne, H. Hanks, P. T. Stratton & C. Hamilton. (Chichester: John Wiley, 2002).

K. A. Crinic & M. T. Greenberg, Minor parenting stresses with young children. *Child Development*, **61** (1990), 1628–37.

D. Glaser, Emotional abuse and neglect (psychological maltreatment): the conceptual framework. *Child Abuse and Neglect*, **26** (2002), 715–30.

R. Goodman, The strengths and difficulties questionnaire: a research note. *Journal of Child Psychology and Psychiatry*, **38** (1997), 581–6.

R. Goodman, H. Meltzer & V. Bailey, The strengths and difficulties questionnaire: a pilot study on the validity of the self-report version. *European Child and Adolescent Psychiatry*, **7** (1998), 125–30.

T. Hobbs, H. Hanks & J. Wynne, *Child Abuse and Neglect. A Clinicians Handbook*. 2nd edn. (Edinburgh: Churchill Livingston, 2002).

D. Jones, *Communicating with Vulnerable Children. A Guide for Practitioners*. (London: Gaskell, The Royal College of Psychiatrists and the Department of Health, 2003).

D. Jones & P. Ramchandani, *Child Sexual Abuse – Informing Practice From Research*. (Oxford: Radcliffe Medical Press, 1999).

V. Sinason (ed). *Attachment, Trauma and Multiplicity. Working with Dissociative Identity Disorder*. (Sussex and New York: Brunner-Routledge, 2002).

M. A. Smith, The effects of low levels of lead on urban children: the relevance of social factors. (Ph.D. Psychology, University of London, 1985).

R. P. Snaith, A. A. Constantopoulos, M. Y. Jardine & P. McGuffin, A clinical scale for the self-assessment of irritability. *British Journal of Psychiatry*, **132** (1978), 164–71.

REFERENCES

Bentovim, A. & Bingley Miller, L. (2001). *The Family Assessment of Family Competence*. Brighton: Pavilion Press.

Brugha, T., Bebington, P., Tennant, C. & Hurry, J. (1985). *The List of Threatening*. Experiences: A subset of 12 life event categories with considerable long-term contextual threat. *Psychological Medicine*, **15**, 189–94. London: The Stationery Office.

Cox, A. & Bentovim, A. (2000). *The Family Pack of Questionnaires and Scales*. Department of Health.

Cox, A. & Walker, S. (2002). *The Home Inventory*. Brighton: Pavilion Press.

Crinic, K. A. & Booth, C. L. (1991). Mothers and fathers perception of daily hassles of parenting across early childhood. *Journal of Marriage and the Family*, **53**, 1043–50.

Crinic, K. A. & Greenberg, M. T. (1990). Minor parenting stresses with young children. *Child Development*, **61**, 1628–37.

Davie, C. E., Hutt, S. J., Vincent, E. & Mason, M. (1984). *The Young Child at Home.* Windsor: NFER–Nelson.

Piccianelli, M., Tessari, E., Bortolomas, M. *et al.* (1997). Efficacy of the alcohol use disorders test as a screening tool for hazardous alcohol intake and related disorders in primary care. *A Validity Study, British Medical Journal,* **514**, 420–4.

Snaith, R. P., Constantopoulos A. A., Jardine, M. Y. & McGuffin, P. (1978). A clinical scale for the self-assessment of irritability. *British Journal of Psychiatry,* **132**, 164–71.

Appendix 23.1. Evidence-based approaches to assist assessments of physical and sexual abuse

- **The Family Pack of Questionnaires and Scales** (Cox & Bentovim, 2000). This includes a set of material with instructions for use. They include those listed below.

- **The Parenting Daily Hassles Scale** (Crinic & Greenberg, 1990; Crinic & Booth, 1991) described the frequency and intensity of common experiences that can be 'a hassle to parents', and can describe areas of pressure felt by the carer to help identify areas where assistance could be provided.

- **The Recent Life Events Questionnaire** (Taken from Brugha *et al.*, 1985) helps to define negative life events over the last 12 months, and significantly whether the respondent thought they have a continuing influence.

- **The Home Conditions Assessment** (Davie *et al.*, 1984) helps make judgements about the context in which the child was living, dealing with questions of safety, order and cleanliness which have an important bearing where issues of neglect are the focus of concern.

- **The Family Activity Scale** (Derived from The Child-Centeredness Scale. Smith, 1985) gives an idea of how child-centred families are and is an important determinant of good child development and has an important link to the profile of parents' capacity to meet the child's needs.

- **The Adult Wellbeing Scale** (Snaith *et al.*, 1978) and **the Alcohol Scale** (Piccinelli *et al.*, 1997) are both important pointers to the individual parent's contribution to significant harm, and also lead to the possibility of referral to adult mental health services. This will assess the level of current mental health problems, requirements for therapeutic work and prospects of change if there are longstanding problems present such as personality disorders which are ordinarily resistant to therapeutic work within the child's timeframe.

- **The HOME Inventory** (Cox & Walker, 2002) assessment through interview and observation provides an extensive profile of the context of care provided for the child and is a reliable approach to assessment of parenting. It gives a reliable account of the parents' capacities to provide learning materials, language stimulation and appropriate physical environment, to be responsive, stimulating, providing adequate modelling variety and acceptance. A profile of needs can be constructed in these areas, and an analysis of how considerable changes would need to be made to meet the specific needs of the significantly harmed child; and the contribution of the environment provided by the parents to the harm suffered. The HOME Inventory has been used extensively to demonstrate change in the family context as a result of intervention, and can be used to assess whether intervention has been successful.

- **The Family Assessment** (Bentovim & Bingley Miller, 2001). The various modules of the family assessment, which include an exploration of family and professional views of the current situation, the adaptability to the child's needs, quality of parenting, various aspects of family relationships and the impact of history provides a standardized evidence based approach to current family strengths and difficulties which have played a role in the significant harm of the child, and also in assessing the capacity for change, and resources in the family to achieve a safe context for the child, and the reversal of family factors which may have played a role in significant harm, and aiding the recovery and future health of the child. The family assessment profile provides it by its qualitative and quantitative information on the parents' understanding of the child's state, and the level of responsibility they take for the significant harm, the capacity of the parents to adapt to the children's changing needs in the past and future, their abilities to promote development, provide adequate guidance, care and manage conflict, to make decisions and relate to the wider family and community. Strengths and difficulties in all these areas are delineated, the influence of history, areas of change to be achieved and the capacities of the family to make such changes.

24

Gender identity disorders

Peggy T. Cohen-Kettenis

Department of Child and Adolescent Psychiatry, Utrecht, The Netherlands

Gender identity disorder: general aspects

Introduction

A newborn does not yet have self-awareness of his or her sex and gender. Such self-awareness evolves gradually in early childhood. Children learn to make consistent and systematic use of genital information as a criterion for the classification of their own and other's sex. Interestingly, long before they do so, they appear to have knowledge about gender stereotypes and display either female or male gender role behaviour. Toy and game preferences as well as preferences for same-sex peers are expressed much earlier than a complete understanding of the various aspects of gender is reached.

Nature as well as nurture play important parts in the shaping of gender role behaviour. Adults and children influence gender development directly by reinforcing or discouraging sex-typed behaviours and indirectly by offering role models. However, from animal and human research, it has been found that sex hormones also play a significant role in the development of sex-typed behaviour and characteristics.

In most cases, sex, gender identity and gender role usually develop in accordance with each other. Sometimes a discrepancy exists between gender identity and role, and biological sex. Parents or children who are confronted with such a divergence often seek professional help. Because the issues in the management of gender identity problems are very different when dealing with children than when dealing with adolescents we will discuss the clinical management of both age groups separately.

A Clinician's Handbook of Child and Adolescent Psychiatry, ed. Christopher Gillberg,
Richard Harrington and Hans-Christoph Steinhausen. Published by Cambridge University Press.
© Cambridge University Press 2005.

Table 24.1. ICD-10 diagnostic criteria for gender identity disorders

Transsexualism (F64.0) has three criteria.
1. The desire to live and be accepted as a member of the opposite sex, usually accompanied by the wish to make his or her body as congruent as possible with the preferred sex through surgery and hormone treatment.
2. The transsexual identity has been present persistently for at least two years.
3. The disorder is not a symptom of another mental disorder or a genetic, intersex, or chromosomal abnormality.

Dual-role transvestism (F 64.1) has three criteria.
1. The individual wears clothes of the opposite sex in order to experience temporary membership in the opposite sex.
2. There is no sexual motivation for the cross-dressing.
3. The individual has no desire for a permanent change to the opposite sex.

Gender identity disorder of childhood (F64.2) has separate criteria for girls and for boys.
For girls
1. The individual shows persistent and intense distress about being a girl, and has a stated desire to be a boy (not merely a desire for any perceived cultural advantages of being a boy) or insists that she is a boy.
2. Either of the following must be present:
   a. persistent marked aversion to normative feminine clothing and insistence on wearing stereotypical masculine clothing
   b. persistent repudiation of female anatomical structures, as evidenced by at least one of the following
      (i) an assertion that she has, or will grow, a penis
      (ii) rejection of urination in a sitting position
      (iii) assertion that she does not want to grow breasts or menstruate.
3. The girl has not yet reached puberty
4. The disorder must have been present for at least 6 months

For boys
1. The individual shows persistent and intense distress about being a boy, and has a desire to be a girl, or, more rarely, insists that he is a girl.
2. Either of the following must be present:
   a. preoccupation with stereotypic female activities, as shown by a preference for either cross-dressing or simulating female attire, or by an intense desire to participate in the games and pastimes of girls and rejection of stereotypical male toys, games and activities.
   b. persistent repudiation of male anatomical structures, as evidenced by at least one of the following repeated assertions:
      1. that he will grow up to become a woman (not merely in the role)
      2. that his penis or testes are disgusting or will disappear
      3. that it would be better not to have a penis or testes
3. The boy has not yet reached puberty
4. The disorder must have been present for at least 6 months

Other gender identity disorders (F64.8) has no specific criteria.
Gender identity disorder, unspecified (F64.9) has no specific criteria.
Either of the previous two diagnoses could be used for those with an intersexed condition.

Definitions and classification

The distress resulting from conflicting gender identity and sex of assignment is often referred to as gender dysphoria. Gender dysphoric individuals may have various diagnoses in the current classification systems. ICD-10 provides five diagnoses in the field of gender identity disorders (see Table 24.1). Criteria differ between children and adults. Transsexualism is an extreme gender identity disorder (GID), which is still in the ICD, but has disappeared from the DSM. In DSM IV gender identity disorder is viewed as basically one disorder that could develop along different routes and could have various levels of intensity. DSM-IV criteria for children have been criticized, because:

- children do not have to express a desire to be of the opposite sex to meet the A criterion (cross-gender identification)
- a discomfort with gender role is given the same diagnostic significance as discomfort with one's biological sex, implying that children that are gender deviant but do not want to be of the opposite sex and do not have an aversion to their own sex characteristics can meet GID criteria
- for boys, aversion to rough-and-tumble play is identified as a symptom of a disorder, whereas it may be seen as a non-pathological factor that only predisposes to its development
- the child's observed distress should not solely stem from rejection or harassment because of its gender atypicality.

Concern with pathologizing healthy functioning gender-atypical children has been an important reason for some to promote that the diagnosis of GID for children should be removed from DSM in its current form. These criticisms should make clinicians aware that referred children may be cross-gendered in some, but not all, possible aspects and that one should be cautious in classifying a child as having a GID on the basis of mere gender-atypical behaviour. Depending on the outcome of the diagnostic process, clinical management may vary from intensive interventions to counseling activities.

In the last decade, the terms transgenderism and transgenderists are increasingly used by lay people and professionals. Originally, the terms were used by individuals living lives 'in-between' sex-typical heterosexual men and women. Now they are used as an umbrella term for all types of individuals that do not completely identify with members of their own biological sex (Tables 24.1, 24.2).

Epidemiology

No epidemiological studies exist that provide data on the prevalence of childhood GID. In a behavioural genetic study of 314 child and adolescent twins it was estimated that the prevalence is 2.3 per cent (Coolidge, Thede & Young, 2002). This number may be influenced because twins are more likely than other fetuses to be subject to intrauterine stress. Furthermore, one should bear in mind, that most

Table 24.2. DSM-IV criteria for gender identity disorder

A. A strong and persistent cross-gender identification (not merely a desire for any perceived cultural advantages of being the other sex).

In children, the disturbance is manifested by four (or more) of the following:

(1) repeatedly stated desire to be, or insistence that he or she is, the other sex

(2) in boys, preference for cross-dressing or simulating female attire; in girls, insistence on wearing only stereotypical masculine clothing

(3) strong and persistent preferences for cross-sex roles in make-believe play or persistent fantasies of being the other sex

(4) intense desire to participate in the stereotypical games and pastimes of the other sex

(5) strong preference for playmates of the other sex

In adolescents and adults, the disturbance is manifested by symptoms such as a stated desire to be the other sex, frequent passing as the other sex, desire to live or be treated as the other sex, or the conviction that he or she has the typical feelings and reactions of the other sex.

B. Persistent discomfort with his or her sex or sense of inappropriateness in the gender role of that sex.

In children, the disturbance is manifested by any of the following: in boys, assertion that his penis or testes are disgusting or will disappear or assertion that it would be better not to have a penis, or aversion toward rough-and-tumble play and rejection of male stereotypical toys, games, and activities; in girls, rejection of urinating in a sitting position, assertion that she has or will grow a penis, or assertion that she does not want to grow breasts or menstruate, or marked aversion toward normative feminine clothing.

In adolescents and adults, the disturbance is manifested by symptoms such as preoccupation with getting rid of primary and secondary sex characteristics (e.g. request for hormones, surgery, or other procedures to physically alter sexual characteristics to simulate the other sex) or belief that he or she was born the wrong sex.

C. The disturbance is not concurrent with a physical intersex condition.

D. The disturbance causes clinically significant distress or impairment in social, occupational, or other important areas of functioning.

Code based on current age:

302.6 Gender identity disorder in children

302.85 Gender identity disorder in adolescents or adults

Specify if (for sexually mature individuals):

Sexually attracted to males

Sexually attracted to females

Sexually attracted to both

Sexually attracted to neither

302.6 Gender identity disorder not otherwise specified

This category is included for coding disorders in gender identity that are not classifiable as a specific gender identity disorder. Examples include:

(1) Intersex conditions (e.g. androgen insensitivity syndrome or congenital adrenal hyperplasia) and accompanying gender dysphoria

(2) Transient, stress-related cross-dressing behaviour

(3) Persistent preoccupation with castration or penectomy without a desire to acquire the sex characteristics of the other sex

prepubertal children with GID are more likely to become homosexual than transsexual (see below). This means that the number of 2.3 per cent almost certainly overestimates the percentage of GID children that will be 'persisters' in adulthood (that is the prevalence of pre-transsexuals is probably lower).

Prevalence estimates of transsexualism among adolescents and adults (that is 15 years and above) are usually based on the number of transsexuals, treated at major centres, or on responses of psychiatrists to surveys. The numbers vary widely across studies. In the first years of transsexual treatment, very low prevalences were reported (between 1 : 100 000 and 1 : 400 000). More recent studies indicated higher prevalences: between 1 : 3000 and 1 : 30 000. These differences probably reflect differences in methodology and differences between countries in treatment availability, in criteria for treatment eligibility.

Sex ratio

The majority of the prepubertal children attending gender clinics are boys. The boy to girl ratios are about 6:1 in Canada, 3:1 in the Netherlands and 4:1 in the UK. The sex ratio of adolescents at the three gender clinics, however, approaches a 1:1 relationship. It might be that a small but equal number of the boys and girls with GID that were seen in childhood apply for sex reassignment (SR) relatively early in life. In adulthood, sex ratios again are about 3:1. It may be that higher numbers of girls with GID will later seek SR than boys. The higher rates of boys seen in childhood in the UK and Canada may reflect a greater anxiety of parents about male effeminacy. This idea is supported by a study showing that children with GID are seen at significantly lower ages than in the Netherlands.

Correspondence between childhood GID and transsexualism

Not all children with GID will seek SR after puberty, as childhood GID is more strongly related to homosexuality than to transsexualism. In a combined sample of (partly non-clinical) boys with GID from six North-American follow-up studies, 6 per cent of 99 boys had a transsexual outcome. This is probably an underestimation of the true numbers. In two clinical samples of boys and girls with GID, 20–23 per cent appeared to be still gender dysphoric after puberty or wanted/already applied for SR. But even when the clinical studies more correctly estimate the true numbers, a clinician meeting a child with GID is far more likely seeing a future homosexual person than a future transsexual. This is something they should bear in mind.

Clinical picture

Children

In children, signs of a developing GID may be apparent as early as 2 years. As soon as they are able to talk, they may state repeatedly that they are or will later become members of the opposite sex, show cross-gender preferences and behaviour and show unhappiness when they are not allowed to act on these preferences. Older, still prepubertal, children often stop talking about their cross-gender feelings and may, out of shame, show less cross-gender behaviours.

Boys with GID are usually interested primarily in girls' toys, and girls' games and activities. They usually dislike rough-and-tumble play. In fantasy play they like to take female roles, such as princess or fairy. Almost all boys with GID have a strong preference for girls as playmates. When growing up, it may be difficult to maintain their friendships with girls. Boys with GID are teased or bullied frequently, especially when they grow older. This increases the risk of developing social or other problems. Many boys express distress about their male body. They may hide their genitals, when they are nude, and pretend to have girls' genitals. More often than not, they sit down when urinating. Young boys sometimes believe that their penis will automatically fall off when they grow up and that they will grow breasts like their mothers.

Girls with GID are equally early as boys in showing cross-gendered behaviour and interests. Parents report that their daughters always disliked typically feminine clothing and jewellery. The girls with very short haircuts are mistaken regularly for boys. Cross-gendered girls are interested in playing with boys' toys such as moving objects or construction play. They love sports, ball games in particular, and rough-and-tumble play. They often prefer to play outside. Boys are their preferred playmates. Like in boys without GID, the friendships of girls with GID seem to be more focused on common activities and interests than on sharing feelings. As cross-gender behaviour is much more accepted in girls than in boys, the girls may be quite popular among boys, when they are good in sports and have pleasant personalities. As a result, girls with GID are less ostracized and teased than boys with GID. Some girls try to move in typical boyish ways or make an effort to speak with a low-pitched voice. Girls with GID can be very distressed about being a girl and having a female body. They may put handkerchiefs or other objects in their underpants to pretend they have a penis. Occasionally, they make attempts at urinating in a standing position, for instance against trees when playing outside in gardens or parks. For them, the idea that they will have breasts and menstruate when they grow up is usually abhorrent.

Adolescents

Adolescents with extreme forms of GID have usually been children with GID. After elementary school, some do not make much change in their behaviour or appearance and start high school in the opposite gender role when they are referred to a clinic. When they grow older, some fall in love and have sexual relationships with same-sex peers. Sexuality ranges from having crushes at a great distance from the person involved to actual dating and sexual activity. Sexually active youngsters invariably exclude involvement of their primary sex characteristics from their love-making. Another group consists of adolescents who try to adjust to gender typical norms until their problem become evident in other ways. They wear gender-neutral or gender-typical clothing, a gender-typical hairstyle and behave as inconspicuously as possible. In the fearful and cautious youngsters, the gender identity disorder is not always easily observable from their behaviour or appearance.

Adolescents who do not fulfil all criteria for GID are a heterogeneous group. They may

- have a SR request but are ambivalent about it
- have a strong SR wish during the intake phase, but change their minds later
- have no real SR request, but are merely confused about their gender feelings
- have questions regarding their gender identity that is secondary to other psychopathology (e.g. pervasive developmental disorder).

Aetiology

Subtypes of GID and its relevance for aetiological theories

GID is not a homogeneous phenomenon. It has been proposed repeatedly to subdivide adults with GID in mostly two categories. One category is referred to as early-onset, core, primary, nuclear, homosexual (attracted to persons of the same biological sex). The other category is referred to as late-onset, non-core, secondary, fetishistic, non-homosexual (not attracted to persons of the same biological sex). Research findings support such a distinction. It seems that there are at least two subtypes of transsexuals that follow different developmental routes. The early-onset group has been extremely cross-gendered from early in life, never had any sexual interest in cross-dressing, is attracted to same-sex, heterosexual partners, pursues SR relatively early in life and has no major psychological problems before treatment. The other group has been more stereotypical with regard to gender role behaviours as a child, is (or used to be) aroused sexually when cross-dressing, and is attracted to the opposite sex. This group applies for SR after having tried to live relatively long in the social role of their biological sex. Some even marry and have children. Psychologically they are less stable than the first group, which could be a consequence of their living in this role, or be caused by other factors.

Like adults, children also vary in type and intensity of cross-genderedness. As has been noted above, most children with GID do not become transsexual, but a substantial minority does. So one would expect that children with GID could be classified in at least two subgroups: the pre-homosexual and pre-transsexual children with GID. It is not yet possible to predict which children will, and which will not, become transsexuals. It is even less clear which children with GID will develop gender problems other than transsexualism (e.g. transvestism). And to complicate things further, not all adult transsexuals (e.g. the late-onset transsexuals) have been children with a full-blown GID. Theories and supporting evidence thus refer to subgroups that developed a variety of gender identity disorders. The work that is done on children largely refers to children with GID that develop into homosexuals or early-onset transsexuals. The work that has been done on adults refers to both early- and late-onset transsexuals who had a complete or incomplete GID in childhood.

Psychological and psychobiological theories

The determinants of cross-gender development are still largely unknown. Many psychological factors have been declared responsible for GID development. The single factor theories are generally far too simplistic to explain GID. Recent theories include multiple cumulative risk factors. Although they are primarily developed to explain childhood GID, they may also explain certain forms of GID in adolescence or adulthood. It is assumed that some of the risk factors must converge during a critical period of development in order to cause a GID.

In one influential current theory anxiety (about self-value) is seen as a core component of GID development. Cross-gender identification, not necessarily with the opposite sex parent, allows a child to feel more secure, safe or valued. Two conditions have to be fulfilled to develop the feeling that being the other sex is more secure or safe. First, children need to be in so much emotional distress that they must seek a solution to survive. This distress may be produced by general (psychological or biological) factors related to the child's temperament, parental characteristics or both. Secondly, during a sensitive developmental period, when the child is developing a coherent sense of self, specific (psychological or biological) factors create a situation in which the resulting anxiety induces cross-gender behaviour.

Thus, according to this theory, a cross-gender identity may be reached through different pathways, and a broad range of factors may contribute to the disorder. Some studies on the proposed factors have corroborated elements of the theory, others, however, did not.

Evidence: parent-related factors in children with GID

Psychopathology in parents of gender-disordered children may be a general predisposing factor, because it might influence their possibilities to set limits, even lead to encouragement of cross-genderedness, hamper effective problem solving between parents and make parents less emotionally available. The anxiety that this unavailability creates might bring the child to 'seek solutions' in the direction of wanting to be the opposite sex. In some studies elevated levels of psychopathology have indeed been found. There is, however, no overwhelming evidence that one particular disorder primarily exists among parents with GID children.

A specific factor, paternal (emotional) distance from their cross-gendered sons, as measured by recalled shared father–son time, appeared to exist to some extent, but it is unclear whether this characteristic is a cause or a consequence of the feminine development of the boy. The wish for a daughter, among clinicians often expected to be an important, even sole, determinant in boys with GID, does not occur more often among mothers with feminine boys than among other mothers.

Evidence: child-related factors in children with GID

An anxious temperament of the child has been put forward as a general predisposing factor that makes the child constitutionally vulnerable to developing GID. Parent reports on the CBCL, a widely used parent questionnaire to measure emotional and behavioural problems at home, show that children with GID do have a pre-dominance of internalizing, as opposed to externalizing, behavioural difficulties. However, when tested in experimental conditions they do not respond physiologically in a typically anxious way. So anxious reaction patterns do not seem to be present on all levels of functioning in children with GID.

Children with GID are different from children without GID with regard to rough-and-tumble play. Boys tend to avoid it; girls often show a clear preference for sports and romping. Prenatal brain exposure to testosterone is probably related to this specific child-related factor.

The appearance of the children may trigger feelings and reinforcement patterns in parents that affect the child's gender development in a specific way. Boys with GID are indeed rated as more attractive, beautiful and handsome, and pretty than other boys, and less all-boy, masculine and rugged. Girls with GID were judged to look more handsome, masculine, rugged and tomboyish than control girls. Morphological features of the face may have accounted for the findings.

Biological theories

The process of sexual differentiation, of becoming male or female, not only refers to the formation of the internal and external genitals. The brain too undergoes a differentiation into male or female. Pre- or perinatal exposure of the brain to sex hormones leads to more permanent changes in its development and therefore in behaviour. A supposed discrepancy between genital differentiation, on the one hand, and brain sexual differentiation, on the other has been invoked as a major factor in the development of the most extreme form of GID, transsexualism.

To test the assumption that prenatal sex hormones have an influence on the development of transsexualism, biomedical research on transsexualism has addressed the following areas: (i) Individuals with abnormal prenatal endocrine history, such as congenital adrenal hyperplasia (CAH). Individuals with this syndrome have adrenal glands secreting large amounts of androgens. Prenatal exposure to high levels of androgens masculinize the external genitals in 46XX individuals, and also influence various sex-related behaviours; (ii) sexual dimorphic brain nuclei and (iii) sex-related cognitive abilities, functional cerebral asymmetry and handedness. From these fields comes increasing, but still largely indirect, evidence that the brains of certain types of cross-gendered individuals have been prenatally exposed to atypical levels of sex hormones. However, such exposure alone is probably not enough to develop a cross-gender identity.

For men, another mechanism, the progressive immunization of mothers to H–Y antigens, has been proposed. Though the existing empirical data are in line with such a mechanism, direct evidence for this mechanism is again still lacking.

A recent twin study in a combined group of children and adolescents suggests that GID has a genetic component. In the study, the genetic component accounted for 62 per cent of the variance, and the non-shared environment (e.g. prenatal hormones, trauma) for 38 per cent. This leaves 0 per cent to the shared environment (the family). However, this is only one study, conducted with a non-clinical sample. Also, one should bear in mind that the sample consisted partly of children with GID, who for a large part will be pre-homosexual. This implies that the numbers may be different when only adolescents and adults would be included. Yet it is the first non-retrospective study pointing towards genetic influences in GID development.

Clinical management of gender problems in children

Diagnosis

When children with gender problems are referred for diagnosis, clinicians first have to assess whether a child actually meets the criteria for GID. In extreme cases this will not be a very difficult task. However, children may take a position anywhere between 'typical for boys' or 'typical for girls' on various dimensions (see Table 24.3). When not only the current situation is taken into account, the picture can be even more complex. Cross-gender profiles may change over time because of true changes or be the result of the growing awareness of older children of the social undesirability of cross-gender behaviour. Especially when children do not state they want to be of the opposite sex and do not report an aversion to their bodies, it can be hard to know whether their cross-gender behaviour and preferences are manifestations of gender dysphoria or just atypical, albeit still in the normal range. But even if all information is accessible, no easy algorithm exists that can help us infer a diagnosis of GID from a cross-gender profile.

Table 24.3. Dimensions of cross-genderedness: a conceptual aid for clinicians

	(typical for) boys	(typical for) girls
Identity statements	|................................|	
Identification figures	|................................|	
Wants sex characteristics of	|................................|	
Rough-and-tumble play	|................................|	
Peer preference	|................................|	
Prefers dressing in clothes of	|................................|	
Role and fantasy play	|................................|	
Toy preference	|................................|	
Play, games and activities preference	|................................|	
Mannerisms/speech	|................................|	

Furthermore, it is worthwhile to try to find out whether family- or child factors reported in the literature are operating in an individual case. Of course, the ultimate significance of most reported factors as actual determinants of GID is not (yet) known. However, even if they are no determinants of the GID, they may have a negative effect on the child's development. So it may be useful to focus psychological interventions on such factors, even if they do not 'cure' the GID.

A third goal of the clinician in the diagnostic phase is to put the information about the child's cross-genderedness in a broader perspective. This means that more general aspects of the child's functioning also have to be evaluated, such as cognitive level, social–emotional functioning and school performance. Poor functioning of children in these areas may help the clinician to interpret certain cross-gender behaviours. For instance, a boy who often plays with (younger) girls, with girls' toys and plays girls' games may do so not because he is unhappy about being a boy. Instead, limited cognitive abilities and immaturity may make him no match for other boys.

Besides a GID, other psychopathology may be present. The relationship between such pathology and the gender problem can take any form. First, cross-gender symptoms may primarily be a component of another disorder (e.g. pervasive developmental disorder). Secondly, other disorders, such as ADHD or Tourette syndrome, may exist that are entirely unrelated to the GID. Such disorders can, however, undermine a boy's social status making him more prone to flee into the less threatening girls' world. Thirdly, certain disorders or problems may be a consequence of the GID (e.g. anorexia in girls). Treatment will very much depend on the assumed relationship between the GID and the other psychopathology.

The broader perspective not only includes the child's functioning but comprises family functioning as well. Family functioning may have a direct impact on the child's gender feelings and behaviour or generate negative feelings on the part of the child. For instance, parental conflicts, due to differences in emotional reactions to the child's cross-gender behaviour, may cause feelings of guilt. For similar reasons it is relevant to know about attitudes of the wider environment towards the cross-gender behaviour of the child.

In sum, proper understanding of the extent of the gender problem itself, the child's development and current functioning, the functioning of the family, and the attitudes of the child's wider environment, is necessary when making a decision as to what type of interventions will benefit the child.

Differential diagnosis

The earlier mentioned subtypes of children referred to a division based on psycho-sexual outcome (homosexual or transsexual). Such a classification can thus far only be made retrospectively. Yet there is heterogeneity within the young children who show cross-gender behaviour. Children with milder forms of cross-genderedness are probably only seen in clinics when they have homophobic parents. The children who are referred to clinics usually show a fair amount of cross-gender behaviours and interests. But whether all these children need clinical attention is debatable, as even in this group there will be children who show 'statistical deviations from the gender norm'. Within the clinically referred children, the following subgroups can be distinguished.

- First, there are children that develop symptoms in reaction to a life event or traumatic experience, such as parental divorce. The onset can be as early as in the 'true' GID group but is usually later. Before the event, gender behaviour was usually not atypical. In our experience, such cross-gender behaviours are less pervasive (e.g. only fantasy play and cross-dressing) and sometimes already decrease before treatment has started.

- Secondly, there are boys that dislike typical boys' games and activities, rarely play with boys, but do not dislike their bodies and do not excessively identify with girls. They seem to play with girls because they are incapable of maintaining relationships. Juvenile unmasculinity is the term used to characterize the behaviour of this group. It has been suggested that boys in this group belong to the healthy functioning gender atypical boys that need little clinical attention. A similar phenomenon does not seem to exist in girls.

- Thirdly, on rare occasions one may encounter boys that are not particularly feminine in their behaviour and preferences, but like to wear female (nylon and silk) undergarments. Like in the first group, this attraction to soft fabrics may emerge after certain life events. Wearing soft clothes appears to have a calming and comforting effect.

- Lastly, there are children with intersex conditions (that is with discrepancies between sex chromosomes, gonads and/or genitals) that may show the same cross-gender behaviour, interests, identification and anatomic dysphoria as other children with GID. When DSM-IV is used, these children cannot be given a GID diagnosis because intersexuality is an exclusion criterion. Despite the fact that the etiology is probably different, treatment (that already varies greatly within the group of non-intersex children with a GID diagnosis) will not be very different from treatment given to non-intersex children with GID.

Diagnostic procedure

The information needed to make a treatment plan can be assembled in four to five sessions, but may take longer in complex cases. After the first session where parents and child are seen together and separately, a session with the child alone, and each parent alone will be needed. At the first session the motive to come to the clinic is discussed. Parents are interviewed shortly about the development and behaviour of the child and their own responses to this behaviour. Also, the parents' expectations of the assessment and possible treatment are discussed and the procedure is explained. The child is asked what the assessment means to him or her, a working alliance is created, and some first information regarding the gender problem is gathered.

In the next sessions the (gender) development and current functioning of the child is discussed in depth with the parents, and behaviours, preferences and statements of the child that are referred to in the DSM IV are addressed. Also, specific attention is paid to the parents' own family history and any gender issues that might have played a role in their lives. Furthermore, feelings of both parents on their child's cross-gender behaviour, their child-rearing practices, and marital or family conflicts regarding the cross-gender behaviour are explored. When family dynamics seem to greatly influence the child's gender problem and family therapy is considered, a family therapist should also see the family. Psychological testing is part of the procedure, because it gives useful information that cannot be gathered easily in another way.

Instruments

Besides the clinical interview a few instruments are available to assess the extent of cross-genderedness of the child (Appendix 24.1). For young children with GID, who tend to be more cognitively confused about gender than children without GID a gender labelling or gender constancy task can be used, in order to test their knowledge of the gender concept. When assessing playmate preference it may be helpful to have sets of photographs of a young boy and girl. Children do not need advanced verbal skills for this task. They only have to indicate their favourite playmate by pointing their finger to the selected picture. Play and games questionnaires are rather culture sensitive. It is not possible to use instruments

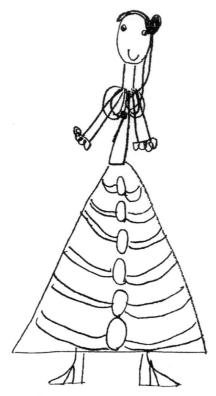

Fig. 24.1.   First drawing of a 7-year old boy with GID.

that have been mostly developed in the US in other countries, without any adaptation.

Besides giving information about object preference, the play observation creates the opportunity to observe the children's mannerisms and gestures. If a boy, indeed, makes many feminine gestures, it becomes understandable why he is an easy target for teasing, even when he is not open about his cross-gender preferences to other children.

Children with GID tend to draw opposite sex persons first. They also tend to draw the opposite sex person taller and with more detail than the same-sex person (Figs. 24.1–24.4). However, as the rates are far from 100 per cent, the value of this measure lies more in the qualitative than in the quantitative information.

Historic and current interventions

Ethics of intervention

Moral or religious motives have led some therapists to treat cross-gendered children in order to prevent homosexuality. Others treat children with GID, because they feel

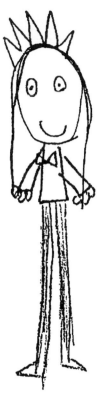

Fig. 24.2.   Second drawing of a 7-year-old boy with GID.

that having a psychiatric disorder is inherently stressful and needs clinical attention. There is, however, strong opposition to such treatment rationales. It is felt that (i) attempts to prevent homosexuality are unethical, because homosexuality is not a psychiatric disorder, (ii) there is no evidence whatsoever that treatment actually prevents homosexuality and (iii) GID in children is not necessarily a psychiatric disorder (if one disagrees with the current DSM criteria). This resistance is directed more toward therapeutic interventions of children who have 'mild' forms of GID and do not express discomfort with their bodies and do not have a desire to be of the opposite sex than towards children with 'extreme' forms of GID. Relatively little dispute exists regarding the prevention of transsexualism, though evidence about the effectiveness of treatment in preventing adult transsexualism is also virtually non-existent.

Among those who consider treatment of children with GID justified, short-term treatment goals depend on the etiological theories of gender identity disorder. Clinicians who consider GID to be the result of an underlying developmental psychopathology and/or a defence to deal with distress, which is generated by early life experiences, will aim at modifying the supposed causal and/or perpetuating

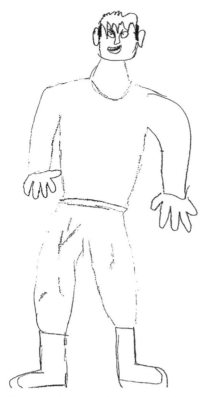

Fig. 24.3.   First drawing of an 8-year-old girl with GID.

factors. In doing so they will try to attain a gender identity change. If they regard GID as a result of inappropriate learning experiences, their aim will be to extinguish cross-gender behaviours and reinforce same-gender behaviours and skills (e.g. athletic skills in boys), assuming that these changes imply a cross-gender identity. Although the aetiological explanations of these clinicians differ, all assume that changing a cross-gender identity is possible, even in extreme cases. Clinicians that consider childhood cross-gender identity and behaviour primarily as manifestations of later homosexuality and do not consider homosexuality a psychiatric disorder will not try to change gender identity and cross-gendered behaviour *per se*. These therapists will rather focus on acceptance of the child's cross-genderedness by parents and child, and try to support the child in establishing a healthy self-esteem and adequate coping mechanisms.

Independent of theoretical background most clinicians will agree that GID may lead to severe distress for parents and children. Such distress may come from social ostracism, non-GID psychiatric or family problems, or intense unhappiness about one's sex characteristics and being a boy or a girl. The suffering should be alleviated under all circumstances.

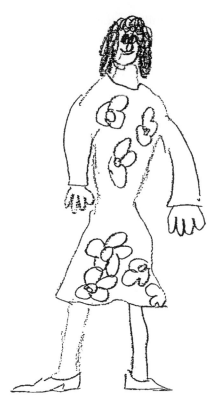

Fig. 24.4.   Second drawing of an 8-year-old girl with GID.

Behaviour therapy

The primary target of behaviour therapists has been the cross-gender behaviour of boys (as there is virtually nothing published about behaviour therapy of girls with GID). Their techniques included reinforcement of gender-typical behaviour during therapy sessions and extinction of cross-gender behaviour, gradual shaping of gender-typical behaviour and desensitizing fear of failure. Mediation therapy has also been used. The same-sex parent (or other same-sex role models within the family) was encouraged to invest time in positive play and interaction with the child. Self-monitoring techniques were used with older children.

Psychoanalytic therapies

Treatment with psychoanalytic psychotherapy, psychoanalysis or other forms of individual psychodynamic psychotherapy has been reported in a great number of case studies. Depending on their theoretical orientation and assessment of the literature on GID, therapists have formulated a wide range of treatment goals. Their focus obviously was on the assumed underlying child or family pathology in order to influence the cross-gender identity. The assumed causal factors in much of the psychotherapy literature were not always similar to the factors that are mentioned in the research literature as potentially contributing to GID.

Combined approaches

As aetiology of GID is still largely in the dark and probably multi-factorial, some therapists do not consider cross-gender identity change as a primary objective. Instead of aiming directly at gender identity change, they focus on developmental processes that may have negatively influenced the child. They also stress the importance of recognition and non-judgemental acceptance of the gender identity problem. This treatment model concentrates on amelioration of emotional, behavioural and relationship difficulties, on breaking the secrecy around GID, and on activation of the child and family's interest in exploring impediments in development (e.g. mourning processes, insufficient separation/individuation). In order to attain these therapeutic interventions such as individual, family and group therapy and social and educational interventions are used. All these activities are integrated into a comprehensive management plan. In some cases, the interventions diminish or solve the gender problem, in others they do not. When child and family appear to function reasonably well, a counseling contact can be offered to the parents, because parents often find it hard to deal with certain practical or emotional matters. This approach allows the clinician to remain involved in the development of a child with GID.

When a child is seen for an individual therapy, parents are always counselled separately. In these sessions the question how they should react to the child's cross-gender behaviour invariably comes up. It is beneficial for children, especially as they grow older, to be able to have social relationships with both boys and girls. In order to have a good time when they play with same-sex peers, it is also necessary that they have at least a few common interests. Because this does not come naturally, children with GID need some encouragement to play with same sex peers. Children could be stimulated to develop broader, perhaps neutral, interests than dolls (in case of boys) or soccer (in case of girls). With regard to cross-dressing setting limits in place and time can be recommended. Allowing cross-dressing only at home and/or at certain times may serve several purposes. For instance, in certain neighburhoods, children would meet much aggression when seen cross-dressed. To keep the cross-dressing away from the eyes of others protects the child from being harassed. If children tend to completely lose themselves in their fantasies, a restriction of cross-dressing keeps them in the reality of their daily world. When the rationale for this restriction is explained, children are much better able to understand why this happens to them, and are thus more compliant. Entirely forbidding children to cross-dress may not work out very well. Parents who completely forbid their children to have opposite sex toys or -clothes often discover that their children manage to get what they want without telling their parents.

Parent organizations

In a few European countries parent organizations exist. They organize educational or supportive meetings for parents, and offer information through the Internet. Because the threshold for these meetings is low, many parents seek contact with this organization before coming to a clinic. They not only provide services for parents and families, but also have contacts with schools. As a result of their activities (often in the national media), teachers are now more aware of the phenomenon and feel more comfortable handling the daily matters they are confronted with. Some schools now have developed 'anti-teasing programmes' to prevent teasing and bullying of gender atypical children.

Treatment effectiveness

Despite the many treatment approaches, controlled studies do not exist. It is therefore still unclear whether (an extreme) GID in childhood can truly be cured. Whether homosexuality or transsexualism can be prevented by psychological interventions before puberty also remains to be demonstrated. Nothing is known about the relative effectiveness of various treatment methods. According to some clinicians, gender identity is more malleable in very young (<6 years) children, whereas in adolescence and adulthood a cross-gender identity is virtually impossible to change. Whether the changes of gender identity that are reported in the literature are the result of the described psychological interventions, of maturation only or of a combination is not known. However, even if there are no short-term or long-term changes in gender identity, many children with GID could profit from psychological interventions. Without treatment, the children are at high risk for the development of problems such as disturbed social relationships, depression, school problems as a consequence of difficulties with concentration, or low self-esteem.

Considering the absence of sound studies providing support for any physical and psychosocial treatment for childhood GID and the ethical problems that would go with such treatment, clinicians should be very cautious with interventions aimed at curing GID *per se*, except in controlled research trials. It might well be that well-meaning therapies in fact hurt the patients and hinder their gender identity development.

Clinical management of gender problems in adolescents

Diagnosis

Most cross-gendered adolescents come to clinics with a straightforward wish for sex reassignment, but some have more open questions regarding their identity. In the diagnostic phase, the gender problem and potential underlying or related problems have to be examined comprehensively. There are no medical instruments that reliably show who is a transsexual and who is not, and psychometrically sound psychological instruments to measure transsexualism do not exist either. Yet it is extremely important not to misdiagnose and thus mistreat applicants for SR. So, in order to make a diagnosis, mental health professionals are largely dependent on the information given by the applicants and their parents. Because of the importance of the decision to be made, the diagnostic procedure is extensive and takes time (see below).

The recommended procedure in the Standards of Care of the International Harry Benjamin Gender Dysphoria Association (HBIGDA), an international professional organization in the field of transsexualism, is to come to the SR decision in various steps. In the first phase, an applicant has to fulfil ICD or DSM criteria for gender identity disorder or transsexualism. The next phase includes three elements, which is sometimes labelled triadic therapy. The elements consist of a real-life experience in the desired role, hormones of the desired gender, and surgery to change the genitals and other sex characteristics.

The first (diagnostic) phase

Procedure

In this phase, information must be obtained from both the adolescent and the parents on various aspects of the general and psychosexual development of the adolescent. Information is also needed about current cross-gender feelings and behaviour, current school functioning of the child, peer relations, and family functioning. With regards to sexuality, the subjective meaning of cross-dressing, the type of cross-dressing, sexual experiences, sexual behaviour and fantasies, sexual attractions, and body image have to be explored.

This diagnostic phase not only focuses on gaining information. In order to prevent unrealistically high expectations as regards their future lives, the adolescent also has to be informed thoroughly about the possibilities and limitations of sex reassignment and other kinds of treatment. This information should be given soon after the first sessions. The way a patient responds to the reality of SR can also be informative diagnostically.

Instruments

Most instruments that measure aspects of gender identity disorder have been developed for adults. Specific instruments that can be used for adolescents with GID are scarce (Appendix 24.2). Some experience exists with the Utrecht Gender Dysphoria Scale, which is a short questionnaire dealing with the distress persons feel when confronted in daily life with the fact that they belong to their biological sex (Appendix 24.3). As can be expected most non-transsexuals score close to the minimum score, which is 12. Most transsexuals score close to the maximum score, which is 60. Problematic applicants in terms of eligibility for SR and in terms of treatment tend to score in the middle range of the scale. The body image scale simply lists 30 physical characteristics. The respondent indicates his/her (dis-) satisfaction with each body part on a five-point scale. They can also express a wish to change the particular body part. Like children, adolescents with GID also tend to draw an opposite sex person first. However, the draw-a-person test is used for its qualitative rather than quantitative information.

Differential diagnosis

As noted before, not all transgendered adolescents have a clear and explicit wish for SR. Some may simply be confused regarding aspects of their gender. For example, young male homosexuals may have a history of stereotypical feminine interests and cross-dressing. In some cases they mistake their homosexuality for a GID, despite a drastic postpubertal reduction or disappearance of their cross-gender interests and activities. In ego-dystonic homosexuals, it is not confusion but lack of acceptance of their homosexuality that makes them consider SR a solution to their problem.

Transvestic fetishism occurs in heterosexual or bisexual male adolescents who become sexually aroused by cross-dressing. Boys with transvestic fetishism may also be confused about their wish to cross-dress. Usually, they hope that SR will 'solve' their sexual excitement when cross-dressed.

Dual-role transvestism occurs when someone wears opposite sex clothes to experience temporary, but not permanent, membership of the opposite sex, without a sexual motivation for the cross-dressing. In adolescents it is hard to know whether this is a permanent situation or just an experimental phase of someone who will eventually seek SR.

In very rare cases a wish for SR exists in persons who prefer to be sexless, but have no cross-gender identity, such as Scoptic syndrome patients. They want to be rid of their sex organs, but do not wish to acquire the sex characteristics of the other sex.

Individuals with transient stress-related cross-dressing may mistake their interest in cross-dressing for a need for SR. This may also happen in patients suffering from severe psychiatric conditions (e.g. schizophrenia), accompanied by delusions of belonging to the opposite sex.

Some individuals with gender problems do not seek complete SR. Instead they try to integrate masculine and feminine aspects of the self and only want hormones or some form of surgery.

The second phase: triadic therapy

The desirability of sex reassignment for adolescents

The desirability of SR as a resolution for the psychological suffering of transsexuals, irrespective of age, has been controversial since the first sex change operations were performed. Many psychotherapists feel that one should try to help transsexuals to resolve emotional conflicts underlying their wish for sex change by no other means than psychotherapy. However, the existing case reports do not provide convincing evidence for complete and long-term reversal of cross-gender identity by means of psychotherapy.

Outcome studies on extremely gender-dysphoric SR applicants, who have been randomly assigned to either SR or psychotherapeutic treatment, and with very long-term follow-ups, do not exist. Considering the lack of motivation for psychotherapy of most transsexuals, one may wonder whether it will ever be possible to conduct such studies. The absence of evidence that psychotherapy is the treatment of choice has led clinicians to look for other solutions to the problem. Because a once firmly established cross-gender identity appeared virtually impossible to change, the only rational solution to the problem seemed to be the adaptation of the sex characteristics to the cross-gender identity. This solution was supported by the results of studies showing no apparent psychological disturbance in transsexuals, which would make SR a hazardous enterprise. This does not mean that psychopathology would be completely absent in an unselected sample of transsexuals. It has become clear that transsexualism is a heterogeneous phenomenon, and that psychopathology is more likely in some subtypes (e.g. late-onset group) than in others. Young applicants are more likely to belong to the early onset group. It is therefore likely that their psychological functioning is relatively favourable.

Because transsexualism is not necessarily associated with psychopathology, an extreme cross-gender identity in most individuals seems to be fixed after puberty, and psychological treatments are not particularly successful in solving the problems of these individuals, SR seems to be the treatment of choice for very gender dysphoric adults. However, even if one agrees with SR as a (palliative) treatment form for adult transsexuals, one could argue that adolescents should never be allowed to start (the hormonal part of) SR, because they are still in a rapidly changing developmental process. Currently, clinicians are faced with increasing numbers of youngsters who powerfully express that they find their lives unbearable without hormonal interventions.

One argument in favour of early hormone treatment is that an eventual arrest in emotional, social and intellectual development can be warded off more successfully when the ultimate cause of this arrest has been taken care of. Another is that early hormone treatment might be beneficial in adolescents because their secondary sex characteristics have not yet fully developed. Young male-to-female transsexuals (MFs) will, as adults, pass much more easily as females when they have never grown a beard or developed a low voice. If the bodily changes of puberty are not interrupted and a child still wants SR in adulthood, major physical interventions will be required to remove the unwanted physical characteristics. Yet, despite these obvious advantages, early hormone treatment for adolescents with GID touches sensitive strings. In the absence of evidence that transsexualism can be treated in adolescence by psychotherapy alone, and that transsexualism is necessarily associated with severe psychopathology and the presence of the arguments in favour of early treatment, a few centres have started, in carefully selected cases, with hormonal therapy before adulthood.

Psychological interventions

Persons who are merely gender-confused or whose wish for SR seems to originate from factors other than a genuine and complete cross-gender identity are served best by psychological interventions. Such interventions may help them to better understand and cope with gender issues, and to try out alternative solutions to their problem, such as part-time cross-gender living.

For individuals who want to explore their options for coping with gender dysphoria, group therapy has also been advocated. The information coming from members who are in different phases of understanding their gender problem, and the support in finding ways to deal with the problem seems to be particularly beneficial to group members.

Family therapy may help to solve conflicts between family members rather than intrapsychic conflicts. These conflicts are quite common in cross-gendered adolescents. For instance, it happens regularly that a transsexual adolescent wants to be more open about his or her condition than the other family members. Conversely, when they already live permanently in the opposite gender role, parents fear aggressive reactions when friends who are not informed, discover the truth.

Psychotherapy, combined with pharmacotherapy (low doses of lithium carbonate), has been reported to be successful in cases of Scoptic syndrome, because the medication made patients more amenable to psychotherapy. In-patient treatment in psychiatric hospitals may be needed for persons suffering from severe psychiatric conditions. The psychiatric disorder must have been treated properly by medication or otherwise the request for SR will have to be re-evaluated. In the case of adolescents with severe psychiatric co-morbidity, hormone therapy will not be prescribed before adulthood, even if the adolescent is transsexual and has recovered from the psychiatric illness. The efficacy of all these interventions, however, has not been investigated in formal outcome studies.

Psychotherapy is not only useful for applicants that do not fulfil GID criteria. For transsexual adolescents, the first (diagnostic) phase is lengthy and intensive. Besides gathering information to make the diagnosis, any relevant issue that comes up in the first phase has to be explored. This means that the diagnostic phase often contains therapeutic elements. Patients need time to reflect on any unresolved personal issues or doubts regarding SR before embarking on somatic treatment. It is paramount that any form of psychotherapy offered to GID patients is supportive. The more the patient is confronted with doubts on the part of the therapist, the less chance he/she has to explore own doubts if they exist. Therapists also need to be knowledgeable about hormone treatment, surgery, and the legal consequences of the treatment to compare the SR solution in a balanced way with other options for living with the gender problem (e.g. part-time living in the opposite role). Other issues that may come up in the first phase are anxieties concerning the loss of family or friends, uncertainties whether passing in the opposite role is feasible and whether it will be possible to have satisfying intimate relationships, support when 'coming out'.

When hormone treatment has started, psychotherapy may still be of use. Some patients indeed have to deal with loss, or negative reactions from the environment. Others can only work on certain personal issues after they no longer need to worry about their masculinizing or feminizing bodies. For these reasons, some clinics offer post-surgical psychotherapy. Whether patients accept this depends largely on the individual needs of the patient and the quality of earlier therapist-patient contact.

Real life experience

In the real life experience (RLE) phase, applicants have to live permanently in the role of the desired sex, if they were not already doing so. Significant persons have to be informed about the impending changes. The underlying idea of this requirement is that applicants should have had ample opportunity to appreciate in fantasy or in vivo the familial, interpersonal, educational and legal consequences of the gender role change. During the RLE phase cross-sex hormone treatment is usually started. Feelings of dysphoria generally decline as a result of both the first bodily changes and the possibility to live in the new social role. During the real-life experience the social transformation is a major focus of the discussions, when an adolescent starts to live in the desired role after the diagnostic phase. This is obviously less the case when they already lived in the desired role before applying for SR.

Physical interventions: hormone treatment

A diagnosis of GID alone is not sufficient for the decision to start the next treatment phase (RLE and hormones). Despite the fact that formal criteria are applicable to an individual patient, the actual extremeness of the GID may vary. With regard to adolescents only applicants for SR that have from very early on (toddlerhood) shown a clear and extreme cross-gender identification in all social environments and want both to adopt the social role of the other sex and SR should be eligible for SR.

But even extremely cross-gender identified youngsters may not be able to handle the drastic life changes that accompany SR. Thus one should take potential risk factors into account when making decisions on the eligibility of early interventions.

For adolescents, the Guidelines of the Royal College of Psychiatrists, as well as the HBIGDA Standards of Care, make a distinction between three stages of physical interventions:

- the fully reversible interventions
- partially reversible interventions
- irreversible interventions.

Fully reversible interventions

As soon as pubertal changes have begun, adolescents with extreme forms of GID may be eligible for puberty-delaying hormones. However, they should be able to make an informed decision about pubertal delay. Therefore, it is preferable if they experience the onset of puberty, at least to the second phase of pubertal development, Tanner Stage Two.

Allowing adolescents with GID to take puberty delaying hormones is justified by two goals. One is to gain time to further explore the gender identity and other developmental issues in psychotherapy. The second is to make passing easier if the adolescent continues to pursue SR. GID adolescents eligible for any form of hormone treatment are required to meet the following criteria:

- throughout childhood the adolescent has demonstrated an intense pattern of cross-gender behaviours and -identity
- gender discomfort has significantly increased with the onset of puberty
- the family consents and participates in the therapy.

Puberty delaying hormone treatment should not be viewed as a first step of the cross-sex treatment, but as a diagnostic help. Therefore, a period of cross-gender living, the RLE, is not required necessarily, when only these hormones are taken. It is difficult to give a general rule for the start of the RLE, as the personalities and life circumstances of adolescents are so different. Some wait until they are 16 and have graduated from school. They start the RLE when they start to take cross-sex hormones, because they want to look 'really convincing' at the moment of their social role change. Some think, correctly, that they already look convincing enough and begin living in the desired role even before they have started with puberty-delaying hormones.

Partially reversible interventions

Adolescents eligible for cross-sex hormone therapy (estrogens for MFs or androgens for FMs) usually are around 16 or older. In many countries 16-year olds are legal adults for medical decision-making. Although parental consent is not required, it is preferred, as adolescents need the support of their parents in this complex phase of their lives.

Mental health professional involvement, for a minimum period of 6 months, is another eligibility requirement for hormonal interventions of adolescents. The objective of this involvement is that treatment is thoughtfully and recurrently considered over time.

Irreversible interventions

Surgery is not carried out prior to adulthood. The Standards of Care emphasize that the 'threshold of 18 should be seen as an eligibility criterion and not an indication in itself for active intervention'. If the RLE supported by the cross-sex hormones has not resulted in a satisfactory social role change or if the patient is not satisfied with or is ambivalent about the hormonal effects, the applicant should not be referred for surgery.

Effects of fully reversible interventions

Lutein hormone-releasing hormone (LHRH) agonists block further progress of puberty. These compounds bind so strongly to the pituitary that the secretion of luteinizing hormone (LH) and follicle-stimulating hormone (FSH) no longer takes place. Eventually the gonadal production of sex steroids discontinues and a prepubertal state is (again) induced.

Adolescents that have gone into puberty at a very young age or have started with LHRH agonists at a relatively late age will already have developed certain secondary sex characteristics. Some cannot be reversed by hormone treatment. Because facial hair growth is very resistant to anti-androgen therapy, additional mechanic hair removal techniques may sometimes be necessary. Speech therapy is sometimes needed, because the vocal cords will not shorten once they have grown, and the MF has to learn to use his voice in a female fashion. Surgical techniques to shorten the vocal cord exist but are as yet rarely employed, because there are still concerns about the safety and effectiveness of such voice modification techniques.

Effects of partially reversible interventions

To induce female sex characteristics in MFs (such as breasts and a more female-appearing body shape due to a change of body fat around waist, hips, shoulders and jaws) oestrogens are used. Other physical effects are decreased: upper body strength, softening of the skin, a decreased testicular size and fertility, and less frequent, less firm erections.

In female-to-male transsexuals (FMs), androgens are used for the induction of male body features, such as a low voice, facial and body hair growth, and a more masculine body shape. Other physical changes are a mild breast atrophy and clitoral enlargement, though the size will never reach the size of a penis by means of androgen treatment only. Reversible changes are increased upper body strength, weight gain and decreased hip fat.

Effects of irreversible interventions

In MFs, female-looking external genitals are created by means of vaginoplasty, clitoroplasty and labiaplasty. In cases of insufficient responsiveness of breast tissue to oestrogen therapy, breast enlargement may also be performed. After surgery, intercourse is possible. Arousal and orgasm are also reported post-surgically, though the percentages differ between studies.

For FMs, a mastectomy is often performed as the first surgery to successfully pass in the desired role. When skin needs to be removed, this will result in fairly visible scar tissue. Considering the still continuing improvements in the field of phalloplasty, some FMs do not want to undergo genital surgery until they have a clear reason for it or choose to have a neoscrotum with a testical prosthesis with or without a metaidoioplasty, which transforms the hypertrophic clitoris into a microphallus. Other genital procedures may include removal of the uterus and ovaries. Whether FMs can have sexual intercourse using their neo-penis depends on the technique and quality of the phalloplasty. Although some patients who had a metaidoioplasty report that they are able to have intercourse, the hypertrophic clitoris usually is too small for coitus. In most cases, the capacity for sexual arousal and orgasm remains intact.

Results of sex reassignment

Many follow-up studies have been carried out to evaluate the effectiveness of SR. Most studies concern treatment effects in adult groups. Success percentages in relatively recent studies are 87 per cent for MFs and 97 per cent for FMs, but outcomes differ greatly between studies. This is probably due to methodology, number of subjects and outcome criteria. Postoperative regret to the point of a second role reversal is estimated to be 1–2 per cent. From studies on adult transsexuals it seems that psychopathology, poor social support and physical appearance may be the pretreatment factors that are most likely associated with poor postoperative functioning. In the few follow-up studies on adolescent transsexuals there were no participants with regrets, gender dysphoria had virtually disappeared, and psychologically and socially the adolescents functioned fairly favourably. This is probably because adolescents with severe psychopathology and poor social support are not allowed to start treatment before adulthood and because they very easily pass in their new social role.

Legal age limits

In many countries that derive their law from Napoleon's Code Civil of 1804, the birth certificate is the source for all other personal documents. Therefore it is essential to change the sex in this document to endow a person with the full rights of his/her new gender. In Anglo-American countries it is easier to adopt a new first name. However, registration of official documents is not centralized. As a result, a person can be male according to one and female according to another document. Nowadays, many countries either have specific laws or administrative solutions, implying that SR has become a fairly well-accepted treatment.

The current guidelines for the treatment of adolescents with GID which distinguish between three types of physical interventions (wholly reversible, partly reversible and irreversible ones) do not give defined ages for the physical interventions. Only for surgery the age of 18 is mentioned, as this is the age of legal adulthood in many Western countries. The rationale of this age limit is somewhat arbitrary. Outside Europe and the US the ages of legal maturity vary between 16 in Iceland and Nepal to 21 in many African and Latin American countries, while some countries do not even have a fixed age. Though the fixed age limits are an attempt to protect children from maltreatment, in the case of adolescents with GID it often seems to work against them. The age of psychological and somatic maturity varies largely interindividually. Adhering to such limits would severely hamper the development of a mature adolescent and may even facilitate fast routine decision making when a still immature 18 year old wants to have surgery. Adolescents are probably better protected when all those involved in their treatment closely observe the Guidelines of The Royal College of Psychiatrists and The Harry Benjamin Gender Dysphoria, and extensively discuss and weigh up the pros and cons of SR for an individual patient.

SUGGESTED READING

P. T. Cohen-Kettenis & F. Pfafflin, *Making Choices. Transgenderism and intersexuality in childhood and adolescence.* (Thousand Oaks, CA: Sage Publications, 2003).

F. L. Coolidge, L. Thede & S. E. Young, The heritability of gender identity disorder in a child and adolescent twin sample. *Behaviour Genetics*, **32** (2002), 251–7.

D. Di Ceglie & D. Freedman (eds.), *A Stranger in my own Body. Atypical Gender Identity Development and Mental Health.* (London: Karnac Books, 1998).

D. Di Ceglie, C. Sturge & A. Sutton, *Gender Identity Disorders in Children and Adolescents: Guidelines for Management.* Council Report CR63. (London: Royal College of Psychiatrists, London, 1998).

S. Golombok & R. Fivush, *Gender Development.* (New York: Cambridge University Press, 1994).

R. Green, *The 'Sissy Boy Syndrome' and the Development of Homosexuality.* (New Haven: Yale University Press, 1987).

G. Herdt, *Third Sex, Third Gender. Beyond the Dimorphism in Culture and History.* (New York: Zone Books, 1994).

W. Meyer (Chairperson), W. O. Bockting, P. T. Cohen-Kettenis *et al.*, *Standards of Care for Gender Identity Disorders of The Harry Benjamin International Gender Dysphoria Association (HBIGDA)*, Sixth Version. *International Journal of Transgenderism*, **5** (2001), http://www.symposion.com/ijt/soc_2001/index/htm.

M. Rottnek (ed.), *Sissies and Tomboys. Gender Noncomformity and Homosexual Childhood.* (New York: New York University Press, 1999).

B. Wren, Early physical intervention for young people with atypical gender identity development. *Clinical Child Psychology and Psychiatry*, **5** (2000), 220–31.

K. J. Zucker & S. J. Bradley, *Gender Identity Disorder and Psychosexual Problems in Children and Adolescents.* (New York, London: Guilford Press, 1995).

Appendix 24.1. Instruments to measure gender understanding, gender identity and gender role behaviour for children younger than 12 with GID

Instruments for children under 6 only:

Name of the instrument	Authors	Source
Gender labelling task	Leinbach, M. D. & Fagot, B. I. (1986)	*Sex Roles*, **5**, 655–66.
Gender constancy task, consisting of subtasks regarding: – gender labelling – gender stability – gender consistency	Slaby, R. G. & Frey, K. S. (1975)	*Child Development*, **52**, 849–56.

Instruments for all children under 12:

Name of the instrument	Authors	Source
Gender identity interview	Zucker, K. J. & Bradley, S. (1995)	Guilford Press.
Gender preference interview	Cohen-Kettenis, P. T. & Pfäfflin, F.	Sage Publications, in press
Free play test (except for 'mature' 11–12 year olds)	Zucker, K. J., Bradley, S. J., Doering, R. W. & Lozinsky, J. A. (1985)	*Journal of the American Academy of Child and Adolescent Psychiatry*, **24**, 710–19.
Draw-a-person test	Rekers, G. A., Rosen, A. C. & Morey, S. M. (1990)	*Perceptual and Motor Skills*, **71**, 71–9.

(cont.)

Appendix 24.1. (*cont.*)

Parent questionnaires for children under 6

Name of the instrument	Authors	Source
Preschool activities inventory	Golombok, S. & Rust, J. (1993)	*Psychological Assessment*, **5**, 131–6, 1993

Parent questionnaires for children under 12

Name of the instrument	Authors	Source
– Child behaviour and attitude questionnaire	Bates, J. E., Bentler, P. M. & Thompson, S. K. (original version) (1973)	*Child Development*, **44**, 591–8.
– Child behaviour and attitude questionnaire – male and female version	Meyer-Bahlburg, H. F. L., Sandberg, D. E., Yager, T. J., Dolezal, C. L. & Ehrhardt, A. A. (revised version) (1994)	*Journal of Psychology and Human Sexuality*, **6**, 19–39.
Child game participation questionnaire	Bates J. E. & Bentler, P. M. (original version) (1973) Meyer-Bahlburg, H. F. L., Sandberg D. E., Dolezal, C. L. & Yager, T. J. (revised version) (1994)	*Developmental Psychology*, **9**, 20–7. *Journal of Abnormal Child Psychology*, **22**, 643–60.
Play activity questionnaire	Finegan, J. A., Niccols, G. A., Zacher, J. E. & Hood, J. E.	*Archives of Sexual Behavior*, **20**, 393–408.
Gender identity questionnaire	Elisabeth, P. H. & Green, R. modified by Zucker, K. J. & Bradley, S. J. (1995)	Guilford Press.

Appendix 24.2. Instruments to measure gender dysphoria, and body image for adolescents with GID

Name of the instrument	Authors	Source
Utrecht Gender Dysphoria Scale (see Appendix 24.3)	Cohen-Kettenis, P. T. & Van Goozen, S. H. M. (1997)	*Journal of the American Academy of Child and Adolescent Psychiatry*, **36**, 263–71.
Body image scale	Lindgren, T. W. & Pauly, I. B. (1975)	*Archives of Sexual Behavior*, **4**, 639–56.
Draw-a-person test	Rekers, G. A., Rosen, A. C. & Morey, S. M. (1990)	*Perceptual and Motor Skills*, **71**, 771–9.

Appendix 24.3. *Utrecht Gender Dysphoria Scale (FM adolescent version).* **Response categories are: agree completely, agree somewhat, neutral, disagree somewhat, disagree completely. Items are scored from 1–5, except for items 1,2,4,5,6,10,11,12, which are scored form 5–1**

1. I preferably behave like a boy.
2. Every time someone treats me like a girl I feel hurt.
3. I love to live as a girl.
4. I continuously want to be treated like a boy.
5. A boy's life is more attractive for me than a girl's life.
6. I feel unhappy because I have to behave like a girl.
7. Living as a girl is something positive for me.
8. I enjoy seeing my naked body in the mirror.
9. I like to behave sexually as a girl.
10. I hate menstruating because it makes me feel like a girl.
11. I hate having breasts.
12. I wish I had been born as a boy.

Index

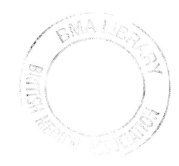